two drugs if you're uncertain of their compatibility. Check appropriate references or with a pharmacist to be sure.

	isoproterenol	kanamycin	lactated Ringer's	lidocaine	metaraminol	methicillin	methylprednisolone	mezlocillin	moxalactam	multiple vitamin infusion	nafcillin	netilmicin	norepinephrine	0.9% NSS	oxacillin	oxytocin	penicillin G potassium	phytonadione	piperacillin	polymyxin B sulfate	potassium chloride	procainamide	sodium bicarbonate	tetracycline	thiamine	ticarcillin	tobramycin	vancomycin	verapamil	vitamin B complex with C	
							24						24	24	8		8	24			4		24	4			24	24			albumin
			24										24										24					48			amikacin
24			24	24	24	24							24			24		24	24			24			24			24		aminophylline
	8											24				1						24			24					amino acid injection
		24										48								24	48				48					ampicillin
		24										24										24					48			bretylium
												24				1	24			24					24					calcium gluconate
												24													24					carbenicillin
												24													24					cefamandole
	48							24				24								24					24		24	24		cefazolin
												24								24					24					cefoxitin
												24													24					cephalothin
24	24		24	24			24			48		24	24			24	24		24	24			24				24	24	48	chloramphenicol
24	24		24			24						24			24			24				24					24	24		cimetidine
												4																	4	corticotropin (ACTH)
24	24		24	6	6	24	24	24	24			6	6	24		24		24		24		24	24		24	24	24	24	24	dexamethasone
24			24	24	24			24	24	24		24	24			24		24		24		24	24			24			24	dextrose 5% in water
24				24			24	24				24		24								24							24	dextrose 5% in R.L.
24	24	24	24				24	24	24			12	24		24	24		24		24		24	24		48		24			dextrose 5% in 0.45% NSS
												24																		dextrose 5% in 0.9% NSS
24			24	24								24	24							24					24					diphenhydramine
24	48	24	24			18						48	24							24		24								dobutamine
	24	2										24																24		dopamine
	18											24										24								epinephrine
			24									24																24		erythromycin lactobionate (IV)
												24										24						24		gentamicin
24			24			24						6			24					24								24		heparin sodium
	24			4								24					24			24								24		hydrocortisone Na succinate
	24																											48		insulin (regular)
	24											24																24		isoproterenol
	24											24																24		kanamycin
24	24		24		24					24	24	24				24		24		24		24			24	48	24	24	24	lactated Ringer's
	24											24										24	24					48		lidocaine
	24											24										24						24		metaraminol
	24											6																24		methicillin
	24											24										24						24		methylprednisolone
												6		6																mezlocillin
	24											24																24		moxalactam
	24									24		24				4						24	24					24		multiple vitamin infusion
	24											24										24						24		nafcillin
	24										24																	24		netilmicin
													24															24		norepinephrine
24	24		24	24	6		6	24	24	24			8		24		24		24	24	24	24		24	48		24	24	24	0.9% NSS
	24											8										24						24		oxacillin
	24											24										24						24		oxytocin
	24			24			4					24										24						24		penicillin G potassium
												24																24		phytonadione
	24											24								24								24		piperacillin
												24																24		polymyxin B sulfate
	24									24		24				24			24			24						24		potassium chloride
	24											24																24		procainamide
	24	24							24			24	24	24		24		24		24								24		sodium bicarbonate
	24									24		24				24												24		tetracycline
																														thiamine
	48											24																24		ticarcillin
	24											48																24		tobramycin
																												24		vancomycin
24			24	48	24	24						24	24	24	24		24		24			24			24	24	24		24	verapamil
	24																											24		vitamin B complex with C

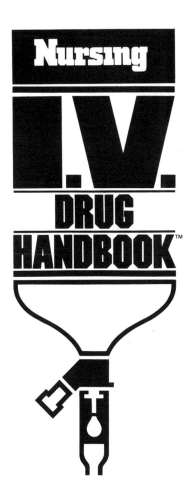

Nursing

I.V.
DRUG
HANDBOOK™

Fourth Edition

Springhouse Corporation
Springhouse, Pennsylvania

STAFF

Executive Director, Editorial
Stanley Loeb

Editorial Director
Matthew Cahill

Clinical Director
Barbara F. McVan, RN

Art Director
John Hubbard

Senior Editor
Michael Shaw

Drug Information Editor
George J. Blake, RPh, MS

Clinical Project Editor
Joanne Patzek DaCunha, RN, BS

Editors
Kate Cassidy, Stephen Daly, Peter Johnson

Clinical Editors
Patricia Holmes, RN, BSN; Beverly Ann Tscheschlog, RN

Copy Editors
Jane V. Cray (supervisor), Nancy Papsin

Designers
Stephanie Peters (associate art director), Matie Anne Patterson (senior designer)

Art Production
Robert Perry (manager), Anna Brindisi, Donald Knauss, Tom Robbins, Robert Wieder

Typography
David C. Kosten (director), Diane Paluba (manager), Elizabeth Bergman, Joyce Rossi Biletz, Phyllis Marron, Robin Rantz, Valerie Rosenberger

Manufacturing
Deborah C. Meiris (manager), T.A. Landis, Jennifer Suter

Production Coordination
Colleen Hayman

Editorial Assistants
Maree DeRosa, Beverly Lane, Mary Madden

Indexer
Janet M. Hodgson

The clinical procedures described and recommended in this publication are based on research and consultation with nursing, medical, and legal authorities. To the best of our knowledge, these procedures reflect currently accepted practice; nevertheless, they can't be considered absolute and universal recommendations. For individual application, all recommendations must be considered in light of the patient's clinical condition and, before administration of new or infrequently used drugs, in light of latest package-insert information. The authors and the publisher disclaim responsibility for any adverse effects resulting directly or indirectly from the suggested procedures, from any undetected errors, or from the reader's misunderstanding of the text.

CONTENTS

CONTRIBUTORS AND CONSULTANTS

At the time of publication, the contributors and consultants held the following positions.

Contributors

Sharon Aboulafia, RN, MSN, CCRN, CNA Clinical Coordinator, Intensive Care Units, St. Luke's/Roosevelt Hospital, New York

Jean Marie Amabile-Michiels, RN, BSN, MA, MSN Assistant Professor of Nursing, Gwynedd-Mercy College, Gwynedd Valley, Pa.

Arlene Androkites, RN, BSN, CPNP Pediatric Oncology Nurse Practitioner, Dana-Farber Cancer Institute, Boston

Jeanne L. Bernosky, RN,C, MSN Part-time Staff Nurse, Holy Redeemer Hospital; Former Nurse Educator, Holy Family College, Philadelphia

Laura J. Burke, RN, MSN Cardiovascular Clinical Nurse Specialist, Aurora Health Care, Inc., Milwaukee

Regina Blumenstein Butler, RN Hematology Nurse, Hemophilia Nurse Coordinator, Children's Hospital of Philadelphia

Joanne Patzek DaCunha, RN, BS Clinical Editor, Springhouse Corporation, Springhouse, Pa.

Jeanette Dunn, RN, BSN Quality Assurance Coordinator, Fair Acres Geriatric Center, Media, Pa.

Vivian Fineman, RN, BSN, CGC Staff Nurse, Gastrointestinal Department, Hospital of the University of Pennsylvania, Philadelphia

Hebe Hearn Jungkind, RN,C, BS, BSN, MSN Coordinator, Maternal-Child Health Nursing, Abington (Pa.) Memorial Hospital School of Nursing

Rosemarie Marinaro, RN, BSN Nursing Staff Development Instructor, Department of Public Health, Philadelphia

Michael J. McNamee, RN, MPS, CEN, CNA Emergency Room Staff Nurse, St. Joseph's Hospital and Medical Center, Paterson, N.J.

Patricia E. Meehan, RN, BSN Nurse Epidemiologist, National Institutes of Health, Clinical Center, Bethesda, Md.

Doris A. Millam, RN, MS, CRNI, I.V. Therapy Clinician, Holy Family Hospital, Des Plaines, Ill.

Lynne M. Patzek Miller, RN,C Clinical Systems Manager, Doylestown (Pa.) Hospital

Chris Platt Moldovanyi, RN, MSN, CDE Director of Nursing Education— Operating Room, Cleveland Clinic Foundation

Ralph O. Morgan, Jr., CRNA, MS Curriculum Coordinator, Graduate Program of Nurse Anesthesia, Medical College of Pennsylvania, Philadelphia

Camille A. Marano Morrison, RN, MSN Neuroscience Clinical Nurse Specialist, Mount Sinai Hospital, Hartford, Conn.

Karen T. O'Connor, RN, MSN Special Projects Coordinator, Department of Nursing, Fox Chase Cancer Center, Philadelphia

Janet N. Pavel, RN, AD Nursing Director, Blood Services, Department of Transfusion Medicine, National Institutes of Health, Rockville, Md.

Frances W. Quinless, RN, PhD, CCRN Chairperson, Department of Nursing Education and Services, College of Medicine and Dentistry of New Jersey, Newark

Cecilia E. Shaw, RN,C, BSN, OCN Clinical Supervisor/Research Coordinator, Cancer Care Associates, Tulsa

Karen N. Shine, RN, MPAH Quality Assurance/Risk Management Coordinator, Dana-Farber Cancer Institute, Boston

Jacqueline Solomon, RN, MS, CCRN Associate Professor, College of Nursing, University of New Mexico, Albuquerque

Audrey Stephan, RN, MSN Assistant Professor of Nursing, Bergen Community College, Paramus, N.J.

Carralee A. Sueppel, RN, CURN Clinical Nursing Specialist I, Urology Nursing Division, University of Iowa Hospitals and Clinics, Iowa City

Julie N. Tackenberg, RN, MA, CNRN Nurse Coordinator, Arizona Comprehensive Epilepsy Program, University Medical Center, Tucson

Janet D'Agostino Taylor, RN, MSN Pulmonary Rehabilitation Clinical Specialist, St. Elizabeth's Hospital, Boston

Patricia A. Varvel, RN,C, MS Nurse Manager, Obstetrics, St. Luke's Episcopal Hospital, Houston

Nancy Baptie Walrath, RN, BSN, CGC Director, Gastroenterology, Daniel Freeman Memorial and Marina Hospitals, Inglewood, Calif.

Joni Walton, RN, MSN, RRT Clinical Nurse Specialist, Vanderbilt University Hospital, Nashville

Patricia Watterson Wells, RN, MSN Pediatric Rheumatology Clinical Nurse Specialist, Duke University Medical Center and University of North Carolina at Chapel Hill, Durham

Lorie Rietman Wild, RN, MN Medical Surgical Clinical Nurse Specialist, University Hospital, Seattle

Lana M. Wilhelm, RN, BSN, CNSN Director, Home Care/Nutritional Support, The University Hospital/St. Louis University Medical School, St. Louis

Clinical consultants

Linda B. Chitwood, RN, MSN, CRNA Freelance Nurse-Anesthetist, Memphis

Sande Jones, RN,C, MSN, MSEd Nursing Education Specialist, Mount Sinai Medical Center, Miami Beach

Diane Foley Osborne, RN, CEN Staff Nurse, McLeod Regional Medical Center, Florence, S.C.

Ann M. Plunkett, RN Apheresis Specialist, National Institutes of Health, Bethesda, Md.

Donald A. St. Onge, RN, MSN Pulmonary Clinical Nurse Specialist, Allegheny General Hospital, Pittsburgh

Beverly Tscheschlog, RN Clinical Consultant, Ottsville, Pa.

Special thanks to the following, who contributed to past editions: Ruth Ann Benfield, RN, MSN, CS; Glen E. Farr, PharmD; Bridget A. Haupt, PharmD; David W. Hawkins, PharmD; Nina E. Jakobowski, RPh, PharmD; Jan-Elian Markind, BS, RPh; Doris A. Millam, RN, MS, CRNI; Janet McCombs, RPh, PharmD; J. Neil McFarland, RPh, BSPh; Louise S. Parent, PharmD; David Pipher, RPh, PharmD; Doris M. Sherpinsky, BS, RPh; Joel Shuster, RPh, PharmD.

FOREWORD

Proficiency in managing I.V. drug therapy is vital for professional confidence. In any hospital, 75% to 85% of the patients are likely to receive I.V. therapy. And among patients receiving such therapy, 75% require one or more I.V. drugs daily. Additionally, more nurses are administering I.V. drugs in home and office settings.

Every year, as the pharmacopeia of I.V. drugs expands, the relevant body of knowledge increases. For each drug you encounter, you need precise information on indications, dosage, preparation, administration techniques, interactions, and incompatibilities. And you need clear instructions in order to prevent such complications as extravasation, infection, hypersensitivity, phlebitis, and occluded catheters. If complications do occur during or after therapy, instructions on how to respond should be readily available.

Fortunately, the *Nursing I.V. Drug Handbook, Fourth Edition,* provides quick access to the hundreds of thousands of crucial details that make safe and effective administration of I.V. drugs possible.

The major portion of the book provides an encyclopedia of information on all currently available I.V. preparations. Entries are listed alphabetically by generic name. Brand names appear under generic names (the index includes both brand and generic names for your convenience). Each entry receives ample coverage in a standard, easy-to-read format. Besides medications, this section discusses blood products, amino acid solutions, dextrose solutions, colloid and crystalloid solutions, and fat emulsions. It covers investigational drugs as well as investigational uses of approved drugs.

The information in each drug entry is organized under standard headings. *Pharmacokinetics* describes the drug's distribution, metabolism, excretion, and action. *Mechanism of Action* describes how the drug achieves its therapeutic effects. *Indications & Dosage* gives the indications for I.V. use of the drug, with dosages for adults and children. It outlines appropriate dosage adjustments, such as those made for patients with renal impairment. *Contraindications & Cautions* tells what conditions contraindicate use of the drug and when to be especially careful in administering the drug. *Preparation & Storage* tells how the drug is supplied, how to store it, what its shelf life is, and how to reconstitute or dilute it, as appropriate. *Administration* gives specific instructions for delivering the drug by appropriate method: direct injection, intermittent infusion, and continuous infusion. Rates are provided when available. *Incompatibility* tells what medications should not be mixed with the drug in direct combination. *Adverse Reactions* lists life-threatening and other potential reactions. *Interactions* tells the effects of mixing the drug with other medications. *Effects on Diagnostic Tests* describes how the drug may alter test results or render them unreliable.

Special Considerations, the final heading, covers key nursing concerns not included elsewhere. If appropriate, this section starts with treatment of an overdose. It may also provide tips on patient monitoring, on how to modify therapy for special patients, and on patient teaching.

You'll also find a pregnancy risk rating with each entry and, where appropriate, the controlled substance schedule. The pregnancy risk category identifies a drug's potential for causing birth defects. It's based on Food and Drug Administration (FDA) ratings, package inserts, and well-respected drug references. Five categories (A, B, C, D, and X) distinguish different levels of risk.

The controlled substance schedule is an FDA classification for drugs with a high potential for abuse. Schedule I drugs, such as heroin and LSD, have high abuse potential and no accepted medical use in the United States. Schedule II, III, IV, and V drugs have progressively declining potentials for abuse, and you will encounter them in your work.

The handbook also contains an Overview of I.V. Drug Administration. Here you'll find basic information about drug preparation and storage, along with more than 40 illustrations detailing I.V. administration methods and I.V. equipment. You'll learn how to recognize and manage complications and how to prevent their occurrence.

In the handbook's appendices, you'll find charts and tables covering such valuable topics as the major components of electrolyte solutions, how to convert units of measure, how to identify and treat toxic drug reactions, how to prevent and treat drug extravasation, and detailed instructions for home I.V. therapy.

The inside front cover contains a compatibility chart of 60 commonly used I.V. drugs. The inside back cover features nomogram charts for adults and children to help you calculate drug dosages.

In sum, the *Nursing I.V. Drug Handbook, Fourth Edition,* provides accurate, detailed information in a concise, easy-to-read format. Prepared by practicing nurses and pharmacists, this comprehensive guide contains everything you need to administer I.V. therapy competently and safely.

DORIS A. MILLAM, RN, MS, CRNI
I.V. Therapy Clinician
Holy Family Hospital
Des Plaines, Ill.

Overview of I.V. drug administration

Over the past 50 years, I.V. therapy has undergone dramatic changes, evolving from a fledgling treatment to a widely practiced, continuously expanding one. In fact, over the past 25 years, the use of I.V. antibiotic therapy has grown rapidly, following the discovery of cephalosporins.

Recent landmarks

Intermittent I.V. therapy has become widely used because it allows drug administration at any desired interval by direct injection (I.V. push) or dilution of the drug with 50 to 100 ml of 0.9% sodium chloride or dextrose 5% in water.

After the introduction of the Continuflo add-a-line I.V. tubing system, drugs for intermittent infusion could be mixed into minibags for large volume dilution and hung piggyback fashion, allowing the nurse maximum control of flow rate and freeing her from prolonged bedside administration. During the 1980s, alternate methods of intermittent administration, such as the syringe pump, have become available.

Currently, up to 50% of all drugs administered in hospitals are given intravenously as more and more antibiotic, antineoplastic, and cardiovascular drugs have become available. Today, the I.V. route is being used to deliver thrombolytic drugs, which dramatically improve prognosis for patients with coronary thrombosis, and histamine$_2$ (H$_2$) receptor antagonists that prevent ulcers. Furthermore, the I.V. route is being used increasingly to deliver anticonvulsant drugs.

Why the upsurge?

I.V. therapy has continued to expand because I.V. drugs permit more rapid and effective treatment of the critically ill. Also, more paramedics are now qualified to give I.V. drugs, and more nurses are trained to perform venipuncture. Although some hospitals still restrict I.V. injection and cannula insertion to the medical staff, most now depend on nurses to perform these services.

Improved equipment

A large selection of convenient I.V. delivery devices is readily available today. The flexible plastic cannula, for instance, is now the preferred device for continuous I.V. therapy. Such devices are also more comfortable for patients and, because infiltration is less likely, increase the margin of safety.

Another device, the heparin lock—an injection cap locked onto a plastic cannula—facilitates intermittent I.V. therapy. Injection caps allow innumerable needle sticks, and easy-to-use heparin and saline flushes prevent clogging of the cannula between injections.

Additional devices, such as electronic infusion pumps, controllers, and syringe pumps, now deliver precisely controlled doses and infusion rates. I.V. tubing with backcheck valves largely prevents drug mixing in piggyback systems, and I.V. filters eliminate particulate matter, bacteria, and air bubbles.

A greater margin of safety
Furthermore, I.V. drugs have a greater margin of safety today. This can be attributed to manufacturers' quality control programs, FDA requirements, and pharmacist preparation of I.V. drugs in most hospitals. Detailed drug labels also promote safety.

ADVANTAGES OF I.V. THERAPY

Compared with oral, S.C., or I.M. administration, I.V. administration possesses many advantages. For instance, it provides immediate and predictable therapeutic effects, making it the preferred route for emergency use. It also eliminates absorption problems, allows accurate titration of doses, reduces administration pain, and provides other advantages.

Eliminates absorption problems
Because I.V. drugs don't need to be absorbed, distribution occurs within seconds of delivery and is predictable. In contrast, oral drug absorption is slower and may be erratic or incomplete. Some oral drugs are unstable in gastric juices and digestive enzymes or irritate gastric mucosa. Even after S.C. or I.M. administration, absorption may be erratic because of impaired tissue perfusion or excessive adipose tissue.

I.V. drugs also circumvent first-pass metabolism, ensuring maximum drug bioavailability. In contrast, oral drugs must pass through the liver, where significant amounts are eliminated before reaching the bloodstream. As a result, only a small fraction of some oral drugs reaches the systemic circulation unchanged. First-pass metabolism may also be

so rapid and extensive (such as with lidocaine) that it precludes oral administration. This explains why an equipotent I.V. dose is much smaller than an oral dose.

Allows accurate titration
I.V. administration allows superior titration of drug doses. Because absorption isn't an issue, an effective dose can be delivered by adjusting concentration and administration rate.

Reduces pain
I.V. administration avoids the pain of I.M. or S.C. injection. Although venous irritation can occur with rapid delivery of some I.V. drugs, pain threshold is much higher in veins than in muscle and subcutaneous tissues. Besides, venous irritation can be reduced by further dilution of the I.V. solution, whereas I.M. and S.C. drugs can be diluted by only a few milliliters.

Other advantages
The I.V. route also provides an alternative when the oral route is inaccessible or contraindicated, such as when a patient is unconscious, uncooperative, or N.P.O. And if an adverse reaction occurs, the I.V. route permits immediate cessation of drug delivery, which may stop the reaction or prevent its exacerbation.

DISADVANTAGES OF I.V. THERAPY

As with other routes of administration, the I.V. route has certain possible disadvantages. These include incompatibility, difficulty in gaining vascular access, immediate onset of adverse and hypersensitivity reactions, and iatrogenic complications.

Incompatibility

Incompatibility refers to an undesirable chemical or physical reaction between a drug and a solution or between two or more drugs. It can occur when drugs are mixed together in a syringe or in I.V. solutions or when an I.V. drug is given piggyback via an existing I.V. line. Typically, the commonly used I.V. solutions are compatible with most I.V. drugs. However, the more complex the solution, the greater the risk of incompatibility. I.V. solutions with bivalent cations, such as calcium, have a higher incidence of such incompatibilities. For example, lactated Ringer's and Ringer's injection can present mixing problems. Such problems are also common with nutritional solutions, alcohol, and mannitol.

The following factors influence I.V. drug compatibility:

• *Drug concentration.* A chemical reaction can't occur unless drugs come in contact. Thus, the higher the concentration, the greater the risk of an ion interaction. For example, aminophylline is incompatible with some I.V. drugs at high concentrations but not at low ones.

• *Duration in solution.* The duration of chemical reactions varies, ranging from 1 second to several days. The longer the contact, the greater the risk of incompatibility. That's one reason why I.V. drugs should be mixed just before use and discarded if not used within 24 to 48 hours. (Another reason is contamination.)

• *Temperature.* Low temperatures preserve drug stability. In fact, reaction rates double each time the temperature rises by 18° F. (10° C.). Although most I.V. drugs and solutions remain stable for up to 48 hours when refrigerated, many may be kept longer provided the cold temperature remains constant. Nev-

ertheless, fungal or bacterial contamination may occur unless the solution contains preservatives.

• *pH.* A drug added to an I.V. solution may change the solution's pH and the drug's stability. Antibiotics, for instance, are especially affected by a pH below 4.0 or above 8.0. Adding calcium raises alkalinity and may cause drug decomposition.

• *Order of mixing drugs.* This is especially important when adding electrolytes to nutritional solutions.

• *Light.* Some solutions must be shielded from light to prevent degradation. For example, nitroprusside must be covered even during infusion.

When combining I.V. drugs or piggybacking an I.V. drug into patent I.V. tubing, refer to a compatibility chart. (See *I.V. drug compatibility* chart on the inside front cover.) If this information is unavailable, consult the pharmacist concerning the effect of individual pH, buffers, or other stability factors on drug administration.

Incompatibilities may be classified as pharmaceutical or therapeutic. Pharmaceutical incompatibilities are further categorized into chemical or physical incompatibilities. Therapeutic incompatibilities, or drug interactions, refer to synergistic, additive, or antagonistic reactions when two drugs are administered concurrently.

Pharmaceutical incompatibilities

Both chemical and physical pharmaceutical incompatibilities alter the characteristics and activities of one or both drugs or solutions and may alter a drug's therapeutic effect. Usually undetectable, chemical changes occur more commonly than physical ones. Typically, they result from a reaction between acidic or alkaline drugs or solutions with unstable pH. *Chemical* reactions include:

• hydrolysis—a reaction of a compound with water, which splits the compound. Both organic and inorganic salts may undergo hydrolysis, and a precipitate may form. Exposure to light can cause hydrolysis (photolysis), with subsequent discoloration. Photolysis can usually be prevented by storing drugs in light-protected containers.

• reduction—one drug gaining electrons from another drug, causing a change in their chemical characteristics. For example, ferric ions are reduced to more absorbable ferrous ions by ascorbic acid (vitamin C).

• oxidation—the loss of electrons from one drug to another, sometimes causing inactivation. Oxidation-prone drugs include dopamine and isoproterenol. Addition of an antioxidant or storage in amber glass vials minimizes oxidation.

• double decomposition—the simultaneous occurrence of reduction and oxidation. Discoloration may result.

Physical incompatibilities are visible, resulting from physical or chemical reactions with a solution's pH, the solvent, or the container material. These incompatibilities include:

• gas formation—a reaction that results in carbon dioxide release. This may follow the mixing of bicarbonate with strong acids.

• color change—a reaction to an effect on ionization by altered drug pH. Cephalosporins may change color if not used within 24 hours.

Therapeutic incompatibilities
When two drugs are administered together, the effects of either or both drugs may be altered, producing a response that differs from the intended one. Interactions generally take place at the site of drug action. Chloramphenicol, for example, antagonizes the bactericidal action of penicillin. If both drugs are used to treat the same illness, you'll need to administer them separately, at least 1 to 2 hours apart.

Because of the potential for incompatibilities, be sure to follow manufacturer's directions for reconstituting or diluting drugs. Some diluents contain preservatives that may cause incompatibility. And because chemical reactions depend on concentration, add either the most concentrated or the most soluble drug to the I.V. container first. Mix one drug at a time, and observe the admixture before adding subsequent drugs.

Inability to gain vascular access
In an emergency, easily accessible veins may collapse from hypovolemia or vasoconstriction. Vasoconstriction may also increase the risk of bruising and infiltration.

Venipuncture may also be difficult in patients requiring frequent or prolonged I.V. therapy. They may develop small, scarred, inaccessible veins from repeated venipuncture or irritating drugs.

If peripheral access isn't possible, the doctor may select the jugular or subclavian vein. Occasionally, he may use the femoral vein, but inadvertent cannulation of the femoral artery and subsequent intra-arterial injection can cause arterial spasm and gangrene.

If venous cannulation is impossible, drugs are usually given I.M. or S.C., provided the volume is small and the drugs are known to cause little tissue irritation.

Immediate adverse and hypersensitivity reactions
I.V. administration, especially by direct injection, can cause adverse effects whose severity correlates directly with drug concentration and delivery rate. Severe reactions may occur immediately because I.V. administration promptly produces high serum drug levels.

Administering controlled drugs: Taking proper precautions

In the United States, government agencies regulate certain drugs with a high potential for abuse. The FDA classifies controlled substances into five groups: Schedules I to V. You'll never administer Schedule I drugs because these drugs have the highest potential for abuse and aren't accepted for any medical use. But you may administer Schedule II to V drugs. Remember that all scheduled drugs are potentially habit-forming or addictive or both.

● Schedule I: No accepted medical use in the United States, with high potential for abuse: heroin, lysergic acid diethylamide (LSD), mescaline, peyote, and psilocybin.

● Schedule II: High potential for abuse, with severe psychological or physical dependence possible: amobarbital, amphetamine, cocaine, codeine, hydromorphone, meperidine, methadone, methamphetamine, methaqualone, methylphenidate, morphine, opium, oxycodone, oxymorphone, pentobarbital, phenmetrazine, secobarbital, and tetrahydrocannabinol (THC) and derivatives.

● Schedule III: Less abuse potential than drugs in Schedule II: anabolic steroids, barbituric acid derivatives (except those listed in Schedule IV), benzphetamine, chlorphentermine, glutethimide, mazindol, methyprylon, paregoric, and phendiametrazine.

● Schedule IV: Less abuse potential than drugs in Schedule III: barbital, benzodiazepine and derivatives, chloral hydrate, diethylpropion, ethchlorvynol, ethinamate, fenfluramine, meprobamate, methohexital, paraldehyde, phenobarbital, and phentermine.

● Schedule V: Less abuse potential than drugs in Schedule IV: diphenoxylate compound and expectorants with codeine.

Before administering any controlled substance, take these precautions:
● Check hospital policy for special procedures.
● Sign out, on the narcotics form, any drugs removed from the narcotics cabinet and remember to relock the narcotics cabinet after removing the needed drugs.
● Follow the proper disposal procedures if drug is not completely used.
● Never leave any drug lying on the counter.

Hypersensitivity to I.V. drugs, though uncommon, can occur at any time. And if a patient is hypersensitive to one drug, he may also be hypersensitive to other chemically similar drugs (cross-sensitivity). Penicillin and its synthetic derivatives are the drugs most likely to produce anaphylaxis, the most severe hypersensitivity reaction. Hypersensitivity results from an antigen-antibody reaction or cell-mediated immunity. The drug binds to tissue proteins, which act as the antigen, and stimulates the immune system to form antibodies. Once antibodies are formed, the patient is sensitized, and subsequent exposure to the drug will provoke an allergic response. In anaphylaxis, an antigen-antibody reaction causes massive release of histamine, which acts on target organs and tissues, producing symptoms within minutes of drug administration.

An allergic reaction may be delayed for several days or even weeks after the drug has been administered. Symptoms include sudden fever, joint swelling, rash, hives, and hematologic changes. Always stay alert for hypersensitivity when giving I.V. drugs.

An idiosyncratic reaction, another type of adverse drug effect, occurs in patients with an inherent inability to tolerate certain chemicals. A tranquilizer, for instance, could cause excitation rather than sedation in some patients.

Iatrogenic complications

Other disadvantages of I.V. therapy include the risk of developing iatrogenic infections, such as human immunodeficiency virus (HIV) infection and hepatitis. Necrosis may develop from infiltration. Venous irritation and phlebitis may also occur.

Certain drugs also carry the potential for abuse (see *Administering controlled drugs: Taking proper precautions*) or cause birth defects (see *Rating drug risk in pregnancy*).

PREPARATION

Although nurses prepare drugs routinely in emergency and intensive care units, pharmacy technicians prepare most I.V. drugs. These technicians receive special training, which helps to minimize the risk of error in drug preparation. Also, the physical setup and tight quality control in the pharmacy unit promote a bacteria-free environment and prevent incompatibilities and contamination.

When preparing drugs, pharmacy admixture units use a laminar flow hood (a filtering system that draws outside air through the hood's filter to remove virtually all airborne bacteria). The filtered air flows horizontally from the back to the front of the hood in uniform parallel streams, preventing nonsterile room air from entering the hood area. In addition, the pharmacy technician wears a protective gown, cap, and gloves.

When antineoplastic drugs are

Rating drug risk in pregnancy

The FDA has established five pregnancy risk categories (A, B, C, D, and X) that indicate a drug's potential for causing birth defects. Although the FDA hasn't assigned a risk category for all drugs in this handbook, the available data has been evaluated for each unrated drug. Such drugs have been assigned a risk category using FDA guidelines.

The FDA defines pregnancy risk categories as follows:
- A: Controlled studies show no risk. Adequate studies in pregnant women have failed to demonstrate risk to the fetus.
- B: No evidence of risk in humans. Either animal findings show risk and human findings do not; or, if no adequate human studies have been done, animal findings are negative.
- C: Risk cannot be ruled out. Human studies are lacking, and animal studies are either positive for fetal risk or are also lacking. However, potential benefits may justify the potential risk.
- D: Positive evidence of risk to the fetus. Nevertheless, potential benefits may outweigh potential risks.
- X: Contraindicated in pregnancy. Studies in animals or humans have shown fetal risk, which clearly outweighs any benefits.

---

prepared, a biological containment cabinet is used to minimize exposure to potential carcinogens and teratogens.

When preparing I.V. drugs, be sure to check the diluent for incompatibility and whether the drug requires filtration. Also remember to inspect the solution for particles and cloudiness. After reconstitution, be sure to check for incompatibility when adding the drug to a large volume parenteral solution—more likely with drugs or I.V. solutions with a high or low pH. Keep in mind that most drugs are moderately acidic, but that some are alkaline, including heparin, aminophylline, ampicillin sodium, and sodium bicarbonate.

If you're mixing a drug into a minibag or minibottle of 0.9% sodium chloride or dextrose 5% in water, you may use the solution in the minicontainer as the diluent. Be sure to inspect it, discarding any solution that appears cloudy or contains particles. Some solutions change color after several hours. Ask the pharmacist if it's safe to use a discolored solution.

Reconstituting powder

Many I.V. drugs are supplied in powder (lyophilized) form requiring reconstitution with such diluents as 0.9% sodium chloride, sterile water for injection, or dextrose 5% in water. To reconstitute such drugs, follow these directions:
• Draw up the amount and type of diluent specified by the manufacturer.
• Aseptically clean the drug vial's rubber stopper.
• Insert the needle with syringe containing diluent into the stopper at a 45- to 60-degree angle. This minimizes coring or breaking off of rubber pieces, which then float inside the vial.
• Mix thoroughly by shaking the vial or rolling it between your palms several times. If the drug doesn't dissolve within a few seconds, let it stand for 10 to 30 minutes. If necessary, invert the vial several times to help dissolve the drug. Don't shake too vigorously; some drugs may froth.
• To remove large particles of undissolved drug as well as pieces of rubber (from inadvertent coring of vials) and glass from broken ampules, aspirate the diluted drug from the container into a syringe with a

disposable, 5-micron filter needle, which traps large particles. Now remove the filter needle and place a new needle on the syringe for injection into a large volume parenteral solution or directly into the patient's vein. If you're injecting the drug directly into the vein, use a 21G, 22G, or 23G winged infusion set.

When using only part of a vial, remember to label it with the date and time of reconstitution, the concentration (for example, 5 mg equals 1 ml), and the person's initials who prepared the drug.

Diluting liquid

Liquid drugs are available in single-dose ampules, multidose vials, prefilled syringes, and disposable cartridges with attached needles, which are inserted into reusable plastic or metal holders. Liquid drugs don't need reconstitution. However, before use, they do commonly require dilution.

Preparing specialized drug containers

Some drugs are available in a *double-chambered vial* that contains powder in the lower chamber and a diluent in the upper one. To combine the contents, apply pressure to the rubber stopper on top of the vial to dislodge the rubber plug separating the compartments. The diluent then mixes with the drug in the bottom chamber.

Additive vials of drug can be attached directly to administration tubing. If the additive vial contains lyophilized drug, first reconstitute the drug and thoroughly mix the solution. You may then infuse the drug directly from the vial.

Adding drugs to I.V. bottles and bags

To add drugs to *I.V. bottles,* first clean the rubber stopper or latex diaphragm of vented bottles with alcohol or povidone-iodine solution. Insert the 19G or 20G needle into the bull's eye center. Then invert the bottle twice to ensure thorough mixing. After adding the drug, remove the latex diaphragm and insert the administration spike in the same area.

To add drugs to *plastic I.V. bags* (large or minibags), begin by inserting a 19G or 20G 1" (2.5-cm) needle into the clean latex medication port. (Short small-gauge needles may not instill the drug completely if the injection port extends from the top of the bag.) Now thoroughly mix the I.V. bag by grasping both ends and quickly inverting the bag twice; don't squeeze or shake the bag.

Adding drugs to infusing solutions

If you have a choice, don't add drugs to an already infusing I.V. solution because of the risk of altering drug concentration. But if you must, be sure the primary solution container is at least two-thirds full to provide adequate drug dilution. To add the drug, first clamp the I.V. tubing, and take down the container. Then with the container in an upright position, add the drug.

To add the drug to a *nonvented bottle,* first remove the air filter from the administration set and the needle from the syringe. Then insert the syringe into the air inlet port, inject the drug, and replace the air filter. For a *vented bottle,* clean the rubber stopper, insert the needle through the stopper, and inject the drug. For an *I.V. bag,* after cleaning the rubber injection port, inject the drug.

Whenever you take down the container, first close the control clamp to prevent air from entering the system. After injecting the drug into the container, invert the container at least twice to ensure thorough mixing of the drug and solution.

Labeling solution containers

Large volume parenterals and minibags and bottles prepared by the pharmacy unit have an attached label that displays the patient's full name and room number, the date, the name and amount of the I.V. solution and additive drugs, and other vital information. However, if you're preparing an admixture, you may use printed labels with space for the patient's name, room number, additive drugs, and dosage. You may also need to use time strip labels that include the patient's name and room number, and the infusion rate (in milliliters per hour, drops per minute, or both). Time strips can be added to I.V. drugs prepared in the pharmacy also. Coordinate information on time strip labels to the tubing calibration (varies with brand of I.V. tubing). Time strip labels help determine whether the correct volume of I.V. solution has been infused over the specified time.

PRECAUTIONS BEFORE ADMINISTRATION

Before administering any I.V. solution, you'll need to examine the label and solution and determine if, according to your institution's policy, a filter is needed. You'll also need to verify the doctor's order and the administration rate, and check for incompatibilities.

Examining the label and solution

If the solution has been refrigerated, remove it 1 hour before administration. Cold solutions may cause vasoconstriction and patient distress. They also release oxygen, resulting in minute air bubbles, which may trigger the air detection alarm on electronically controlled infusion devices.

Examine the solution label. Check the dose, volume, type of solution, date of preparation (shouldn't be over 24 hours old), patient's name and room and hospital number, administration time, and infusion rate.

Hold the container up to a good light. Does the solution contain any floating particles? Is it cloudy or abnormally discolored? Observe bottles for cracks or chips. Don't use a solution that's cloudy or contains particles or a container that's damaged. If the solution is discolored, ask the pharmacist if it's safe to use.

Using a filter

Be sure you know your hospital's guidelines for filter use. Hospital policies vary widely, ranging from no filter use to filtering of every I.V. drug and solution. Add-on or in-line filters, generally 0.22-micron, can remove all bacteria, air, and particles.

Most commonly, filtration is used for total parenteral nutrition (TPN), central line infusions, and such drugs as lyophilized antibiotics, which may contain particles in solution. For critically ill patients and those receiving long-term I.V. drug therapy, filters protect against bacterial contamination of the I.V. line and harmful effects of particulate accumulation. Filters may also protect against granulomas of the lungs and other organs, sometimes associated with long-term I.V. therapy. Some studies suggest that filters help prevent phlebitis.

Special filters are used when administering blood components. Both single and multiple use filters are available.

Determining flow rate and infusion rate

Keep in mind that I.V. solution sets deliver fluids at varying amounts per drop. If the doctor orders a rate in drops per minute, make sure that he knows which set calibration is being used. To avoid confusion, request rates in milliliters per hour. (The number of drops per milliliter appears on the set package.) Be sure the doctor's initial order specifies the desired rate for large volume solutions and for smaller volumes containing drugs when delivery time is recommended. Piggyback solutions may not have a delivery time specified; they're normally diluted in 50 to 100 ml and delivered over 30 to 60 minutes. Keep-vein-open rate should fall between 20 and 50 ml per hour.

To calculate an I.V. flow rate, consider the amount of solution, set calibration (number of drops that equal 1 ml), and infusion duration. (See *Calculating flow rates.*)

To calculate the infusion rate when administering I.V. drugs, you'll need to know the drug concentration in the infusion fluid, the dose to be administered per unit of time, and the drop factor of the administration set (refer to the chart in *Calculating flow rates*). Then follow these steps:

● Convert all amounts to the same units of measure, such as all times to minutes, all volumes to milliliters, and all weights to milligrams.

● If an infusion rate is ordered in mg/kg or μg/kg, find the dose in milligrams or micrograms by multiplying the ordered dose by the patient's weight in kilograms.

● Calculate the infusion rate by using the equation:

$$\text{Drug dose} \times \frac{1}{\text{drug concentration}} \times \text{drip factor} = \text{infusion rate}$$

The drug concentration — usually written as g, mg, μg/ml — is in re-

Calculating flow rates

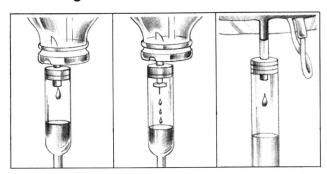

When calculating the flow rate of I.V. solutions, remember that the number of drops required to deliver 1 ml varies with the type of administration set used and the manufacturer. The illustration on the left shows a standard (macrodrip) set, which delivers from 10 to 20 drops/ml. The illustration in the center shows a pediatric (microdrip) set, which delivers about 60 drops/ml. The illustration on the right shows a blood transfusion set, which delivers about 10 drops/ml.

To calculate the flow rate, it is necessary to know the calibration of the drip rate for each manufacturer's product. As a quick guide, refer to the chart below. Use this formula to calculate specific drip rates.

$$\frac{\text{Volume to be infused (in ml)}}{\text{time of infusion (in min)}} \times \text{drip factor (in drops/ml)} = \text{flow rate (drops/min)}$$

		ORDERED VOLUME					
		500 ml/ 24 hr or 21 ml/hr	1,000 ml/ 24 hr or 42 ml/hr	1,000 ml/ 20 hr or 50 ml/hr	1,000 ml/ 10 hr or 100 ml/hr	1,000 ml/8 hr or 125 ml/hr	1,000 ml/6 hr or 166 ml/hr
ADMINISTRA- TION SET	DROPS/ ML	DROPS/MINUTE TO INFUSE					
Macrodrip Abbott	15	5	10	12	25	31	42
Baxter Healthcare	10	3	7	8	17	21	28
Cutter	20	7	14	17	34	42	56
IVAC	20	7	14	17	34	42	56
McGaw	15	5	10	12	25	31	42
Microdrip Various manu- facturers	60	21	42	50	100	125	166

ciprocal (inverted) form. If the drug dose appears in mg/minute, the drug concentration in mg/ml (the reciprocal is ml/mg) and the drip factor in gtt/ml, the equation can be expressed as:

$$mg/min \times ml/mg \times gtt/ml = gtt/min$$

For example, suppose the doctor's order specifies that 2 g of lidocaine be added to 500 ml of dextrose 5% in water. The drug concentration, therefore, is:

$$\frac{2\ g}{500\ ml} = \frac{2,000\ mg}{500\ ml} = \frac{4\ mg}{1\ ml}$$

The reciprocal of this concentration is 1 ml/4 mg. The drug is to be infused at 2 mg/min (the drug dose), using a microdrip set that delivers 60 mcgtt/ml (the drip factor). Substitute these numbers in the infusion rate equation:

$$\frac{2\ mg}{1\ min} \times \frac{1\ ml}{4\ mg} \times \frac{60\ mcgtt}{1\ ml} = \frac{30\ mcgtt}{min} \text{(infusion rate)}$$

For patients receiving large-volume parenterals (fluids given to maintain hydration or to replace fluids or electrolytes), you may have to convert the infusion rate to the volume administered over a period of time, such as 1 hour, 8 hours, or 24 hours. How you perform the calculations depends on how the original orders were written and how the institution requires orders to be written for large-volume parenterals. The calculations will vary, depending on whether you need to know the flow rate, the volume per hour, or the volume per shift or day.

To convert the infusion rate over a period of time, use this formula:

$$\frac{\text{Volume of fluid}}{\text{time in hours}} = X\ ml/hour$$

Checking for incompatibility

Before giving any I.V. drug for the first time, find out if it's to be given with another drug or I.V. solution. To avoid incompatibility with drugs given intermittently or by direct injection, first flush the primary tubing or heparin lock with 0.9% sodium chloride or dextrose 5% in water or with any other compatible solution.

What if a drug is to be given piggyback and is incompatible with the primary solution? Try these alternatives:
● Temporarily stop the primary I.V. solution and flush the line with 0.9% sodium chloride. Infuse the piggyback drug, then flush the line again.
● Insert a heparin lock elsewhere.
● Add a T-connector to the distal end of the tubing, flush the T-connector, and give the piggyback drug via the injection port of the T-connector while the primary infusion continues. (A T-connector allows simultaneous or intermittent administration at the same site.)

Remember, too, that drugs may be compatible if not mixed in the same solution or if once mixed, they're infused within a specified time. (Most incompatibility charts don't specify degrees of incompatibility that result from mixing in I.V. tubings or containers.) Ask the pharmacist if drugs can be safely piggybacked in tubing of a continuously infusing I.V. or with a T-connector. If no compatibility data exist, *always administer drugs separately.*

ADMINISTRATION METHODS

I.V. fluids and drugs are given by direct injection, intermittent infusion, or continuous infusion by various devices. (See *Understanding I.V.*

therapy devices, pages xx to xxvii and *Comparing central venous catheters,* pages xxviii to xxxi for more information about types of drug delivery devices.) Most fluids are infused continuously, whereas drugs can be given by any of the three methods.

Direct injection
Using direct injection, a single drug dose may be given or multiple doses may be delivered intermittently at scheduled intervals. Adverse reactions occur most commonly with direct injection because of high drug concentrations. Dilution for direct injection is usually 10 ml and shouldn't exceed 25 ml. Because direct injection exerts more pressure on the vein than other methods, it also carries a greater risk of infiltration in patients with fragile veins.

A high concentration of an I.V. drug may be injected directly into a vein, a heparin lock, or the tubing of an infusing I.V. line. If the drug isn't compatible with the I.V. solution, be sure to flush the line before injecting the drug. To do so, clamp the primary line and then instill 0.9% sodium chloride infusion through the injection port. Inject the drug into the port's rubber stopper and flush the line again.

Intermittent infusion
The most common and flexible I.V. method, intermittent infusion is used to administer drugs over short periods at varying intervals, achieving peak and trough levels that optimize therapeutic effectiveness. This infusion may be used to deliver a small volume (25 to 250 ml) over several minutes or a few hours. It may be delivered via a winged infusion set, an intermittent injection cap (heparin lock), existing peripheral or central venous line, implanted venous

access device, or syringe pump.

Continuous infusion
This infusion method permits carefully regulated drug delivery over a prolonged period. Sometimes an initial loading dose is given to reach peak serum levels quickly before beginning continuous infusion.

Continuous infusion enhances the effectiveness of some drugs, such as lidocaine and heparin. It may be administered through an existing peripheral I.V. line or a central venous line.

Infusion controllers and pumps
These electronic devices permit accurate, on-time delivery of fluids and drugs. They allow immediate changes in flow rate, decrease the number of hands-on infusion checks, prevent overly rapid infusion, reduce the incidence of severe infiltration, and maintain cannula patency. (See *Comparing controllers and pumps,* page xxxii, for a summary of the differences between these types of devices.)

Infusion controllers and pumps are used for certain drugs, especially aminophylline, antibiotics, antifungal agents, fibrinolytic agents, heparin, high-dose potassium chloride, lidocaine, oxytocin, and vasopressors. They're also employed for drug infusion in all infants and children. Other uses include TPN, infusion for patients with restricted fluid intake or multiple vein problems, and infusion for patients in whom position changes (from walking, sitting, or raising the arms) may change or stop the I.V. flow rate.

Controllers and pumps may also be used to overcome other common problems. These include exceedingly slow I.V. rates, which allow blood backup from venous pressure; small-gauge cannulas; small, scarred, nar-

(Text continues on page xxvi.)

Understanding I.V. therapy devices

DEVICE	HOW TO USE

Direct injection

Winged infusion set
Short hubless steel needle with wings and extension tubing can be attached to a syringe or I.V. tubing. Used for I.V. push, short-term I.V. drug or fluid therapy, and for withdrawing blood samples from small veins.

After flushing the tubing to eliminate air, insert the needle into any accessible vein, aspirate blood, and slowly inject the drug.

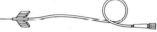

Intermittent injection device (heparin lock)
Used as a direct injection device or can be attached to any peripheral or central venous catheter for intermittent injection or infusion.

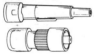

Prime injection cap with sterile fluid, then attach cap to venous access device. (Some needles and cannulas have preattached injection caps.) Inject saline or heparin flush to maintain patency. Before use, flush with 0.9% sodium chloride if heparin is incompatible with primary infusion. Attach I.V. tubing to 1″ 20G (or smaller) needle, insert into cap, then tape in place.

Intermittent infusion

Piggyback Continu-Flo add-a-line system
Tubing with backcheck valve and Y injection port uses existing peripheral I.V. line for intermittent delivery of drugs or solution in minibottles or bags.

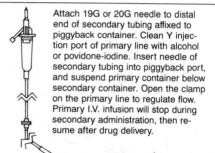

Attach 19G or 20G needle to distal end of secondary tubing affixed to piggyback container. Clean Y injection port of primary line with alcohol or povidone-iodine. Insert needle of secondary tubing into piggyback port, and suspend primary container below secondary container. Open the clamp on the primary line to regulate flow. Primary I.V. infusion will stop during secondary administration, then resume after drug delivery.

Volume-control set
In-line graduated fluid chamber uses existing peripheral I.V. line for administration of drugs or fluids in a small volume of diluent; especially suitable for children.

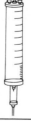

Prime set with I.V. fluid and clean the injection port on top of chamber with alcohol or povidone-iodine. Inject drug into port. Agitate chamber gently to disperse the medication. Next, fasten tubing below chamber to 20G needle and into primary line injection port. Open clamp on primary line to regulate infusion rate. Infusion stops when delivery is complete. Refill volume chamber for each dose.

SPECIAL CONSIDERATIONS

● With this device, blood return is clearly visible, wings allow easy needle grip, and sharp, thin needle is easy to insert. Also, tubing changes are easily made at extension tubing hub, vein wall damage is less, and infusion rate is more easily controlled than with syringe and needle.
● Extravasation occurs easily because needle is nonflexible. Tape in place without obscuring needle tip to observe for extravasation.
● Stabilize on armboard for long-term use.

● Clean latex cap with alcohol or povidone-iodine before each use.
● If not routinely used, flush at least once daily to prevent clogging.
● Change I.V. site according to hospital policy.
● Cap is resealable with multiple injections.

● Heparin lock can be used instead of keep-vein-open I.V.
● Because of less drug-vein contact, heparin lock is less likely to cause phlebitis.
● Allows patient freedom of movement between infusions.

● Permits infusion of most drugs with primary solutions because of minimal mixing of primary and secondary solutions. Before next dose, backflow primary fluid into secondary tubing to remove any air.
● Backcheck valve prevents backflow into primary container.
● Change tubings according to hospital policy.
● Rate of primary I.V. may need adjustment after secondary container empties.

● Volume-control set may be attached in piggyback manner to primary I.V. set or connected directly onto I.V. cannula. May be used as continually flowing device by clamping air vent tubing on volume-control set.
● Set is available with or without in-line filter.

● Check for incompatibilities. Avoid simultaneous infusion if primary infusion of I.V. solution or drugs (or both) is incompatible with piggyback drug.
● Flush entire set after administration to remove drug in distal tubing.

(continued)

Understanding I.V. therapy devices *(continued)*

DEVICE	HOW TO USE

Multiple-lumen peripheral catheter (Arrow Twin-Cath)
Multiple-lumen over-the-needle catheter designed for peripheral placement or blood sampling. Two separate lumens prevent mixing of infusates within the catheter.

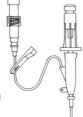

After readying the puncture site, prepare the catheter by flushing the proximal port through the injection cap. Perform a venipuncture, remove the introducer needle, and attach a stopcock, injection cap, or connecting tubing to the distal hub. Next, check the proximal lumen hub. Aspirate for blood from the proximal port. Flush, then attach the proximal hub to the desired connecting line.

Controlled Release Infusion System (CRIS)
Secondary administration system delivers drugs via a reconstituted vial.

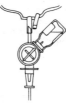

Spike reconstituted vial directly onto a CRIS adapter attached to primary I.V. tubing. Valve on the adapter allows primary solution to enter and flush out the vial, which then delivers drug and solution into tubing.

Central venous catheters (Groshong, Hickman, multiple lumen)
Silastic or polyurethane catheter is inserted into jugular or subclavian vein and terminated in superior vena cava. Used for intermittent infusion of drugs and withdrawal of blood samples. Drugs and solutions may be simultaneously delivered in double and triple lumen catheters; especially suited for long-term and multiple therapies.

Clean injection cap attached to hub of lumen with alcohol or povidone-iodine. To deliver drug, insert needle with I.V tubing into cap. After direct injection or infusion, flush line with saline or heparin.

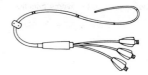

Click-Lock I.V. system
This device has two components: a transparent housing that contains a recessed needle and a diaphragm-covered port that fits into the needle housing. Used to piggyback an existing I.V. line into a heparin lock, a central line, or an existing peripheral line with regular tubing.

To use with a regular I.V. line, first attach the Click-Lock extension tubing to the tubing from the I.V. container. Fill the extension tubing with solution, expel the air, and attach it to the I.V. catheter. Next, attach the piggyback I.V. set tubing to the Click-Lock housing unit. Run solution through the set. Slide the needle housing over the injection port in the extension tubing until they lock.

SPECIAL CONSIDERATIONS

● May be used to infuse incompatible drugs.
● Don't allow flush solution to go beyond the catheter tip when flushing the proximal port.

● When using the proximal port for blood sampling, temporarily shut off the distal port.
● Acetone may weaken the catheter and cause leakage.

● Requires minimal amount of diluent to prepare solution (good for fluid-restricted patients).
● Some drugs require transfer to an empty sterile vial with additional diluent.

● Check for compatibility with primary infusion.
● System eliminates need for minibags, minibottles, and secondary tubing.

● Central venous catheters must be inserted by a doctor, have a greater potential for infection than peripheral line catheters, and require heparin or saline flushes after each use. Initial cost is higher than for peripheral catheters.
● With this device, there's a greater risk of life-threatening complications, such as air embolism and cardiac tamponade (not a risk with peripheral catheters). Air elimination filtration may be needed to lower risk of air emboli.
● Must use sterile technique.
● Groshong and Hickman catheters may be tunneled under skin, don't dislodge easily, and are comfortable for the patient. However, they may require surgical insertion and removal if used long-term.
● Central venous catheters allow administration of highly osmolar fluids and irritating drugs because of high volume blood flow in vena cava.
● On multiple lumen tubes, mark lumen used for drug delivery.
● Teach the patient how to administer medication using this device.
● May stay in place weeks, months, or even years if no complications.

● This system helps to minimize accidental disconnection, prevent contamination, and avoid needle sticks.
● With a Click-Lock in place, blood samples can be drawn from a central line using a Vacutainer setup. After drawing blood, flush the central line with 0.9% sodium chloride solution, then instill 2.5 ml of heparin flush solution (10 units/ml).
● Aseptic technique is critical.

(continued)

DEVICE	HOW TO USE
Syringe pump Prefitted and labeled in the pharmacy, syringe (5 to 60 ml) is used for intermittent infusion. A microbore tubing is attached to the syringe and a needle to the distal end.	After removing air by automatic pump priming, insert needle into a continuous I.V. or a heparin lock. Then start pump to mechanically deliver drug over ordered time interval. If ordered, place multiple doses in syringe. An alarm sounds when dose is infused or syringe is empty.

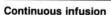

Implanted venous access device (Chemo-Cath, Hickman, Infuse-a-Port, Life Port, MediPort, Port-a-Cath, Q-Port, Strato-Port, and others) Totally implanted port with self-sealing septum is attached to a Silastic catheter that terminates in the superior vena cava or other body cavity. Most commonly used for chemotherapy or other long-term therapies. Injections are made into portal through skin.	Using sterile gloves and aseptic technique, clean skin over the portal with alcohol or povidone-iodine. Insert 21G or 22G Huber needle (noncoring) attached to syringe or tubing into middle of portal until rigid back of port is palpable. Aspirate blood return to confirm needle placement, then infuse drug. Afterward, flush port with saline and heparin and remove needle.

Continuous infusion

Existing peripheral I.V. An indwelling plastic cannula can be placed in any accessible peripheral vein to maintain peripheral I.V. line.	After cleaning the site with povidone-iodine or alcohol, perform a venipuncture. Then place the cannula and stylet into the vein. Blood return indicates correct placement. Remove the stylet and attach I.V. tubing that's been flushed with fluid to remove any air. Tape the tubing in place, and regulate the flow of infusion.

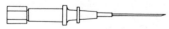

Central venous catheter (Groshong, Hickman, multiple lumen) Silastic or polyurethane catheter is inserted into jugular or subclavian vein and terminated in superior vena cava for continuous infusion of drugs into a central line. Drugs and solutions may be simultaneously delivered in double and triple lumen catheters; especially suited for long-term and multiple therapies.	First, clean injection cap attached to hub of lumen with alcohol or povidone-iodine. To deliver drug, insert needle with I.V. tubing into cap. After infusion, cap the lumen and flush line with saline or heparin.

SPECIAL CONSIDERATIONS

- Syringe pumps are portable and lightweight. They easily attach to clothing of ambulatory patients.
- A disadvantage is the pump's inability to accept more than 60 ml of drug with solution.
- Small drug volumes increase risk of phlebitis.

- May be difficult to palpate portal when entering system (especially if patient is obese).
- Requires sterile technique.
- Leave capped extension tubing and Huber needle in place for repeated injections.
- Life-threatening complications, such as air embolism and cardiac tamponade, are less common than with central venous lines.
- Risk of infection is low because device is sealed inside body.

- Device requires only once monthly heparin flush between treatments; dressing changes not required.
- Sealed under the skin, this device is cosmetically acceptable because body image and activity aren't affected. However, acceptance is poor if patient is averse to needles.
- Device requires surgical insertion. More expensive than other central lines.
- Teach patient how to give medication.

- A peripheral I.V. line is easy to insert and causes less vein trauma than a winged infusion set. It also involves less risk of thrombophlebitis and infiltration.
- If possible, establish I.V. line in large arm veins. Hand veins are more easily irritated by continuous drug therapy. Leg and feet veins aren't usually used because of the potential for thrombophlebitis.

- For special considerations, see central venous catheters listing on page xxiii of this chart.

(continued)

DEVICE	HOW TO USE

Supplemental equipment

Extension tubing
Small-bore tubing
extending 6″ to 12″
(15.2 to 30.5 cm)
attaches to any I.V. tubing.

Remove air from the tubing before attaching to venipuncture device.

I.V. loop
Horseshoe-shaped connector made
of small-bore tubing fits between the
venipuncture device and I.V. tubing.

Remove air from the tubing before attaching the loop to the venipuncture device.

T-connector
Small-bore extension
tubing, 3″ to 6″ long,
equipped with an
injection site located
near its luer-lock
adapter.

After removing air from the tubing, attach the luer end to the venipuncture device and the opposite end to the I.V. tubing. Then, another I.V. needle can be inserted into the latex injection cap.

Flow regulator
Rate selector positioned
between venipuncture
device and I.V. tubing
delivers a specified number
of milliliters per hour.

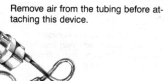

Remove air from the tubing before attaching this device.

---

row veins from long-term I.V. therapy or phlebitis; kinked I.V. tubing or tubing compressed or twisted from the patient lying on it; or a kinked cannula in a positional I.V. with cannula tip resting in a flexion area.

Electronic infusion devices sound an alarm when they detect an occlusion, air in the line (on some models), completion of infusion, low battery power, pump malfunction, and a host of other problems. Some devices detect infiltration and can administer piggyback drugs as well as a primary I.V. In fact, some pumps control up to 10 infusions simultaneously.

Specialized pumps, such as pa-

- Unlike large-bore tubing, extension tubing allows a smaller loop tubing to adjoin the venipuncture device.

- Allows I.V. tubing to be changed away from the insertion site, reducing the risk of contamination.

- Enables I.V. tubing to be changed away from the insertion site.
- Stabilizes the venipuncture device.

- Useful for simultaneous administration of fluids and drugs, this device often eliminates the need for insertion of a second venipuncture device.

- Added injection site can serve as an intermittent infusion device, for example, a heparin lock while the primary I.V. solution infuses.

- Flow regulators help ensure correct delivery of I.V. fluids.
- Less accurate than infusion pumps

or controllers, flow regulators are most reliable with inactive patients.

tient-controlled analgesia (PCA) pumps and ambulatory and implanted pumps, incorporate additional features as well.

PCA pumps

PCA pumps allow the patient to control I.V. delivery of analgesics (usually morphine) and maintain optimal serum levels. The device con-

sists of an infusion pump (joined to a timing unit) with a syringe that delivers a continuous maintenance dose of an analgesic at a controlled rate. By pressing a button attached to a cord, the patient can trigger drug delivery. The timing unit prevents overdose by imposing a lock-

(Text continues on page xxx.)

Comparing central venous catheters

CATHETER	DESCRIPTION	INDICATIONS
Short-term, single-lumen catheter	• Polyvinylchloride (PVC) or polyurethane • Approximately 8″ (20.3 cm) • Lumen gauge varies	• Short-term I.V. access • Emergency access • Patient who requires only one lumen
Short-term, multi-lumen catheter	• PVC or polyurethane • Double, triple, or quadruple lumens exiting at ¾″ (1.9 cm) intervals • Lumen gauges vary	• Short-term central venous (CV) access • Patient with limited insertion sites who needs multiple infusions
Groshong catheter	• Silicone rubber • Approximately 35″ (88.9 cm) long • Closed end with pressure-sensitive two-way valve • Dacron cuff • Available with single or double lumen	• Long-term CV access • Patient with heparin allergy
Hickman catheter	• Silicone rubber • Approximately 35″ long • Open end with clamp • Dacron cuff 11¾″ (29.8 cm) from hub • Single lumen or multilumen	• Long-term CV access • Home I.V. therapy

ADVANTAGES AND DISADVANTAGES	SPECIAL CONSIDERATIONS
Advantages: • Easily inserted at bedside • Easily removed • Stiffness aids central venous pressure (CVP) monitoring *Disadvantages:* • Limited functions • PVC is thrombogenic • PVC irritates inner lumen vessel • Needs to be changed every 3 to 7 days	• Minimize patient motion. • Assess frequently for signs of infection and clot formation.
Advantages: • Easily inserted at bedside • Easily removed • Stiffness aids CVP monitoring • Allows infusion of multiple solutions through the same catheter, even incompatible solutions *Disadvantages:* • Limited functions • PVC is thrombogenic • PVC irritates inner lumen vessel • Needs to be changed every 3 to 7 days	• Know gauge and purpose of each lumen. • Use the same lumen for the same task, for example, total parenteral nutrition (TPN) or blood sampling.
Advantages: • Less thrombogenic • Pressure-sensitive two-way valve eliminates frequent heparin flushes • Dacron cuff anchors catheter and prevents bacterial migration *Disadvantages:* • Requires surgical insertion • Tears and kinks easily • Blunt end makes it difficult to clear substances from tip	• Two surgical sites require dressing after insertion. • Handle catheter gently. • Check the external portion frequently for kinks or tears. • Repair kit is available. • Remember to flush with enough saline solution to clear catheter, especially after drawing or administering blood.
Advantages: • Less thrombogenic • Dacron cuff prevents excess motion and organism migration • Clamp eliminates need for Valsalva maneuver *Disadvantages:* • Requires surgical insertion • Open end • Requires doctor for removal • Tears and kinks easily	• Two surgical sites require dressing after insertion. • Handle catheter gently. • Observe frequently for kinks or tears. • Repair kit is available. • Clamp catheter any time it becomes disconnected or open, using nonserrated clamp.

(continued)

Comparing central venous catheters *(continued)*

CATHETER	DESCRIPTION	INDICATIONS
Broviac catheter	• Identical to Hickman except smaller inner lumen	• Long-term CV access • Patient with small central vessels (pediatric, elderly)
Hickman-Broviac catheter	• Hickman and Broviac catheters combined	• Long-term CV access • Patient who needs multiple infusions
Long-line catheter	• Silicone rubber • 20″ (50.8 cm) long; available in 16G, 18G, and 20G	• Long-term CV access • Patient with poor central access • Patient at risk for fatal complications from central insertion • Patient who needs CV access but faces or has had head and neck surgery

out time (usually 5 to 10 minutes) between doses. Used for acute or chronic pain, the pump may be especially useful in postoperative and terminal cancer patients.

With the PCA pump, better pain control may result in fewer postoperative complications and shorter recovery time because immediate drug delivery promotes patient compliance with coughing, deep breathing, and ambulation. Compared to conventional analgesic administration, the PCA pump reduces the need for analgesics.

Recently, a disposable, nonelectronic, nonbattery PCA and drug administration device has become available. The device contains an infuser and a patient-controlled module that's worn like a wristwatch. The lightweight, disposable infuser uses an inflatable reservoir (balloon) to deliver the drug at a constant rate. The elastomeric balloon serves as a storage chamber and provides energy for drug infusion. As the balloon deflates, pressure on the fluid produces a prolonged, constant flow. The infuser leads into the watchlike module, which is attached to an I.V. line.

ADVANTAGES AND DISADVANTAGES	SPECIAL CONSIDERATIONS
Advantages: ● Smaller lumen *Disadvantages:* ● Small lumen may limit its uses ● Single lumen	● Check hospital policy before drawing or administering blood or blood products.
Advantages: ● Double-lumen Hickman catheter allows sampling and administration of blood ● Broviac lumen delivers I.V. fluids, including TPN *Disadvantages:* ● Requires surgical insertion ● Open end ● Requires doctor for removal ● Tears and kinks easily	● Know purpose and function of each lumen. ● Label lumens to prevent confusion.
Advantages: ● Peripherally inserted ● Easily inserted at bedside with minimal complications ● May be inserted by trained registered nurse in some states *Disadvantages:* ● Catheter may occlude smaller peripheral vessels ● May be difficult to keep immobile ● Single lumen ● Long path to CV circulation	● Check frequently for signs of phlebitis and thrombus formation. ● Insert catheter above the antecubital fossa. ● Use armboard if necessary. ● Catheter may alter CVP measurements.

The patient requests analgesia by pushing a button on the module. No more than 0.5 ml of solution can be delivered in 6 minutes (the time required by the infuser to refill the reservoir). This device combines economical drug control with patient convenience.

Ambulatory infusion pumps

Ambulatory infusion pumps are small, battery-operated, portable, and programmable devices designed for outpatient use. The drug is contained in a prefilled, sterilized cassette (50 to 100 ml), which is maintained in a locked compartment. Alarms warn the user of low residual volume, low battery power, or mechanical failure. Ambulatory pumps may be used for continuous delivery of antineoplastic drugs. The delivery tubing from the pump is attached to a peripheral, central venous, or arterial line or to an intraperitoneal port.

Implanted pumps

The Infusaid pump, an implanted delivery system, can be used to deliver heparin and fluorouracil. The disc-shaped pump has two chambers separated by a titanium bellows: an inner chamber that's used to deliver the drug into the catheter and an outer sealed chamber that contains the power supply. The entire device is implanted subcutaneously. A Silastic catheter inserted into a vein is connected to the pump. The pump itself has a 50-ml volume and a set rate of 3 to 6 ml/day; it requires refilling every 8 to 16 days. Pump re-

fills and side port injections are performed by percutaneous injection into a self-sealing septum.

Completely sealed within the body, the implanted pump reduces the risk of complications, provides continuous and precise drug flow, and can deliver high drug concentrations to a target organ. However, a surgeon must place the pump, and locating the target site for injections can be difficult. The pump is also expensive.

SITE CARE

You'll perform site care primarily to prevent infection. But such care also allows routine observation to detect phlebitis, extravasation, and venous irritation.

Initial access

Before choosing an initial access site, find out how long I.V. therapy is expected to last, if the prescribed drug causes venous irritation, and if repeated venipuncture may be necessary.

Site selection

Some I.V. drugs cause local irritation and pain immediately or after several hours of infusion. These drugs include high-dose potassium chloride (40 mEq or more), calcium, phenytoin sodium, diazepam, nafcillin sodium, erythromycin, dactinomycin, penicillin G potassium and sodium, amino acid and hypertonic dextrose solutions, multivitamins, and some antineoplastic drugs.

To minimize irritation, select larger arm veins. Avoid veins in the hand or inner arm, which are smaller and have thinner walls. However, if you anticipate long-term I.V. therapy, start an I.V. in hand veins and proceed upward. Then, if possible, alternate extremities and change them routinely or at the first sign of inflammation; this allows reuse of veins and longer therapy. Central venous lines may be used when venous access is limited or long-term therapy is required.

Use sites in flexion areas, such as the bend of the wrist and elbow, only as a last resort. Such sites increase patient discomfort, make an even flow rate difficult to maintain, and heighten the risk of cannula blockage and subsequent clotting.

Aseptic technique
Thorough hand-washing is essential before any I.V. insertion procedure, dressing or tubing change, drug injection, or discontinuation of therapy. After selecting the vein site, you'll also need to aseptically clean the patient's skin, first shaving or clipping any excessively hairy access area. (Some experts believe that shaving predisposes the skin to bacterial contamination so check hospital policy.) Next apply povidone-iodine (10% iodine), starting at the venipuncture site and working outward in a circle for about 2″ (5 cm). In allergic patients, use alcohol. After the iodine dries, wipe the site with alcohol to facilitate vein visualization.

Securing the site
Insert the cannula (see *Inserting an over-the-needle catheter,* pages xxxiv and xxxv, and *Inserting an intermittent I.V. device,* page xxxvi) and cover the site with a sterile dressing—an adhesive bandage and tape or transparent semi-occlusive dressings. In restless, active, or confused patients or in children, place a protective net sleeve over the site to further protect the dressing and tubing against dislodgment (see *Securing an I.V. catheter,* pages xxxviii and xxxix, and *Applying a transparent occlusive dressing,* page xl).

Dealing with venous irritation
Check the site several times daily for venous irritation. If the patient complains of pain, you may need to increase drug dilution (if not contraindicated by fluid restrictions), reduce the flow rate, place warm or cold packs over the site (depending on hospital policy), or add a buffer (ask the pharmacy if buffering with sodium bicarbonate is feasible). The solution may have been made more acidic by a drug additive.

Add heparin to the solution (1,000 to 5,000 units per liter), as ordered. Heparin helps prevent thrombophlebitis and is especially beneficial for nutritional support solutions. Finally, you may need to remove the I.V. and start a new one in a larger vein.

Existing peripheral I.V. line
Before entering a peripheral line, clean the injection Y ports on the I.V. tubing with povidone-iodine or alcohol. Use a new needle for each insertion into a Y port and take special care to prevent contamination of the tubing's distal end during tubing changes and to the tubing spike during solution changes.

Keep the site dry and the dressing intact. If the dressing becomes soiled, loose, or wet, remove it and clean the cannula site with povidone-iodine, working outward in concentric circles from the site. Apply a new dressing to the clean, dry site. If the cannula isn't fully inserted, be careful not to advance it further into the vein because microorganisms can travel into the bloodstream with the cannula.

To ensure patency of an existing I.V., check the flow rate. If it's sluggish, raise the solution or squeeze the tubing near the site, after clamp-

Inserting an over-the-needle catheter

Before you begin, assemble the following supplies: an I.V. start pack containing a tourniquet, an alcohol swab, a povidone-iodine ampulet and ointment, two 2″ × 2″ gauze sponges, tape, an adhesive bandage strip or transparent occlusive dressing, and an insertion site label; a warm, moist cloth; extra alcohol swabs; an over-the-needle catheter; an extension set; an armboard; and a stockinette. Also, obtain the I.V. solution to be infused, hang the container, and attach and prime the extension set tubing. Remember that you must wear gloves anytime there's a chance of contamination from the patient's blood or body fluids.

1. Check the patient's identification bracelet against the name on the order and solution bottle. Explain the procedure. Then wash your hands. If the patient is immunocompromised, use povidone-iodine soap.

2. Distend the patient's metacarpal veins by applying the tourniquet about 8″ to 10″ (20 to 25 cm) above the approximate site, as shown. If the veins don't distend, apply a blood pressure cuff and inflate it to a few points below the patient's diastolic pressure. Or tap the vein gently, and have the patient open and close his fist or hang his arm over the side of the bed.

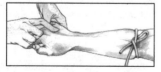

If veins fail to distend, have the patient hold a warm, moist compress in his hand. When the veins are adequately distended, choose one of the most distal sites for the insertion.

3. Clean the site with alcohol swabs. Start at the center of the site and wipe outward in a circular motion. Continue cleaning until the last swab comes away clean.

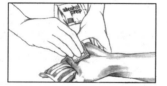

4. Repeat this procedure using povidone-iodine. (If the patient is allergic to iodine, skip this step. Just scrub the site with alcohol for 1 full minute.) Use a gauze sponge, either plain or soaked with alcohol, to wipe off the excess for better visualization.

5. Hold the skin and selected vein taut below the site to stabilize the vein.

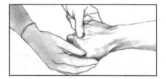

6. Insert the catheter by the indirect or direct method. To use the indirect method (preferred for small veins), first pierce the skin with the catheter's bevel up and at a 15- to 20-degree angle.

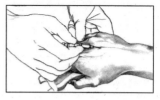

To use the direct method (preferred for large veins), thrust the catheter through the skin and into the vein with one quick motion.

7. Lessen the angle and gently advance the catheter. You should feel resistance when it reaches the vein wall. As you advance the catheter into the vein, you should feel a "popping" or "giving way" sensation. Watch for blood return in the flashback chamber.

8. Once you see blood return or feel the vein wall give way, advance the catheter about ¼" farther to ensure that the catheter itself (not just the introducer needle) has entered the vein. Then remove the tourniquet.

9. Withdraw the needle, as shown. Advance the catheter up to the hub or until you meet resistance.

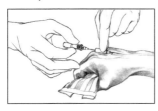

10. Attach the I.V. tubing to the hub.

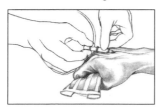

11. Begin the infusion slowly, checking to see that the line is patent.

12. Check the skin above the insertion site for signs of infiltration or hematoma formation, such as swelling or discoloration.

ing off the tubing. Forcing fluid through the cannula under mild pressure increases patency.

If position changes greatly alter the flow rate, use an armboard to limit flexion of the extremity. To prevent many positional problems, insert cannulas with tips away from flexion areas and, when feasible, use shorter cannulas (¾" to 1¼" [1.9 to 3.2 cm]). Or if hospital policy permits, aspirate and irrigate the cannula with 1 ml of 0.9% sodium chloride.

Existing central venous line
Aseptic technique is vital for delivering drugs by an I.V. line connected directly to the hub of the central line or by injection into a heparin-locked central line port. Because central lines are usually in place for extended periods, they're especially vulnerable to catheter-related infections. If the heparin lock must be changed or the tubing disconnected, clamp the line temporarily to prevent possible air aspiration. Also, remember to change injection caps at least once weekly. Upon completion of drug therapy, flush the heparin lock port with 5 to 10 ml of 0.9% sodium chloride, then follow with 250 units of heparin in at least 2.5 ml of 0.9% sodium chloride.

COMPLICATIONS

Administration of I.V. drugs always carries the risk of complications, including hypersensitivity, extravasation, infection, and phlebitis.

Hypersensitivity
Before giving any drug for the first time, ask the patient about known allergens, including food and pollen as well as any family history of allergies. Patients with a personal or

Inserting an intermittent I.V. device

You may use a ready-made, all-in-one intermittent infusion device, or you can fashion your own by combining a plastic I.V. catheter, an extension set, and an injection cap, as shown here. With an extension set, the device is manipulated less during drug administration and heparin flushes, thus reducing trauma.

An intermittent device filled with a heparin solution maintains venous access in patients receiving drugs intermittently. (Some hospitals use sodium chloride solution with or in place of heparin solution.) The device also minimizes the risk of fluid overload and electrolyte imbalance, increases patient comfort and mobility, and reduces patient anxiety as well as cost.

Barring complications, the device can remain in place for 72 hours when used with a sterile transparent occlusive dressing. If you use a gauze dressing, it should be changed every 24 hours.

Begin by gathering the following supplies: an I.V. start pack containing a tourniquet, alcohol swabs, povidone-iodine ampulet and ointment; two 2″ x 2″ gauze sponges, tape, an adhesive bandage strip or a transparent occlusive dressing, and an insertion site label; a plastic catheter; an injection cap; an extension set; a cartridge containing 100 units/ml heparin flush solution; and a cartridge syringe.

1. Check the patient's identification bracelet against the name on the order, then explain the procedure to him. Wash your hands with povidone-iodine soap. Attach the injection cap to the distal end of the extension set and prime it with heparin or sodium chloride solution. Clean the site and insert the catheter.

2. Attach the primed injection cap and extension set to the catheter hub.

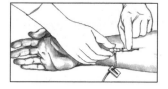

3. Swab the injection cap port with alcohol. Insert the syringe containing the heparin flush solution and

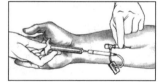

aspirate, checking for blood return. Then slowly inject 1 ml of heparin. Check the site for signs of infiltration. If the I.V. line is patent, tape the catheter securely in place.

4. According to institutional policy, apply a small amount of povidone-iodine ointment to the site (unless the patient is allergic to iodine).

5. Cover the site with either an adhesive bandage strip or a transparent occlusive dressing. Loop the extension set tubing and tape the device in place.

   Record the date, time, your name, and type and size of catheter on the dressing or insertion site label.

6. Cover the site with a stockinette to protect it.

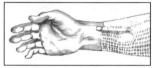

7. To keep the device patent when no medication is being given, flush it every 8 hours with 1 ml of heparin flush (concentration of 10 to 100 units/ml, depending on the device you use).

family history of allergies are most likely to develop drug hypersensitivity. In infants under 3 months, consider especially the mother's allergy history because maternal antibodies can be present in her infant. However, hypersensitivity is far less common in infants and children than in adults.

After giving an I.V. drug, remain with the patient for 5 to 10 minutes to detect any signs of hypersensitivity. If the patient's receiving the drug for the first time, subsequently check on him every 5 to 10 minutes. Otherwise, check the patient every 30 minutes after your initial assessment for a hypersensitivity reaction.

At the first sign of hypersensitivity, discontinue the drug and notify the doctor. Remember, immediate severe reactions are life-threatening. Stay alert for anaphylaxis, the most serious form of drug reaction. Initiate and assist in emergency treatment.

Extravasation

Not always preventable, extravasation may stem from venous irritation from prolonged catheter placement. In elderly patients, it may result from thin, fragile veins.

The risk of extravasation rises when the cannula remains in the vein over 2 days, when the tip is positioned near extremity flexion areas, and when the catheter is insecurely inserted into the vein. Patient movement may cause the cannula to retract from the vein.

Extravasation of a small amount of an isotonic solution or a nonirritating drug usually causes only mild discomfort, requiring routine comfort measures, such as application of warm soaks. However, extravasation of vesicant drugs, such as various antineoplastic drugs and sympathomimetics, can cause severe local tissue damage. Such damage may prolong healing, cause infection and disfigurement, and lead to loss of function and possibly amputation. (See *Prevention and emergency treatment of extravasation,* page 578.)

Be aware that blood return doesn't always indicate the absence of infiltration. Use of a small cannula in a small vein or with low venous pressure may not allow blood return. Also, if the tip of the cannula is pressed against the vein wall, blood return may be impossible.

Another common misconception is that infiltration always causes a hard lump. This may happen if the cannula tip is completely out of the vein wall. However, infiltration may produce a flat, diffuse swelling if fluid leaks out of the vein slowly, as it may, for example, if the cannula tip partially erodes the vein wall.

Keep in mind, too, that the patient may not always experience coldness or discomfort with extravasation. Coldness may be felt with extravasation during rapid administration but only rarely during slow administration. Discomfort results from irritating solutions and drugs, especially if they extravasate during a high flow rate infusion.

If you suspect extravasation, stop the I.V. at once and elevate the patient's arm. Subsequent treatment varies with the extravasated drug and hospital policy.

Infection

Besides causing local infection, I.V. therapy can cause hepatitis and, rarely, HIV infection.

Hepatitis B

Hepatitis B isn't easily transmitted in the general population; however, health care workers in frequent contact with body fluids have a much

Securing an I.V. catheter

When you're certain that the I.V. line is patent, tape the catheter in place.

1. To use the chevron method of taping, first place a ¼" wide strip of tape, sticky side up, under the catheter hub. Next, crisscross the tape over the hub, toward the fingers. Finally, place another strip of tape over the hub.

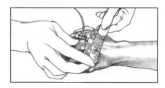

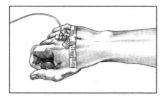

2. As institutional policy dictates, apply a small amount of povidone-iodine ointment to the site, unless the patient is allergic to iodine.

3. Cover the insertion site with a sterile bandage strip as shown at top of next column.

4. Loop and tape the tubing so it won't catch on the patient's clothing or bedclothes, which could injure the vein or disconnect the tubing from the catheter.

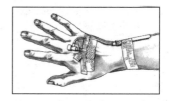

5. Record the following information on the insertion site label or tape: date, time, your name, and type and size of catheter. Attach the label to the site.

---

higher risk of acquiring this viral infection. Hepatitis B can be transmitted by blood, mucus, semen, saliva, and tears; the virus can survive for several days on inanimate objects. Use the same precautions with blood and body fluids of hepatitis B patients as you would with AIDS patients.

Nurses who administer I.V. drugs and solutions should receive hepatitis B vaccine. This vaccine is effective for at least 5 years and produces antibodies in 95% of those vaccinated, effectively preventing hepatitis B in high-risk individuals.

HIV infection
The cause of AIDS, HIV infection can occur after accidental needle stick, although the risk is small. However, you should treat all patients as potentially infected with HIV and take appropriate precautions. (See *Preventing transmission of hepatitis and AIDS,* page xli.)

Local infection
I.V. sites aren't easily infected, but the risk of infection rises with poor insertion technique, a soiled or wet insertion site, or severe postinfusion phlebitis. Aseptic technique can prevent infection during tubing and dressing changes. Proper taping of the I.V. device prevents movement

6. If the insertion site is over an area of flexion, use an armboard to immobilize the site. First, cover the armboard with absorbent paper so the patient's arm won't stick to it when he perspires. Then position his hand over the end of the armboard, as shown. The wrist should be flexed at 20 degrees, and the knuckle joints flexed at 45 to 60 degrees. Cup the palm slightly, and position the thumb as it would be to pinch something. Never flatten the hand on the armboard; immobilizing it in a nonfunctional position could cause nerve damage.

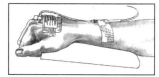

7. To tape the armboard to the arm, first double-back the tape so the adhesive side won't be next to the patient's skin. Then tape the armboard as shown, making sure it's not too tight, which could restrict blood flow and cause clotting or infiltration.

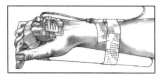

8. Cover the site with a stockinette or stretch net to protect it and prevent pulling on the I.V. tubing.

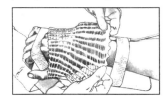

9. In your nurses' notes, record the date and time of insertion, the type and size of the catheter, the insertion site, and your name.

10. Remember that the site should be changed every 48 to 72 hours to reduce the risk of complications.

---

that may carry pathogens into the bloodstream.

If you observe purulent drainage at the insertion site when removing the catheter, consider the possibility of infection. Obtain a specimen of the drainage for culture and sensitivity testing, then apply an antibiotic ointment to the site.

Suspect sepsis if the patient has fever and chills. Obtain two or three blood samples for culture testing. Chills and fever may occur without evidence of phlebitis or other vein problems. If a positive blood culture can't be attributable to any other source, suspect the I.V. line as the infection source. Incidence increases with use of multiple lines.

Staphylococcus aureus and *Staphylococcus epidermidis* are the most common causative organisms. Others include *Klebsiella pneumoniae, Proteus mirabilis, Pseudomonas aeruginosa,* enterococcus, *Escherichia coli,* and *Candida albicans.*

Phlebitis

Postinfusion phlebitis is a major and common complication of I.V. therapy. It's commonly associated with drugs or solutions having a low pH or high osmolality. Other contributing factors include vein trauma during insertion, use of too small a vein or too large a needle

Applying a transparent occlusive dressing

Sterile transparent occlusive dressings are proven timesavers in I.V. therapy. This type of dressing can be left on an I.V. site for up to 72 hours (barring complications) without being changed. That's quite different from the maximum 24 hours for a standard gauze dressing or bandage strip. Because the dressing is changed less often, catheter manipulation is reduced, decreasing the risk of infiltration and phlebitis.

The transparent dressing allows you to assess the site as often as necessary without disturbing the dressing. Because site inspection is easier, you can detect complications earlier. The dressing helps prevent infection by keeping water and bacteria out while allowing water vapor to escape. To begin, gather the following supplies: an I.V. start pack, extra alcohol swabs, and a transparent occlusive dressing.

1. Check the patient's identification bracelet and explain the procedure. Then wash your hands with povidone-iodine soap and apply gloves.

2. Remove the old dressing, and assess the site for tenderness, redness, and swelling.

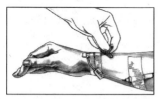

3. Clean the site with alcohol swabs, starting at the center and wiping outward in a circular motion until the last swab comes away clean.

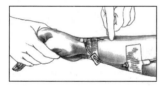

4. Repeat this procedure using a povidone-iodine swab or ampulet (unless the patient is allergic to iodine). Use a gauze sponge to blot the excess solution.

5. According to institutional policy, apply a small dab of povidone-iodine ointment (unless contraindicated).

6. Check to see that the I.V. device is taped securely.

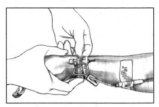

7. Write the date, time, size, and type of I.V. device, and your initials on the dressing. Use the tab to peel the dressing halfway away from its paper backing. Place half the dressing on one side of the catheter.

8. Pull off the remaining backing while "pinching" the dressing over the catheter. Smooth the rest of the dressing in place. Document the procedure and your assessment of the site in your nurses' notes.

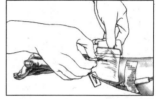

or cannula, and prolonged use of the same infusion site.

More common after continuous infusions, phlebitis can follow any infusion or even injection of a single drug. Typically, it develops 2 to 3 days after vein exposure to the drug or solution. In fact, 35% to 50% of patients develop phlebitis if an I.V. cannula remains in place for 3 days or longer. Distal veins develop phlebitis more rapidly than the larger veins close to the heart.

Drugs given by direct injection generally don't cause phlebitis when administered at the correct dilution and rate. However, phenytoin and diazepam, which are frequently given by this method, can cause phlebitis after one or more injections at the same site. Some piggybacked I.V. drugs are more irritating than others, including erythromycin, achromycin, nafcillin sodium, vancomycin, and amphotericin B. Addition of 250 to 1,000 ml of diluent lessens the risk of irritation but may not obviate the need to change the I.V. site every 24 hours. Large doses of potassium chloride (40 mEq/liter or more), amino acids, dextrose solutions (10% or more), and multivitamins can also cause phlebitis.

Mechanical phlebitis can result from motion and pressure of the cannula and also from particles in drugs and I.V. solutions. Filter needles and I.V. filters can reduce this risk.

To detect phlebitis, inspect the I.V. site several times daily. Use transparent dressing or minimal adhesive tape so the skin site is visible distal to the cannula tip. At the first sign of redness or tenderness, move the I.V. cannula to a different site, preferably on the opposite extremity. (See *Detecting phlebitis,* page xlii.) To ease patient discomfort, apply warm packs or soak the extremity in warm water.

Preventing transmission of hepatitis and AIDS

To guard against possible contamination from hepatitis and HIV-infected blood, take the following precautions:
● Avoid accidental needle sticks after venipuncture.
● Don't recap, bend, break, or otherwise manipulate needles, syringes, and blades. Dispose of sharp instruments in a rigid, sealable container in the patient's room. Be especially careful to avoid leaving needles and sharp instruments in bedclothes or on tables or floors. All sharp instruments are potential hazards.
● Wear gloves when touching blood and body fluids, mucous membranes, or any broken skin area on any patient; when performing venipuncture and other vascular access procedures; and when handling items or surfaces soiled with blood or body fluids. Keep in mind that gloves protect against contamination from open wounds, but torn or pierced gloves are no longer safe — they offer no protection against needle sticks and accidental cuts.
● Wear gowns when clothing may be soiled with body fluids, blood, or excretions. Protect your eyes with goggles and your face with a mask against splattering blood, secretions, or body fluids.
● Clean blood or fluid spills promptly, using 1 part bleach (5.25% sodium hypochlorite) to 10 parts water.
● Wash your hands immediately if contaminated with blood, secretions, or excretions and after removing gloves, gowns, and other protective apparel.

To help prevent phlebitis, the pharmacist can alter drug osmolality and pH. However, the cardinal preventive measures include expert venipuncture technique, proper at-

Detecting phlebitis

If detected early, postinfusion phlebitis can be treated effectively. If undetected, it can cause local infection, severe discomfort, and sepsis.

Skin tenderness over the cannula tip marks the first sign of phlebitis. As platelets aggregate at the damage site and a thrombus begins to form, histamine, bradykinin, and serotonin are released. Subsequently, increased blood flow to the injury site and thrombus formation at the vein wall cause redness, tenderness, and slight edema. If the cannula isn't removed, the vein wall becomes hard and tender and may develop a red streak 2″ to 6″ (5 to 15.2 cm) long. If untreated, phlebitis may produce exudate at the I.V. site, accompanied by elevated WBC count and fever. Degrees of phlebitis may be classified as follows:

1+ Painful I.V. site; absence of erythema, swelling, induration, or a palpable venous cord.

2+ Painful I.V. site; some erythema, some swelling, or both; absence of induration or a palpable venous cord.

3+ Painful I.V. site; erythema, swelling with induration or a palpable venous cord less than 3″ (7.6 cm) above site.

4+ Painful I.V. site; erythema, swelling, induration, and a palpable venous cord greater than 3″ above site.

---

tention to dilution and administration rates, frequent observation of the I.V. site to permit prompt intervention, and prompt change of the I.V. insertion site.

DOCUMENTATION

Documentation is required for all administered drugs as well as for those that couldn't be administered. To save time, prevent error, and maintain legibility, many hospitals use computerized drug administration forms that list the hospital number, patient's name and room number, dose and volume of the drug, diluent used, schedule of dosing times, and the date.

In addition, you'll record on an I.V. flow sheet or in the nurses' notes the date and time of drug administration, the signature of the person giving the drug, infusion starting date and time, solution name, device and needle gauge inserted in the vein, the insertion site, the venipuncturist's name, the administration rate, and any additives, including their dosage.

You'll also record the number of attempts required to start the I.V., including reasons for any change of site, such as extravasation, phlebitis, occlusion, patient removal of cannula, or routine change according to hospital policy. Include details of any problems with I.V. flow or site condition.

The medication administration record allows for quick review of medications the patient has received. Always remember to record the drug given. And if it wasn't given, circle the indicated time and sign your name.

Also chart on an intake and output record all large-volume parenteral solutions, including those containing drug admixtures. (See *Exploring legal issues.*)

Exploring legal issues

State laws differ concerning the practice of I.V. therapy by nurses. Some states have no specific rulings; others include policy statements in nursing practice acts or issue joint statements with state medical societies, hospital associations, and other health agencies. No state prohibits nurses from performing I.V. therapy, but a few states specify limits.

Standards of practice
Increasing numbers of institutions and agencies are establishing standards of practice for I.V. therapy — detailed nursing actions based on policy. These are used as criteria for safe, competent I.V. therapy and help guarantee high-quality nursing. For example, the Intravenous Nurses Society (INS) standards of practice are applied by many hospitals when formulating I.V. therapy policies and procedures. The Centers for Disease Control also serves as a source for I.V. therapy practice recommendations.

Hospital policies
The hospital has the ultimate responsibility to ensure that nurses perform I.V. procedures knowledgeably and safely. Written hospital policies should cover all aspects of I.V. therapy.

Policies that vary most markedly among hospitals are those involving I.V. drugs the nurse may administer. Some hospitals allow the nurse to administer any I.V. drug; others place restrictions on narcotics, antineoplastics, and emergency drugs. Before administering any I.V. drug, be sure to know the dose and effect, administration rate, incompatibilities, adverse reactions, interactions, and contraindications.

Hospital policies require nurses to fully document administration of I.V. drugs and I.V. therapy procedures. I.V. drugs are generally recorded on a preprinted medication administration record, which lists all drugs a patient receives.

A FINAL WORD

I.V. therapy has obvious benefits — it's the quickest and most effective route for drug treatment. But keep in mind that drug administration by this route requires constant watchfulness for potential problems, ranging from drug incompatibility to hypersensitivity reactions.

I.V. Drugs, Solutions, and Blood Products

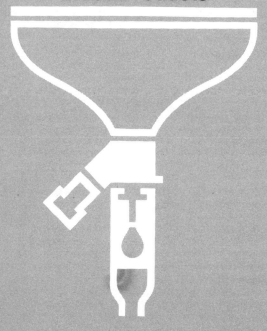

acetazolamide sodium
Diamox♦

Pregnancy Risk Category: C

PHARMACOKINETICS
Distribution: throughout body tissues and, in unknown quantities, across the placenta. Highest concentrations found in erythrocytes, plasma, and kidneys; lesser amounts in liver, muscle, eyes, and CNS. Drug doesn't accumulate in tissues.
Metabolism: not metabolized.
Excretion: by renal tubular secretion and passive reabsorption, with 70% to 100% excreted unchanged in urine in 24 hours. Not known if drug appears in breast milk.
Action: onset, 2 minutes; peak plasma level, 15 minutes; duration, 4 to 5 hours.

MECHANISM OF ACTION
This carbonic anhydrase inhibitor decreases production of aqueous humor, thus reducing intraocular pressure 50% to 60%. By inhibiting renal tubular secretion of hydrogen ions, it increases excretion of sodium, potassium, bicarbonate, and water, thus producing an alkaline diuresis.

INDICATIONS & DOSAGE
• Acute angle-closure glaucoma.
Adults: 500 mg initially, then 125 to 250 mg q 4 hours. *Children:* 5 to 10 mg/kg q 6 hours.
• Edema. *Children:* 5 mg/kg or 150 mg/m² once daily for 1 to 2 days, alternated with a drug-free day.

CONTRAINDICATIONS & CAUTIONS
• Contraindicated in sulfonamide sensitivity because of a heightened risk of hypersensitivity.
• Use cautiously in hepatic or renal disease because of an enhanced risk of hepatotoxicity or nephrotoxicity.
• In chronic pulmonary disease, use cautiously because of increased risk of respiratory acidosis.
• Give cautiously in diabetes mellitus because acetazolamide may raise glucose levels and in gout and renal calculi because drug may exacerbate these conditions.

PREPARATION & STORAGE
Available as a powder in a 500 mg vial. Reconstitute with 5 ml of sterile water for injection, preferably just before use. Alternately, refrigerate the reconstituted drug and use within 24 hours.

ADMINISTRATION
Direct injection: Using a 21G or 23G needle, inject 100 to 500 mg/ minute into a large vein.
Intermittent infusion: not recommended.
Continuous infusion: not recommended.

INCOMPATIBILITY
Incompatible with multivitamins.

ADVERSE REACTIONS
Life-threatening: bone marrow suppression (rare).
Other: anorexia, confusion, drowsiness, fever, transient myopia, nausea, minimal paresthesias, polyuria, pruritus, vomiting.

INTERACTIONS
Amphetamines, antimuscarinics, procainamide, quinidine, tricyclic antidepressants: enhanced or prolonged effects of these drugs because alkaline urine decreases their excretion.
Amphotericin B, corticosteroids, corticotropin, diuretics: heightened risk of hypokalemia.

Unmarked trade names available in the United States only.
♦Also available in Canada.   ♦♦Available in Canada only.

Cardiac glycosides: increased risk of toxicity in hypokalemic patients.

Lithium, phenobarbital: reduced effects because alkaline urine promotes their excretion.

Mannitol, urea: increased diuresis and reduced intraocular pressure.

Methenamine compounds: inactivated by alkaline urine.

Salicylates: increased elimination because of alkaline urine and enhanced risk of salicylate toxicity because of systemic acidosis.

EFFECTS ON DIAGNOSTIC TESTS

$PaCO_2$, plasma bicarbonate: possible reduced levels.

Serum ammonia, bilirubin, chloride, glucose, uric acid: possible increased levels.

Serum potassium, urine citrate: possible elevated levels.

Urine calcium, glucose, urobilinogen: possible increased levels.

Urine 17-hydroxycorticosteroids: possible false-positive results with Glenn-Nelson technique.

Urine protein: because of alkaline urine, false-positive results with bromphenol blue reagent and sulfosalicylic acid; heat and acetic acid; and nitric acid ring test.

SPECIAL CONSIDERATIONS

• Give drug under continuous medical supervision. I.V. administration reduces intraocular pressure rapidly.

• Carefully monitor intake and output and serum electrolytes, especially potassium.

• Monitor arterial blood gases (ABGs) of patients with chronic obstructive pulmonary disease (COPD) for respiratory acidosis.

• Monitor diabetic patient carefully for hyperglycemia and glycosuria.

---

acyclovir sodium (acycloguanosine)
Zovirax♦

Pregnancy Risk Category: C

PHARMACOKINETICS

Distribution: extensive, in tissues and body fluids, including brain, kidney, liver, lung, muscle, spleen, uterus, vaginal mucosa and secretions, cerebrospinal fluid, and herpetic vesicular fluid. Acyclovir sodium crosses the placenta.

Metabolism: partly in liver.

Excretion: in urine by glomerular filtration and renal tubular secretion, with 80% to 95% excreted unchanged in 24 hours. Plasma concentration follows a biphasic decline: initial phase half-life lasts up to 15 minutes; terminal phase, 2 to 3½ hours. Drug may appear in breast milk.

Action: peak serum level, at end of standard 1-hour infusion.

MECHANISM OF ACTION

Cells infected with herpes simplex virus (HSV) take up acyclovir and convert it to its active form, acyclovir triphosphate, which inhibits replication of viral DNA. Acyclovir is active against Herpesviridae, including HSV-I and HSV-II, varicella-zoster virus, Epstein-Barr virus, herpesvirus simiae (B virus), and cytomegalovirus.

INDICATIONS & DOSAGE

• Mucocutaneous HSV-I and HSV-II infections in immunocompromised patients with normal renal function. *Adults:* 5 mg/kg q 8 hours for 1 week. *Infants and children under age 12:* 250 mg/m^2 q 8 hours for 1 week.

• Initial herpes genitalis in nonimmunocompromised patients with normal renal function. *Adults:* 5 mg/kg q 8 hours for 5 days. *Infants and children under age 12:* 250 mg/m^2 q 8 hours for 5 days.

• Herpes simplex encephalitis. *Adults:* 10 mg/kg q 8 hours for 10 days. *Children ages 6 months to 12 years:* 500 mg/m^2 q 8 hours for 10 days.

• Varicella zoster in immunocompromised patients.
Adults: 10 mg/kg q 8 hours for 7 days (with normal renal function). *Children under age 12 years:* 500 mg/m^2 q 8 hours for 7 days.
Note: Dosage in renal failure is based on creatinine clearance. For adults, give 2.5 mg/kg q 24 hours if clearance is less than 10 ml/min.; 5 mg/kg q 24 hours if it's 10 to 25 ml/min.; 5 mg/kg q 12 hours if it's 25 to 50 ml/min.; and 5 mg/kg q 8 hours if clearance exceeds 50 ml/min.

CONTRAINDICATIONS & CAUTIONS
• Contraindicated in acyclovir hypersensitivity.
• Use cautiously in patients with a previous CNS reaction to cytotoxic drugs or with neurologic abnormalities because of a heightened risk of adverse neurologic effects.
• Also use cautiously in renal impairment or dehydration because of an increased risk of nephrotoxicity.

PREPARATION & STORAGE
Available as a powder supplied in 10 ml sterile vials (equivalent to 500 mg of acyclovir). Store at 59° to 77° F. (15° to 25° C.). Reconstitute in 10 ml of sterile water for injection or in a combination of bacteriostatic water with benzyl alcohol. This yields a concentration of 50 mg/ml. (In a neonate, don't reconsti-

tute with bacteriostatic water containing benzyl alcohol because of an increased risk of toxicity.)

If refrigerated, the reconstituted solution may form a precipitate, which dissolves when warmed to room temperature. Once reconstituted, the drug should be used within 12 hours.

For intermittent infusion, dilute reconstituted drug with commercially available electrolyte and glucose solutions and use within 24 hours. Dilute with at least 70 ml for a concentration of 7 mg/ml or less. Greater concentrations can cause phlebitis.

ADMINISTRATION
Direct injection: not recommended.
Intermittent infusion: Administer over no less than 1 hour using an intermittent infusion device or an I.V. line containing a free-flowing, compatible solution. Shorter infusion time risks nephrotoxicity.
Continuous infusion: not recommended.

INCOMPATIBILITY
May precipitate when combined with parabens. Also incompatible with biological or colloidal solutions.

ADVERSE REACTIONS
Life-threatening: cerebral edema, coma, renal failure.
Other: blood dyscrasias, diaphoresis, encephalopathy, headache, hematuria, hypotension, renal failure (with rapid infusion), inflammation or phlebitis at injection site, nausea, rash or hives.

INTERACTIONS
Interferon, intrathecal methotrexate: possible neurologic abnormalities.
Nephrotoxic drugs: heightened risk of nephrotoxicity.

Probenecid: prolonged serum half-life.

Zidovudine: possible neurotoxicity.

EFFECTS ON DIAGNOSTIC TESTS

BUN, serum creatinine: elevated levels, possibly from nephrotoxicity.
Serum alkaline phosphatase, SGOT, SGPT: elevated levels.

SPECIAL CONSIDERATIONS

• Carefully monitor intake and output. Because maximum drug concentration occurs in kidneys during first 2 hours of infusion, be sure to maintain adequate hydration and urine output during this period.
• Observe for fungal and bacterial superinfection with prolonged use.
• Acyclovir can be removed by hemodialysis.

adenosine
Adenocard

Pregnancy Risk Category: C

PHARMACOKINETICS

Distribution: Drug is rapidly removed from the systemic circulation, presumably by erythrocytes and vascular endothelial cells. The plasma half-life has been estimated at less than 10 seconds.
Metabolism: Once taken up into the body pool of nucleosides, drug is utilized in a variety of ways. May be converted to inosine and adenosine monophosphate.
Excretion: unknown.
Action: immediate.

MECHANISM OF ACTION

Adenosine acts on the atrioventricular (AV) node to slow conduction and inhibit reentry pathways.

INDICATIONS & DOSAGE

• Conversion of paroxysmal supraventricular tachycardia (PSVT) to sinus rhythm. *Adults:* 6 mg I.V. by rapid bolus injection (over 1 to 2 seconds). If PSVT is not eliminated in 1 to 2 minutes, give 12 mg by rapid I.V. push. Repeat 12 mg dose if necessary.

Note that adenosine is useful for treating PSVT associated with accessory bypass tracts (Wolff-Parkinson-White syndrome).

CONTRAINDICATIONS & CAUTIONS

• Contraindicated in patients with known hypersensitivity to the drug.
• Also contraindicated in patients with atrial flutter, atrial fibrillation, and ventricular tachycardia because the drug is ineffective in the treatment of these dysrhythmias.
• Because it decreases conduction through the AV node, adenosine may briefly induce a first-, second-, or third-degree heart block. For this reason, it is contraindicated in patients with second- or third-degree heart block or sick sinus syndrome, unless the patient has an artificial pacemaker. Because the drug has a very short half-life, these effects are usually transient; however, patients who develop significant block after a dose of adenosine should not receive additional doses.
• More than half of the patients in clinical trials developed new dysrhythmias at the time adenosine was used to convert to normal sinus rhythm. These effects were usually transient and included sinus bradycardia or tachycardia, atrial premature contractions, various degrees of AV block, premature ventricular contractions, and skipped beats.

PREPARATION & STORAGE
Supplied in vials containing 6 mg/2 ml. Store at controlled room temperature (59° to 86° F. [15° to 30° C.]). Do not refrigerate.

Observe solution for crystals, which may appear if solution has been refrigerated. If crystals are visible, gently warm solution to room temperature. Do not use solutions that aren't clear. Discard unused drug because it lacks preservatives.

ADMINISTRATION
Direct injection: Rapid I.V. injection is necessary for drug action. Administer directly into a vein if possible; if using an I.V. line, employ the most proximal port and follow the injection with a rapid saline flush to hasten drug delivery to systemic circulation.
Intermittent infusion: not recommended.
Continuous infusion: not recommended.

INCOMPATIBILITY
Do not mix with other drugs.

ADVERSE REACTIONS
Life-threatening: asystole, heart block.
Other: apprehension, back pain, blurred vision, burning sensation, chest pain, chest pressure, dizziness, dyspnea, facial flushing, groin pressure, headache, heaviness in arms, hyperventilation, hypotension, light-headedness, metallic taste, nausea, neck pain, numbness, palpitations, sweating, tightness in throat, tingling in arms.

INTERACTIONS
Carbamazepine: possible higher-degree heart block.
Dipyridamole: may potentiate the drug's effects, and smaller doses may be necessary.

Methylxanthines: may antagonize the drug's effects. Patients receiving theophylline or caffeine may require higher doses or may not respond to adenosine therapy.

EFFECTS ON DIAGNOSTIC TESTS
None reported.

SPECIAL CONSIDERATIONS
• Single doses over 12 mg are not recommended.
• Explain the procedure to the patient, and warn that facial flushing may occur.
• Most adverse reactions are self-limiting because adenosine has an extremely short plasma half-life. Bolus dosages of 6 or 12 mg usually do not elicit systemic hemodynamic effects.
• Give drug only under medical supervision with continuous monitoring of EKG.
• When appropriate, ask the patient to attempt vagal maneuvers such as the Valsalva maneuver before administering adenosine.
• Adenosine has been administered intravenously to patients with bronchial asthma, and no problems have been reported. However, the potential for bronchoconstriction exists. Inhaled adenosine will cause bronchoconstriction in patients with asthma, but not in healthy patients.
• Adenosine must reach the systemic circulation in sufficient quantity to provide an adequate therapeutic effect. Therefore, rapid I.V. bolus injection is necessary.
• Because the drug is not metabolized or excreted, impaired hepatic or renal function should have no effect on efficacy or duration of action of adenosine.
• Don't confuse this drug with adenosine phosphate (Cobalasine, Kay-

sine), a vasodilator used to treat complications of stasis dermatitis.
• Early clinical studies revealed that 60% of patients responded to 6 mg of adenosine or less within 1 minute of bolus injection, and 92% of patients responded to doses of 12 mg or less.
• Some experimental evidence shows that high concentrations of adenosine may induce chromosomal damage. However, the clinical significance of this finding is not known.

alfentanil hydrochloride
Alfenta

Controlled Substance Schedule II
Pregnancy Risk Category: C

PHARMACOKINETICS
Distribution: rapidly dispersed into body tissues and across blood-brain barrier, with 92% bound to plasma proteins. Drug readily crosses placenta.
Metabolism: in liver.
Excretion: primarily by liver. Inactive metabolites and less than 1% of unchanged drug are excreted in urine. Drug appears in breast milk.
Action: onset, within 1 minute for analgesia and 1 to 2 minutes for loss of consciousness; duration, 5 to 10 minutes for analgesia and 10 minutes to regain consciousness.

MECHANISM OF ACTION
Alfentanil acts as an agonist at stereospecific opioid receptor sites in the CNS. As a result, the drug alters the perception of pain and the emotional response to it.

INDICATIONS & DOSAGE
• Adjunct to anesthesia for surgery lasting 45 minutes or more. *Adults:* 130 to 245 mcg/kg.

• Maintenance of anesthesia. *Adults in surgery lasting more than 30 minutes:* 20 to 75 mcg/kg, then 5 to 15 mcg/kg as needed; or infusion of 0.5 to 4 mcg/kg/minute. *Adults in surgery lasting 30 minutes or less:* 8 to 20 mcg/kg, then 3 to 5 mcg/kg as needed. *Children:* 30 to 50 mcg/kg, then 10 to 15 mcg/kg as needed; or infusion of 0.5 to 1.5 mcg/kg/minute.

CONTRAINDICATIONS & CAUTIONS
• Contraindicated in hypersensitivity to fentanyl derivatives.
• Use cautiously in patients with head injury, increased intracranial pressure (ICP), or intracranial lesions. Drug may make neurologic assessment findings unreliable and may raise ICP by causing hypoventilation and hypercarbia.
• Also use cautiously in bradydysrhythmias because drug may induce or exacerbate dysrhythmias; in hepatic impairment because of lengthened half-life, prolonged duration, and increased drug concentration at receptor sites; in hypothyroidism because of an increased risk of respiratory depression and prolonged CNS depression; in pulmonary dysfunction or poor pulmonary reserve because of possible further decline in respiratory drive and increase in airway resistance; and in compromised cardiac reserve because of a magnified risk of severe bradycardia and hypotension.
• Because decreased metabolism prolongs drug effect, administer carefully in obese, elderly, or pediatric patients.

PREPARATION & STORAGE
Available in ampules containing 2, 5, 10, or 20 ml at a concentration of 500 mcg/ml. Drug may be injected full-strength using a tuberculin or 1

ml syringe. For continuous infusion, dilute in 0.9% sodium chloride, dextrose 5% in water, dextrose 5% in 0.9% sodium chloride, or Ringer's lactate. Store undiluted drug between 59° and 86° F. (15° and 30 ° C.); avoid freezing. Protect from light.

ADMINISTRATION
Only staff trained in administering I.V. anesthetics and managing their potential adverse effects should give this drug.
Direct injection: Over 90 seconds to 3 minutes, inject undiluted drug into I.V. tubing of a free-flowing, compatible solution.
Intermittent infusion: not recommended.
Continuous infusion: Using an I.V. piggyback, infuse diluted drug at ordered rate through tubing containing a free-flowing, compatible solution.

INCOMPATIBILITY
No incompatibilities reported.

ADVERSE REACTIONS
Life-threatening: bronchospasm, cardiac arrest, laryngospasm, respiratory depression or arrest.
Other: blurred vision, bradycardia, bradypnea, dyspnea, dysrhythmias, excitement or delirium, hypotension, muscle rigidity, nausea, postoperative depression, urticaria.

INTERACTIONS
Antihypertensives: potentiated hypotensive effects.
Erythromycin: possible decreased clearance and prolonged or delayed respiratory depression.
Hepatic enzyme inhibitors: possible decreased plasma clearance and prolonged alfentanil effect.
MAO inhibitors: increased risk of hypertension, hypotension, and tachycardia if taken within 14 days.

Nalbuphine, naloxone, pentazocine: decreased alfentanil effects.
Neuromuscular blocking drugs: prevention or reversal of muscle rigidity.
Nitrous oxide: possible cardiovascular depression.
Other CNS depressants: deepened CNS and respiratory depression.

EFFECTS ON DIAGNOSTIC TESTS
Serum amylase, lipase: elevated levels.

SPECIAL CONSIDERATIONS
• *Treatment of overdose:* Reverse effects with naloxone, then give symptomatic care. For apnea, administer oxygen and provide mechanical ventilation. Use positive-pressure ventilation via bag or mask. For hypotension, give I.V. fluids and vasopressors. For muscle rigidity, give a neuromuscular blocking drug.
• Closely monitor respiratory, cardiovascular, and neurologic systems during and after surgery.
• Discontinue drug 10 to 20 minutes before surgery ends.
• The patient who develops tolerance to other opioids may become tolerant to alfentanil as well.
• Alfentanil induces a shorter period of respiratory depression than other fentanyl derivatives. Respiratory depression may cause carbon dioxide retention, increasing cerebrospinal fluid pressure.
• The patient may need analgesics shortly after surgery.

alpha₁-proteinase inhibitor (human)
Prolastin

Pregnancy Risk Category: C

COMPOSITION
Prepared from pooled human plasma that has been tested for hepatitis and human immunodeficiency virus and found to be negative, this drug contains alpha₁-proteinase inhibitor, the deficient protein in alpha₁-antitrypsin deficiency. It also contains small amounts of other plasma proteins, including alpha₂-plasmin inhibitor, alpha₁-antichymotrypsin, C1-esterase inhibitor, haptoglobin, antithrombin III, alpha₁-lipoprotein, and albumin.

MECHANISM OF ACTION
Increases alpha₁-antitrypsin levels in plasma and the lungs' epithelial lining, thus preventing panacinar emphysema from worsening.

INDICATIONS & DOSAGE
• Replacement therapy for patients with congenital alpha₁-antitrypsin deficiency and signs of panacinar emphysema. *Adults:* 60 mg/kg once weekly.

CONTRAINDICATIONS & CAUTIONS
• Use cautiously in patients with circulatory overload because the colloidal solution increases plasma volume.
• Pediatric safety and efficacy have not been established.

PREPARATION & STORAGE
Available in single-dose vials containing 500 or 1,000 mg of alpha₁-proteinase inhibitor. The package includes a vial of sterile water for injection (20 ml for 500 mg and 40 ml for 1,000 mg), a double-ended transfer needle, and a filter needle. Refrigerate package before use.

To reconstitute, bring vials to room temperature and follow manufacturer's directions. Use within 3 hours. Dilute with 0.9% sodium chloride, if necessary.

ADMINISTRATION
Direct injection: Inject directly into vein at a rate of at least 0.08 ml/minute.
Intermittent infusion: not recommended.
Continuous infusion: not recommended.

INCOMPATIBILITY
No incompatibilities reported, but don't mix with other drugs or solutions.

ADVERSE REACTIONS
Life-threatening: none reported.
Other: dizziness, fever, transient leukocytosis, light-headedness.

INTERACTIONS
None reported.

EFFECTS ON DIAGNOSTIC TESTS
None reported.

SPECIAL CONSIDERATIONS
• Although treated to minimize viral transmission, alpha₁-proteinase inhibitor still possesses a small risk of transmitting severe infection, such as hepatitis and AIDS.
• Educate the patient about AIDS, and encourage immunization against hepatitis B in the HBsAg-negative patient.

Unmarked trade names available in the United States only.
♦ Also available in Canada.   ♦♦ Available in Canada only.

alprostadil
(prostaglandin E₁)
Prostin VR Pediatric♦

Pregnancy Risk Category: not applicable

PHARMACOKINETICS
Distribution: in plasma.
Metabolism: pulmonary, with up to 80% metabolized by oxidation on first pass through lungs.
Excretion: primarily by the kidneys, as metabolites, within 24 hours.
Action: onset, 1½ to 3 hours in acyanotic congenital heart disease, 15 to 30 minutes in cyanotic heart disease; peak effect, 3 hours in coarctation of aorta, 1½ hours in interruption of aortic arch, 30 minutes in cyanotic heart disease; duration, length of infusion. Ductus usually begins to close 1 or 2 hours after end of infusion.

MECHANISM OF ACTION
Inhibits platelet aggregation and produces vasodilation by acting directly on vascular smooth muscle. By relaxing the smooth muscle of the ductus arteriosus, it prevents the closure that normally occurs 10 to 15 hours after birth.

INDICATIONS & DOSAGE
• Temporary maintenance of ductus arteriosus patency until surgery can be performed. *Neonates:* 0.05 to 0.1 mcg/kg/minute, not to exceed 0.4 mcg/kg/minute. When therapeutic response is achieved, reduce dosage to lowest level that maintains it.
Note: Patients with low values of partial pressure of oxygen (PO₂) respond best.

CONTRAINDICATIONS & CAUTIONS
• Contraindicated in neonates with respiratory distress syndrome because a patent ductus can cause circulatory overload.
• Use cautiously in neonates with bleeding disorders because drug inhibits platelet aggregation.

PREPARATION & STORAGE
Dilute 1 ml (500 mcg/ml) in 250 ml of 0.9% sodium chloride or dextrose 5% in water. This yields a concentration of 2 mcg/ml. Store solution at 36° to 46° F. (2° to 8° C.). Don't freeze. Use prepared solution within 24 hours.

ADMINISTRATION
Only staff trained in pediatric intensive care should give this drug.
Direct injection: not recommended.
Intermittent infusion: not recommended.
Continuous infusion: Using a continuous-rate pump, infuse drug through large peripheral or central vein or through umbilical artery catheter placed at level of ductus arteriosus.

INCOMPATIBILITY
No incompatibilities reported.

ADVERSE REACTIONS
Life-threatening: apnea, bradycardia, cardiac arrest, cerebral bleeding, congestive heart failure, damage to ductus and pulmonary aorta, disseminated intravascular coagulation, hypotension, respiratory distress, seizures, sepsis, tachycardia, ventricular fibrillation, weakened aorta wall.
Other: anemia, cortical proliferation of long bones, diarrhea, fever, flushed face and arms, hyperbilirubinemia, hyperirritability, hypoglycemia, hypokalemia, hypothermia, lethargy, vomiting.

INTERACTIONS
None reported.

EFFECTS ON DIAGNOSTIC TESTS
Serum bilirubin: elevated levels.
Serum glucose: reduced levels.
Serum potassium: elevated or reduced levels.

SPECIAL CONSIDERATIONS
• *Treatment of overdose:* Discontinue drug and begin supportive therapy.
• Drug must be given before ductus closes to maintain patency.
• Monitor respiratory status during treatment and keep resuscitation equipment readily available. Apnea usually occurs in first hour in 10% to 12% of neonates weighing under 2 kg at birth.
• Keep neonate on cardiac monitor and check arterial pressures frequently via umbilical artery catheter, auscultation, or Doppler transducer. Expect to reduce infusion rate if hypotension or fever develops. Expect to discontinue drug if apnea or bradycardia occurs.
• Reposition catheter if flushing occurs.
• Infusion may continue during cardiac catheterization.
• Drug may be given by intraaortic or intraarterial infusion.
• Monitor PO_2 values.

---

alteplase
(recombinant alteplase, tissue plasminogen activator)
Activase

Pregnancy Risk Category: C

PHARMACOKINETICS
Distribution: in plasma.
Metabolism: in liver.
Excretion: 86% in urine, 5% in feces. Serum half-life ranges from 3 to 5 minutes. Not known if drug appears in breast milk.
Action: onset, rapid; duration, short.

MECHANISM OF ACTION
Binds to fibrin in thrombi and converts plasminogen into plasmin, thus initiating local fibrinolysis and limited systemic proteolysis.

INDICATIONS & DOSAGE
• Destruction of coronary artery thrombi in acute myocardial infarction. *Adults 143 lb (65 kg) and over:* 100 mg over 3 hours, with 60 mg given in first hour (6 to 10 mg in first 1 to 2 minutes), 20 mg in second hour, and 20 mg in third hour. Don't exceed dosage; 150 mg has been linked with intracranial bleeding. *Adults under 143 lb:* 1.25 mg/kg over 3 hours, with 60% of dose given in first hour (10% in first 1 to 2 minutes) and balance over next 2 hours.
• Lysis of acute pulmonary emboli. *Adults:* 100 mg over 2 hours.

CONTRAINDICATIONS & CAUTIONS
• Contraindicated in patients with internal bleeding, aneurysm, arteriovenous malformation, bleeding diathesis, history of cerebrovascular accident, brain tumor, CNS surgery or trauma in previous 2 months, or systolic blood pressure above 179 mm Hg or diastolic blood pressure above 109 mm Hg.
• Use cautiously in patients with acute pericarditis, cerebrovascular disease, diabetic hemorrhagic retinopathy, significant hepatic disease, risk of left heart thrombus (as in mitral stenosis with atrial fibrillation), marked hypertension, subacute bacterial endocarditis, septic thrombo-

phlebitis, or an occluded arterio-venous cannula at an infected site.
• Also use cautiously in patients over age 75; within 10 days after GI or genitourinary bleeding, major surgery, or trauma; and during oral anticoagulant therapy.
• Safety and efficacy in children not established.

PREPARATION & STORAGE

Available as lyophilized powder in 20 mg and 50 mg vials. Store at room temperature or refrigerate. Reconstitute just before injection. Using an 18G needle, reconstitute to 1 mg/ml by adding 20 or 50 ml of preservative-free, sterile water for injection, provided by manufacturer. (Don't use bacteriostatic water for injection.) Aim diluent at lyophilized cake and expect slight foaming. Let vial stand for several minutes.

If necessary, dilute drug to 0.5 mg/ml in glass bottles or PVC bag. For 20 ml vial, add 20 ml of 0.9% sodium chloride or dextrose 5% in water; for 50 ml vial, add 50 ml. Avoid undue agitation. Diluted solution remains stable for 8 hours at room temperature.

ADMINISTRATION

Direct injection: not recommended.
Intermittent infusion: not recommended.
Continuous infusion: Infuse diluted solution at recommended rate.

INCOMPATIBILITY

Do not mix with other drugs.

ADVERSE REACTIONS

Life-threatening: accelerated idioventricular rhythm, anaphylaxis, premature ventricular contractions, uncontrolled bleeding, ventricular tachycardia.
Other: fever, headache, hypotension, nausea, sinus bradycardia, urticaria.

INTERACTIONS

Drugs altering platelet function (such as aspirin and dipyridamole): increased risk of bleeding during and after infusion.

EFFECTS ON DIAGNOSTIC TESTS

Coagulation and fibrinolytic tests: altered results.

SPECIAL CONSIDERATIONS

• Drug must be given within 6 hours after onset of symptoms.
• If possible, obtain coagulation studies (prothrombin time, partial thromboplastin time, fibrin split products) before starting alteplase therapy.
• If unable to stop severe bleeding with local pressure, discontinue alteplase and heparin infusions.
• Avoid I.M. injections because of high risk of bleeding into muscle. Also avoid turning and moving the patient excessively during infusion.
• Monitor EKG because transient dysrhythmias result from reperfusion after coronary thrombolysis. Keep atropine or lidocaine available to treat dysrhythmias.
• To prevent new clot formation, give heparin during or after alteplase infusion, if ordered.
• Avoid venipuncture and arterial puncture during therapy because of the increased risk of bleeding. If arterial puncture is necessary, select a site on an arm and apply pressure for 30 minutes afterward. Also use pressure dressings, sandbags, or ice packs on recent puncture sites to prevent bleeding.

amikacin sulfate
Amikin♦

Pregnancy Risk Category: D

PHARMACOKINETICS
Distribution: in most extracellular fluids, including serum, ascitic, pericardial, pleural, synovial, lymphatic, peritoneal, and abscess. Drug crosses the placenta. Low levels appear in cerebrospinal fluid.
Metabolism: not metabolized.
Excretion: by glomerular filtration, with 70% to 95% recovered in urine in 24 hours. Low levels appear in breast milk. Serum half-life can extend up to 100 hours.
Action: peak plasma levels, 45 minutes to 2 hours.

MECHANISM OF ACTION
This semisynthetic aminoglycoside inhibits protein synthesis by binding to the 30S ribosomal subunit. As a result, DNA is misread, resulting in nonfunctional protein.

Amikacin acts against such aerobic bacteria as gram-negative *Acinetobacter, Citrobacter, Enterobacter, Escherichia coli, Klebsiella, Proteus, Providencia, Pseudomonas aeruginosa, Salmonella, Serratia,* and *Shigella.* Susceptible gram-positive bacteria include *Staphylococcus aureus* and *S. epidermidis.*

INDICATIONS & DOSAGE
• Septicemia, peritonitis, and severe burn, bone, joint, respiratory tract, skin, and soft tissue infections caused by susceptible organisms.
Adults and children with normal renal function: 15 mg/kg/day in divided doses q 8 to 12 hours for 7 to 10 days, not to exceed 1.5 g daily.
Adults and children with renal impairment: loading dose, 7.5 mg/kg.

Subsequent dosage based on serum levels and degree of impairment. *Neonates with normal renal function:* initially, 10 mg/kg, then 7.5 mg/kg q 12 hours.

CONTRAINDICATIONS & CAUTIONS
• Contraindicated in aminoglycoside hypersensitivity.
• Give cautiously in dehydration and renal impairment because of an increased risk of toxicity; in 8th cranial nerve damage because of the risk of ototoxicity; and in myasthenia gravis or Parkinson's disease because drug can cause neuromuscular blockade.
• Give cautiously to premature infants, neonates, and the elderly because of an increased risk of toxicity.

PREPARATION & STORAGE
Supplied as a 50 mg/ml concentration in 2 ml vials, as a 250 mg/ml concentration in 2 ml and 4 ml vials, and as 2 ml disposable syringes.

For infusion, add 500 mg of amikacin to 100 to 200 ml of 0.9% sodium chloride; dextrose 5% in water; dextrose 5% and 0.22%, 0.45%, or 0.9% sodium chloride; Ringer's lactate; or dextrose 5% and Plasmalyte 56, Plasmalyte 148, Normosol-M, or Normosol-R. All solutions remain stable for 24 hours at room temperature. Yellowing of solution doesn't indicate loss of potency.

ADMINISTRATION
Direct injection: Using a 21G to 23G needle, inject drug into an I.V. line containing a free-flowing, compatible solution. Give over 3 to 5 minutes to prevent neuromuscular blockade. Drug may also be injected into vein using an intermittent infusion device.

Intermittent infusion: Using a 21G to 23G needle, infuse diluted drug over 30 to 60 minutes in children and adults, over 1 to 2 hours in infants.
Continuous infusion: not recommended.

INCOMPATIBILITY
Incompatible with amphotericin B, cephalothin, cephapirin, heparin, phenytoin, thiopental, and vitamin B complex with C. Manufacturer recommends that amikacin not be mixed with any drug.

ADVERSE REACTIONS
Life-threatening: encephalopathy, nephrotoxicity.
Other: auditory and vestibular ototoxicity, hypersensitivity, neuromuscular blockade, neurotoxicity, peripheral neuritis.

INTERACTIONS
Aminoglycosides, amphotericin B, cisplatin, and methoxyflurane: increased risk of nephrotoxicity.
Cephalosporins, loop diuretics: heightened risk of ototoxicity.
Neuromuscular blocking agents: possible potentiated effects.
Parenteral penicillins: possible synergistic effect against certain organisms or amikacin inactivation.

EFFECTS ON DIAGNOSTIC TESTS
BUN, serum alkaline phosphatase, bilirubin, LDH: elevated levels.
Creatinine clearance: increased.
RBC count: possibly high or low.
SGOT, SGPT: increased levels.
Urine specific gravity: reduced.

SPECIAL CONSIDERATIONS
• *Treatment of overdose:* Use hemodialysis or peritoneal dialysis to remove drug, if ordered. Exchange transfusions may be considered for neonates.

• Obtain specimens for culture and sensitivity tests before first dose; therapy may begin before results are available.
• Evaluate patient's hearing before and during treatment.
• Be alert to loss of balance in ambulatory patients.
• Obtain periodic peak and trough levels, and adjust dosage as ordered. Normal peak is 15 to 30 mcg/ml; normal trough, 5 to 10 mcg/ml. Higher levels accompany toxicity; lower levels, fever. (Trough is drawn before next dosage; peak is drawn 30 minutes after dosage.)
• Obtain periodic BUN and creatinine levels to assess renal function.
• Keep patient well hydrated to reduce risk of nephrotoxicity; measure intake and output. Monitor urine for decreased specific gravity.
• Observe patient for fungal and bacterial superinfection with prolonged use.
• May contain sulfites.

---

amino acid injection
amino acid solution
Aminess, Aminosyn♦, Branch Amine, FreAmine III♦, HepatAmine, NephrAmine, Novamine, ProcalAmine, RenAmin, Travasol♦, TrophAmine

Pregnancy Risk Category: C

COMPOSITION
Amino acid injection and solution provide various concentrations of parenteral nutrients, including essential and nonessential amino acids, nitrogen, electrolytes, and calories. They supply nitrogen in a readily assimilable form. Solutions vary in amount of protein and nitrogen, os-

---

molarity, and electrolyte concentration. Nonprotein calories are usually provided as dextrose and, to a lesser extent, as glycerin, fructose, alcohol, or fat.

Special solutions can be prepared by the pharmacy for patients with specific nutrient requirements or intolerance to the components of conventional solutions. For example, solutions are available for patients with renal or hepatic failure.

INDICATIONS & DOSAGE

• Prevention of nitrogen loss or negative nitrogen balance when patient can't get adequate nutrition orally; when gastric feeding or ostomy is impossible or undesirable (as in GI disorders or surgery); in such hypermetabolic conditions as burns, sepsis, or severe trauma; and in anorexia nervosa, coma, hepatic insufficiency, or neoplastic disease.
Adults: 1 to 1.5 g/kg daily. *Children:* 2 to 3 g/kg daily. Dosage adjustment must be based on nitrogen balance and body weight corrected for fluid balance.

CONTRAINDICATIONS & CAUTIONS

• Contraindicated in severe uncorrected electrolyte or acid-base imbalance because of possible exacerbation; in hypersensitivity to any solution component; in inborn error of amino acid metabolism; in hyperammonemia, which could worsen; or in reduced blood volume, which can lead to acid-base imbalance.
• General amino acid solutions are contraindicated in renal failure, severe hepatic disease, hepatic coma, and encephalopathy.
• Special solutions for hepatic failure and encephalopathy and metabolic stress are contraindicated in anuria.

• Hyperosmolar solutions are contraindicated in intracranial or intraspinal hemorrhage because fluid overload can exacerbate the condition.
• Use cautiously in cardiac disease because of possible fluid overload; in diabetes because of increased insulin requirements; and in children, especially those with renal failure.

PREPARATION & STORAGE

Available in bottles containing 250 to 1,000 ml. Add dextrose 5% to 70% in water, electrolytes, trace elements, and vitamins, as needed. When modifying solutions, use strict aseptic technique, follow manufacturer's instructions, and administer within 24 hours. Discard any remaining solution.

Use only clear solution; hold up to light to find particulates or evidence of damaged container.

ADMINISTRATION

Direct injection: not recommended.
Intermittent infusion: not recommended.
Continuous infusion: Infuse solution based on patient tolerance, usually over 8 hours. In severely debilitated patients or those requiring long-term parenteral nutrition, administer solutions containing more than 12.5% dextrose (hypertonic solution) via subclavian catheter into the superior vena cava. In moderately debilitated patients, administer solutions mixed with dextrose 5% or 10% in water via peripheral route.

INCOMPATIBILITY

Incompatible with bleomycin. Because of the high risk of incompatibility with other substances, add only required nutritional products.

ADVERSE REACTIONS

Life-threatening: anaphylaxis, seizures, septicemia (from contaminated solution).
Other: abdominal pain, chills, dehydration (from hyperosmotic solution), edema at injection site, electrolyte imbalance, fatty liver, flushing, glycosuria, hyperammonemia, hyperglycemia, hypoglycemia (rebound), metabolic acidosis or alkalosis, nausea, tissue sloughing, vomiting.

INTERACTIONS

Tetracyclines: possible reduced protein-sparing effect.

EFFECTS ON DIAGNOSTIC TESTS

None reported.

SPECIAL CONSIDERATIONS

• If you're giving total parenteral nutrition (TPN) solution, don't add anything to it except electrolytes, vitamins, and trace elements without first asking a pharmacist. Use strict aseptic technique when adding.
• When solution is used in TPN, monitor serum electrolytes, glucose, BUN, and renal and liver function studies. If glycosuria occurs, expect to give insulin.
• Begin with a 5% to 10% dextrose concentration and gradually increase to hypertonicity (greater than 12.5% dextrose), if needed.
• If flow rate lags behind ordered rate, don't try to catch up by increasing rate beyond original order.
• Check infusion site frequently. Change peripheral I.V. site every 48 hours to prevent irritation and infection.
• Take the patient's temperature every 4 hours because fever may indicate sepsis. If patient has fever or chills, replace I.V. tubing and bottle and send them to the laboratory for culture.
• Monitor the patient for signs of fluid overload.
• Notify doctor of all adverse reactions. He may reduce infusion rate, change to a different brand of solution, or order a new catheter insertion site.

aminocaproic acid
Amicar♦

Pregnancy Risk Category: C

PHARMACOKINETICS

Distribution: throughout intravascular and extravascular compartments. Readily penetrates RBCs and tissues and probably crosses placenta. Apparently, the drug isn't bound to plasma proteins.
Metabolism: not metabolized.
Excretion: in urine by glomerular filtration and reabsorption within 12 hours, largely unchanged. Not known if drug appears in breast milk.
Action: peak level variable.

MECHANISM OF ACTION

Inhibits fibrinolysis—and thus clot dissolution—by inhibiting plasminogen activator substances and, to a lesser degree, by blocking antiplasmin activity.

INDICATIONS & DOSAGE

• Life-threatening hemorrhage caused by systemic hyperfibrinolysis associated with complications of cardiac surgery and portacaval shunt; cancer of the lung, prostate, cervix, or stomach; abruptio placentae; hematologic disorders, such as aplastic anemia; and urinary fibrinolysis associated with severe trauma, shock, and anoxia. *Adults:* initially, 4 to 5

g, then 1 to 1.25 g hourly. Alternately, continuous infusion of 1 g/hour for about 8 hours to maintain plasma level of 130 mcg/ml. Maximum dosage, 30 g/day. *Children:* 100 mg/kg or 3 g/m² body surface area during first hour, then continuous infusion of 33 mg/kg/hour or 1 g/m²/hour. Maximum dosage, 18 g/m²/day.
• Subarachnoid hemorrhage. *Adults:* 1 to 1.5 g hourly.

CONTRAINDICATIONS & CAUTIONS

• Contraindicated in active intravascular clotting associated with possible fibrinolysis and bleeding as a primary disorder.
• Also contraindicated in disseminated intravascular coagulation unless used with heparin. Otherwise, the drug could cause potentially fatal thrombi.
• Use cautiously in cardiac disorders because of possible hypotension and bradycardia; in renal disorders because drug may accumulate and cause renal damage; in hepatic disease because the cause of bleeding may be more difficult to diagnose; and in patients predisposed to thrombosis.
• Also use cautiously in upper urinary tract bleeding because glomerular capillary thrombosis or clots in the renal pelvis and ureter could cause intrarenal obstruction.

PREPARATION & STORAGE

Available in 250 mg/ml solutions containing 5 g (20 ml) or 24 g (96 ml) with benzyl alcohol. Further dilute with 0.9% sodium chloride, dextrose 5% in water, Ringer's solution, or sterile water for injection. (Don't use sterile water for injection when patient has subarachnoid hemorrhage.) Store at 59° to 86° F. (15° to 30° C.); avoid freezing.

ADMINISTRATION

Direct injection: not recommended.
Intermittent infusion: not recommended.
Continuous infusion: Slowly infuse 4 to 5 g of diluted drug during first hour. Then infuse 1 g/hour to maintain serum level of 130 mcg/ml.

INCOMPATIBILITY

Incompatible with fructose solution.

ADVERSE REACTIONS

Life-threatening: none, when patient is in hyperfibrinolytic state.
Other: acute renal failure (reversible), bradycardia, conjunctival injection, cramping, diarrhea, dizziness, headache, hypotension, malaise, myopathy, nasal congestion, nausea, prolonged menstruation with cramping, rash, rhabdomyolysis, thrombophlebitis, tinnitus.

INTERACTIONS

Oral contraceptives, estrogens: hypercoagulability resulting from increased clotting factors.

EFFECTS ON DIAGNOSTIC TESTS

Serum aldolase, CPK, SGOT: possible elevated levels.
Serum potassium: possible increased levels, especially in renal impairment.

SPECIAL CONSIDERATIONS

• Drug shouldn't be given without a definitive diagnosis or positive test results for hyperfibrinolysis or hyperplasmia.
• Guard against thrombophlebitis by using proper technique for needle insertion and positioning.
• Keep in mind that rapid infusion may induce hypotension and bradycardia.
• Contains benzyl alcohol.

amiodarone hydrochloride
Cordarone♦

Pregnancy Risk Category: C

PHARMACOKINETICS
Distribution: rapid and widespread throughout body tissues. Crosses blood-brain barrier and placenta.
Metabolism: extensively metabolized, probably in liver and possibly in intestinal lumen.
Excretion: in feces, primarily unchanged. The metabolite N-desethylamiodarone is eliminated through bile. Drug appears in breast milk. Serum half-life averages 25 days after single dose, longer after multiple doses.
Action: onset, minutes to hours; duration, about 6 hours when given over 30 to 60 minutes.

MECHANISM OF ACTION
A group III antiarrhythmic, amiodarone prolongs the refractory period and repolarization. It also antagonizes alpha and beta responses to catecholamine stimulation.

INDICATIONS & DOSAGE
● Ventricular and supraventricular dysrhythmias, including those caused by hypertrophic cardiomyopathy, atrial flutter and fibrillation, ventricular tachycardia, chronic stable angina, and recurrent supraventricular tachycardia (including Wolff-Parkinson-White syndrome), only when these don't respond to other antiarrhythmics. *Adults:* loading dose, 5 to 10 mg/kg by I.V. infusion via central line, then 10 mg/kg/day for 3 to 5 days.

CONTRAINDICATIONS & CAUTIONS
● I.V. use is investigational. To minimize risk, use lowest effective dose. Pediatric dosage not established.
● Contraindicated in amiodarone hypersensitivity, severe sinus bradycardia, and second- and third-degree atrioventricular (AV) block.
● Use cautiously in preexisting pulmonary disease and in the elderly because of possibly fatal cardiopulmonary effects.
● Patient must be closely monitored during loading phase.

PREPARATION & STORAGE
Store at room temperature and protect from light.

ADMINISTRATION
Direct injection: Give initial bolus of 5 to 10 mg/kg; may be repeated in 15 minutes.
Intermittent infusion: not recommended.
Continuous infusion: investigational; follow protocols.

INCOMPATIBILITY
Incompatible with quinidine gluconate.

ADVERSE REACTIONS
Life-threatening: bradycardia, dysrhythmias, hepatic dysfunction, hypotension, pulmonary toxicity (fibrosis, pneumonitis).
Other: congestive heart failure, constipation, corneal microdeposits, diplopia, epididymitis, extrapyramidal symptoms, fatigue, headache, hyperthyroidism, hypothyroidism, malaise, nausea, nystagmus, peripheral neuropathy, photosensitivity, thrombocytopenia, tremors, weakness, vomiting.

INTERACTIONS
Anticoagulants: increased prothrombin time (may last for months).

Beta blockers, calcium channel blockers: potentiated AV block, bradycardia, sinus arrest.

Digoxin, phenytoin: toxicity resulting from increased serum levels of these drugs.

Disopyramide, mexiletine: prolonged QT interval and, rarely, torsade de pointes.

Flecainide: possible impaired metabolism.

Inhalation anesthetics: potentiated hypotension and atropine-resistant bradycardia.

Potassium-depleting diuretics: increased risk of dysrhythmias associated with hypokalemia.

Procainamide, quinidine: toxicity resulting from elevated serum levels of these drugs, prolonged QT interval and, rarely, torsade de pointes.

Sodium iodide ^{131}I: reduced thyroid uptake.

EFFECTS ON DIAGNOSTIC TESTS

Antinuclear antibody titer: possible increase.

EKG: prolonged QT segments, altered T-wave configuration.

Platelet count: reduced.

Prothrombin time: prolonged.

Serum alkaline phosphatase, SGOT, SGPT: elevated levels.

Thyroid function tests: reduced serum T_3, increased serum T_4 and thyroid-stimulating hormone levels.

Thyroid imaging tests: reduced uptake of sodium iodide ^{123}I and sodium pertechnetate Tc 99m.

SPECIAL CONSIDERATIONS

• *Treatment of overdose:* Give symptomatic and supportive care. Monitor EKG and blood pressure. If needed, give an I.V. beta-adrenergic antagonist (such as isoproterenol) or assist with transvenous pacemaker insertion to treat bradycardia. Infuse I.V. fluids and place in Trendelen-

burg position to correct hypotension. Also give an I.V. vasopressor or inotropic drugs (such as norepinephrine or dopamine) to improve tissue perfusion. Hemodialysis and peritoneal dialysis are *not* helpful.

• Obtain baseline ophthalmologic data. Monitor for dry eyes, halo vision, and photophobia. Recommend a sunscreen or sunglasses.

• Obtain baseline pulmonary function tests. Assess respiratory system for pulmonary toxicity.

• Monitor EKG status continuously for AV block, bradycardia, paradoxical dysrhythmias, and prolonged QT segments.

• Monitor thyroid and liver function tests.

ammonium chloride

Pregnancy Risk Category: B

PHARMACOKINETICS

Distribution: throughout body in circulating plasma. Not known if drug crosses placenta.

Metabolism: in liver, where ammonium ions are metabolized to urea and hydrochloric acid.

Excretion: in urine. Not known if drug appears in breast milk.

Action: onset, 15 to 60 minutes; duration, 1 to 3 days.

MECHANISM OF ACTION

This systemic acidifier increases free hydrogen ions (H^+), which then react with bicarbonate ions to form water and carbon dioxide. Chloride anions then combine with bases in extracellular fluid, displacing bicarbonate and causing acidosis. After 1 to 3 days, the kidneys increase ammonium production and chloride ion excretion to compensate for sodium loss.

INDICATIONS & DOSAGE
● Metabolic alkalosis caused by chloride loss from vomiting, gastric suction, pyloric stenosis, or gastric fistula drainage; diuretic-induced chloride depletion. *Adults:* Dosage reflects severity of alkalosis and patient tolerance. It's calculated by amount of chloride deficit and estimated in milliequivalents. First, establish patient's estimated fluid volume. To do this, multiply 20% of body weight in kilograms by serum chloride level. For example, in a patient weighing 70 kg with a chloride level of 94 mEq/ml, multiply 14 by 94 for a dosage of 1,316 mEq. One liter of 2.14% solution provides 400 mEq of NH_4^+ and Cl^- ions.

CONTRAINDICATIONS & CAUTIONS
● Contraindicated in hypersensitivity to drug; in severe hepatic disease; and in hepatic coma.
● Also contraindicated in primary respiratory acidosis because of the risk of developing systemic acidosis.
● Use cautiously in pulmonary insufficiency and edema because of possible changes in arterial blood gas levels.

PREPARATION & STORAGE
Prepare diluted solution by adding 1 or 2 vials (100 or 200 mEq) of aqueous ammonium chloride to 500 or 1,000 ml of 0.9% sodium chloride for injection. Also available as prepared solution in a 500 ml bottle containing 2.14 g/dl (0.4 mEq/ml).

Solution may crystallize if stored at low temperature. Crystals will dissolve when solution is placed in warm water.

ADMINISTRATION
Direct injection: not recommended.
Intermittent infusion: not recommended.

Continuous infusion: Infuse diluted solution at no more than 5 ml/minute to avoid pain, toxic effects, and local irritation. Infuse the 2.14% solution at 0.9 to 1.3 ml/minute (but always under 2 ml/minute). Start infusion at half the calculated rate to determine patient tolerance.

INCOMPATIBILITY
Incompatible with alkalis and their carbonates; strong oxidizing agents, such as potassium chloride; and dimenhydrinate, levorphanol tartrate, methadone, and warfarin.

ADVERSE REACTIONS
Life-threatening: dysrhythmias.
Other: anorexia, bradycardia, coma, confusion, diarrhea, drowsiness, excitement, fatigue, glycosuria, headache, hyperventilation, hypokalemia, hyponatremia, Kussmaul's respirations, nausea, thirst, tonic seizures, twitching.

INTERACTIONS
Antidepressants, ephedrine, methadone, salicylates: reduced effects.
Spironolactone: increased effects.

EFFECTS ON DIAGNOSTIC TESTS
Serum potassium: decreased levels.

SPECIAL CONSIDERATIONS
● *Treatment of overdose:* Discontinue drug and give potassium chloride I.V. or sodium bicarbonate for acidosis. Resuscitate if necessary. Signs of overdose include asterixis, bradycardia, dysrhythmias, coma, Kussmaul's respirations, pallor, local or generalized twitching, sweating, tonic seizures, and vomiting.
● If metabolic alkalosis results from continuous acid loss from stomach, an inhibitor of acid secretion (such as an H_2 antagonist) may be useful.

Unmarked trade names available in the United States only.
♦Also available in Canada.   ♦♦Available in Canada only.

• Assess for pain at infusion site and adjust rate if necessary.
• To prevent acidosis, determine serum electrolyte levels throughout therapy.
• Monitor input and output, edema, weight, and urine pH during therapy. Expect diuresis for the first 2 days.
• Assess respiratory pattern frequently.

amobarbital sodium
Amytal Sodium♦

Controlled Substance Schedule II
Pregnancy Risk Category: B

PHARMACOKINETICS
Distribution: rapidly dispersed throughout body tissues, with highest concentration in liver and brain. Drug crosses placenta.
Metabolism: slowly metabolized to an inactive metabolite by hepatic microsomal enzymes.
Excretion: in urine and, less commonly, in feces. Inactive metabolites are excreted as conjugates of glucuronic acid. Drug appears in breast milk. After I.V. bolus, plasma concentration follows biphasic decline: first phase of half-life is about 40 minutes; second phase averages 20 to 25 hours.
Action: onset, 1 to 5 minutes; duration, 3 to 6 hours, depending on dose and distribution rate.

MECHANISM OF ACTION
Probably interferes with impulse transmission from the thalamus to the cerebral cortex.

INDICATIONS & DOSAGE
• Agitation in psychoses, insomnia, seizures, and status epilepticus. I.V. route typically used only in emergencies; dosage varies by patient.
Adults and children over age 6 when used as sedative or anticonvulsant: 65 to 500 mg, not to exceed 1 g/day.
Children age 6 and under when used as sedative or anticonvulsant: 3 to 5 mg/kg or 125 mg/m².

CONTRAINDICATIONS & CAUTIONS
• Contraindicated in liver impairment from cirrhosis, drug or alcohol abuse, or lengthy exposure to hepatic carcinogens.
• Also contraindicated in patients with a history of acute intermittent or variegate porphyria because of possible aggravation of symptoms.
• Use especially cautiously in patients with a history of drug abuse.
• Also use cautiously in elderly or debilitated patients because of possible excitement, depression, or confusion; in renal impairment, uremia, or shock because of prolonged or intensified hypnotic effects; in cardiac disease because of adverse circulatory effects, especially with overly rapid administration; in pulmonary disease because of possible ventilatory depression; in asthma because of heightened risk of a hypersensitivity reaction; in hyperthyroidism or hyperkinesis because of possible exacerbation of symptoms; in borderline hyperadrenalism because of reduced effect of exogenous hydrocortisone and endogenous cortisol; in acute or chronic pain because of induced paradoxical reaction; and in hypertension because drug may cause hypotension.

PREPARATION & STORAGE
To prepare the standard 100 mg/ml (10%) injection, dissolve 250 or 500 mg of sterile powder in 2.5 or 5 ml, respectively, of sterile water for injection. Rotate the ampule to facilitate mixing; don't shake. If solution

becomes cloudy after 5 minutes, discard; the drug breaks down in solution or on exposure to air. Drug also precipitates if diluent pH is 9.2 or less. Give within 30 minutes of reconstitution.

ADMINISTRATION
Direct injection: Give 1 to 5 ml, depending on dose needed. Don't exceed a rate of 100 mg/minute (1 ml of a 10% concentration) for adults and 60 mg/m²/minute (0.6 ml of a 10% concentration) for children. Avoid extravasation, which can cause necrosis.
Intermittent infusion: not recommended.
Continuous infusion: not recommended.

INCOMPATIBILITY
Incompatible with cefazolin, cephaloridine, cephalothin, chlorpromazine, cimetidine, clindamycin, droperidol, isoproterenol, metaraminol bitartrate, methyldopa, norepinephrine bitartrate, penicillin G, pentazocine lactate, propiomazine, succinylcholine, tetracycline, and thiamine.

ADVERSE REACTIONS
Life-threatening: bronchospasm, cardiac arrest, respiratory arrest.
Other: agitation, apnea, ataxia, bradycardia, circulatory collapse, confusion, constipation, diarrhea, drowsiness, edema, epigastric pain, fever, hallucinations, hyperkinesia, hypersensitivity, hypotension, hypoventilation, lethargy, nausea, nightmares, rash, syncope, severe subcutaneous tissue necrosis, vomiting.

INTERACTIONS
Anticonvulsants: worsened lethargy and motor disturbances.
Ascorbic acid: increased excretion.

Calcium channel blockers: excessive hypotension.
Corticosteroids, digitoxin, tricyclic antidepressants: increased metabolism.
Divalproex sodium, valproic acid: possible enhanced CNS adverse effects.
Doxycycline: decreased half-life of doxycycline.
Guanadrel, guanethidine, loop diuretics: possible new or worsened orthostatic hypotension.
Haloperidol, maprotiline, primidone: possible change in frequency or pattern of epileptiform seizures.
Hypnotics, muscle relaxants, tranquilizers, other CNS depressants: potentiated hypnotic and sedative effects.
Hypothermia-producing drugs: heightened risk of hypothermia.
Ketamine: increased risk of hypotension and respiratory depression.
MAO inhibitors: possible prolonged barbiturate effects.
Metronidazole: decreased antimicrobial effect.
Mexiletine: reduced plasma concentration.
Oral anticoagulants: decreased response to these drugs because barbiturates promote hepatic microsomal enzyme activity and enhance metabolism of oral anticoagulants.
Oral contraceptives and estrogens: decreased therapeutic effect of hormonal agents.
Phenmetrazine: Decreased weight-reducing effect.

EFFECTS ON DIAGNOSTIC TESTS
Liver function tests: possible increased retention of sulfobromophthalein.
Phentolamine test: false-positive results.

SPECIAL CONSIDERATIONS
• *Treatment of overdose:* Signs of toxicity include clammy skin, coma, cyanosis, hypotension, and pupillary constriction. If overdose occurs, maintain airway and, if needed, provide ventilatory support. Monitor vital signs and fluid balance. For shock, give fluids and follow standard care measures; for hypotension, give vasopressors, as ordered. In normal renal function, forced diuresis may help remove drug; hemodialysis or hemoperfusion may enhance removal.
• Give drug only to hospitalized patients under close observation and respiratory monitoring. Keep resuscitation equipment available.
• Dependence and severe withdrawal symptoms may follow long-term therapy. When discontinuing drug after prolonged use, withdraw over 5 to 6 days to prevent withdrawal symptoms and rebound rapid eye movement (REM) stage of sleep.
• Monitor prothrombin time carefully when patient starts or ends anticoagulant therapy. Anticoagulant dose may need adjustment.
• Barbiturates potentiate narcotic effect. If given during labor, reduce narcotic dose to lessen risk of neonatal respiratory depression.
• When patient's receiving hypnotic dose, remove cigarettes, assist him in walking, and raise bed rails, especially if he's elderly. Morning hangover commonly occurs with hypnotic dose because of disrupted REM sleep.
• Don't give drug within 24 hours of liver function tests.

amphotericin B
Fungizone♦

Pregnancy Risk Category: B

PHARMACOKINETICS
Distribution: to joints, kidneys, lungs, liver, muscle, and spleen, with 90% to 95% protein-bound. Drug is poorly distributed to aqueous humor, bone, brain, and pancreas. Drug may cross placenta.
Metabolism: mechanism unknown.
Excretion: eliminated slowly in urine, with 40% removed in 7 days; 2% to 5% of dose excreted in biologically active form. Initial phase half-life is 24 to 48 hours; second phase half-life, 15 days.

MECHANISM OF ACTION
Binds to sterols in fungal cell walls, changing cell permeability and allowing leakage of potassium and other cellular constituents.

INDICATIONS & DOSAGE
• Systemic fungal infections: aspergillosis, blastomycosis, coccidioidomycosis, cryptococcosis, disseminated moniliasis, histoplasmosis, and phycomycosis. *Adults and children:* therapy usually begun with dose of 0.25 mg/kg infused over 6 hours (if tolerated, may be infused over 2 to 4 hours). Initially, a test dose of 1 mg in 20 ml of dextrose 5% in water is infused over 20 to 30 minutes. Patient's vital signs should be monitored q 30 minutes for 4 hours. Dosage is increased gradually, depending on patient tolerance and infection's severity, to a maximum of 1 mg/kg/day. Dosage must never exceed 1.5 mg/kg/day. If discontinued for 1 week or more, therapy resumes with initial dose and gradually in-

creases as described. Therapy may last for months.

CONTRAINDICATIONS & CAUTIONS
• Contraindicated in patients with known hypersensitivity unless infection is life-threatening and susceptible only to this drug.
• Use only for hospitalized patients (under close supervision) with confirmed diagnosis of potentially fatal fungal infection. Use cautiously in renal impairment.

PREPARATION & STORAGE
For 50 mg vial, reconstitute with 10 ml of sterile water for injection (not bacteriostatic). Shake until solution clears. Further dilute in 50 ml of dextrose 5% in water with a pH above 4.2. Final concentration will be 0.1 mg/ml.

Store concentrate at room temperature for 24 hours or refrigerate for 1 week. When diluted, use drug promptly. Protect from light until ready to hang.

ADMINISTRATION
Direct injection: not recommended.
Intermittent infusion: not recommended.
Continuous infusion: Administer 250 ml of diluted solution over 3 to 4 hours. Any in-line filter should have a pore diameter larger than 1 micron. Because of severe adverse reactions, remain with home care patient during entire infusion.

INCOMPATIBILITY
Incompatible with amikacin, calcium chloride, calcium gluceptate, carbenicillin disodium, chlorpromazine, cimetidine, diphenhydramine, edetate calcium disodium, gentamicin, kanamycin, metaraminol, methyldopa, oxytetracycline, penicillin G potassium, penicillin G sodium, poly-myxin B, potassium chloride, prochlorperazine mesylate, Ringer's lactate, 0.9% sodium chloride, streptomycin, tetracycline hydrochloride, and verapamil.

ADVERSE REACTIONS
Life-threatening: Abnormal renal function including azotemia, hypokalemia, hyposthenuria, and renal tubular acidosis. Rare reactions include acute liver failure, cardiac arrest (after rapid injection), hypotension, ventricular fibrillation, and anaphylactoid reactions.
Other: Most common—anorexia, diarrhea, dyspepsia, epigastric cramps, fever, headache, hypomagnesemia, malaise, muscle and joint pain, nausea, normochromic or normocytic anemia, pain or thrombophlebitis at injection site, shaking chills, vomiting, and weight loss. Less common—agranulocytosis, coagulation defects, hearing loss, leukopenia, neurologic toxicity, rash, and thrombocytopenia.

INTERACTIONS
Antineoplastics, nephrotoxic antibiotics, potassium-depleting diuretics: increased risk of nephrotoxicity.
Carbonic anhydrase inhibitors, corticosteroids, corticotropin: severe hypokalemia.
Cardiac glycosides: increased risk of toxicity.
Flucytosine: possible increased antifungal effects.
Nondepolarizing neuromuscular blockers: enhanced effect resulting from hypokalemia.
Potassium-depleting diuretics: possible worsened hypokalemia.

EFFECTS ON DIAGNOSTIC TESTS
• None reported.

SPECIAL CONSIDERATIONS

• Assess I.V. site for signs of thrombophlebitis. Rotate I.V. sites regularly.
• Adding a small amount of heparin to solution may lessen risk of thrombophlebitis.
• Giving small doses I.V. of an adrenal corticosteroid just before or during administration of this drug may reduce febrile reaction.
• Protect drug from light during administration.
• Monitor vital signs every 30 minutes for 4 hours during initial therapy. Fever may appear 1 to 2 hours after start of infusion; it should subside within 4 hours after stopping drug.
• Monitor intake and output, reporting any change in urine appearance or volume. Renal damage is usually reversible if therapy stops at first sign of dysfunction.
• Monitor serum potassium and magnesium levels and expect to administer supplements if serum levels are low. Monitor hemoglobin and hematocrit for anemia.
• Antihistamines, antipyretics, corticosteroids, and antiemetics may be ordered prophylactically to relieve adverse reactions.
• Obtain weekly liver and kidney function studies. If BUN level exceeds 40 mg/dl or serum creatinine level exceeds 3 mg/dl, drug may be discontinued until kidney function improves. Drug also may be discontinued if serum levels of alkaline phosphatase or bilirubin rise.
• Advise patient to use a soft toothbrush and to employ dental floss and toothpicks with caution; possible myelosuppression may predispose him to gingival infection or bleeding.
• Observe patient for fungal and bacterial superinfection with prolonged use.

ampicillin sodium
Omnipen-N♦, Polycillin-N, Totacillin-N

Pregnancy Risk Category: B

PHARMACOKINETICS
Distribution: readily distributed to most body tissues and bone. Normally poor distribution to eye, brain, and cerebrospinal fluid improves when inflammation is present. Drug crosses placenta and appears in cord blood and amniotic fluid.
Metabolism: partially, in liver.
Excretion: largely by glomerular filtration and renal tubular secretion. Small amounts appear in bile and breast milk. Elimination half-life averages about 1 hour; in neonates and patients with renal impairment, 10 to 24 hours.
Action: peak serum level, immediately after 15-minute infusion.

MECHANISM OF ACTION
Ampicillin, an aminopenicillin, joins with penicillin-binding proteins in susceptible bacteria, inhibiting cell-wall synthesis. The drug acts against nonpenicillinase-producing strains of *Staphylococcus aureus, Staphylococcus epidermidis,* groups A, B, C, and G streptococci, *Streptococcus pneumoniae, Streptococcus viridans,* and some strains of enterococci.

Susceptible gram-negative bacteria include *Bordetella pertussis, Eikenella corrodens, Legionella, Pasteurella multocida, Gardnerella vaginalis, Branhamella catarrhalis, Neisseria gonorrhoeae, N. meningitidis, Haemophilus influenzae, Escherichia coli, Proteus mirabilis, Salmonella,* and *Shigella.* Susceptible anaerobic bacteria include strains of *Actinomyces, Arachnia, Bifidobacterium, Eubacterium, Fusobacterium,*

Propionibacterium, Clostridium tetani, C. perfringens, Peptococcus, Peptostreptococcus, Lactobacillus, and *Campylobacter fetus.*

INDICATIONS & DOSAGE

• Systemic, respiratory tract, skin, GI, and acute urinary tract infections. *Adults:* 0.5 to 2 g q 4 to 6 hours. *Children:* 25 to 50 mg/kg q 6 hours.
• Meningitis. *Adults:* 1 to 2.5 g q 3 to 4 hours for 3 days, then given I.M. or P.O. *Children:* 12.5 to 50 mg/kg q 3 to 4 hours for 3 days, then given I.M. or P.O.
Note: Adjust dosage in renal failure. In adult patients with a creatinine clearance less than or equal to 10 ml/minute, increase dosage interval to q 12 hours.

CONTRAINDICATIONS & CAUTIONS

• Contraindicated in penicillin or cephalosporin hypersensitivity.
• Also contraindicated in infectious mononucleosis because of the high risk of maculopapular rash.
• Use cautiously in the elderly and patients with renal impairment. Dosage may need to be reduced.

PREPARATION & STORAGE

Supplied in vials containing 125 mg, 250 mg, 500 mg, 1 g, and 2 g. Reconstitute by adding 5 ml of sterile water for injection to 125, 250, or 500 mg vial; 7.5 ml to 1 g vial; or 10 ml to 2 g vial. Dilute for infusion with 50 or 100 ml 0.9% sodium chloride, dextrose 5% in water, dextrose 5% and 0.45% sodium chloride, invert sugar 10% and water, ⅙ M sodium lactate, Ringer's lactate, or sterile water for injection. Concentration of the drug shouldn't exceed 30 mg/ml. Solution remains stable for 1 hour in dextrose 5% in water and for up to 8 hours in other solutions when refrigerated.
When frozen, drug is stable for 30 days. Allow solution to thaw for 8 hours before administration.

ADMINISTRATION

Direct injection: Inject reconstituted drug into a large vein or cannula over 10 to 15 minutes. After injection, flush cannula with 0.9% sodium chloride.
Intermittent infusion: Give diluted solution through I.V. piggyback or cannula over 30 to 60 minutes.
Continuous infusion: not recommended.

INCOMPATIBILITY

Incompatible with amikacin, amino acid solutions, chlorpromazine, dextran solutions, dopamine, erythromycin lactobionate, 10% fat emulsions, fructose, gentamicin, heparin sodium, hetastarch, hydrocortisone sodium succinate, kanamycin, lidocaine hydrochloride, lincomycin, oxytetracycline, polymyxin B, prochlorperazine edisylate, sodium bicarbonate, streptomycin, and tetracycline hydrochloride.

ADVERSE REACTIONS

Life-threatening: acute interstitial nephritis, bone marrow depression (anemia, eosinophilia, leukopenia, thrombocytopenia, thrombocytopenic purpura).
Other: bacterial or fungal superinfection, diarrhea, glossitis, nausea, pseudomembranous colitis, stomatitis, thrombophlebitis, vein irritation, vomiting.

INTERACTIONS

Allopurinol: increased risk of rash.
Aminoglycosides: reduced serum levels.
Clavulanic acid, sulbactam sodium: enhanced bactericidal effects.

Unmarked trade names available in the United States only.
♦Also available in Canada.   ♦♦Available in Canada only.

Methotrexate: diminished excretion.
Oral contraceptives: reduced effectiveness.
Probenecid: decreased ampicillin excretion.

EFFECTS ON DIAGNOSTIC TESTS

Serum uric acid: false elevations with copper chelate method.
SGOT, SGPT: possible elevated levels.
Total conjugated estriol, conjugated estrone, estradiol, estriol-glucuronide: possible reduced levels in pregnancy.
Urine glucose: false-positive results when tested with cupric sulfate (Benedict's solution, Clinitest).

SPECIAL CONSIDERATIONS

• Check for previous penicillin or cephalosporin hypersensitivity before first dose. Negative history doesn't rule out future allergic reaction.
• Obtain specimens for culture and sensitivity testing before first dose. Therapy may start before results are available.
• Intermittent infusion reduces risk of vein irritation. Change I.V. site every 48 hours.
• Monitor hematologic and renal function studies during therapy.
• Monitor for signs of bacterial or fungal superinfection.
• If diarrhea persists during therapy, collect stool specimens to rule out possible pseudomembranous colitis.
• Discontinue drug if acute interstitial nephritis, bone marrow depression, or pseudomembranous colitis develops.
• Use Clinistix or Tes-Tape for urine glucose determinations to prevent spurious results.

ampicillin sodium/ sulbactam sodium

Unasyn

Pregnancy Risk Category: B

PHARMACOKINETICS

Distribution: widely distributed in body fluids and tissues. Brain and cerebrospinal fluid penetration increase with meningeal inflammation. Drug crosses placenta.
Metabolism: ampicillin partly metabolized in liver; sulbactam metabolism unknown.
Excretion: in normal renal function, 75% to 85% excreted unchanged in urine, primarily by glomerular filtration and renal tubular secretion. Serum half-life is about 1 hour. Drug appears in breast milk.
Action: peak serum level, immediately after 15-minute infusion.

MECHANISM OF ACTION

Inhibits bacterial cell-wall synthesis by joining with penicillin-binding proteins. Addition of sulbactam, a beta-lactamase inhibitor, makes the compound effective against many beta-lactamase–producing bacteria that are normally resistant to ampicillin alone. Susceptible aerobic cocci include *Acinetobacter caloaceticus, Bacteroides fragilis, Enterobacter,* enterococci, *Escherichia coli, Klebsiella, Neisseria gonorrhoeae, Proteus mirabilis, Staphylococcus aureus, Staphylococcus epidermidis, Staphylococcus soprophyticus, Staphylococcus pyogenes, Streptococcus pneumoniae,* and *Streptococcus viridans.* Sulbactam alone ineffective except against *N. gonorrhoeae.*

INDICATIONS & DOSAGE

• Peritonitis and gynecologic, skin, and skin structure infections caused by susceptible organisms. *Adults:* 1.5 g (1 g ampicillin, 0.5 g sulbactam) to 3 g (2 g ampicillin, 1 g sulbactam) q 6 hours, not to exceed 4 g/day of sulbactam.

Note: Dosage in renal failure is based on creatinine clearance. In adult patients, give 1.5 to 3 g q 6 to 8 hours if creatinine clearance exceeds 29 ml/minute; 1.5 to 3 g q 12 hours if it's 15 to 29 ml/minute; or 1.5 to 3 g q 24 hours if it's 5 to 14 ml/minute.

CONTRAINDICATIONS & CAUTIONS

• Contraindicated in penicillin, cephalosporin, or sulbactam hypersensitivity; also in mononucleosis because of an increased risk of maculopapular rash.

• Use cautiously in the elderly and in patients with renal impairment. Dosage may need reduction.

• Safety and efficacy in children have not been established.

PREPARATION & STORAGE

Available in 1.5 g and 3 g vials. Also available in piggyback vials. Reconstitute with sterile water for injection to yield a concentration of 375 mg/ml. For infusion, immediately dilute reconstituted solution with compatible diluent to yield 3 to 45 mg/ml.

Storage times reflect diluent and concentration. Using sterile water for injection or 0.9% sodium chloride injection, a 45 mg/ml solution remains stable for 8 hours at 77° F. (25° C.) and for 48 hours at 39° F. (4° C.); a 30 mg/ml solution remains stable for 72 hours at 39° F.

Using dextrose 5% in water, a 30 mg/ml solution is stable for 2 hours at 77° F. and for 24 hours at 39° F.

Using Ringer's lactate, a 45 mg/ml solution remains stable for 8 hours at 77° F. and for 24 hours at 39° F.

Other compatible diluents include dextrose 5% and 0.45% sodium chloride or 10% invert sugar.

ADMINISTRATION

Direct injection: Inject reconstituted drug into large vein or cannula over at least 10 to 15 minutes. Then flush with 0.9% sodium chloride.

Intermittent infusion: After diluting reconstituted drug (usually in 100 ml of solution), infuse over 15 to 30 minutes.

Continuous infusion: not used.

INCOMPATIBILITY

Incompatible with amikacin, amino acid solutions, chlorpromazine, dextran solutions, dopamine, erythromycin lactobionate, 10% fat emulsions, fructose, gentamicin, heparin sodium, hetastarch, hydrocortisone sodium succinate, kanamycin, lidocaine hydrochloride, lincomycin, oxytetracycline, polymyxin B, prochlorperazine edisylate, sodium bicarbonate, streptomycin, or tetracycline hydrochloride.

ADVERSE REACTIONS

Life-threatening: acute interstitial nephritis, anaphylaxis, bone marrow depression (anemia, eosinophilia, leukopenia, thrombocytopenia, thrombocytopenic purpura).

Other: abdominal distention, bacterial or fungal superinfection, chest pain, chills, diarrhea, dysuria, edema, erythema, facial swelling, fatigue, flatulence, glossitis, headache, local reactions (pain, thrombophlebitis), malaise, mucosal bleeding, nausea, pruritus, pseudomembranous colitis, rash, substernal pain, tightness in throat, urine retention, vomiting.

INTERACTIONS

Allopurinol: increased risk of rash.

Aminoglycosides: reduced serum levels. Administer separately.
Methotrexate: diminished excretion.
Oral contraceptives: reduced effectiveness.
Probenecid: decreased ampicillin and sulbactam excretion.

EFFECTS ON DIAGNOSTIC TESTS

Basophils, eosinophils, lymphocytes, monocytes, platelets: increased counts.
BUN, serum alkaline phosphatase, creatinine, LDH, SGOT, SGPT: elevated levels.
Hematocrit, hemoglobin level, RBC count: decreased.
Serum albumin, total protein: reduced levels.
Serum uric acid: false elevations with copper chelate method.
Urine glucose: false-positive results when tested with cupric sulfate (Benedict's solution, Clinitest).

SPECIAL CONSIDERATIONS
● Check patient history for previous penicillin or cephalosporin hypersensitivity before administering first dose. Negative history doesn't rule out the possibility of future allergic reaction.
● Obtain specimens for culture and sensitivity testing before administering first dose. Therapy may start before results of tests are known.
● If diarrhea persists during therapy, collect stool specimens to rule out possible pseudomembranous colitis.
● Discontinue drug if acute interstitial nephritis, bone marrow depression, or pseudomembranous colitis develops.
● Observe patient for fungal and bacterial superinfection with prolonged use.
● Patients with renal impairment must be monitored frequently for

signs of toxicity resulting from high serum drug concentration.
● Hemodialysis removes ampicillin and probably sulbactam.

---

amrinone lactate
Inocor

Pregnancy Risk Category: C

PHARMACOKINETICS
Distribution: not fully understood, but probably throughout body tissues, with 10% to 49% bound to plasma proteins. Not known if drug crosses placenta or blood-brain barrier.
Metabolism: in liver, which produces several metabolites from acetylation, glucuronidation, and glutathione addition.
Excretion: primarily in urine, with 10% to 40% excreted unchanged in 24 hours. In rapid I.V. administration, serum half-life averages almost 4 hours. In controlled infusion for congestive heart failure (CHF), it's about 6 hours. Not known if drug appears in breast milk.
Action: onset, 2 to 5 minutes; peak level, 10 minutes; duration, 30 minutes to 2 hours.

MECHANISM OF ACTION
A noncatecholamine, nonglycoside cardiotonic drug, amrinone produces a positive inotropic effect by increasing cellular levels of cyclic adenosine monophosphate through phosphodiesterase inhibition. It also acts as a vasodilator. The resultant declines in central venous pressure, pulmonary capillary wedge pressure, and systemic and peripheral vascular resistance reduce preload and afterload.

INDICATIONS & DOSAGE

• Short-term management of CHF (primarily in patients unresponsive to cardiac glycosides, diuretics, and vasodilators). *Adults:* initially, 0.75 mg/kg given over 2 to 3 minutes, followed by 200 mg in 250 ml of 0.9% sodium chloride given at 5 to 10 mcg/kg/minute. If needed, additional bolus of 0.75 mg/kg can be given 30 minutes after therapy starts. Maximum daily dosage, 10 mg/kg. Steady-state plasma level should be maintained at 3 mcg/ml.

CONTRAINDICATIONS & CAUTIONS

• Contraindicated in hypersensitivity to amrinone and to sulfites.
• Contraindicated in acute myocardial infarction or ischemic coronary artery disease *without CHF* because experience is lacking; in severe aortic or pulmonary valve disease because surgery is required to relieve the obstruction; and in hypertrophic subaortic stenosis because of aggravated outflow tract obstruction.

PREPARATION & STORAGE

Available in 20 ml ampules of clear yellow solution containing 5 mg/ml. Protect ampules from light and store at room temperature. Don't use if solution discolors or precipitates. Administer undiluted or dilute in 0.45% or 0.9% sodium chloride. Concentrations of 1 to 3 mg/ml remain stable for 24 hours.

ADMINISTRATION

Direct injection: Over 2 to 3 minutes, inject diluted or undiluted drug into vein or I.V. tubing containing a free-flowing, compatible solution. Avoid extravasation. After injection, flush tubing and cannula with 0.9% sodium chloride.
Intermittent infusion: not recommended.

Continuous infusion: Dilute only with sodium chloride solution to 1 to 3 mg/ml. May be piggybacked into line close to insertion site containing dextrose 5% in water. Infusion rate is usually controlled by pump at 5 to 10 mcg/kg/minute.

INCOMPATIBILITY

Incompatible with furosemide, glucose, bicarbonate, and dextrose-containing solutions.

ADVERSE REACTIONS

Life-threatening: anaphylaxis, dysrhythmias, thrombocytopenia.
Other: abdominal pain, anorexia, burning at injection site, chest pain, diarrhea, fever, hepatotoxicity, hypotension, nausea, vomiting.

INTERACTIONS

Cardiac glycosides: increased inotropic effect.
Disopyramide: excessive hypotension.

EFFECTS ON DIAGNOSTIC TESTS

None reported.

SPECIAL CONSIDERATIONS

• *Treatment of overdose:* Reduce infusion rate and treat hypotension symptomatically.
• Carefully monitor fluid and electrolyte levels, hepatic and renal function, and platelet count. Expect to decrease dosage if platelet count drops below 150,000/mm^3.
• During infusion, check vital signs every 5 to 15 minutes. If blood pressure drops, slow or stop infusion and notify doctor.
• Because amrinone may increase ventricular response rate, patients with atrial fibrillation or flutter may require concomitant therapy with cardiac glycosides.

amsacrine
(acridinyl, anisidide, m-AMSA, NSC-249992)

Investigational drug available only from National Cancer Institute
Pregnancy Risk Category: C

PHARMACOKINETICS
Distribution: throughout all tissues, except brain. Highest concentrations occur in liver and kidneys.
Metabolism: in liver, which produces several metabolites.
Excretion: primarily in bile; also in urine. Plasma level follows biphasic decline; initial phase half-life is 12 minutes; second phase, 2½ hours.
Action: onset, duration; unknown.

MECHANISM OF ACTION
Amsacrine has broad-spectrum antineoplastic, antiviral, and immunosuppressive effects. Although its mechanism of action isn't fully understood, this acridine dye derivative may inhibit DNA synthesis.

INDICATIONS & DOSAGE
• Treatment of acute myelocytic leukemia, breast cancer, carcinomas, chronic lymphocytic leukemia, Hodgkin's disease and non-Hodgkin's lymphoma, liposarcoma, melanoma, ovarian cancer, and refractory acute myelocytic leukemia. *Adults and children:* 10 to 150 mg/m² daily (based on toxicity) over 1 hour or as continuous 24-hour infusion. May be given weekly or monthly.

CONTRAINDICATIONS & CAUTIONS
• Contraindicated in electrolyte imbalance, heart disease, and severe hepatic disease.

PREPARATION & STORAGE
To avoid mutagenic, teratogenic, and carcinogenic risks when giving drug, use a biological containment cabinet and avoid contact with skin. Wear mask and gloves. If solution comes in contact with skin or mucosa, immediately wash thoroughly with soap and water. Correctly dispose of needles, syringes, ampules, vials, and any unused drug.

Amsacrine is available as a unit containing a 2 ml ampule and 20 ml vial. Ampule contains 50 mg/ml of drug in 1.5 ml of fluid. The 20 ml amber vial contains 13.5 ml of 0.0353M L-lactic acid diluent. Reconstitute by mixing contents of both containers. Use a glass syringe because the reconstituted drug can dissolve plastic. Before reconstitution, the drug is stable at room temperature. Afterward, it's stable at room temperature for 48 hours only.

Dilute reconstituted drug in at least 100 ml/m² of dextrose 5% in water before administering, to prevent severe phlebitis. For continuous infusion, dilute reconstituted drug in at least 500 ml dextrose 5% in water to a concentration no greater than 1 mg/ml, to avoid phlebitis. It's safe to use plastic once the drug's diluted with dextrose 5% in water.

ADMINISTRATION
Direct injection: not recommended.
Intermittent infusion: Inject through a central venous line, if possible, to prevent phlebitis and avoid extravasation. Use a separate I.V. line and avoid membrane-type in-line filters. Infuse over 1 hour.
Continuous infusion: Give 24-hour dose in two 12-hour bottles via a separate I.V. line. Don't prepare in advance or interrupt infusion.

INCOMPATIBILITY
Incompatible with chloride-containing solutions.

ADVERSE REACTIONS
Life-threatening: dysrhythmias secondary to metabolic abnormality; leukopenia; thrombocytopenia.
Other: allergic reactions (rare), alopecia, cardiac toxicity, hepatotoxicity, hyperbilirubinemia, hypokalemia, nausea, phlebitis, seizures, stomatitis, vomiting.

INTERACTIONS
None reported.

EFFECTS ON DIAGNOSTIC TESTS
Liver function tests: elevated values.

SPECIAL CONSIDERATIONS
• Use cardiac monitoring during and for 1 hour after infusion. If significant dysrhythmias develop, stop infusion and notify doctor.
• Monitor serum electrolyte levels during infusion.
• WBC nadir occurs in about 10 days for single-dose schedule.
• May color urine orange.
• Doctor must be approved by National Cancer Institute (NCI) to use this drug and must report all adverse reactions to NCI.

---

anistreplase (anisoylated plasminogen-streptokinase activator complex; APSAC)
Eminase

Pregnancy Risk Category: C

PHARMACOKINETICS
Distribution: not fully characterized. The production of plasmin from plasminogen by the activated complex can take place in the bloodstream or clot; the reaction is more efficient within the clot but both contribute to fibrinolysis.
Metabolism: unknown. Half-life of circulating drug is 94 minutes.
Excretion: no information available.
Action: reperfusion occurs 45 minutes after administration.

MECHANISM OF ACTION
Anistreplase is derived from *Lys*-plasminogen and streptokinase. It is formulated into a fibrinolytic enzyme plus activator complex with the activator temporarily blocked by an anisoyl group. The drug is activated in vivo by a nonenzymatic process that removes the anisoyl group. The active *Lys*-plasminogen-streptokinase activator complex is progressively formed in the bloodstream or within the thrombus; it acts as plasminogen to form plasmin, which produces fibrinolysis in coronary arterial clots. This promotes lysis of coronary artery thrombi and results in reperfusion of ischemic myocardium.

INDICATIONS & DOSAGE
• Lysis of coronary artery thrombi following acute myocardial infarction.
Adults: 30 units I.V. over 2 to 5 minutes. Administer by direct injection.

CONTRAINDICATIONS & CAUTIONS
• Anistreplase is contraindicated in patients with active internal bleeding, history of cerebrovascular accident, recent (within the past 2 months) intraspinal or intracranial surgery or trauma, aneurysm, arteriovenous malformation, intracranial neoplasm, or known bleeding diathesis.
• Administer cautiously in patients for 10 days following major surgery, trauma (including cardiopulmonary resuscitation), or GI or GU bleeding.

• Administer cautiously in patients with cerebrovascular disease or hypertension (systolic $\geq$ 180 mm Hg or diastolic $\geq$ 110 mm Hg); in mitral stenosis or atrial fibrillation or other condition that may lead to left heart thrombosis; in acute pericarditis or subacute bacterial endocarditis; in septic thrombophlebitis; in patients age 75 and older; in diabetic hemorrhagic retinopathy; and in patients receiving anticoagulants.

PREPARATION & STORAGE
Available in vials containing 30 units. Store the drug in the refrigerator at 36° to 46° F. (2° to 8° C.). Reconstitute the drug by slowly adding 5 ml of sterile water for injection. Direct the stream against the side of the vial, not at the drug itself. Gently roll the vial to mix the dry powder and water. To avoid excessive foaming, don't shake the vial. The reconstituted solution should be colorless to pale yellow. Inspect for particulate matter. Do not dilute reconstituted solution.

If the drug is not administered within 30 minutes of reconstituting, discard the vial.

ADMINISTRATION
Direct injection: Inject the drug over 2 to 5 minutes into an I.V. line or vein.
Intermittent infusion: not recommended.
Continuous infusion: not recommended.

INCOMPATIBILITY
Do not mix with other drugs.

ADVERSE REACTIONS
Life-threatening: anaphylactoid reactions (rare), dysrhythmias, intracranial hemorrhage.
Other: bleeding, conduction disorders, delayed (2 weeks after therapy) purpuric rash, flushing, GI bleeding, gum/mouth hemorrhage, hematomas, hematuria, hemoptysis, hypotension, itching, urticaria.

INTERACTIONS
Heparin, oral anticoagulants, and drugs that alter platelet function (including aspirin and dipyridamole): may increase the risk of bleeding.

EFFECTS ON DIAGNOSTIC TESTS
Blood studies: anistreplase will cause marked increases in thrombin time, activated partial thromboplastin time, and prothrombin time and marked decreases in circulating plasminogen and fibrinogen. In vitro coagulation tests will be affected by the presence of anistreplase. This can be attenuated if blood samples are collected in the presence of aprotinin (2,000 to 3,000 kallikrein inhibiting units/ml).

SPECIAL CONSIDERATIONS
• Anistreplase is derived from human plasma. No cases of hepatitis or human immunodeficiency virus (HIV) infection have been reported to date. The manufacturing process is designed to purify the plasma used in the preparation of the drug.
• As with other thrombolytics, drug must be given within 6 hours after onset of symptoms.
• Avoid I.M. injections because of the high risk of bleeding into muscle. Also avoid turning and moving the patient excessively.
• To prevent new clot formation, administer heparin during or after anistreplase infusion, if ordered.
• Monitor for reperfusion dysrhythmias, including sinus bradycardia, accelerated idioventricular rhythm, ventricular tachycardia, or premature

ventricular contractions. Have emergency treatment readily available.

• Avoid venipuncture and arterial puncture during therapy because of the increased risk of bleeding. If arterial puncture is necessary, select a compressible site (such as an arm) and apply pressure for 30 minutes afterward. Also use pressure dressings, sandbags, or ice packs on recent puncture sites to prevent bleeding.

• Teach the patient signs of internal bleeding (including hematemesis, hematuria, and black, tarry stools). Tell him to report these immediately.

• Advise the patient about proper dental care techniques to avoid excessive gum trauma.

• Don't mix anistreplase with other drugs.

anti-inhibitor coagulant complex
Autoplex T, Feiba VH Immuno

Pregnancy Risk Category: C

COMPOSITION
Prepared from pooled human plasma that has been tested for hepatitis and human immunodeficiency virus and found to be negative, this drug contains varying amounts of clotting factor precursors, activated clotting factors, and factors of the kinin-generating system.

INDICATIONS & DOSAGE
Drug controls hemorrhage in hemophilia A patients who have a Factor VIII inhibitor level above 10 Bethesda units. Patients with a level of 2 to 10 Bethesda units may receive the drug if they have severe hemorrhage or respond poorly to Factor VIII infusion.

• Joint hemorrhage. *Adults and children:* 50 to 100 units/kg q 12 hours until improvement occurs.

• Mucous membrane hemorrhage. *Adults and children:* 50 units/kg q 6 hours, increasing to 100 units/kg q 6 hours if hemorrhage continues. Maximum daily dose, 200 units/kg.

• Soft tissue hemorrhage. *Adults and children:* 100 units/kg q 12 hours. Maximum daily dose, 200 units/kg.

• Other severe hemorrhages. *Adults and children:* 100 units/kg q 12 hours (occasionally, q 6 hours).

CONTRAINDICATIONS & CAUTIONS
• Contraindicated in fibrinolysis and disseminated intravascular coagulation (DIC) because the drug heightens the risk of intravascular clotting.

• Use cautiously in infants because hepatitis, if contracted, causes higher mortality in them than in adults.

• Also use cautiously in hepatic disease because of the increased risk of hepatotoxicity if hepatitis is contracted.

PREPARATION & STORAGE
Available in a package containing a vial of dry concentrate, a vial of sterile water for injection, a double-ended transfer needle, and a filter needle. Refrigerate vials before use.

To reconstitute, bring vials to room temperature and follow manufacturer's instructions. If drawing more than 1 vial into a syringe, use a new filter needle for each vial.

Don't refrigerate after reconstitution. Use Autoplex T within 1 hour and Feiba VH Immuno within 3 hours; otherwise, the patient will become hypotensive because of increased prekallikrein activator.

ADMINISTRATION
Direct injection: Inject Autoplex T directly into vein at an initial rate of 2 ml/minute, increasing to 10 ml/minute based on patient tolerance. Stop administration if the patient develops a headache, flushing, or change in pulse or blood pressure. Resume at a slower rate when symptoms disappear.

Inject Feiba VH Immuno no faster than 2 units/kg/minute.
Intermittent infusion: not recommended for Autoplex T. For Feiba VH Immuno, follow the manufacturer's directions for using the administration set. Be sure to use a standard blood filter. Infuse no faster than 2 units/kg/minute.
Continuous infusion: not recommended.

INCOMPATIBILITY
No incompatibilities reported, but don't mix with any other drugs or solutions.

ADVERSE REACTIONS
Life-threatening: anaphylaxis.
Other: chest pain, cough, dyspnea, flushing, headache, pulse and blood pressure changes.

INTERACTIONS
None reported.

EFFECTS ON DIAGNOSTIC TESTS
Coagulation tests: results may not correlate with clinical response.

SPECIAL CONSIDERATIONS
• Although treated to minimize viral transmission, anti-inhibitor coagulant complex still possesses a small risk of transmitting severe infection, such as hepatitis and AIDS.
• Educate the patient about AIDS, and encourage immunization against hepatitis B in the HBsAg-negative patient.
• Before therapy, verify that the patient has a diagnosed clotting deficiency caused by Factor VIII inhibitors.
• Be alert for signs of intravascular coagulation, such as dyspnea, chest pain, cough, and pulse and blood pressure changes. If such signs appear, stop the infusion and monitor for DIC. Laboratory indicators of DIC include prolonged thrombin, prothrombin, and activated partial thromboplastin times; reduced fibrogen levels and platelet count; and the presence of fibrin split products.

---

ascorbic acid (vitamin C)
Cenolate, Cevalin

Pregnancy Risk Category: A
(C if recommended allowance exceeded)

PHARMACOKINETICS
Distribution: throughout body tissues, especially liver, leukocytes, glandular tissue, and ocular lenses, with about 25% bound to proteins. Vitamin crosses placenta. Fetal levels are two to four times higher than maternal levels.
Metabolism: mainly in liver.
Excretion: unchanged, in urine. Vitamin appears in breast milk.
Action: onset, 15 to 60 minutes; duration, until deficiency resolves—usually in about 3 days.

MECHANISM OF ACTION
Vitamin is needed for collagen formation and tissue repair. It's involved in oxidation-reduction reactions throughout the body.

INDICATIONS & DOSAGE
• Vitamin C deficiency (scurvy). *Adults:* 100 to 250 mg once daily, b.i.d., or t.i.d. *Pregnant or lactating women:* 60 to 80 mg daily, not to exceed 1 g/ day. *Children:* 100 to 300 mg once daily, b.i.d., or t.i.d. *Infants:* 50 to 100 mg daily.
• Prevention of vitamin C deficiency during hemodialysis. *Adults:* 100 to 200 mg daily.
• Severe burns. *Adults and children:* usually 1 to 2 g daily.
• Idiopathic methemoglobinemia. *Adults and children:* 300 to 600 mg daily in divided doses.
• Total parenteral nutrition. *Adults:* 100 to 500 mg daily I.V. supplementation.

CONTRAINDICATIONS & CAUTIONS
• Use cautiously in glucose-6-phosphate dehydrogenase deficiency and in renal failure.
• Avoid high doses during pregnancy because of the risk of scurvy in neonates.
• Also avoid high doses in hyperoxaluria because of the risk of calculi.

PREPARATION & STORAGE
Available in 100 mg/ml, 200 mg/ml, 250 mg/ml, and 500 mg/ml parenteral formulations. Refrigerate if required by the manufacturer. Solution remains stable at room temperature for 96 hours. Light exposure darkens drug but doesn't reduce its effectiveness. If required, dilute drug in 50 to 100 ml of compatible solution.

ADMINISTRATION
Direct injection: Slowly inject into vein over 2 to 3 minutes. Alternately, inject into I.V. tubing containing a compatible solution. Avoid rapid injection, which may cause transient dizziness or faintness.

Intermittent infusion: Infuse diluted drug over 20 to 30 minutes.
Continuous infusion: Add drug to compatible I.V. solution.

INCOMPATIBILITY
Incompatible with aminophylline, bleomycin, cefazolin, cephapirin, chlorothiazide, conjugated estrogens, erythromycin lactobionate, nafcillin, sodium bicarbonate, and warfarin. May be incompatible with chloramphenicol and hydrocortisone.

ADVERSE REACTIONS
Life-threatening: none reported.
Other: abdominal cramps, diarrhea, drowsiness, fatigue, flushing, headache, heartburn, insomnia, leg swelling, nausea, necrotic skin lesions, urticaria (with doses exceeding 1 g/ day), vomiting.

INTERACTIONS
Barbiturates, primidone, salicylates: possible increased ascorbic acid excretion.
Cellulose sodium phosphate: ascorbic acid metabolized to oxalate.
Deferoxamine: possible enhanced tissue iron toxicity.
Disulfiram: interference with disulfiram-alcohol interaction.
Heparin: reduced anticoagulant effect.
Mexiletine: accelerated excretion.
Oral anticoagulants: possible decreased effects.
Tobacco: increased ascorbic acid requirements.

EFFECTS ON DIAGNOSTIC TESTS
Alterations occur with large doses.
Occult blood test: false-negative results.
Serum bilirubin, urine sodium: possible reduced levels.
Serum LDH, SGOT, SGPT: altered results with autoanalyzer.

Urine calcium: elevated levels.
Urine glucose: false-positive results using Benedict's solution; false-negative results using glucose oxidase method.
Urine oxalate: may raise levels.
Urine pH: possible decline.

SPECIAL CONSIDERATIONS
• Therapeutic value of ascorbic acid is controversial when used for acne, anemia, burns, cancer, common cold, depression, fractures, hemorrhage, infections, infertility, and pressure sores.
• Prolonged use of high doses may increase metabolism.
• Infiltration may cause local tissue irritation and damage. Frequently assess I.V. site.
• Hemodialysis can remove vitamin.
• May contain sulfites.

asparaginase (colaspase, L-asparaginase)
Elspar, Kidrolase♦♦

Pregnancy Risk Category: C

PHARMACOKINETICS
Distribution: minimal outside vascular compartment. Drug doesn't cross blood-brain barrier.
Metabolism: unknown.
Excretion: minimal. Drug isn't excreted in urine. Initial half-life is 4 to 9 hours; terminal half-life, about 1 to 5 days.
Action: onset, immediate in plasma; duration, 23 to 33 days (active enzyme can be detected in plasma).

MECHANISM OF ACTION
Derived from *Escherichia coli*, this enzyme depletes neoplastic cells of exogenous asparagine, thus inhibiting the DNA and protein synthesis essential for neoplastic cell survival.

INDICATIONS & DOSAGE
• Induction phase of acute lymphocytic leukemia (in combination therapy). *Adults and children:* 1,000 IU/kg/day for 10 days.
• Induction phase of acute lymphocytic leukemia (as sole agent). *Adults and children:* 200 IU/day for 28 days, followed by 6,000 IU/m^2/day for 5 days, then by 20,000 IU/m^2 once weekly for 2 weeks.
  Dosage varies with protocol.

CONTRAINDICATIONS & CAUTIONS
• Contraindicated in asparaginase hypersensitivity and in patients with past or current pancreatitis.
• Also contraindicated in chicken pox, herpes, or recent exposure to these viral illnesses because of the risk of severe, generalized disease.
• Use with caution in diabetes mellitus because of elevated serum glucose levels; in gout or a history of urate stones because of increased serum uric acid levels; in hepatic impairment because of a heightened risk of hepatotoxicity; and in infection because of an enhanced risk of generalized disease.

PREPARATION & STORAGE
Use extreme caution when preparing or giving drug to avoid mutagenic, teratogenic, and carcinogenic risks. Use a biological containment cabinet and avoid contact with skin. Wear mask and gloves. If solution comes in contact with skin or mucosa, immediately wash thoroughly with soap and water. Correctly dispose of needles, syringes, vials, and any unused drug.
  Asparaginase is available in 10,000 IU vials, which are stable for 2 years at room temperature, 4 years

if refrigerated. Reconstitute drug with 2 to 5 ml of 0.9% sodium chloride (without a preservative) or sterile water for injection. Drug may be clear or slightly cloudy. Dilute in dextrose 5% in water or 0.9% sodium chloride within 8 hours after reconstitution.

ADMINISTRATION
Direct injection: not recommended.
Intermittent infusion: Start new I.V. site in distal vein to allow for successive venipunctures, if necessary, using a 23G or 25G butterfly needle. Give drug through side port of rapidly infusing dextrose 5% in water or 0.9% sodium chloride solution.
Continuous infusion: not recommended.

INCOMPATIBILITY
No incompatibilities reported.

ADVERSE REACTIONS
Life-threatening: anaphylaxis.
Other: anorexia, drowsiness, hepatotoxicity, hyperglycemia, immunosuppression, lethargy, malaise, nausea, pancreatitis, renal failure.

INTERACTIONS
Corticosteroids, corticotropin: enhanced hyperglycemic effect, increased risk of neuropathy, altered erythropoiesis.
Cyclophosphamide, cytarabine: impaired activation or detoxification.
Methotrexate: heightened risk of hepatotoxicity and therapeutic antagonism or synergism.
Other immunosuppressants: increased therapeutic and adverse effects.
Vincristine: impaired detoxification, enhanced hyperglycemic effect, heightened risk of neuropathy, altered erythropoiesis.

EFFECTS ON DIAGNOSTIC TESTS
BUN, serum alkaline phosphatase, ammonia, bilirubin, cholesterol, gamma globulin, glucose, uric acid: possible elevated levels.
Partial thromboplastin time, platelet count, prothrombin time: possible increase in first 3 weeks.
Serum albumin, calcium, fibrinogen: possible reduced levels.
SGOT, SGPT: possible elevated levels.
Thyroid function tests: reduced serum T_4 levels and increased thyroxine-binding globulin index.

SPECIAL CONSIDERATIONS
• Skin testing and desensitization are mandatory before first dose or if more than 1 week has elapsed between treatments. Life-threatening hypersensitivity occurs in 20% to 35% of patients. For skin test, inject 2 IU intradermally at least 1 week before first asparaginase dose, and observe injection site for at least 1 hour for flare or wheal. If skin test is positive or if patient was previously treated with asparaginase, desensitize by gradually increasing I.V. doses until reaching ordered daily dose (provided no allergic reaction occurs). A negative skin test doesn't rule out future allergic reactions. Keep emergency equipment nearby.
• Incidence of hypersensitivity is lower with daily dosage schedule than with weekly one. Risk of hypersensitivity rises with repeated courses of therapy.
• Resistance to cytotoxic effects of asparaginase develops rapidly.
• Drug has low therapeutic index; therapeutic effects aren't likely without some signs of toxicity.
• Obtain liver function tests before and during therapy. Teach patient to recognize signs of hepatic impair-

ment: jaundice, dark orange urine, and clay-colored stools.
• Adequate hydration, alkalinization of urine, and possibly allopurinol administration will reduce risk of uric acid nephropathy.
• If the patient's taking an antidiabetic or antigout drug, he may require an increased dosage because asparaginase raises serum glucose and uric acid levels.
• Women shouldn't breast-feed while taking drug because of potential adverse effects on infant.
• Observe the patient for signs of CNS toxicity or thromboembolism. Be especially alert for dyspnea and chest pain, which may indicate pulmonary embolism.

atenolol
Tenormin

Pregnancy Risk Category: C

PHARMACOKINETICS
Distribution: minimally protein bound (5% to 15%).
Metabolism: not metabolized.
Excretion: primarily renal. Over 85% of an I.V. dose is excreted in the urine within 24 hours.
Action: peak levels occur within 5 minutes after I.V. administration; elimination half-life is 6 to 7 hours.

MECHANISM OF ACTION
The mechanism whereby atenolol, a beta$_1$ (cardioselective) adrenergic blocking agent, improves survival in patients with myocardial infarction (MI) is unknown. It also reduces the frequency of ventricular premature beats, reduces chest pain, reduces myocardial oxygen consumption (in most cases), and reduces post-infarct cardiac muscle enzyme elevation.

INDICATIONS & DOSAGE
• To reduce cardiovascular mortality and risk of reinfarction in hemodynamically stable patients who have survived the acute phase of an MI.
Adults: 5 mg I.V., followed by another 5 mg I.V. 10 minutes later. Initiate oral therapy 10 minutes after the final I.V. dose in patients who tolerate the full I.V. dose. Give 50 mg P.O., followed by another 50 mg 12 hours later. The patient should then be given 50 mg b.i.d. for at least 6 to 9 days, or until discharge from the hospital. If not contraindicated, therapy may sometimes be continued for 1 to 3 years.

CONTRAINDICATIONS & CAUTIONS
• Contraindicated in patients with sinus bradycardia, heart block greater than first degree, cardiogenic shock, and overt cardiac failure. Also contraindicated in patients with acute MI accompanied by cardiac failure that is not effectively and promptly controlled by furosemide 80 mg I.V. (or equivalent therapy).
• Contraindicated in patients with a history of bronchospastic disease. However, the relative selectivity of atenolol for beta-1 receptors may allow the drug to be used with caution, depending upon the doctor's clinical judgment. Have a bronchodilator (preferably a beta-2 stimulant) available.
• There appears to be no basis for treating patients with systolic blood pressure <100 mm Hg or heart rate <50 beats/minute.
• Use cautiously in diabetic patients. Beta-adrenergic blocking agents may block some hypoglycemic symptoms.
• Use cautiously in patients with congestive heart failure (CHF) controlled by digitalis or diuretics. Intrinsic sympathetic stimulation is necessary to support circulatory function in CHF,

and excessive beta blockade may exacerbate heart failure.

PREPARATION & STORAGE

Available in 10 ml ampules containing 5 mg atenolol. Store the drug at room temperature (59° to 86° F. [15° to 30° C.]) and protect from light. Dilute with 0.9% sodium chloride, dextrose 5% in water, or sodium chloride and dextrose injection. Dilutions are stable for 48 hours.

ADMINISTRATION

Direct injection: Administer over at least 5 minutes into a large vein.
Intermittent infusion: not recommended.
Continuous infusion: not recommended.

INCOMPATIBILITY

Do not mix with other drugs.

ADVERSE REACTIONS

Life-threatening: bronchospasm, cardiac arrest, cardiogenic shock (all are rare).
Other: bradycardia, dysrhythmias, heart block, hypotension.

INTERACTIONS

Inhalational anesthetics (such as ether or trichlorethylene), calcium channel blockers (such as verapamil), digitalis glycosides (such as digoxin): possibly enhanced cardiac depressant effects.
Sympathomimetics (such as dobutamine hydrochloride or isoproterenol hydrochloride): counteract the effects of atenolol.

EFFECTS ON DIAGNOSTIC TESTS

None reported.

SPECIAL CONSIDERATIONS

• Administration of I.V. atenolol should be restricted to a critical care area such as the coronary care unit (CCU).
• During the acute phase of MI, beta-adrenergic blocker therapy should supplement standard CCU treatment.
• I.V. atenolol affords a rapid onset of the protective effects of beta-adrenergic blockade against reinfarction. The I.V. route is preferred during the acute postinfarct period because there is some evidence that gastric absorption of orally administered atenolol may be delayed in the early phase of MI. This may be a result of physiologic changes accompanying MI or secondary to decreased GI motility caused by morphine administration. However, oral therapy alone may still provide benefits.
• Administer the drug as soon as the patient's eligibility is established and his hemodynamic condition has stabilized. Reduction of mortality appears to be most significant during the first 24 hours after infarct.
• During administration, monitor the patient's blood pressure, heart rate, and EKG. Discontinue the drug if significant hypotension or bradycardia occurs.
• Closely monitor patients suspected of having thyroid disease. Beta-adrenergic blocking agents may mask some of the signs of hyperthyroidism (such as tachycardia).
• Patients with borderline blood pressure (<120 mm Hg systolic) or who are more than age 60 years may not respond adequately to atenolol therapy.
• If the patient cannot tolerate I.V. atenolol, he may still be a candidate for oral therapy. Clinical trials suggest giving 100 mg of atenolol daily P.O. (either as 50 mg b.i.d. or 100 mg once a day) for at least 7 days.
• Dosage adjustments may be required in patients with renal failure.

atracurium besylate
Tracrium♦

Pregnancy Risk Category: C

PHARMACOKINETICS
Distribution: into extracellular space by a mechanism that's not well understood. Drug crosses placenta and is 82% protein-bound.
Metabolism: rapid, by enzymatic pathways (nonoxidative ester hydrolysis catalyzed by nonspecific esterases) and nonenzymatic pathways via Hofmann elimination (chemical degradation).
Excretion: in urine and bile, with a small fraction unchanged. About 90% of drug is eliminated in 7 hours. Not known if drug appears in breast milk.
Action: onset, dose-related; 0.4 to 0.5 mg/kg produces maximum relaxation in 3 to 5 minutes; duration, 20 to 35 minutes for effects to start subsiding and 60 to 70 minutes for them to end.

MECHANISM OF ACTION
A competitive, nondepolarizing neuromuscular blocker, atracurium produces muscle relaxation by blocking acetylcholine's effect at the myoneural junction. This action prevents muscle depolarization and leads to short-term paralysis.

INDICATIONS & DOSAGE
• Facilitation of endotracheal intubation and muscle relaxation during surgery or mechanical ventilation. Dosage must be individualized; guidelines appear below.
Adults: initially, 0.4 to 0.5 mg/kg (represents double the dose needed for nearly complete neuromuscular blockade); maintenance dose of 0.08 to 0.10 mg/kg, as needed, depends on response to peripheral nerve stimulation or observation of muscle tone recovery, spontaneous breathing, coughing, or if patient bucks endotracheal tube.
Children age 1 month to 2 years: initially, 0.3 to 0.4 mg/kg. Frequent maintenance doses may be needed.

CONTRAINDICATIONS & CAUTIONS
• Contraindicated in patients hypersensitive to the drug.
• Use cautiously in patients who have a history of severe anaphylactic reaction, asthma, or disorders exacerbated by substantial histamine release.
• Also use cautiously in patients with bronchogenic carcinoma and such neuromuscular diseases as myasthenia gravis and Eaton-Lambert syndrome because atracurium potentiates neuromuscular blockade.
• Use cautiously in hypotension because the condition may be exacerbated; and in hyperthermia because the drug's duration of action may be intensified or prolonged.
• Use cautiously in pulmonary impairment because the drug deepens respiratory depression.
• Also use cautiously in patients with electrolyte imbalance or dehydration, which may alter drug action.

PREPARATION & STORAGE
Atracurium is available in 5 and 10 ml ampules. Each milliliter contains 10 mg of drug. Dilute the drug with dextrose 5% in water or 0.9% sodium chloride for intermittent or continuous infusion. Refrigerate at 36° to 46° F. (2° to 8° C). Don't freeze.

ADMINISTRATION
Only staff trained in giving I.V. anesthetics and managing adverse reactions should give this drug.

Unmarked trade names available in the United States only.
♦Also available in Canada.   ♦♦Available in Canada only.

Direct injection: Inject rapidly into an I.V. line containing a free-flowing, compatible solution.

Intermittent infusion: Infuse diluted drug into I.V. line containing a compatible solution, as needed, during procedure.

Continuous infusion: After direct injection, give a 0.02% to 0.05% solution at 7.5 mcg/kg/minute during procedure.

INCOMPATIBILITY
Incompatible with alkaline solutions because of drug's acid pH.

ADVERSE REACTIONS
Life-threatening: anaphylaxis.
Other: bradycardia, hypotension, increased bronchial secretions, tachycardia, wheezing.

INTERACTIONS
Aminoglycoside antibiotics, lithium, magnesium, procainamide, quinidine: potentiated neuromuscular blockade.

Antimyasthenics, edrophonium: antagonism of atracurium effects.

Calcium salts: reversed atracurium effects.

Depolarizing neuromuscular blocking agents: enhanced neuromuscular blockade.

Doxapram: possible masking of residual effects if used after atracurium.

Inhalation anesthetics: potentiated atracurium effects by all except nitrous oxide. Halothane enhances atracurium effects the least; enflurane, the most.

Opioid analgesics: possible worsened respiratory depression and hypotension.

EFFECTS ON DIAGNOSTIC TESTS
None reported.

SPECIAL CONSIDERATIONS
• *Treatment of overdose:* symptomatic. Maintain a patent airway and assist breathing, as needed. Administer fluids and vasopressors for hypotension and edrophonium, neostigmine, or pyridostigmine for neuromuscular blockade. Usually reverses in 8 to 10 minutes.

• Keep emergency resuscitation equipment available at all times.

• Size of initial dose depends on degree of muscle relaxation required and whether drug will be combined with inhalation anesthetics or narcotics. When possible, use a peripheral nerve stimulator to assess depth of blockade and to determine subsequent doses.

• Reduce drug dose by 33% if used with isoflurane or enflurane and by 10% if used with halothane.

• Maintenance doses have no cumulative effect on duration of neuromuscular blockade if recovery is allowed to begin before their administration.

atropine sulfate

Pregnancy Risk Category: C

PHARMACOKINETICS
Distribution: throughout body tissues and across the blood-brain barrier and placenta.

Metabolism: in liver, into several metabolites, including tropine acids and esters; 18% of drug binds to serum albumin.

Excretion: mainly in urine, with small amounts in feces and expired air and trace amounts in breast milk. Serum half-life is 2 to 3 hours.

Action: onset, 2 to 4 minutes; duration, 4 to 6 hours.

MECHANISM OF ACTION

An anticholinergic, atropine binds to postganglionic receptors and blocks acetylcholine, thereby obstructing vagal effects on the sinoatrial node and increasing heart rate. Atropine also increases conduction through the atrioventricular node. The drug has antimuscarinic effects on bronchial and intestinal smooth muscle.

INDICATIONS & DOSAGE

• Symptomatic bradycardia. *Adults:* 0.5 mg q 5 minutes until desired heart rate is reached (usually 80 beats/minute). Maximum total dose, 2 mg; minimum dose, 0.5 mg. Lower dose could cause paradoxical bradycardia by vagal stimulation.
• Ventricular asystole in advanced life support. *Adults:* 1 mg q 5 minutes. *Adolescents and children:* 0.02 mg/kg (in children, minimum 0.1 mg; maximum 1 mg) q 5 minutes, if needed. In adolescents, maximum total dose is 2 mg.
• Blocked muscarinic effects of anticholinesterase agents. *Adults:* 0.6 to 1.2 mg for each 0.5 to 2.5 mg of neostigmine methylsulfate or each 10 to 20 mg of pyridostigmine bromide. *Neonates:* 0.02 mg/kg for each 0.04 mg/kg of neostigmine methylsulfate.
• Antidote for anticholinesterase toxicity. *Adults:* initially, 1 to 2 mg, then 2 mg q 5 to 60 minutes until symptoms subside. In severe cases, initial dose may be as much as 6 mg q 5 to 60 minutes, as needed.

CONTRAINDICATIONS & CAUTIONS

• Because the drug may raise intraocular pressure, it is contraindicated in glaucoma, except for cases of open-angle glaucoma being treated with miotics.
• Also contraindicated in myasthenia gravis, obstructive uropathy, and unstable cardiovascular status caused by acute hemorrhage.
• Patients sensitive to other belladonna alkaloids or salicylates may show atropine intolerance.
• In benign prostatic hypertrophy, other obstructive uropathy, and autonomic neuropathy, administer carefully because the drug may cause urine retention.
• In obstructive GI disease, intestinal atony, paralytic ileus, and ulcerative colitis, give carefully because of impaired motility.
• Use cautiously in children with brain damage because CNS effects may be exacerbated; in Down's syndrome because of abnormal pupillary dilation and tachycardia; in reflux esophagitis because of increased reflux; in fever because of possible suppressed sweat gland secretions; in hepatic or renal impairment because of decreased drug metabolism or excretion; in hypertension and pregnancy-induced hypertension because the condition may be aggravated; in hyperthyroidism because of the risk of severe tachycardia; and in xerostomia because drug may further decrease salivary flow. Use cautiously in tachycardia that threatens to cause cardiac decompensation.

PREPARATION & STORAGE

Available in single-dose ampules of 0.4 mg/ml, 0.5 mg/ml, and 0.4 mg/ 0.5 ml; in single-dose vials of 0.4 mg/ml, 1 mg/ml, and 1.2 mg/ml; in multidose 20 ml vials of 0.4 mg/ml; and in prefilled syringes containing 0.5 and 1 mg of drug. Store at room temperature.

ADMINISTRATION

Direct injection: Inject prescribed amount of undiluted drug into vein or I.V. tubing over 1 to 2 minutes.

Intermittent infusion: not recommended.
Continuous infusion: not recommended.

INCOMPATIBILITY
Incompatible with alkalides, bromides, iodides, isoproterenol, metaraminol bitartrate, methohexital, norepinephrine, pentobarbital sodium, and sodium bicarbonate.

ADVERSE REACTIONS
Life-threatening: aggravated atrioventricular block, anaphylaxis, ventricular fibrillation, ventricular tachycardia.
Other: anhidrosis, ataxia, bloating, blurred vision, coma, confusion, constipation, cycloplegia, delirium, dizziness, drowsiness, dry mouth, fever, flushing, headache, increased intraocular pressure, insomnia, lightheadedness, local irritation at injection site, mydriasis, nausea, nervousness, photophobia, rash, restlessness, tachycardia, urinary hesitancy and urine retention, urticaria, vomiting, weakness.

INTERACTIONS
Alphaprodine, antihistamines, antiparkinson drugs, buclizine, disopyramide, meperidine, orphenadrine, quinidine: intensified antimuscarinic effects.
Antimyasthenics: possible further reduction in intestinal motility.
Antipsychotics, benzodiazepines, glutethimide, phenothiazines, tricyclic antidepressants: intensified antimuscarinic effects.
Cholinesterase inhibitors: blocked miosis.
Cyclopropane: heightened risk of ventricular dysrhythmias.
Digoxin: possible elevated serum levels.
Ketoconazole: reduced absorption.

MAO inhibitors: intensified atropine action, blocked atropine detoxification.
Methotrimeprazine: possible extrapyramidal effects.
Opioids: increased risk of severe constipation, paralytic ileus.
Potassium chloride (wax-matrix preparations): increased risk of GI lesions.
Urinary alkalinizers: delayed excretion of atropine.

EFFECTS ON DIAGNOSTIC TESTS
EKG: possible bradycardia or tachycardia.
Gastric acid secretion test: antagonized pentagastrin and histamine action.

SPECIAL CONSIDERATIONS
• *Treatment of overdose:* symptomatic. Give fluids for shock, diazepam for CNS irritability, pilocarpine for mydriasis, and hyperthermia blanket for cold. Catheterize patient to prevent urine retention. Provide respiratory support and possibly give physostigmine to treat delirium, hallucinations, coma, or supraventricular tachycardia.
• Monitor blood pressure closely to evaluate drug tolerance.
• Initial drug bolus may cause bradycardia, which usually resolves in 1 to 2 minutes.
• Monitor EKG for patients receiving drug for bradycardia or heart block. Watch for heart rate exceeding 100 beats/minute, increased premature ventricular contractions, and ventricular tachycardia. Notify doctor if these occur.
• Encourage fluids and provide mouth care when appropriate.
• Assess for urine retention by monitoring intake and output. Palpate patient's bladder every 4 hours.

• When assessing a patient with CNS injury who has received atropine, realize that patient's pupil size is not a reliable diagnostic sign.

azacytidine (5-azacytidine, ladakamycin, mylosar, NSC-102816)

Investigational drug available only from National Cancer Institute
Pregnancy Risk Category: C

PHARMACOKINETICS
Distribution: throughout most body tissues and fluids.
Metabolism: not known.
Excretion: mainly in urine but also in feces, sputum, and vomitus. Not known if drug appears in breast milk.
Action: peak serum level, 12 hours (for full cytotoxicity); duration, several days.

MECHANISM OF ACTION
Disrupts transcription of nucleic acid into proteins; also inhibits pyrimidine synthesis by blocking orotidylic acid decarboxylase. Drug acts in S phase of cell cycle.

INDICATIONS & DOSAGE
• Refractory acute myelogenous leukemia. *Adults:* 200 mg/m^2/day for 10 days. *Children:* 50 to 200 mg/m^2/day for 10 days as tolerated.

CONTRAINDICATIONS & CAUTIONS
• Contraindicated in patients with hepatic metastases or a serum albumin level below 3 g/dl.

PREPARATION & STORAGE
Supplied in 100 mg vials. Refrigerate unopened vials at 36° to 46° F.

(2° to 8° C.). Reconstitute with 19.9 ml of sterile water for injection to yield a 5 mg/ml solution. To avoid hydrolysis at room temperature, use within 30 minutes, following hospital protocol. For dilution, add one-eighth of total daily dosage to 50 to 250 ml of dextrose 5% in water, lactated Ringer's solution, or 0.9% sodium chloride. Specific amount of diluent depends on the patient's age and hydration and cardiac status. Solution remains stable for about 3 hours but decomposes by 10% in 1 to 2 hours. Optimum stability occurs at pH 6.5 to 7.

ADMINISTRATION
Direct injection: not recommended.
Intermittent infusion: not recommended.
Continuous infusion: Infuse the 50 to 250 ml solution over 3 hours. Then replace with a freshly prepared solution and infuse over 3 hours. Repeat for duration of therapy.

INCOMPATIBILITY
Incompatible with highly acidic or basic solutions, which cause drug degradation.

ADVERSE REACTIONS
Life-threatening: myelosuppression.
Other: CNS toxicity (myalgia, weakness, and lethargy progressing to drowsiness, stupor, and coma), diarrhea, fever, hepatotoxicity, hypophosphatemia, hypotension, muscle cramps, nausea, phlebitis, rash, renal toxicity (azotemia), vomiting.

INTERACTIONS
Etoposide (VP-16): intensified adverse reactions, especially prolonged pancytopenia.
Hydroxyurea: worsened and abrupt myelosuppression.

Unmarked trade names available in the United States only.
♦ Also available in Canada.   ♦ ♦ Available in Canada only.

EFFECTS ON DIAGNOSTIC TESTS
Serum transaminase: increased levels.

SPECIAL CONSIDERATIONS
• Continuous infusion tends to produce less nausea and vomiting than bolus injection. Start an antiemetic regimen 24 to 48 hours before therapy begins.
• Report adverse reactions to National Cancer Institute.
• Monitor blood pressure before therapy and at least every 30 minutes during infusion. If systolic pressure falls below 90 mm Hg, stop infusion and notify doctor immediately.
• Monitor temperature, CBC, and liver function tests.
• Notify doctor if patient develops muscular pain or weakness; may indicate neurotoxicity.

---

azlocillin sodium
Azlin

Pregnancy Risk Category: B

PHARMACOKINETICS
Distribution: readily distributed into bile, bone, bronchial and wound secretions, serum, urine, and other tissues. CNS penetration is poor when meninges aren't inflamed. Drug crosses placenta; it's 25% to 45% protein-bound.
Metabolism: only about 15% metabolized in the liver.
Excretion: 50% to 70% excreted unchanged in urine within 24 hours by renal tubular secretion and glomerular filtration; 20% to 25% excreted unchanged in bile. Low concentrations appear in breast milk. Elimination half-life is 55 to 70 minutes.

Action: peak level, immediately after infusion.

MECHANISM OF ACTION
Inhibits bacterial cell-wall synthesis in susceptible organisms. Its spectrum of activity includes such gram-positive aerobic bacteria as non–penicillinase-producing strains of *Staphylococcus aureus, Staphylococcus epidermidis,* groups A, B, C, and G streptococci, *Streptococcus pneumoniae, Streptococcus viridans,* and some enterococci.

Susceptible gram-negative aerobic bacteria include *Neisseria meningitides, N. gonorrhoeae, Haemophilus influenzae,* some strains of *Escherichia coli, Morganella morganii, Proteus mirabilis, P. vulgaris, Providencia rettgeri, Salmonella, Shigella, Citrobacter, Enterobacter, Klebsiella, Serratia, Pseudomonas aeruginosa, Moraxella,* and some species of *Flavobacterium.* Susceptible anaerobic bacteria include some strains of *Actinomyces, Bifidobacterium, Clostridium, Eubacterium, Lactobacillus, Peptococcus, Peptostreptococcus, Propionibacterium, Bacteroides, Fusobacterium,* and *Veillonella.*

INDICATIONS & DOSAGE
• Severe infections caused by susceptible organisms. *Adults:* 200 to 300 mg/kg/day divided q 4 to 6 hours; or 3 g q 4 hours.
• Uncomplicated infections caused by susceptible organisms. *Adults:* 100 to 125 mg/kg/day divided q 6 hours; or 2 g q 6 hours.
• Pulmonary infection in cystic fibrosis. *Children:* 75 mg/kg q 4 hours. Maximum dosage, 24 g/day. *Note:* Dosage in renal failure must be reduced in adult patients whose creatinine clearance is less than 30 ml/minute.

CONTRAINDICATIONS & CAUTIONS
- Contraindicated in penicillin or cephalosporin hypersensitivity.
- Use cautiously in hematopoietic, liver, or renal impairment because of an increased risk of toxicity or adverse reactions.
- Also use cautiously in fluid and electrolyte imbalance because hypokalemia can occur.
- Use cautiously in patients with a history of GI disorders, especially ulcerative colitis, regional enteritis, or antibiotic-associated colitis, because of increased risk of pseudomembranous colitis.
- Use cautiously in bleeding disorders because drug may cause platelet dysfunction and hemorrhage.
- Use cautiously in patients on restricted sodium diet; drug contains approximately 2.2 mEq of sodium per gram.

PREPARATION & STORAGE
Available in vials and infusion bottles containing 2 g, 3 g, or 4 g of drug. Store vials at room temperature for up to 24 hours. Reconstitute each gram with 10 ml of sterile water for injection, dextrose 5% in water, or 0.9% sodium chloride. Shake vigorously, if necessary, to dissolve drug. Solution should be clear and colorless.

Dilute reconstituted drug with such compatible solutions as dextrose 5% in water, dextrose 5% and 0.22% or 0.45% sodium chloride, Ringer's lactate, or 0.9% sodium chloride.

ADMINISTRATION
Direct injection: Over 5 minutes or more, inject ordered dose into intermittent infusion device or I.V. line containing a free-flowing, compatible solution. To minimize vein irritation, don't exceed rate of 100 mg/ml.

Intermittent infusion: Over 30 minutes, give 50 to 100 ml of diluted solution, using an intermittent infusion device or an I.V. line containing a free-flowing, compatible solution.
Continuous infusion: not recommended.

INCOMPATIBILITY
Incompatible with aminoglycosides.

ADVERSE REACTIONS
Life-threatening: anaphylaxis, pseudomembranous colitis.
Other: abnormal body odor, abnormal platelet aggregation, bacterial or fungal superinfection, bleeding (in renal impairment), diarrhea, erythema, flatulence, hypernatremia, hypokalemia, nausea, pain, phlebitis, seizures, stomatitis, thrombophlebitis, transient chest discomfort, unpleasant taste, vein irritation, vomiting.

INTERACTIONS
Anticoagulants, anti-inflammatory analgesics, salicylates, other platelet aggregation inhibitors, thrombolytics: heightened risk of severe hemorrhage.
Chloramphenicol, erythromycin, sulfonamides, tetracycline: possible interference with bactericidal effects of azlocillin.
Hepatotoxic drugs: increased risk of hepatotoxicity.
Probenecid: reduced azlocillin excretion.
Vecuronium: possible prolonged neuromuscular blockade.

EFFECTS ON DIAGNOSTIC TESTS
BUN, serum alkaline phosphatase, bilirubin, creatinine, LDH, sodium: increased levels.
Partial thromboplastin time, prothrombin time: prolonged.
SGOT, SGPT: elevated levels.

Urine potassium: increased levels.
Serum potassium: decreased levels.
Serum uric acid: decreased levels.
Urine and serum protein: possible false-positive results because of reduced serum uric acid.

SPECIAL CONSIDERATIONS
• Check for previous penicillin or cephalosporin hypersensitivity before first dose. Negative history doesn't rule out future allergic reaction.
• Obtain specimens for culture and sensitivity testing before first dose. Therapy may start before results are available.
• If diarrhea persists during therapy, collect stool specimens to rule out possible pseudomembranous colitis.
• Monitor renal, hepatic, and hematologic function. Also monitor serum potassium levels for hypokalemia and give supplements, as ordered.
• Watch for prolonged bleeding time or for evidence of bleeding.
• Dosage may need adjustment in cystic fibrosis because of increased tubular secretion, and in elderly patients because of reduced tubular secretion.
• Drug doesn't affect protein tests using biuret reagent (Albustix, Albutest).
• Drug can be removed by hemodialysis.
• Observe for signs of fungal and bacterial superinfection with prolonged use.

---

aztreonam
Azactam

Pregnancy Risk Category: B

PHARMACOKINETICS
Distribution: widely distributed in fluids and tissues, with 40% to 60% protein-bound. Cerebrospinal fluid concentration is higher when meninges are inflamed. Drug crosses placenta.
Metabolism: 6% to 16% of drug is metabolized to inactive metabolites by hydrolysis of beta-lactam ring.
Excretion: in urine, primarily as unchanged drug, by glomerular filtration and renal tubular secretion. Drug appears in breast milk. Serum half-life averages about 90 minutes in normal renal function.
Action: peak level, 2 to 3 minutes; duration, 6 to 8 hours.

MECHANISM OF ACTION
A narrow-spectrum, bactericidal monobactam antibiotic, aztreonam joins with penicillin-binding protein (PBP-3) to inhibit bacterial cell-wall synthesis. It's effective against many gram-negative aerobic bacteria, including *Neisseria meningitidis, N. gonorrhoeae, Haemophilus influenzae, Branhamella catarrhalis, Citrobacter diversus, Enterobacter agglomerans, Escherichia coli, Hafnia alvei, Klebsiella pneumoniae, Morganella morganii, Proteus mirabilis, P. vulgaris, Providencia, Serratia marcescens, Salmonella, Shigella, Pasteurella multocida,* and *Pseudomonas aeruginosa.*

Aztreonam exerts little or no effect against gram-positive aerobic bacteria, anaerobic bacteria, *Chlamydia,* fungi, *Mycoplasma,* or viruses. As a result, it's usually combined with other antibiotics for life-threatening infections.

INDICATIONS & DOSAGE
• Infections of the respiratory or genitourinary tract, bone, skin, and soft tissues caused by susceptible organisms. *Adults with normal renal function:* 1 to 2 g q 6 to 12 hours. Maximum daily dosage, 8 g. *Adults with creatinine clearance of 10 to 30 ml/minute/1.73 m²:* initially, 1 to

2 g, then 0.5 to 1 g q 6 to 12 hours.
Children: pediatric dosage not established; however, 30 to 50 mg/kg q 6
to 12 hours is reportedly effective.

CONTRAINDICATIONS & CAUTIONS

• Contraindicated in patients hypersensitive to aztreonam. Use cautiously in patients hypersensitive to
such beta-lactam antibiotics as penicillins, cephalosporins, cephamycins,
1-oxa-beta-lactams, and carbape-
nems.
• Use cautiously in the elderly and
in patients with renal impairment.
• Also use cautiously in hepatic cirrhosis because of prolonged drug
half-life.

PREPARATION & STORAGE

Available in 15 ml vials or 100 ml
piggyback infusion bottles containing 500 mg, 1 g, or 2 g of drug. For
direct injection, add 6 to 10 ml of
sterile water for injection to vial and
shake well. For infusion, add at least
3 ml sterile water for each gram of
drug. Dilute with 50 to 100 ml of
0.9% sodium chloride, dextrose 5%
in water, dextrose 5% in 0.9% sodium chloride injection, or Ringer's
lactate. Solutions reconstituted with
0.9% sodium chloride or sterile
water retain potency for 48 hours at
room temperature and for 7 days if
refrigerated. Slight pink tint doesn't
affect potency.

Before reconstitution, store at
room temperature. After reconstitution, promptly use any solution over
2% concentration and discard the
unused amount.

ADMINISTRATION

Direct injection: Using a 21G to
23G needle, inject reconstituted drug
over 3 to 5 minutes into vein or I.V.
line containing a free-flowing, compatible solution.

Intermittent infusion: Over 20 to 60
minutes, infuse into I.V. tubing of a
free-flowing, compatible solution or
give using a volume-control device.
If you're using a volume-control device, final dilution shouldn't exceed
2% (20 mg/ml).
Continuous infusion: not recommended.

INCOMPATIBILITY

Incompatible with nafcillin, cephradine, and metronidazole. Should not
be mixed with any drug.

ADVERSE REACTIONS

Life-threatening: anaphylaxis.
Other: bacterial or fungal superinfection, chills, confusion, diarrhea,
EKG changes, eosinophilia, fever,
hypotension, pseudomembranous colitis, rash, seizures, thrombophlebitis, vomiting.

INTERACTIONS

*Aminoglycosides, beta-lactam anti-
biotics, clavulanic acid, clindamycin:* synergistic effect on many
gram-negative aerobic bacteria.
Probenecid: slower renal tubular secretion of aztreonam.

EFFECTS ON DIAGNOSTIC TESTS

BUN, serum creatinine, LDH: tran-
siently elevated levels.
Coombs' test: false-positive findings.
*Partial thromboplastin time, pro-
thrombin time:* possible prolonged
duration.
*Serum alkaline phosphatase,
SGOT, SGPT:* transiently elevated
levels.
Urine glucose: false-positive results
when tested with cupric sulfate
(Benedict's solution, Clinitest).

SPECIAL CONSIDERATIONS

• Check for previous antibiotic hypersensitivity. Negative history

---

Unmarked trade names available in the United States only.
♦ Also available in Canada.   ♦ ♦ Available in Canada only.

doesn't rule out future allergic reaction.
- Obtain specimens for culture and sensitivity testing before first dose. Therapy may start before results are available.
- Monitor for phlebitis at infusion site, pseudomembranous colitis, and hypersensitivity.
- If diarrhea persists during therapy, collect stool specimens to rule out possible pseudomembranous colitis.
- Monitor BUN and creatinine levels during therapy. Patients with renal dysfunction or elderly patients may require dosage adjustments.
- Monitor liver function studies during therapy. Cirrhotic patients on extended, high-dose regimen may require dosage reduction.
- Use Clinistix or Tes-Tape for urine glucose determinations to prevent spurious results.
- Observe patient for fungal and bacterial superinfection with prolonged use.
- Hemodialysis and peritoneal dialysis can remove drug.

---

benzquinamide hydrochloride
Emete-Con

Pregnancy Risk Category: C

PHARMACOKINETICS
Distribution: throughout body tissues, with highest concentrations in liver and kidneys. Drug is 55% to 60% bound to plasma proteins. Not known if drug crosses placenta.
Metabolism: rapidly and almost completely metabolized (90% to 95%) in liver, producing 10 to 12 metabolites.
Excretion: 5% to 10% removed unchanged in urine and remainder excreted in bile, feces, and urine as metabolites within 72 hours. Serum half-life is 40 minutes. Not known if drug appears in breast milk.
Action: onset, usually within 15 minutes; duration, 3 to 4 hours.

MECHANISM OF ACTION
Inhibits nausea and vomiting by depressing the brain's chemoreceptor trigger zone. Drug may also stimulate respiration during anesthesia.

INDICATIONS & DOSAGE
- Prevention and management of nausea and vomiting from anesthesia and surgery. *Adults:* 25 mg or 0.2 to 0.4 mg/kg as a single dose by slow I.V. injection. Subsequent doses should be given I.M.
- Prevention and control of acute hypotension during anesthesia (investigational). *Adults:* 10 to 15 mg by slow I.V. injection.
Note: Dosages may be reduced for elderly or debilitated patients.

CONTRAINDICATIONS & CAUTIONS
- Contraindicated in benzquinamide hypersensitivity.
- Also contraindicated in cardiovascular disease and in patients receiving preanesthetic or cardiovascular drugs because of the risk of possible dysrhythmias and sudden hypertension.
- Not recommended for pediatric use.

PREPARATION & STORAGE
Available in vial containing 50 mg of drug. Reconstitute with 2.2 ml of sterile water for injection to yield 2 ml solution containing 25 mg/ml of drug. After reconstitution, drug remains potent for 14 days at room temperature. Store in light-resistant containers.

ADMINISTRATION
Direct injection: Aspirate desired dose from vial and inject directly into a vein or I.V. tubing containing a free-flowing, compatible solution. Give 1 ml over 30 to 60 seconds.
Intermittent infusion: not recommended.
Continuous infusion: not recommended.

INCOMPATIBILITY
Incompatible with chlordiazepoxide, diazepam, pentobarbital sodium, phenobarbital sodium, secobarbital sodium, and thiopental sodium. May precipitate if reconstituted with 0.9% sodium chloride for injection.

ADVERSE REACTIONS
Life-threatening: acute hypertension, premature ventricular contractions.
Other: abdominal cramps, anorexia, atrial fibrillation, blurred vision, dizziness, drowsiness, dry mouth, excitement, extrapyramidal symptoms, fatigue, fever, flushing, headache, hiccups, hypertension, hypotension, insomnia, nausea, nervousness, premature atrial contractions, rash, restlessness, salivation, shivering, sweating, tremors, urticaria, vomiting, weakness.

INTERACTIONS
Epinephrine, other vasopressors: increased hypertensive effect. Lower doses may prevent sudden rise in blood pressure.

EFFECTS ON DIAGNOSTIC TESTS
None reported.

SPECIAL CONSIDERATIONS
• *Treatment of overdose:* In overdose, signs of CNS stimulation (restlessness, excitement, and hypertension) occur with those of CNS depression (drowsiness, fatigue, and hypotension). Provide supportive measures as needed. Atropine may be helpful. Dialysis offers little benefit because drug binds to plasma proteins.
• Monitor blood pressure during administration.
• Drug may be given prophylactically if emesis could jeopardize surgical outcome or harm patient.
• Drug may mask signs of overdose and may thwart diagnosis of intestinal obstruction or brain tumor.

benztropine mesylate
Cogentin♦

Pregnancy Risk Category: C

PHARMACOKINETICS
Distribution: throughout the body, especially in CNS, cardiovascular system, GI tract, and urinary smooth muscle. Drug crosses placenta.
Metabolism: minimal in liver.
Excretion: most excreted unchanged or as metabolites in urine. Small amounts appear in breast milk.
Action: onset, within a few minutes; duration, 24 hours.

MECHANISM OF ACTION
Although this cholinergic blocker's action isn't fully understood, the drug probably acts by decreasing acetylcholine activity in the basal ganglia.

INDICATIONS & DOSAGE
• Arteriosclerotic, idiopathic, or postencephalitic parkinsonian syndrome. *Adults:* 1 to 2 mg daily. Maximum dose, 6 mg/day until symptomatic relief is obtained.

- Drug-induced extrapyramidal symptoms. *Adults:* 1 to 4 mg once daily or b.i.d.
- Acute dystonic reactions. *Adults:* initially, 1 to 2 mg I.V. daily, then 1 to 2 mg P.O. b.i.d. Dosage adjusted as needed and tolerated. *Children age 3 and older:* individualized dosage.

CONTRAINDICATIONS & CAUTIONS

- Contraindicated in hypersensitivity to benztropine.
- Also contraindicated in tardive dyskinesia because symptoms may worsen.
- Use cautiously in the elderly and in patients with dementia because of possible impaired memory and increased risk of confusion and psychosis; in glaucoma because of elevated intraocular pressure; in alcoholism and CNS disorders because of possible anhidrosis leading to hyperthermia; and in hepatorenal impairment because of possible toxic effects.
- Also use cautiously in cardiac instability or dysrhythmias because of a heightened risk of dysrhythmias; in hypertension or myasthenia gravis because of possible aggravation; and in patients with a history of extrapyramidal reactions because of possible intensified symptoms.
- In intestinal obstruction, give carefully because of decreased GI tone and motility.
- In prostatic hypertrophy or urine retention, administer carefully because urine retention may worsen.
- Not recommended for children under age 3.

PREPARATION & STORAGE

Supplied in 1 mg/ml concentration. Store in light-resistant container at room temperature. For intermittent infusion, dilute in 50 to 100 ml of a compatible solution.

ADMINISTRATION

Direct injection: Aspirate solution from ampule. Over 3 to 5 minutes, inject into vein or into I.V. tubing containing a free-flowing, compatible solution.
Intermittent infusion: Give diluted solution over 15 to 30 minutes.
Continuous infusion: not recommended.

INCOMPATIBILITY

No incompatibilities reported.

ADVERSE REACTIONS

Life-threatening: none reported.
Other: anhidrosis, blurred vision, confusion, constipation, depression, dilated pupils, disorientation, dizziness, dry mouth, dysuria, hallucinations, hyperthermia, lethargy, memory impairment, nausea, nervousness, paralytic ileus, paresthesias, photophobia, psychosis, rash, sedation, tachycardia, urine retention, vomiting.

INTERACTIONS

Alcohol, other CNS depressants: deepened CNS depression.
Amantadine, antihistamines, procainamide, quinidine: additive anticholinergic effects.
Carbidopa-levodopa, levodopa: possible increased efficacy of levodopa.
Haloperidol, MAO inhibitors, phenothiazines, tricyclic antidepressants: additive anticholinergic effects.

EFFECTS ON DIAGNOSTIC TESTS

None reported.

SPECIAL CONSIDERATIONS

- *Treatment of overdose:* Give physostigmine salicylate 1 to 2 mg S.C.

or I.V., as ordered. Repeat dose in 2 hours, if necessary.
- I.V. route rarely used because of small difference in onset time compared to I.M. route.
- Full drug effects may not occur for 2 to 3 days.
- Monitor heart rate and EKG for tachycardia; input and output for anhidrosis and urine retention; and temperature.
- Be alert for signs of paralytic ileus: abdominal distention and pain, decreased or absent bowel sounds, and constipation.
- Expect to give lower doses to the elderly, thin patients, and those with arteriosclerosis or parkinsonism.
- Closely monitor patients with a history of mental illness because symptoms may intensify.
- Encourage or perform good mouth care to prevent oral lesions caused by dry mouth.
- Never discontinue drug abruptly. Reduce dosage gradually.

betamethasone sodium phosphate
Betameth, Celestone Phosphate♦, Cel-U-Jec, Selestoject

Pregnancy Risk Category: C

PHARMACOKINETICS
Distribution: rapidly distributed to intestines, kidneys, liver, muscles, and skin. Drug crosses placenta.
Metabolism: primarily in liver, where drug is metabolized to biologically inactive compounds. Lesser amounts metabolized in kidneys and other tissues.
Excretion: by kidneys. Inactive metabolites are excreted as glucuronides and sulfates; small amounts of unmetabolized drug are excreted in urine, negligible amounts in bile. Drug appears in breast milk.
Action: onset, 1 to 5 minutes; duration varies, depending on dosage and time of administration.

MECHANISM OF ACTION
A synthetic glucocorticoid, betamethasone reduces inflammation, mainly by stabilizing leukocyte lysosomal membranes. Betamethasone also suppresses pituitary release of corticotropin, which, in turn, stops adrenocortical production of corticosteroids.

INDICATIONS & DOSAGE
- Severe inflammation or immunosuppression. *Adults:* 0.5 to 9 mg daily. After achieving satisfactory response, reduce dosage gradually and maintain at lowest level that produces therapeutic response.

CONTRAINDICATIONS & CAUTIONS
- Contraindicated in corticosteroid hypersensitivity.
- Use cautiously in hypothyroidism or cirrhosis because drug response may be exaggerated; in hyperthyroidism because of accelerated drug metabolism; in congestive heart failure (CHF), diverticulitis, hypertension, nonspecific ulcerative colitis, peptic ulcer, and psychosis because drug may aggravate these conditions; in cardiac disease and renal impairment because fluid retention may be hazardous; in diabetes mellitus because of possible exacerbation; in glaucoma because of elevated intraocular pressure; in hyperlipidemia because drug may raise serum fatty acid and cholesterol levels; and in hypoalbuminemia because of an increased risk of toxicity.
- Also use cautiously in myasthenia gravis because of worsened weakness; in osteoporosis because of pos-

sible exacerbation; and in uncontrolled viral, fungal, or bacterial infection because drug increases susceptibility to infection and masks symptoms.
• In patients with a history of tuberculosis, administer carefully because drug may reactivate disease.
• Always use cautiously in children because safe and effective dosage hasn't been established. Intracranial pressure may rise, leading to headache, oculomotor or abducens nerve paralysis, papilledema, and vision loss. Long-term use may retard bone growth, whereas high doses may cause pancreatic inflammation or destruction.

PREPARATION & STORAGE
Available in 5 ml multidose vials containing 3 mg/ml. Dilute as needed with dextrose 5% in water, 0.9% sodium chloride, Ringer's lactate, or dextrose 5% in Ringer's or Ringer's lactate. For direct injection, dilute dose in 10 ml; for intermittent infusion, dilute in 50 to 100 ml. Store between 59° and 86° F. (15° and 30° C.); don't freeze. Protect from light.

ADMINISTRATION
Direct injection: Use only in severe or life-threatening conditions and follow with intermittent infusion. Inject diluted dose over 5 to 10 minutes into vein or into I.V. line containing a free-flowing, compatible solution.
Intermittent infusion: Infuse over 20 to 30 minutes into established I.V. line containing a free-flowing, compatible solution.
Continuous infusion: not recommended.

INCOMPATIBILITY
Incompatible with parenteral local anesthetics containing preservatives,

such as parabens or phenols, because betamethasone may flocculate.

ADVERSE REACTIONS
Most adverse reactions are dose- or duration-dependent.
Life-threatening: anaphylaxis.
Other: acne, adrenocortical insufficiency, anorexia, cataracts, delayed wound healing, desquamation, edema, euphoria, fever, fluid and electrolyte imbalance, glaucoma, headache, hyperglycemia, hypertension, hypokalemia, hypotension, increased susceptibility to infection, joint pain, lethargy, myalgia, nausea, peptic ulcers, psychotic behavior, vomiting, weakness, weight loss.

INTERACTIONS
Acetaminophen: increased risk of hepatotoxicity.
Alcohol, NSAIDS: heightened risk of GI hemorrhage.
Anabolic steroids, androgens: increased risk of edema.
Anticholinesterase drugs: further weakness in myasthenia gravis patients.
Barbiturates, phenytoin, rifampin: enhanced glucocorticoid metabolism.
Carbonic anhydrase inhibitors, parenteral amphotericin B: heightened risk of severe hypokalemia.
Ephedrine: increased metabolic clearance of betamethasone.
Estrogen, oral contraceptives: altered betamethasone metabolism.
Ethacrynic acid, furosemide, thiazides, other potassium-depleting drugs: enhanced potassium-wasting effects.
Hepatic enzyme–inducing drugs: decreased betamethasone effect.
Mexiletine: accelerated metabolism.
Neuromuscular blocking agents: enhanced neuromuscular blockade.
Oral anticoagulants: possible increased blood coagulability.

Other immunosuppressants: heightened risk of infection and lymphomas.

Potassium supplements: reduced effects.

Salicylates: decreased effects and magnified risk of GI hemorrhage.

Sodium-containing drugs and foods: possible hypernatremia.

Streptozocin: heightened risk of hyperglycemia.

Toxoids, live or inactivated vaccines: possible diminished response.

EFFECTS ON DIAGNOSTIC TESTS

Basophils, eosinophils, lymphocytes, monocytes: possible reduced counts.

Gonadorelin test: altered results.

Nitroblue tetrazolium test: possible false-positive results.

Platelet and polymorphonuclear counts: increased.

Radioactive iodine tests: increased ^{131}I uptake, ^{123}I uptake, and protein-bound iodine concentration.

Radionuclide brain and bone imaging: decreased uptake of contrast medium.

Serum calcium: reduced levels.

Serum cholesterol, fatty acids, lipids: possible elevated levels.

Serum glucose, sodium: elevated levels.

Serum protein-bound iodine, thyroxine: possible reduced levels.

Serum uric acid: possible elevated or reduced levels.

Skin tests: unreliable response because drug suppresses inflammation.

Urine glucose: possible elevated levels.

SPECIAL CONSIDERATIONS

• Before and during long-term therapy, monitor EKG, blood pressure, chest and spinal X-rays, glucose tolerance tests, serum potassium levels, and hypothalamic and pituitary function tests. Also, periodically check electrolyte levels, CBC, height, weight, and intraocular pressure.

• If patient has a GI disorder, ensure that upper GI studies are performed before therapy.

• Adrenal function recovery may take 1 week after high-dose therapy lasting 1 to 5 days; up to 1 year after prolonged therapy.

• Discontinue drug gradually and as soon as possible.

• Watch for signs of infection.

• Because of betamethasone's hyperglycemic effect, the diabetic patient may require a larger dosage of an antidiabetic drug.

• Because drug increases catabolism, keep in mind that the patient may have greater protein needs.

• May contain sulfites.

---

biperiden lactate
Akineton Lactate♦

Pregnancy Risk Category: C

PHARMACOKINETICS

Distribution: not fully understood, but probably throughout most body tissues.

Metabolism: probably in the liver.

Excretion: mainly in urine, as unchanged drug or metabolites. Not known if drug appears in breast milk.

Action: onset, unknown; duration, unknown.

MECHANISM OF ACTION

By inhibiting acetylcholine's muscarinic effects, biperiden exerts a central cholinergic-blocking effect similar to that of atropine. It relaxes smooth muscle; diminishes GI, bronchial, and sweat gland secretions; and dilates pupils.

Unmarked trade names available in the United States only.
♦Also available in Canada.   ♦♦Available in Canada only.

INDICATIONS & DOSAGE

• Drug-induced extrapyramidal disorders. *Adults:* initially, 2 mg (0.4 ml), repeated q 30 minutes until symptoms subside. Maximum of 4 doses (or 8 mg) over 24 hours.

CONTRAINDICATIONS & CAUTIONS

• Contraindicated in biperiden hypersensitivity.
• Use cautiously in closed-angle glaucoma because drug may raise intraocular pressure; in prostate disorders because of possible urine retention; in debilitated patients or those with tachycardia because drug may cause thyrotoxicosis or decreased cardiac output; and in febrile patients or those exposed to heat because drug decreases ability to sweat.
• Also use cautiously in cardiac instability and dysrhythmias because of a heightened risk of dysrhythmias; in hypertension and tardive dyskinesia because of possible aggravation; in patients with a history of extrapyramidal reactions because symptoms may worsen; in hepatic or renal impairment because of an increased risk of toxicity; in intestinal obstruction because of decreased GI motility and tone; and in myasthenia gravis because of worsened weakness.
• Give the drug cautiously to confused or elderly patients because euphoria, confusion, and agitation may occur.
• Safety and efficacy in children have not been established.

PREPARATION & STORAGE

Available in 1 ml ampules containing 5 mg/ml. Drug is stable at room temperature. Protect from light.

ADMINISTRATION

Direct injection: Using a 21G to 23G needle, inject drug over at least 1 minute into vein or into I.V. tubing containing a free-flowing, compatible solution.
Intermittent infusion: not recommended.
Continuous infusion: not recommended.

INCOMPATIBILITY

No incompatibilities reported.

ADVERSE REACTIONS

Life-threatening: orthostatic hypotension.
Other: agitation, blurred vision, constipation, disorientation, dizziness, drowsiness, dry mouth, euphoria, hematuria, hyperpyrexia, impaired coordination, photophobia, tachycardia, transient psychotic reactions, urine retention.

INTERACTIONS

Anticholinesterase drugs: reduced effects.
Antihistamines, meperidine, phenothiazines, quinidine, tricyclic antidepressants: enhanced anticholinergic effects.
CNS depressants: deepened sedation.

EFFECTS ON DIAGNOSTIC TESTS

None reported.

SPECIAL CONSIDERATIONS

• *Treatment of overdose:* Give vasopressors for persistent hypotension. Provide respiratory support, antipyretics, and fluid replacements. Don't give phenothiazines because they could cause coma. In life-threatening emergency, give physostigmine, as ordered.
• Obtain baseline blood pressure and heart rate. Monitor for hypotension

and tachycardia during and after drug administration. Keep patient in bed during injection and until blood pressure stabilizes. Warn him to change positions slowly.
• Keep patient's room darkened if he experiences photophobia.
• Institute safety precautions if patient becomes confused or disoriented.
• Provide frequent mouth care to relieve dry mouth. Monitor bladder and bowel functions for possible urine retention and constipation.
• Expect the doctor to switch patient to oral form of drug as soon as possible.

---

bleomycin sulfate
Blenoxane♦

Pregnancy Risk Category: D

PHARMACOKINETICS
Distribution: mainly to kidneys, lungs, lymphatic system, peritoneum, and skin. Studies suggest higher concentration in squamous cell carcinoma than in sarcoma. Low concentration in bone marrow probably results from high concentration of bleomycin enzymes. Drug doesn't cross blood-brain barrier.
Metabolism: rapidly deactivated in all normal tissues, especially in liver and kidneys.
Excretion: 60% to 70% excreted unchanged in urine within 24 hours. Terminal half-life is about 2 hours.
Action: onset, immediate; peak serum level, 30 to 60 minutes.

MECHANISM OF ACTION
May inhibit synthesis of DNA, RNA, and proteins by binding directly with DNA; may also break single- and double-stranded DNA.

INDICATIONS & DOSAGE
• Lymphoma, lymphosarcoma, reticulum cell sarcoma; squamous cell carcinomas of aropharynx, buccal mucosa, cervix and vulva, epiglottis, gingiva, head, larynx, lips, mouth, nasopharynx, neck, palate, paralarynx, penis, sinuses, skin, tongue, tonsils; testicular cancer. *Adults and children:* 0.25 to 0.5 units/kg once or twice weekly; or 0.25 units/kg/day by continuous infusion over 4 to 5 days; or 30 to 60 units over 1 to 24 hours.
• Hodgkin's disease. *Adults and children:* 0.25 to 0.5 units/kg once or twice weekly. After tumor is reduced by 50%, 1 unit daily or 5 units weekly.

CONTRAINDICATIONS & CAUTIONS
• Contraindicated in bleomycin hypersensitivity.
• Use cautiously in patients with pulmonary impairment because about 10% develop pulmonary toxicity and about 1% die from pulmonary fibrosis. Elderly patients are also at risk for pulmonary toxicity.
• In hepatic impairment, give carefully because of a heightened risk of hepatotoxicity.
• Patients with creatinine clearance under 35 ml/minute are at risk for toxicity.

PREPARATION & STORAGE
Vials contain 15 units of drug. For direct injection, reconstitute with 1 to 5 ml 0.9% sodium chloride or dextrose 5% in water. For intermittent infusion, dilute in 50 to 100 ml of sterile water for injection, dextrose 5% in water, bacteriostatic water for injection, or 0.9% sodium chloride. For continuous infusion, dilute 24-hour dose in 1 liter of compatible solution; use a glass bottle.

Unmarked trade names available in the United States only.
♦Also available in Canada.   ♦♦Available in Canada only.

Diluted solution stable for 24 hours at room temperature. Because preparation does not contain preservatives, manufacturer recommends use within 24 hours, though it will remain stable for 7 days if refrigerated. Discard unused portion.

ADMINISTRATION
Direct injection: Using a 23G or 25G butterfly needle, inject reconstituted drug over 10 minutes at a new I.V. site.
Intermittent infusion: Using a secondary line, infuse dose into an established line containing a free-flowing, compatible solution.
Continuous infusion: Give diluted solution over 24 hours.

INCOMPATIBILITY
Incompatible with solutions containing divalent and trivalent cations, especially calcium salts and copper, because drug causes chelation. Also incompatible with amino acids, aminophylline, ascorbic acid injection, cephalosporins, diazepam, drugs containing sulfhydryl groups, furosemide, hydrocortisone, methotrexate, mitomycin, penicillin, riboflavin, and terbutaline sulfate.

ADVERSE REACTIONS
Life-threatening: anaphylaxis, interstitial pneumonitis (may be dose-related), pulmonary fibrosis.
Other: alopecia, anorexia, chills, darkened palm skin, desquamation (on hands, feet, and pressure areas), fatigue, fever, fingernail ridging, headache, nausea, pain at injection or tumor site, mild stomatitis, vomiting.

INTERACTIONS
Cisplatin: delayed bleomycin clearance.
General anesthetics: possible rapid pulmonary deterioration.
Methotrexate: reduced effect.

Other antineoplastics: increased bleomycin toxicity.
Vincristine: possible increased susceptibility of cells to bleomycin.

EFFECTS ON DIAGNOSTIC TESTS
Hemoglobin: possible reduced level.
Thrombocytes, WBC: decreased counts.

SPECIAL CONSIDERATIONS
• Because of possible anaphylaxis, give patient (especially one with lymphoma) 1 to 5 units I.M. 4 hours before starting treatment.
• Assess respiratory function carefully before each treatment, especially if patient is at high risk for pulmonary toxicity. Signs include dyspnea, bibasilar crackles, and a nonproductive cough. Patients over age 70 or who receive more than 400 units total dose face an increased risk of toxicity. Up to 10% of patients may experience pneumonitis and up to 1% may die.
• Monitor patient closely during infusion and for 1 hour after.
• Obtain BUN and creatinine clearance measurements, pulmonary function tests, and chest X-rays before and during treatment. Expect to stop the drug if tests show marked deterioration.
• In patients prone to posttreatment fever, give acetaminophen before treatment and for 24 hours after it.
• After treatment, give supplemental oxygen at an FIO_2 no higher than 25% to avoid potential lung damage.
• Warn patient about possible hair loss, which is usually temporary.
• Dialysis may not remove drug.

botulism antitoxin, trivalent equine

Available only through Centers for Disease Control
Pregnancy Risk Category: unknown

PHARMACOKINETICS
Distribution: throughout bloodstream.
Metabolism: not metabolized.
Excretion: unknown.
Action: unknown.

MECHANISM OF ACTION
Antibodies in this treated equine globulin bind to botulism toxins, preventing their further effects.

INDICATIONS & DOSAGE
• Botulism. *Adults:* 7,500 IU of Type A, 5,500 IU of Type B, and 8,500 IU of Type E given at 1:10 dilution. May be repeated in 2 to 4 hours if condition worsens. Same doses can be given I.M. to provide antitoxin reservoir.

CONTRAINDICATIONS & CAUTIONS
• Use cautiously in patients with a history of allergy or sensitivity to equine serum products, or positive skin test to antitoxin.

PREPARATION & STORAGE
Type A supplied as 7,500 IU (2,381 U.S. units); Type B as 5,500 IU (1,839 U.S. units); and Type E as 8,500 IU. Store at 36° to 46° F. (2° to 8° C.). Dilute to 1:10 before use and give at room temperature.

ADMINISTRATION
Direct injection: Using 21G or 23G needle, inject 1:10 dilution at 1 ml/minute.

Intermittent infusion: not recommended.
Continuous infusion: not recommended.

INCOMPATIBILITY
No incompatibilities reported.

ADVERSE REACTIONS
Life-threatening: anaphylaxis.
Other: serum sickness (edematous skin, fever, lymphadenopathy, joint pain, and rash appearing alone or together within 14 days of administration), thermal reaction (chills, slight dyspnea, and high fever 20 to 60 minutes after administration).

INTERACTIONS
None reported.

EFFECTS ON DIAGNOSTIC TESTS
None reported.

SPECIAL CONSIDERATIONS
• Perform skin or eye sensitivity test before giving antitoxin. However, use extreme caution when testing patients with history of allergy or sensitivity to horses or equine serum products. Skin test could be fatal. Don't use eye test in children.
• For skin test, inject 0.1 ml of a 1:100 saline dilution intracutaneously. For eye test, instill 1 drop of a 1:10 saline dilution in one eye and 1 control drop of plain saline solution in the opposite eye.
• If skin tests are positive, administer antitoxin with extreme caution. However, even a negative skin test doesn't rule out allergic reaction.
• Desensitization may be used for sensitive patients. Administer a series of gradually increasing antitoxin doses subcutaneously, as ordered, every 20 minutes. If reaction occurs, stop injections for 1 hour, resuming

with last dose given. Give injection slowly.
• Be prepared to administer 0.3 ml of epinephrine solution (1:1,000), if ordered, before therapy begins. Also keep a syringe of epinephrine solution (1:1,000) on hand throughout testing and therapy.
• Outcome depends largely on how quickly antibodies reach needed concentration. For best results, give antitoxin as soon as possible.
• Observe patient for 24 hours after administration, especially during the first 2 hours.
• Treat urticarial reactions, as ordered, with 0.5 ml epinephrine (1:1,000) I.M. Severe reaction may require corticotropin or cortisone.

bretylium tosylate
Bretylate♦♦, Bretylol

Pregnancy Risk Category: C

PHARMACOKINETICS
Distribution: to tissues of high adrenergic innervation, including sympathetic ganglia, heart, and spleen. Traces concentrate in adrenals. Drug doesn't cross blood-brain barrier. It's 1% to 10% bound to plasma proteins. Not known if drug crosses placenta.
Metabolism: not metabolized.
Excretion: by kidneys, unchanged. Half-life averages 5 to 10 hours but can extend up to 4 days in renal impairment (creatinine clearance of less than 30 ml/minute). Not known if drug appears in breast milk.
Action in ventricular fibrillation: onset, 10 to 15 minutes; duration, 6 to 24 hours average.
Action in ventricular tachycardia: onset, 20 minutes to 6 hours; duration, 6 to 24 hours average.

Onset is occasionally delayed 30 minutes to several hours.

MECHANISM OF ACTION
Although this antiarrhythmic's mechanism of action isn't fully understood, bretylium seems to increase the threshold for ventricular fibrillation by prolonging repolarization. To accomplish this, the drug may block postganglionic sympathetic neurons or deplete catecholamines. This causes an adrenergic blocking action, prolonging repolarization. The drug also may have vasodilating, cardiostimulating, and weak local anesthetic effects.

INDICATIONS & DOSAGE
• Ventricular fibrillation. *Adults:* 5 mg/kg given rapidly and undiluted, then 10 mg/kg q 15 to 30 minutes if needed. Maximum dosage, 30 mg/kg/day.
• Ventricular tachycardia and other ventricular dysrhythmias. *Adults:* 5 to 10 mg/kg over 10 to 30 minutes, repeated after 1 or 2 hours if needed. Maintenance dosage, 5 to 10 mg/kg over 10 to 30 minutes, repeated q 6 hours; or continuous infusion at rate of 1 to 2 mg/minute.

CONTRAINDICATIONS & CAUTIONS
• Contraindicated in digitalis-induced dysrhythmias unless they're life-threatening.
• Use cautiously in patients with impaired cardiac output because of the risk of severe hypotension.
• Reduce dosage in renal impairment because of high risk of toxicity.

PREPARATION & STORAGE
Supplied as single-dose 10 ml ampule containing 500 mg bretylium. For infusion, dilute with at least 50

---

ml of dextrose 5% in water or 0.9% sodium chloride.

Store at 59° to 86° F. (15° to 30° C.). Diluted drug remains stable for 48 hours at room temperature, 7 days if refrigerated.

Prediluted, commercially prepared solutions are also available.

ADMINISTRATION
Direct injection: Using a 20G to 22G needle, inject over about 1 minute into vein or into I.V. line containing a free-flowing, compatible solution.
Intermittent infusion: Infuse ordered dose over 10 to 30 minutes.
Continuous infusion: Give diluted drug at rate of 1 to 2 mg/minute.

INCOMPATIBILITY
Incompatible with nitroglycerin, phenytoin, and procainamide.

ADVERSE REACTIONS
Life-threatening: postural and supine hypotension.
Other: abdominal pain, aching in legs, angina, anorexia, anxiety, bradycardia, chest pressure, confusion, conjunctivitis, depression, diaphoresis, dizziness, dyspnea, emotional lability, facial flushing, frequent bowel movements, generalized tenderness, headache, lethargy, lightheadedness, nausea, paranoid psychosis, rash, renal dysfunction, syncope, transient hypertension, vertigo, vomiting.

INTERACTIONS
Cardiac glycosides: worsened toxicity.
Lidocaine, procainamide, propranolol, quinidine: neutralized inotropic effect, potentiated hypotension.

EFFECTS ON DIAGNOSTIC TESTS
None reported.

SPECIAL CONSIDERATIONS
● Closely monitor EKG, heart rate, pulse, and blood pressure.
● Keep patient supine until he develops tolerance to hypotension. Norepinephrine, dopamine, or volume expanders may be used to raise blood pressure.
● Subtherapeutic doses may cause hypotension.
● Be alert for increased anginal pain in susceptible patients.
● Drug can be removed by hemodialysis.
● Drug used investigationally to treat hypertension.

brompheniramine maleate
Chlorphed, Codimal-A, Dehist, Dimetane-Ten, Histaject Modified, Nasahist B, ND-Stat Revised, Oraminic II

Pregnancy Risk Category: B

PHARMACOKINETICS
Distribution: throughout body tissues and fluids. Drug crosses placenta.
Metabolism: hepatic; undergoes N-dealkylation to form monodesmethylbrompheniramine and didesmethylbrompheniramine, then becomes partially conjugated with glycine.
Excretion: primarily in urine within 24 hours, either unchanged or as metabolites. Small amounts appear in breast milk. Elimination half-life is 12 to 35 hours.
Action: onset, at end of infusion; duration, 3 to 12 hours.

MECHANISM OF ACTION
Brompheniramine apparently competes with histamine for H_1-receptor sites on effector cells. The drug prevents histamine-mediated response but doesn't reverse it.

INDICATIONS & DOSAGE

• Moderate to severe allergic reaction. *Adults:* 5 to 20 mg q 6 to 12 hours. Maximum dosage, 40 mg daily. *Children under age 12:* 0.5 mg/kg/day divided q 6 to 8 hours.

CONTRAINDICATIONS & CAUTIONS

• Contraindicated in neonates and lactating women; in acute asthmatic attacks because of possible thickened secretions and impaired expectoration; and in hypersensitivity to brompheniramine, chemically similar antihistamines, and MAO inhibitors.
• Use cautiously in narrow-angle glaucoma, stenosing peptic ulcer, pyloroduodenal obstruction, symptomatic prostatic hypertrophy, bladder neck obstruction, and hyperthyroidism to prevent worsened symptoms.

PREPARATION & STORAGE

Available in 1 ml ampules containing 10 mg of drug. For direct injection, drug may be diluted in dextrose 5% in water or 0.9% sodium chloride in a 1:10 concentration before use. For intermittent infusion, dilute desired dose with 50 ml dextrose 5% in water or 0.9% sodium chloride.

Store brompheniramine injection away from light and at room temperature. Crystals may form in ampules stored below 32° F. (0° C.) but may be dissolved by warming to 84° F. (29° C.).

ADMINISTRATION

Give drug with patient in recumbent position to ensure safety if hypotension occurs.
Direct injection: Administer undiluted—or diluted in a 1:10 concentration—over 3 to 5 minutes.
Intermittent infusion: Inject into established I.V. line with free-flowing

compatible solution. Infuse over 20 to 30 minutes.
Continuous infusion: not used.

INCOMPATIBILITY

Incompatible with diatrizoate meglumine and diatrizoate sodium combinations and with iodipamide meglumine. Not recommended for use with whole blood.

ADVERSE REACTIONS

Life-threatening: agranulocytosis, anaphylaxis, hemolytic anemia, thrombocytopenia.
Other: blurred vision; chills; confusion; diaphoresis; dry mouth, nose, and throat; euphoria; excitation; fatigue; headache; hypotension; insomnia; irritability; palpitations; paresthesias; rash; respiratory depression; restlessness; sedation; seizures; tachycardia; thickened bronchial secretions; tremors; urinary frequency and difficulty, urine retention; urticaria.

INTERACTIONS

Amantadine, antimuscarinics, haloperidol, ipratropium, phenothiazines, procainamide: increased antimuscarinic effects.
CNS depressants: potentiated CNS depression.
MAO inhibitors: prolonged, intensified anticholinergic and CNS depressant effects.

EFFECTS ON DIAGNOSTIC TESTS

Skin tests for allergies: unreliable findings.

SPECIAL CONSIDERATIONS

• *Treatment of overdose:* Keep in mind that antihistamine overdose may cause fatal CNS depression or stimulation (most likely in children). Treat symptomatically, including artificial respiration, if needed; vaso-

pressors, such as norepinephrine or phenylephrine (do not use epinephrine); and physostigmine to counteract CNS anticholinergic effects. If physostigmine fails to correct seizures, give diazepam. Treat hyperthermia with cold packs or by sponging with tepid water.
• If the patient experiences dry mouth, give sugarless gum, hard candy, or ice chips to counteract the effect.
• Withdraw brompheniramine 4 days before skin tests for allergies to avoid misleading results.
• Drug may mask effects of ototoxic drugs and may also inhibit lactation.

bumetanide
Bumex

Pregnancy Risk Category: C

PHARMACOKINETICS
Distribution: not fully understood. Highest concentrations thought to occur in kidneys, liver, and plasma; lowest concentrations found in heart, lung, muscle, and adipose tissue. Drug probably crosses placenta.
Metabolism: partly in liver to at least five inactive metabolites.
Excretion: 80% excreted in urine as unchanged drug or metabolites by glomerular filtration and possibly by renal tubular secretion; 10% to 20% excreted in feces and bile almost entirely as metabolites. Elimination half-life is 60 to 90 minutes. Not known if drug appears in breast milk.
Action: onset, a few minutes; peak, 15 to 30 minutes; duration, 3 to 4 hours.

MECHANISM OF ACTION
This sulfonamide-type loop diuretic inhibits sodium and chloride reabsorption primarily in the ascending loop of Henle. Although bumetanide's precise mechanism of action is unknown, the drug may affect sodium reabsorption in the proximal tubule but apparently doesn't act on the distal tubule.

INDICATIONS & DOSAGE
• Edema associated with congestive heart failure, hepatic and renal disease, carcinoma, hypertension caused by renal insufficiency, and other conditions. *Adults:* initially, 0.5 to 2 mg. Repeat q 2 to 3 hours, if needed, up to maximum of 10 mg daily.
• Adjunctive treatment to enhance drug or toxin elimination in intoxication: *Adults:* Dosage varies, depending on desired response. Maximum dosage, 10 mg daily.

CONTRAINDICATIONS & CAUTIONS
• Contraindicated in hepatic impairment and severe electrolyte depletion because of an increased risk of dehydration and electrolyte imbalance, possibly leading to hepatic coma and death; in severe renal impairment because of a heightened risk of toxicity; and in bumetanide hypersensitivity.
• Give cautiously to patients with sulfonamide sensitivity because of possible enhanced bumetanide sensitivity.
• Also give cautiously to patients with an increased risk of hypokalemia, such as those with potassium-losing nephropathy or diarrhea-causing conditions, and to patients with ventricular dysrhythmias because bumetanide-induced hypokalemia heightens their risk.
• In gout or hyperuricemia, administer carefully because the drug raises serum uric levels.

• Use cautiously in patients with acute MI because excessive diuresis can precipitate shock.

PREPARATION & STORAGE
Available with premixed preservative in 2 ml (0.25 mg/ml) ampules and 2, 4, and 10 ml (0.25 mg/ml) vials. Drug can be further diluted for I.V. infusion using dextrose 5% in water, 0.9% sodium chloride, or Ringer's lactate solution in both glass and plastic containers. Prepare solution for I.V. infusion within 24 hours of use. Protect drug from light to avoid discoloration.

When large doses are required, use vials to prevent glass particles from broken ampules from entering the solution. If ampules must be used, add a filter to I.V. tubing.

ADMINISTRATION
Direct injection: Using a 21G or 23G needle, inject desired dose of 0.25 mg/ml solution over 1 to 2 minutes.
Intermittent infusion: Give diluted drug through an intermittent infusion device or piggyback into an I.V. line containing a free-flowing, compatible solution. Infuse at ordered rate.
Continuous infusion: not needed.

INCOMPATIBILITY
Incompatible with dobutamine.

ADVERSE REACTIONS
Life-threatening: acute fluid depletion, circulatory collapse, electrolyte depletion, embolism, hypovolemia, vascular thrombosis.
Other: abdominal pain, anorexia, arthritic pain, asterixis, chest pain, confusion, cramps, dehydration, diaphoresis, diarrhea, dizziness, dry mouth, earache, EKG changes, hearing loss, hyperventilation, hypotension, lethargy, leukopenia, musculoskeletal pain, nausea, paresthesias, pruritus, thirst, thrombocytopenia, urticaria, vomiting, weakness.

INTERACTIONS
Aminoglycosides, other ototoxic drugs: heightened risk of ototoxicity.
Amphotericin B: increased risk of hypokalemia and ototoxicity.
Anticoagulants: decreased effect. Adjust dose.
Antihistamines, loxapine, phenothiazines, thioxanthenes, trimethobenzamide: possible masked signs of ototoxicity.
Antihypertensives: potentiated hypotensive effects.
Cardiac glycosides: hypokalemia and an enhanced risk of toxicity.
Corticosteroids, corticotropin: heightened risk of hypokalemia.
Dopamine: enhanced diuresis.
Indomethacin, probenecid: reduced diuresis.
Lithium: toxicity from reduced renal clearance.
Nephrotoxic drugs: magnified risk of nephrotoxicity.
Nondepolarizing neuromuscular blocking drugs: prolonged effects.
Sodium bicarbonate: increased risk of hypochloremic alkalosis.
Sympathomimetics, estrogens: reduced antihypertensive effects.

EFFECTS ON DIAGNOSTIC TESTS
BUN, serum creatinine, uric acid: increased levels.
Hematocrit, hemoglobin level, prothrombin time: elevated or prolonged.
Serum alkaline phosphatase, bilirubin, LDH, SGOT, SGPT: elevated levels.
Serum calcium, magnesium, potassium, sodium: reduced levels.
Serum cholesterol: elevated or reduced levels.
Urine phosphate: increased levels.

WBC count, differential: altered results.

SPECIAL CONSIDERATIONS
• *Treatment of overdose:* Monitor urine output and serum and urine electrolyte levels to determine symptomatic care. Provide replacement fluids and electrolytes, as needed.
• I.V. route is intended to be used when rapid onset is necessary, GI absorption is impaired, or P.O. route is impractical. Whenever possible, I.V. route should be changed to oral as soon as the patient can safely tolerate it.
• May cause hypochloremic metabolic alkalemia.
• Because drug causes potassium loss, give potassium replacements, as needed.
• Monitor blood pressure and serum electrolyte levels, especially potassium.
• Observe for signs of hypokalemia, such as weakness, dizziness, confusion, anorexia, lethargy, vomiting, and cramps.
• May contain benzyl alcohol.

buprenorphine hydrochloride
Buprenex, Temgesic♦♦

Controlled Substance Schedule V
Pregnancy Risk Category: C

PHARMACOKINETICS
Distribution: not fully understood; 96% bound to plasma proteins with concentrations found in liver, brain, and GI tract. Drug crosses the blood-brain barrier but not clear if it crosses the placenta.
Metabolism: hepatic; undergoes N-dealkylation to form norbuprenorphine and then conjugates with glucuronic acid.

Excretion: primarily in feces as free buprenorphine and metabolites and secondarily in urine as conjugated buprenorphine and metabolites. Not known if drug appears in breast milk. Elimination half-life averages 2 minutes for first phase, 11 minutes for second phase, and 132 minutes for last phase.
Action: onset, immediately after administration; peak level, after 2 minutes; duration, 4 to 8 hours.

MECHANISM OF ACTION
How this centrally acting partial opiate agonist achieves its analgesic effects isn't entirely known. These effects may result from binding with opiate receptors at many CNS sites. Buprenorphine possesses narcotic antagonist activity as well. This alters the perception of pain and the emotional response to it. The drug's long duration of action may result from its slow dissociation from receptor sites.

INDICATIONS & DOSAGE
• Relief of moderate to severe pain (postoperative, cancer, trigeminal neuralgia, trauma). *Adults and children age 13 or older:* 0.3 mg q 6 hours, p.r.n. May increase up to 0.6 mg q 4 hours if needed (higher doses haven't proved safe). Continuous infusion of 25 to 250 mcg/hour used experimentally for postoperative pain.
• Reversal of fentanyl-induced anesthesia. *Adults:* 0.3 to 0.8 mg 1 to 4 hours after anesthesia induction and about 30 minutes before end of surgery.

CONTRAINDICATIONS & CAUTIONS
• Contraindicated in buprenorphine hypersensitivity. Avoid use in children under age 13 because pediatric

---

safety and effectiveness haven't been established.

• Also contraindicated in diarrhea caused by poisoning or pseudomembranous colitis because of delayed elimination of toxins.

• Give with extreme caution in respiratory disorders or compromise because of possible decreased respiratory drive and increased airway resistance. In hypothyroidism, myxedema, and adrenocortical insufficiency, use cautiously because of a heightened risk of respiratory depression.

• Give cautiously in head injury, coma, CNS depression, and elevated intracranial pressure because drug may raise cerebrospinal fluid (CSF) pressure and decrease level of consciousness.

• Also give cautiously in narcotic dependence because drug may induce withdrawal symptoms; in hepatic disease because of impaired drug metabolism and excretion; in gallbladder disease because of elevated intracholedochal pressure stimulating contraction of the sphincter of Oddi; and in elderly or debilitated patients and those with severe renal impairment because of reduced renal clearance.

• In patients with a history of drug abuse or emotional instability, administer carefully because of the risk of drug dependence.

• In prostatic hypertrophy, urethral stricture, or recent urinary tract surgery, give buprenorphine cautiously because of possible urine retention.

• In the elderly, give lower doses because of increased sensitivity to the drug and delayed clearance.

PREPARATION & STORAGE

Supplied as 0.324 mg (equivalent to 0.3 mg) buprenorphine in 1 ml preservative-free ampules. Prevent prolonged exposure to light and exposure to temperatures above 104° F. (40° C.) or below 32° F. (0° C.).

Drug can be diluted in dextrose 5% in water, dextrose 5% and 0.9% sodium chloride, or Ringer's lactate and 0.9% sodium chloride. For continuous infusion, dilute with 0.9% sodium chloride to a concentration of 15 mcg/ml.

ADMINISTRATION

Direct injection: Inject over 3 to 5 minutes into an I.V. line containing a free-flowing, compatible solution. Avoid rapid injection to prevent possibly fatal anaphylactoid reaction or cardiopulmonary problems.

Intermittent infusion: not recommended.

Continuous infusion: used experimentally. Using a controller, infuse diluted drug through an I.V. line containing a free-flowing, compatible solution at prescribed rate.

INCOMPATIBILITY

Incompatible with diazepam and lorazepam.

ADVERSE REACTIONS

Life-threatening: anaphylaxis, apnea, respiratory and vascular collapse.

Other: agitation, anxiety, blurred vision, bradycardia, chills, cold and clammy skin, confusion, conjunctivitis, constipation, cyanosis, depression, diaphoresis, diarrhea, diplopia, dizziness, dry mouth, dyspepsia, dysrhythmias, euphoria, flatulence, flushing, headache, hypertension, hypotension, hypoventilation, miosis, nausea, paresthesias, pruritus, sedation, slurred speech, tachycardia, tinnitus, urine retention, vomiting, weakness.

INTERACTIONS

Alcohol, benzodiazepines, general anesthetics, MAO inhibitors, parenteral magnesium sulfate, phenothiazines, sedative-hypnotics, tranquilizers: deepened CNS and respiratory depression, hypotension.

Diazepam (oral): respiratory and cardiovascular collapse.

Naltrexone: reduced buprenorphine effects from blocked opiate receptors.

Narcotic analgesics: reduced analgesia if buprenorphine is given before narcotic; decreased respiratory depression if given after narcotic; increased respiratory depression if given with low narcotic doses.

Phenprocoumon: purpura.

EFFECTS ON DIAGNOSTIC TESTS

Gastric emptying studies: delayed emptying.

Hepatobiliary imaging: misleading results because buprenorphine-induced constriction of the sphincter of Oddi can resemble obstructed common bile duct.

Lumbar puncture: possible increased CSF pressure secondary to respiratory depression–induced carbon dioxide retention.

Serum amylase, lipase: increased levels for up to 24 hours after drug administration.

SPECIAL CONSIDERATIONS

• *Treatment of overdose:* Maintain airway and provide respiratory support. Naloxone may be used to reverse respiratory depression; however, it may not be effective. If ineffective, give 1 to 2 mg/kg of doxapram by I.V. push to stimulate respiration. Administer I.V. fluids and vasopressors as needed to maintain blood pressure.

• Monitor blood pressure and respiratory status frequently for at least 1 hour after administration. Keep resuscitation equipment and naloxone readily available. If respiratory rate drops below 8 breaths per minute, arouse patient to stimulate breathing, and notify the doctor.

• Caution patient to get up slowly and avoid activities that require alertness because dizziness and drowsiness can result.

• Keep in mind that physical and psychological dependence can develop with prolonged use. If dependence develops, withdrawal symptoms may occur up to 14 days after drug is stopped.

• Assess bowel function. Patient may need stool softener.

• Fixed dosage schedule helps to minimize breakthrough pain in chronic conditions.

butorphanol tartrate
Stadol

Pregnancy Risk Category: B
(D for prolonged use or high dose at term)

PHARMACOKINETICS

Distribution: throughout all body tissues with highest concentrations in lungs, spleen, heart, endocrine tissue, blood cells, and fat tissue. Drug crosses placenta; fetal concentrations are one half to one and a half times maternal levels. Cerebral levels are lower than serum levels.

Metabolism: extensively by the liver. Metabolites have no analgesic activity.

Excretion: in urine as unconjugated hydroxybutorphanol (60% to 80%) and unchanged drug (less than 5%) in 72 to 96 hours. Remainder appears in bile and feces and undergoes enterohepatic recycling. Drug

also appears in breast milk. Elimination half-life is 3 to 4 hours.
Action: onset, 1 minute; peak, 4 to 5 minutes; duration, 2 to 4 hours.

MECHANISM OF ACTION
Drug has narcotic agonist and antagonist properties. It binds with opiate receptors at many CNS sites, altering the perception of pain and the emotional response to it.

INDICATIONS & DOSAGE
• Moderate to severe pain from acute and chronic disorders, obstetric analgesia during labor, preoperative sedation. *Adults:* 0.5 to 2 mg q 3 to 4 hours, as needed.

CONTRAINDICATIONS & CAUTIONS
• Contraindicated in butorphanol hypersensitivity; acute respiratory depression; and diarrhea caused by poisoning or pseudomembranous colitis because of delayed toxin removal.
• Avoid use in patients under age 18 because pediatric safety and effectiveness haven't been established.
• Use cautiously in narcotic-dependent patients. Detoxification should precede butorphanol administration.
• In patients with a history of drug abuse or emotional instability, administer the drug carefully because of the risk of dependence.
• Give cautiously in hepatic or renal disease because of a heightened risk of toxicity; in head trauma or increased intracranial pressure (ICP) to avoid the risk of further ICP elevation and the masking of key symptoms; in myocardial infarction or coronary artery disease because of increased cardiac work load; in hypertension, dysrhythmias, and seizures to prevent exacerbation; in hypothyroidism because of deepened respiratory and prolonged CNS de-

pression; and in respiratory compromise to reduce the risk of respiratory depression.
• Also give cautiously in acute abdominal conditions because significant symptoms can be obscured; in recent GI surgery because drug decreases intestinal motility; in inflammatory bowel disease because of possible toxic megacolon; and in prostatic hypertrophy, urethral stricture, or recent urinary tract surgery because of the risk of urine retention.

PREPARATION & STORAGE
Available in single and multiple dose vials and disposable syringes with concentrations of 1 and 2 mg/ml. No dilution needed. Store at room temperature away from light.

ADMINISTRATION
Give drug with patient in recumbent position to minimize hypotension and dizziness.
Direct injection: Inject drug directly into the vein or an established I.V. line over several minutes.
Intermittent infusion: not recommended.
Continuous infusion: not recommended.

INCOMPATIBILITY
Incompatible with dimenhydrinate and pentobarbital sodium.

ADVERSE REACTIONS
Life-threatening: anaphylaxis, cardiac arrest, circulatory collapse, respiratory depression, severe hypotension.
Other: agitation, anxiety, blood pressure fluctuations, blurred vision, clammy skin, confusion, constipation, diaphoresis, diplopia, dizziness, dry mouth, euphoria, floating sensation, flushing, hallucinations, headache, lethargy, nausea, palpita-

tions, rash, sedation, unusual
dreams, urticaria, vomiting.

INTERACTIONS
Alcohol, CNS depressants: additive
effects.
Antihypertensives: potentiated hypo-
tension.
Antimuscarinics: increased risk of
severe constipation, paralytic ileus,
or urine retention.
Antiperistaltic antidiarrheals:
heightened risk of severe constipa-
tion and CNS depression.
Buprenorphine: reduced therapeutic
effects of butorphanol.
Hydroxyzine: enhanced analgesia
and worsened CNS depression and
hypotension.
MAO inhibitors: increased reaction
to butorphanol.
Metoclopramide: reduced effect on
GI motility.
Naloxone: antagonized analgesia and
CNS and respiratory depression.
Naltrexone: blocked therapeutic ef-
fects of butorphanol.
Narcotic analgesics: possible de-
creased analgesia.
Neuromuscular blocking agents:
deepened respiratory depression.
Pancuronium: conjunctival changes.

EFFECTS ON DIAGNOSTIC TESTS
Gastric emptying studies: delayed
gastric emptying.
Lumbar puncture: elevated cerebrospinal fluid pressure secondary to
respiratory depression–induced carbon dioxide retention.

SPECIAL CONSIDERATIONS
• *Treatment of overdose:* Administer
naloxone and monitor cardiopulmonary status. Provide oxygen, respiratory support, I.V. fluids, and
vasopressors.
• Keep in mind that butorphanol can
cause physical and psychological de-

pendence. Abrupt withdrawal after
chronic use produces intense withdrawal symptoms.
• Assess bowel function. Patient
may need a stool softener.
• Rapid I.V. injection can cause severe respiratory depression, hypotension, circulatory collapse, and
cardiac arrest.
• Keep emergency resuscitation
equipment available when giving
drug.

---

calcium chloride
calcium gluceptate
calcium gluconate
Kalcinate

Pregnancy Risk Category: C

PHARMACOKINETICS
Distribution: into extracellular fluid
and then rapidly incorporated into
bone (99%) or divided between intracellular and extracellular fluid
(1%); 45% of serum calcium binds
to plasma proteins. Calcium crosses
placenta, reaching higher levels in
fetal blood than in maternal blood.
Metabolism: not metabolized.
Excretion: mainly removed in feces
as unabsorbed calcium or part of
bile and pancreatic juices. Also filtered by renal glomeruli but reabsorbed in loop of Henle and
convoluted tubules. Small amounts
of calcium appear in urine. Also appears in breast milk and sweat.
Action: onset, immediately after infusion; duration, 30 minutes to 2
hours.

MECHANISM OF ACTION
Maintains integrity of nervous system, muscular, and skeletal function
and cell membrane and capillary

permeability. Essential for coagulation, release and storage of neurotransmitters and hormones, amino acid uptake and binding, vitamin B_{12} absorption, and gastrin secretion.

INDICATIONS & DOSAGE
• Emergency treatment of hypocalcemia. *Adults:* 7 to 14 mEq. *Children:* 1 to 7 mEq. *Infants:* less than 1 mEq. Repeat q 1 to 3 days if needed.
• Hypocalcemic tetany. *Adults:* 4.5 to 16 mEq. *Children:* 0.5 to 0.7 mg/kg t.i.d. or q.i.d. or until tetany is controlled. *Infants:* 2.4 mEq/kg daily in divided doses.
• Hypocalcemia with secondary cardiac toxicity. *Adults:* 2.25 to 14 mEq given while monitoring EKG.
• Advanced cardiac life support. *Adults:* 2.7 mEq calcium chloride, 4.5 to 6.3 mEq calcium gluceptate, or 2.3 to 3.7 mEq calcium gluconate. Repeat p.r.n. *Children:* 0.27 mEq/kg calcium chloride, repeated in 10 minutes if needed.
• Magnesium toxicity. *Adults:* 7 mEq; subsequent doses based on response.
• Transfusion of citrated blood. *Adults:* 1.35 mEq/dl of citrated blood. *Neonates:* 0.45 mEq/dl of citrated blood.

CONTRAINDICATIONS & CAUTIONS
• Contraindicated in cardiac glycoside toxicity and ventricular fibrillation because of an increased risk of dysrhythmias; in hypercalciuria, calcium renal calculi, or hypercalcemia because of possible exacerbation; and in sarcoidosis because hypercalcemia may be potentiated.
• Use cautiously in renal impairment, dehydration, and electrolyte imbalance because of a heightened risk of hypercalcemia. Also use cau-

tiously in cardiac disease because of an increased risk of dysrhythmias.
• Use calcium chloride carefully in cor pulmonale, respiratory acidosis, renal disease, or respiratory failure because of its acidifying effects.

PREPARATION & STORAGE
Calcium chloride comes in a 10 ml ampule, vial, and syringe of 10% solution containing 1.36 mEq calcium/ml. Calcium gluceptate comes in a 5 ml ampule and in 50 and 100 ml bulk containers of a 22% solution containing 0.9 mEq calcium/ml. Calcium gluconate is available in 10 ml ampules and vials and 20 ml vials as a 10% solution containing 0.45 to 0.48 mEq calcium/ml. Calcium salts may be diluted with compatible solutions, including most I.V. and intravenous total parenteral nutrition solutions, before infusion.

Store between 59° and 86° F. (15° and 30° C.), unless otherwise specified by the manufacturer. Use only clear solutions. If crystals are present in calcium gluceptate, discard solution. If crystals are present in calcium gluconate, warm solution to 86° to 104° F. (30° to 40° C.) to dissolve them.

Warm injection to body temperature before administering in nonemergencies.

ADMINISTRATION
Direct injection: Administer slowly through a small needle into a large vein or through an I.V. line containing a free-flowing, compatible solution at a rate not exceeding 1 ml/minute (1.5 mEq/minute) for calcium chloride, 1.5 to 5 ml/minute for calcium gluconate, and 2 ml/minute for calcium gluceptate. Do not use scalp veins in children.
Intermittent infusion: Infuse diluted solution through an I.V. line containing a compatible solution. Maximum

rate of 200 mg/minute suggested for calcium gluceptate and calcium gluconate.

Continuous infusion: Infuse after addition of large volume of fluid at a maximum rate of 200 mg/minute for calcium gluceptate and calcium gluconate.

INCOMPATIBILITY

All three calcium salts are precipitated by carbonates, bicarbonates, phosphates, sulfates, and tartrates. Chelation occurs when calcium salts are mixed with tetracyclines.

Calcium chloride is incompatible with amphotericin B, cephalothin sodium, chlorpheniramine malcate, dobutamine, and magnesium sulfate. Calcium gluceptate is incompatible with cefamandole nafate, cephalothin sodium, magnesium sulfate, prednisolone sodium phosphate, and prochlorperazine edisylate. Calcium gluconate is incompatible with amphotericin B, cefamandole nafate, cephalothin sodium, dobutamine, magnesium sulfate, methylprednisolone sodium succinate, and prochlorperazine edisylate.

ADVERSE REACTIONS

Life-threatening: bradycardia, cardiac arrest, dysrhythmias, hypotension, syncope, vasodilation—all from rapid I.V. injection.
Other: cellulitis, chalky taste, dizziness, drowsiness, hot flashes, irregular heartbeat, nausea, paresthesias, soft tissue calcification, sweating, venous irritation, vomiting.

INTERACTIONS

Cardiac glycosides: dysrhythmias from potentiated inotropic and toxic glycoside effects. Use cautiously.
Nondepolarizing neuromuscular blocking drugs: reversed effects.
Parenteral magnesium sulfate: neutralized effects.

Potassium supplements: dysrhythmias.
Thiazide diuretics: reduced calcium excretion, possibly resulting in hypercalcemia.

EFFECTS ON DIAGNOSTIC TESTS

Plasma 11-hydroxycorticosteroids: transient elevations within 1 hour of calcium chloride administration using Glenn-Nelson technique.
Serum amylase: elevated levels (with calcium chloride).
Serum and urine magnesium: possible false-negative results using Titan yellow method.
Serum phosphate: reduced levels with large doses and prolonged use.

SPECIAL CONSIDERATIONS

• **Treatment of overdose:** If serum calcium levels exceed 12 mg/dl, give 0.9% sodium chloride, I.V. fluids, and furosemide or ethacrynic acid to promote calcium excretion. Closely monitor serum potassium and magnesium levels and EKG to identify complications. If ordered, assist with hemodialysis and administer calcitonin and adrenocorticosteroids.
• Review results of renal function tests before calcium administration.
• Infiltration into intramuscular or subcutaneous tissue may cause burning, sloughing, and necrosis of tissue. If infiltration does occur, discontinue infusion, infiltrate area with 1% procaine and hyaluronidase to reduce vasospasm and dilute calcium, and apply local heat.
• After I.V. injection, keep the patient recumbent briefly.
• Monitor blood pressure and be alert for a moderate drop. In a hypertensive or elderly patient, blood pressure may rise briefly.
• Closely monitor serum calcium levels and possibly EKG. Check

urine calcium levels to help avoid hypercalciuria.
• Hypocalcemia may cause muscle twitching and spasms. Hypercalcemia may cause bradycardia, depressed nervous and neuromuscular function, dysrhythmias, and impaired renal function.

carbenicillin disodium
Geopen, Pyopen♦

Pregnancy Risk Category: B

PHARMACOKINETICS
Distribution: into pleural, peritoneal, synovial, and ascitic fluids; sputum; lymph; and bile. In meningeal inflammation, carbenicillin also reaches cerebrospinal fluid, brain, and eyes. Drug is 29% to 60% bound to plasma proteins and is thought to cross the placenta.
Metabolism: partly by the liver. About 2% to 5% is metabolized by hydrolysis of the penicillin nucleus' beta-lactam ring to penicilloic acid.
Excretion: in urine by tubular secretion and glomerular filtration. Most of the drug is excreted unchanged in 2 to 6 hours, with 79% to 99% excreted within 24 hours. Drug appears in breast milk.
Action: peak levels, after 5 to 15 minutes of infusion.

MECHANISM OF ACTION
A semisynthetic extended-spectrum penicillin, carbenicillin acts systemically against bacteria. By adhering to penicillin-binding proteins, the drug inhibits bacterial cell-wall synthesis. Carbenicillin's extended spectrum of activity includes many gram-positive aerobic bacteria, including nonpenicillinase-producing strains of *Staphylococcus aureus; Staphylococcus epidermidis;* groups A, B, C, and G streptococci; *Streptococcus pneumoniae; Streptococcus viridans;* and some strains of enterococci.

Susceptible gram-negative bacteria include most beta-lactamase–producing strains of *Haemophilus influenzae* and *H. parainfluenzae;* many strains of *Neisseria meningitidis* and *N. gonorrhoeae;* and some strains of *Escherichia coli, Morganella morganii, Proteus mirabilis, P. vulgaris, Providencia rettgeri, Salmonella, Shigella, Citrobacter, Enterobacter, Klebsiella, Serratia, Pseudomonas, Acinetobacter, Moraxella, Pasteurella multocida, Legionella, Bordetella pertussis, Brucella,* and *Gardnerella vaginalis.*

Susceptible anaerobic bacteria include some strains of *Actinomyces, Bifidobacterium, Clostridium, Eubacterium, Lactobacillus, Peptococcus, Peptostreptococcus, Propionibacterium, Bacteroides, Fusobacterium,* and *Veillonella.*

INDICATIONS & DOSAGE
• Severe systemic infection caused by susceptible organisms. *Adults:* 15 to 40 g (maximum) daily divided into doses given q 4 hours. *Children and infants older than 1 month:* 250 to 500 mg/kg by continuous infusion or divided into doses given q 4 to 6 hours. Maximum dosage, 40 g daily. *Neonates weighing less than 2 kg:* 100 mg/kg initially, followed by 75 mg/kg q 8 hours during the first week of life, increasing to 100 mg/kg q 6 hours thereafter. *Neonates weighing more than 2 kg:* 100 mg/kg q 6 hours, starting on 4th day of life.
• Uncomplicated urinary tract infection. *Adults:* 1 to 2 g q 6 hours. *Children and infants older than 1 month:* 50 to 200 mg/kg q 4 to 6 hours.

- Severe urinary tract infection. *Adults:* 200 mg/kg daily by continuous infusion.
- Meningitis caused by *H. influenzae* and *S. pneumoniae*. *Adults:* 30 to 40 g daily by continuous infusion or divided into doses given q 4 hours. *Children and infants older than 1 month:* 400 to 600 mg/kg by continuous infusion or divided into doses given q 4 hours.

Note: Adjust dosage in renal failure. In adult patients with creatinine clearance less than 10 ml/min, give 2 g q 8 to 12 hours, or give usual dose q 24 to 48 hours.

In adult patients undergoing hemodialysis, give 2 g q 4 hours for serious infection. Or give as above with supplemental 750 mg to 2 g after each treatment. In adult patients undergoing peritoneal dialysis, give 2 g I.V. q 8 to 12 hours.

CONTRAINDICATIONS & CAUTIONS

- Contraindicated in penicillin or cephalosporin hypersensitivity.
- Use cautiously in patients with hypersensitivity to other drugs because of possible cross-allergenicity. Also use cautiously in those with bleeding tendencies because of the risk of thrombocytopenia and in those with uremia because of possible nephrotoxicity.
- Carbenicillin contains large amounts of sodium. Use cautiously in patients on sodium-restricted diets.
- Because of a heightened risk of toxicity, use cautiously in neonates and in patients with hepatic or renal impairment or dehydration.
- Give cautiously in hypokalemia because serum potassium levels may decline further.
- In patients with a history of ulcerative colitis, regional enteritis, or antibiotic-associated colitis, administer

carefully because of an enhanced risk of pseudomembranous colitis.

PREPARATION & STORAGE

A white to off-white crystalline powder, carbenicillin requires reconstitution. Add 2 to 3.6 ml of sterile water for injection to each 1 g vial, 4 to 7.2 ml to each 2 g vial, and 7 to 17 ml to each 5 g vial. Shake well.

If you're using a 2 g piggyback unit, reconstitute with 100, 50, or 20 ml sterile water for injection to yield a solution containing 20, 40, or 100 mg/ml, respectively. If you're using a 5 or 10 g piggyback unit, add 50 or 100 ml of sterile water for injection to provide a solution containing 50 or 100 mg/ml.

For direct injection, further dilute each gram with at least 5 ml sterile water for injection after reconstitution. For continuous infusion, add the reconstituted drug to an appropriate solution, such as dextrose 5% in water, 0.45% sodium chloride, Ringer's lactate, or 0.9% sodium chloride. Titrate carefully.

Store carbenicillin powder at room temperature or refrigerate. Reconstituted solutions retain their potency for 24 hours at room temperature and for 72 hours if refrigerated. Discard unused solutions after these periods.

ADMINISTRATION

Direct injection: Inject into vein through an intermittent infusion device or an I.V. line containing a free-flowing, compatible solution. Administer over 3 to 5 minutes to minimize vein irritation. Don't use direct injection in neonates or in patients with severe infection.

Intermittent infusion: Deliver diluted solution through an intermittent infusion device or an I.V. line containing a free-flowing, compati-

ble solution over 30 minutes to 2 hours. In neonates, infuse diluted solution over 15 minutes.
Continuous infusion: Infuse diluted solution over 24 hours. Don't use in neonates.

INCOMPATIBILITY
Carbenicillin inactivates aminoglycoside antibiotics, such as gentamicin, when mixed together. Give at separate sites.

Carbenicillin is incompatible with amphotericin B, bleomycin, colistimethate sodium, chloramphenicol, sodium succinate, lincomycin, streptomycin, and tetracyclines.

ADVERSE REACTIONS
Life-threatening: anaphylaxis.
Other: bacterial and fungal superinfection, bleeding (with high doses), diarrhea, eosinophilia, hypokalemia, leukopenia, nausea, neuromuscular irritability (with high serum levels), neutropenia, pain at injection site, phlebitis, seizures (with exceedingly high serum levels), thrombocytopenia, weakness.

INTERACTIONS
Anticoagulants, indanedione derivatives, NSAIDs, salicylates, sulfinpyrazone, thrombolytics: increased risk of bleeding.
Bacteriostatic drugs (chloramphenicol, erythromycins, sulfonamides, tetracyclines): decreased bactericidal effect of carbenicillin.
Ceftazidime, gentamicin: synergistic effect against *Pseudomonas aeruginosa.*
Probenecid: increased carbenicillin blood levels. Probenecid often given for this purpose.

EFFECTS ON DIAGNOSTIC TESTS
Serum potassium: possible reduced levels.

Serum sodium: elevated levels possible after large doses.
SGOT, SGPT: elevated levels possible, especially in children.

SPECIAL CONSIDERATIONS
• *Treatment of overdose:* Provide symptomatic care and assist with hemodialysis if ordered. Four to six hours of hemodialysis reduces drug's serum half-life by 44% to 70%.
• Before giving drug, check for penicillin or cephalosporin hypersensitivity. Negative history doesn't rule out future allergic reaction.
• Obtain specimens for culture and sensitivity tests before first dose. Therapy can begin before results are available.
• Drug is usually used with another antibiotic. Give carbenicillin at least 1 hour before bacteriostatic drugs.
• In patients with impaired renal function, monitor intake and output and BUN and serum creatinine levels to detect nephrotoxicity.
• Frequently check CBC to spot thrombocytopenia and serum potassium levels to detect hypokalemia.
• Monitor carbenicillin levels closely because seizures may result if blood level is high. Raise bed's side rails if blood levels rise.
• Prolonged therapy may lead to superinfection, especially in elderly, debilitated, or immunosuppressed patients.
• Check cardiac status during therapy. Observe for hemorrhagic complications, especially in patients with renal impairment. Expect dosage adjustment in these patients.
• Change I.V. site every 48 to 72 hours to prevent vein irritation. Also dilute injectable drug to a concentration of 1 g to 20 ml.

carboplatin
Paraplatin♦

Pregnancy Risk Category: D

PHARMACOKINETICS
Distribution: no significant protein binding of the parent compound, but free platinum may irreversibly bind to plasma proteins. Unknown if drug appears in breast milk.
Metabolism: hydrolyzed to form hydroxylated and aquated species.
Excretion: by the kidneys, with 65% eliminated within 12 hours and 71% within 24 hours. Carboplatin exhibits a half-life of 5 hours with possible enterohepatic recirculation. However, platinum from carboplatin is slowly excreted, with a minimum half-life of 5 days.
Action: peak level, at end of infusion.

MECHANISM OF ACTION
Although carboplatin has properties similar to alkylating agents, its precise mechanism of action hasn't been determined. Apparently, it cross-links strands of DNA material, inhibiting DNA synthesis and leading to cell death. Carboplatin also has immunosuppressive, radiosensitizing, and antimicrobial properties.

INDICATIONS & DOSAGE
• Ovarian carcinoma. *Adults:* 360 mg/m^2 on day one q 4 weeks, as indicated. Reduce dose 75% if platelet count falls below 50,000/mm^3 or neutrophil count falls below 500/mm^3.

If creatinine clearance falls between 41 and 59 ml/min, adjust dose to 250 mg/m^2. If creatinine clearance falls between 16 and 40 ml/min, adjust dose to 200 mg/m^2.

CONTRAINDICATIONS & CAUTIONS
• Contraindicated in patients with a history of hypersensitivity to cisplatin, platinum-containing compounds, or mannitol.
• Also contraindicated in severe bone marrow depression or bleeding.
• Use cautiously in patients with creatinine clearance less than 60 ml/min because they may experience more severe bone marrow depression and in patients older than 65 years because they face a greater risk for neurotoxicity. Both types of patients may require dosage adjustments.

PREPARATION & STORAGE
To avoid mutagenic, teratogenic, and carcinogenic risks, exercise extreme caution when preparing or administering carboplatin. Use a biological containment cabinet, wear gloves and mask, and use syringes with Luer-Lok fittings to prevent leakage of drug solution. Also correctly dispose of needles, vials and unused drug, and avoid contaminating work surfaces. Avoid inhalation of dust or vapors and contact with skin or mucous membranes.

Available in vials containing 50, 150, and 450 mg. Immediately before use, reconstitute with dextrose 5% in water, 0.9% sodium chloride, or sterile water for injection to a concentration of 10 mg/ml.

Dilute reconstituted carboplatin with 0.9% sodium chloride injection or dextrose 5% in water.

Store unopened vials at room temperature and protect from light. Once reconstituted and diluted, solution remains stable at room temperature for 8 hours. Because the drug does not contain antibacterial preservatives, discard unused drug after 8 hours.

Do not use needles or intravenous administration sets containing alumi-

num because carboplatin may precipitate and lose potency.

ADMINISTRATION
Direct injection: not recommended.
Intermittent infusion: usually infused over 15 minutes or longer into
vein or with a free-flowing, compatible I.V. solution.
Continuous infusion: not recommended.

INCOMPATIBILITY
No incompatibilities reported.

ADVERSE REACTIONS
Life-threatening: anaphylaxis-like
reaction, bone marrow depression
(thrombocytopenia, leukopenia, neutropenia).
Others: alopecia, anemia, asthenia,
central neurotoxicity, constipation,
diarrhea, electrolyte loss, hypersensitivity, hepatotoxicity, nausea, pain,
peripheral neuropathy, ototoxicity,
vomiting.

INTERACTIONS
*Aminoglycosides, other nephrotoxic
or ototoxic drugs:* increased risk of
nephrotoxicity or ototoxicity.
Myelosuppressive agents: additive
bone marrow suppression.

EFFECTS ON DIAGNOSTIC TESTS
*Serum bilirubin, alkaline phospha-
tase, SGOT:* elevated levels with
high doses of carboplatin.
Serum creatinine, blood urea: elevated levels.

SPECIAL CONSIDERATIONS
• Treat hepatic and hematologic toxicity symptomatically.
• Monitor vital signs during infusion.
• Determine serum electrolytes, creatinine, BUN, CBC, and creatinine

clearance levels before the first infusion and before each course.
• Monitor CBC and platelet count
frequently during therapy and, when
indicated, until recovery. Leukocyte
and platelet nadirs usually occur by
day 21. Levels usually return to
baseline by day 28. Don't repeat
dose unless platelet count exceeds
100,000/mm^3 and neutrophil counts
are above 2,000/mm^3.
• Only one increase in dosage is
recommended. Subsequent doses
should not exceed 125% of starting
dose.
• Carboplatin can produce severe
emesis. Administer antiemetic therapy before carboplatin therapy. Administer a single dose of antiemetic
over 24 hours or divide total dose
over 5 days.
• Patients with anemia resulting
from cumulative doses may require a
transfusion.
• Because of the possibility of infant
toxicity, mothers taking carboplatin
who are breast-feeding should discontinue this practice.
• Have epinephrine, corticosteroids,
and antihistamines available when
administering carboplatin because
anaphylaxis-like reactions may occur
within minutes of administration.
• Advise women of childbearing age
to avoid becoming pregnant during
therapy, and to consult a doctor before becoming pregnant.
• Depending on his condition, patient may require periodic audiometric testing.

---

carmustine (BCNU)
BiCNU♦

Pregnancy Risk Category: D

PHARMACOKINETICS
Distribution: throughout body tissues. Drug crosses the blood-brain barrier and the placenta.
Metabolism: by the liver within 15 minutes of administration. Some metabolites are active.
Excretion: primarily by the kidneys, with 30% removed within 24 hours and 60% to 70% within 96 hours. Lungs excrete 6% to 10% as carbon dioxide; 1% is excreted in feces.
Action: onset, rapid; peak plasma level, at end of infusion.

MECHANISM OF ACTION
This cell-cycle–nonspecific nitrosourea interferes with DNA and RNA synthesis by acting as an alkylating agent.

INDICATIONS & DOSAGE
• Brain and hepatic tumors, Hodgkin's disease, lymphomas, malignant melanoma, multiple myeloma. *Adults and children:* 200 mg/m². Repeat full dose q 6 to 8 weeks if WBC count exceeds 3,000/mm³ and platelet count exceeds 75,000/mm³. Give 140 mg/m² if WBC count falls between 2,000/mm³ and 3,000/mm³, platelet count between 25,000/mm³ and 75,000/mm³. Give 100 mg/m² for lower WBC and platelet counts.

CONTRAINDICATIONS & CAUTIONS
• Contraindicated in carmustine hypersensitivity. Also contraindicated in chicken pox (or recent exposure) and herpes zoster because of the risk of severe generalized disease.

• Use cautiously in myelosuppression, existing infection, and renal, hepatic, or pulmonary impairment because of the increased risk of toxicity or adverse reactions.
• Also use cautiously in smokers and patients with previous radiation (especially to mediastinum) or cytotoxic drug therapy because of an increased risk of pulmonary toxicity.

PREPARATION & STORAGE
Take special precautions during preparation because of the drug's mutagenic, teratogenic, and carcinogenic effects. When preparing drug, wear gloves and mask, use a biological containment cabinet, and prevent work surface contamination. Avoid contact with skin because drug will cause a brown stain. If contact occurs, wash the area immediately and thoroughly. Correctly dispose of all equipment and unused drug.

Drug comes as a powder in 100 mg vials. Before preparation, check for oily film at bottom of vial (sign of decomposition) and discard if present.

Dilute 100 mg with 3 ml of sterile, dehydrated ethyl alcohol supplied by the manufacturer. After dissolving, add 27 ml of sterile water for injection. This produces a clear, colorless solution with a concentration of 3.3 mg carmustine/ml of 10% alcohol. Preparation remains stable for 8 hours at room temperature and for 24 hours if refrigerated. Protect from light. Reconstituted solution may be further diluted with 250 to 500 ml of dextrose 5% in water or 0.9% sodium chloride for infusion. If refrigerated and protected from light, this solution remains stable for 48 hours if prepared in a glass container; solution becomes unstable in plastic I.V. bag. Store in original container, pro-

---

tected from light, at 36° to 46° F. (2° to 8° C.).

ADMINISTRATION
Direct injection: not recommended.
Intermittent infusion: Infuse diluted solution (250 to 500 ml) over 1 to 2 hours. If patient reports pain, dilute drug further or slow infusion.
Continuous infusion: not used.

INCOMPATIBILITY
Incompatible with sodium bicarbonate.

ADVERSE REACTIONS
Life-threatening: myelosuppression (occurs 4 to 6 weeks after administration; lasts 1 to 2 weeks).
Other: alopecia, anemia, anorexia, azotemia (progressive), burning sensation at site during infusion, conjunctival suffusion, decreased kidney size, diarrhea, dysphagia, esophagitis, fever, flushed skin, hepatotoxicity, jaundice, leukopenia, nausea and vomiting (may last 2 to 6 hours), nephrotoxicity, phlebitis, pruritus, pulmonary infiltrates and fibrosis, stomatitis, thrombocytopenia.

INTERACTIONS
Hepatotoxic or nephrotoxic drugs: possible heightened toxic effects.
Myelosuppressants, radiation therapy: further bone marrow suppression.

EFFECTS ON DIAGNOSTIC TESTS
BUN, serum alkaline phosphatase, bilirubin, SGOT: may be elevated.

SPECIAL CONSIDERATIONS
• Treat hypersensitivity symptomatically.
• Check CBC to monitor extent of myelosuppression. Avoid immunizing patient or exposing him to recipients of oral polio vaccine.

• Periodically monitor hepatic and renal function.
• Tell patient to report signs of infection and bleeding.
• Perform baseline pulmonary function tests, then monitor function during therapy. Risk of pulmonary toxicity increases with cumulative doses greater than 1,400 mg/m^2.
• Give antiemetics before carmustine.

cefamandole nafate
Mandol♦

Pregnancy Risk Category: B

PHARMACOKINETICS
Distribution: throughout body tissues, bone, and fluids, including pleural and synovial fluid and bile. Small amounts diffuse into cerebrospinal fluid, even when meninges are inflamed. Drug readily crosses placenta. It's 65% to 75% bound to plasma proteins.
Metabolism: not metabolized.
Excretion: by the kidneys through glomerular filtration and tubular secretion; 60% to 80% is excreted unchanged within 8 hours. Low levels appear in breast milk. Serum half-life varies from 30 to 120 minutes in healthy adults to about 12 to 18 hours in those with renal impairment.
Action: peak level, at end of infusion.

MECHANISM OF ACTION
A semisynthetic second-generation cephalosporin, cefamandole achieves its bactericidal effects by inhibiting mucopeptide synthesis in the bacterial cell wall, promoting osmotic instability. Its broad spectrum of activity includes most gram-positive aerobic cocci, including *Staphylococ-*

cus aureus, Staphylococcus epidermidis, Streptococcus pneumoniae, group A beta-hemolytic streptococci, and group B streptococci.

Susceptible gram-negative aerobic bacteria include many strains of *Citrobacter, Escherichia coli, Klebsiella pneumoniae, Proteus mirabilis, Shigella, Enterobacter,* and *Providencia* and most strains of *Haemophilus influenzae.* Susceptible anaerobic bacteria include *Bacteroides fragilis, Clostridium, Peptococcus,* and *Peptostreptococcus.*

INDICATIONS & DOSAGE
• Severe infection caused by susceptible organisms. *Adults:* 500 mg to 1 g q 4 to 8 hours. *Children age 1 month and older:* 50 to 100 mg/kg in equally divided doses q 4 to 8 hours.
• Severe, life-threatening infections, infections caused by less-susceptible organisms. *Adults:* up to 2 g q 4 hours. *Children age 1 month and older:* 150 mg/kg daily in divided doses q 4 to 8 hours. Maximum dosage, 12 g daily.
• Surgical prophylaxis. *Adults:* 1 to 2 g 30 to 60 minutes before surgery and 1 to 2 g q 6 hours for 24 hours after surgery. *Children age 3 months and older:* 50 to 100 mg/kg 30 to 60 minutes before surgery and 50 to 100 mg/kg q 6 hours for 24 hours after it.
Note: Dosage in renal failure reflects creatinine clearance. *Adults with severe infections:* If creatinine clearance is less than 2 ml/min, dosage is 250 to 500 mg q 12 hours; if 2 to 10 ml/min, 500 to 750 mg q 12 hours; if 10 to 25 ml/min, 500 mg to 1 g q 8 hours; if 25 to 50 ml/min, 750 mg to 1.5 g q 8 hours; if 50 to 80 ml/min, 750 mg to 1.5 g q 6 hours; if more than 80 ml/min, 1 to 2 g q 6 hours. *Adults with life-threatening infections:* if creatinine

clearance is less than 2 ml/min, dosage is 500 mg q 8 hours or 750 mg q 12 hours. If 2 to 10 ml/min, 670 mg q 8 hours or 1 g q 12 hours; if 10 to 25 ml/min, 1 g q 6 hours or 1.25 g q 8 hours; if 25 to 50 ml/min, 1.5 g q 6 hours or 2 g q 8 hours; if 50 to 80 ml/min, 1.5 g q 4 hours or 2 g q 6 hours; if more than 80 ml/min, give usual adult dose.

CONTRAINDICATIONS & CAUTIONS
• Contraindicated in cephalosporin hypersensitivity and given carefully to patients with hypersensitivity to penicillins or other drugs.
• Use cautiously in GI disease (especially colitis) because of an increased risk of pseudomembranous colitis; in renal impairment because of reduced drug excretion; and in patients with a history of bleeding disorders because drug may cause hypoprothrombinemia or hemorrhage.
• Also use cautiously in patients with vitamin K deficiency or predisposition to it.

PREPARATION & STORAGE
Available in 500 mg and 1, 2, and 10 g vials. Before reconstitution, store drug between 59° and 86° F. (15° and 30° C.).

For direct injection, reconstitute with 10 ml of sterile water for injection, dextrose 5% in water, or 0.9% sodium chloride. Reconstitute just before use because carbon dioxide buildup in the syringe can cause leakage.

For intermittent infusion, further dilute with 100 ml of a compatible solution. For continuous infusion, dilute with a larger amount. Compatible solutions include amino acid solutions; dextran; dextrose 5% or 10% in water; 0.9% sodium chloride; dextrose 5% and Ionosol B;

dextrose 5% and Isolyte E; mannitol 5%, 10%, or 20% in water; and ⅙ M sodium lactate. Shake well until dissolved. Solution remains stable for 24 hours at room temperature and for 96 hours if refrigerated.

ADMINISTRATION
Direct injection: Give over 3 to 5 minutes through a large vein or an I.V. line containing a free-flowing, compatible solution.
Intermittent infusion: Give 100 ml over 15 to 30 minutes through an intermittent infusion device or an I.V. line containing a free-flowing, compatible solution.
Continuous infusion: Over 24 hours, infuse solution diluted into appropriate amounts of fluid.

INCOMPATIBILITY
Incompatible with aminoglycosides, calcium gluceptate, calcium gluconate, cimetidine, Isolyte M, and magnesium and calcium ions (including Ringer's injection and Ringer's lactate injection).

ADVERSE REACTIONS
Life-threatening: anaphylaxis.
Other: bacterial and fungal superinfection, diarrhea, dizziness, fatigue, headache, hypoprothrombinemia, leukopenia, malaise, nausea, neutropenia, phlebitis, pseudomembranous colitis, thrombocytopenia, thrombophlebitis, urticaria, vomiting.

INTERACTIONS
Alcohol: disulfiram-like reaction if ingested within 72 hours.
Aminoglycosides, bumetanide, carmustine, colistin, ethacrynic acid, furosemide, polymyxin B, streptozocin, vancomycin: increased risk of nephrotoxicity.
Anticoagulants, thrombolytics: magnified risk of hemorrhage and irreversible platelet damage.
Anti-inflammatory drugs, platelet aggregation inhibitors, sulfinpyrazone: heightened risk of hemorrhage.
Probenecid: reduced cefamandole excretion.

EFFECTS ON DIAGNOSTIC TESTS
BUN, serum creatinine: increased levels.
Coombs' test: positive findings.
Prothrombin time: possibly prolonged.
Serum alkaline phosphatase, LDH, SGOT, SGPT: elevated levels.
Urine glucose: false-positive results when tested with cupric sulfate (Benedict's solution, Clinitest).
Urine protein: false-positive results with acid and denaturization precipitation tests.

SPECIAL CONSIDERATIONS
• Treat overdose symptomatically and supportively.
• Check for previous penicillin or cephalosporin hypersensitivity. Negative history doesn't rule out future allergic reaction.
• Obtain specimens for culture and sensitivity testing before first dose. Therapy may start before results are available.
• Monitor prothrombin time and provide prophylactic vitamin K, if necessary. Check for ecchymosis and easy bruising.
• If diarrhea persists during therapy, collect stool specimens to rule out possible pseudomembranous colitis.
• Monitor BUN and liver enzyme levels and creatinine clearance in patients with potential renal impairment.
• Use Clinistix or Tes-Tape for urine glucose determinations to prevent spurious results.

• Advise patient to avoid alcohol during therapy and 46 to 72 hours after treatment ends.

cefazolin sodium
Ancef♦, Kefzol♦

Pregnancy Risk Category: B

PHARMACOKINETICS
Distribution: widely distributed into body tissues and fluids, including pleural and synovial fluid, bile, and bone. Not readily distributed into cerebrospinal fluid even when meninges are inflamed. Drug crosses the placenta.
Metabolism: not metabolized.
Excretion: in the urine by glomerular filtration and tubular secretion. Sixty percent excreted in 6 hours, 80% to 100% in 24 hours. Drug appears in breast milk in low concentrations. Serum half-life is about 1 to 2 hours.
Action: peak serum level, 1 to 2 hours.

MECHANISM OF ACTION
A semisynthetic first-generation cephalosporin, cefazolin achieves its bactericidal effects by inhibiting mucopeptide synthesis in the bacterial cell wall, promoting osmotic instability. Its spectrum of activity includes many gram-positive aerobic cocci, including *Staphylococcus aureus, Staphylococcus epidermidis, Streptococcus pneumoniae,* group A beta-hemolytic streptococci, and group B streptococci.

INDICATIONS & DOSAGE
• Septicemia, endocarditis, and infections of the respiratory tract, genitourinary tract, skin, soft tissue, biliary tract, bones, and joints caused by susceptible organisms.
Adults: in mild infection, 250 to 500 mg q 8 hours; in moderate to severe infection, 500 mg to 1 g q 6 to 8 hours; in life-threatening infection, 1 to 1.5 g q 6 hours. Maximum daily dosage, 12 g.
• Surgical prophylaxis. *Adults:* 1 g 30 to 60 minutes before surgery; during surgery, 0.5 to 1 g q 2 hours; after surgery, 0.5 to 1 g q 6 to 8 hours for 24 hours. *Children over age 1 month:* 8 to 16 mg/kg q 8 hours or 6 to 12 mg/kg q 6 hours.
Note: Dosage in renal failure reflects creatinine clearance. In adults, if clearance is less than or equal to 10 ml/min, dosage is half usual dose q 18 to 24 hours; if 11 to 34 ml/min, dosage is half usual dose q 12 hours; if 35 to 54 ml/min, dosage is full dose q 8 hours or less frequently; if more than 55 ml/min, give usual adult dose. In children, if clearance is 5 to 20 ml/min, dosage is 2.5 to 10 mg/kg q 24 hours; if 20 to 40 ml/min, 3.125 to 12.5 mg/kg q 12 hours; if 40 to 70 ml/min, 7.5 to 30 mg/kg q 12 hours; if more than 70 ml/min, give usual pediatric dose.

CONTRAINDICATIONS & CAUTIONS
• Contraindicated in hypersensitivity to cephalosporins, penicillins, or penicillin-like products.
• Use cautiously in premature infants and neonates because safety in this age-group hasn't been established.
• Give cautiously in renal disease to prevent toxicity.
• Also give cautiously in patients with a history of ulcerative colitis, regional enteritis, or antibiotic-associated colitis because of an increased risk of pseudomembranous colitis.

PREPARATION & STORAGE

Available in 250 mg, 500 mg, and 1 g vials. To reconstitute, add 2 ml of 0.9% sodium chloride or sterile or bacteriostatic water to the 250 or 500 mg vial, 2.5 ml to the 1 g vial. Shake well. This dilution yields a concentration of 125, 225, and 330 mg/ml, respectively. Further dilute reconstituted Ancef with 5 ml and Kefzol with 10 ml of compatible solution for direct injection.

For intermittent infusion, add reconstituted drug to 50 to 100 ml of compatible solution, such as dextrose 5% in water; dextrose 5% in Ringer's lactate; dextrose 5% in 0.2%, 0.45%, or 0.9% sodium chloride; dextrose 5% and Normosol-M; or dextrose 5% and Ionosol B or Plasma-Lyte.

Reconstituted and diluted drug remains stable for 24 hours at room temperature or for 10 days if refrigerated.

Solutions reconstituted with sterile water or bacteriostatic water or 0.9% sodium chloride injection are stable for 12 weeks when stored at −4° F. (−20° C.). Don't refreeze thawed solutions.

ADMINISTRATION

Don't use a cloudy or precipitated solution.
Direct injection: Inject the solution into a vein over 3 to 5 minutes or into I.V. tubing containing a free-flowing, compatible solution.
Intermittent infusion: Insert a 21G or 23G needle into port of primary tubing, and infuse 50 to 100 ml of solution over 30 minutes.
Continuous infusion: not recommended.

INCOMPATIBILITY

Incompatible with amobarbital sodium, ascorbic acid injection, calcium gluceptate, calcium gluconate, cimetidine, colistimethate sodium, erythromycin gluceptate, kanamycin, oxytetracycline, pentobarbital sodium, polymyxin B, tetracycline hydrochloride, and M.V.I.-12.

ADVERSE REACTIONS

Life-threatening: anaphylaxis.
Other: abdominal cramps, bacterial and fungal superinfection, bloating and diarrhea (moderate to severe), colitis, confusion, dyspepsia, fever, glossitis, headache, malaise, nausea, paresthesias, phlebitis, pseudomembranous colitis, rash, rectal or genital pruritus, tissue sloughing, transient leukopenia, urticaria, vomiting, weight loss.

INTERACTIONS

Bacteriostatic drugs (chloramphenicol, erythromycin, sulfonamides, tetracyclines): additive bactericidal effects against certain organisms.
Loop diuretics (such as furosemide), nephrotoxic drugs (such as aminoglycosides and vancomycin): heightened risk of nephrotoxicity.
Probenecid: increased cefazolin effects.

EFFECTS ON DIAGNOSTIC TESTS

BUN, serum creatinine: increased levels.
Coombs' test: positive results.
Serum alkaline phosphatase, SGOT, SGPT: elevated levels.
Urine creatinine, protein: false-positive results.
Urine glucose: false-positive findings when tested with cupric sulfate (Benedict's solution, Clinitest).

SPECIAL CONSIDERATIONS

• Give epinephrine in an emergency, if needed.
• Check for previous penicillin or cephalosporin hypersensitivity. Neg-

ative history doesn't rule out future allergic reaction.
- Obtain specimens for culture and sensitivity testing before first dose. Therapy may start before results are available.
- Monitor BUN and serum creatinine levels to assess renal function.
- Warn patient that side effects may last for several weeks after drug is discontinued.
- Dialysis may help to remove drug.
- Use glucose oxidase methods (Clinistix, Tes-Tape) for urine glucose determinations to avoid spurious results.
- Observe patient for fungal and bacterial superinfection with prolonged use.

cefmetazole sodium
Zefazone

Pregnancy Risk Category: B

PHARMACOKINETICS
Distribution: drug is 65% bound to plasma proteins at a plasma concentration of 100 mcg/ml. Not known if drug enters cerebrospinal fluid (CSF). High urine concentrations occur within 12 hours.
Metabolism: not substantially metabolized.
Excretion: mainly by tubular secretion. About 85% of a dose is excreted within 12 hours. Mean plasma or serum half-life, 1.2 hours.

MECHANISM OF ACTION
Cefmetazole inhibits cell-wall synthesis, promoting osmotic instability. Usually bactericidal.

INDICATIONS & DOSAGE
- Lower respiratory tract infections caused by *Streptococcus pneumoniae, Staphylococcus aureus* (penicillinase- and non-penicillinase-producing strains), *Escherichia coli,* and *Haemophilus influenzae* (non-penicillinase-producing strains; intra-abdominal infections caused by *E. coli* or *Bacteroides fragilis;* skin and skin-structure infections caused by *S. aureus* (penicillinase- and non-penicillinase-producing strains), *Staphylococcus epidermidis, Streptococcus pyogenes, Streptococcus agalactiae, E. coli, Proteus mirabilis, Klebsiella pneumoniae,* and *B. fragilis. Adults:* 2 g I.V. q 6 to 12 hours for 5 to 14 days.
- Urinary tract infections caused by *E. coli. Adults:* 2 g I.V. q 12 hours.
- Prophylaxis in patients undergoing vaginal hysterectomy. *Adults:* 2 g I.V. 30 to 90 minutes before surgery as a single dose; or 1 g I.V. 30 to 90 minutes before surgery, repeated in 8 and 16 hours.
- Prophylaxis in patients undergoing abdominal hysterectomy. *Adults:* 1 g I.V. 30 to 90 minutes before surgery, repeated in 8 and 16 hours.
- Prophylaxis in patients undergoing Cesarean section. *Adults:* 2 g I.V. as a single dose after clamping cord; or 1 g I.V. after clamping cord, repeated after 8 and 16 hours.
- Prophylaxis in patients undergoing colorectal surgery. *Adults:* 2 g I.V. as a single dose 30 to 90 minutes before surgery. Some doctors follow with additional 2 g doses in 8 and 16 hours.
- Prophylaxis in patients undergoing cholecystectomy (high risk). *Adults:* 1 g I.V. 30 to 90 minutes before surgery, repeated in 8 and 16 hours.
Note: Adult dosage in renal failure is based on creatinine clearance. If clearance is below 10 ml/min, dosage is 1 to 2 g I.V. q 48 hours; if 10 to 30 ml/min, 1 to 2 g I.V. q 24 hours; if 30 to 50 ml/min, 1 to 2 g I.V. q 16 hours; if 50 to 90 ml/min, 1 to 2 g I.V. q 12 hours.

CONTRAINDICATIONS & CAUTIONS

• Contraindicated in hypersensitivity to cefmetazole or cephalosporins.
• Use cautiously in hypersensitivity to penicillin.
• In patients with a history of GI disease (especially colitis), give cautiously because of increased risk of pseudomembranous colitis.
• Give cautiously in renal impairment because of risk of toxicity from prolonged excretion.

PREPARATION & STORAGE

Available in 1 g and 2 g vials. Reconstitute with bacteriostatic water for injection, sterile water for injection, or 0.9% sodium chloride for injection. Shake to dissolve the drug, then let solution stand until clear. Add 3.7 ml to the 1 g vial to make a solution with an average concentration of 250 mg/ml. Add 10 ml to the 1 g vial to make a solution of about 100 mg/ml. Add 7 ml to the 2 g vial to form a solution of 250 mg/ml. Add 15 ml to the 2 g vial to make a solution of 125 mg/ml.

Store powder at controlled room temperature (59° to 86° F. [15° to 30° C.]). Reconstituted solutions are stable for 24 hours at room temperature (77° F., 25° C.) or for 1 week if refrigerated (46° F., 8° C.). Alternatively, solutions may be frozen for up to 6 weeks (− 4° F., − 20° C.). Thaw by gradual warming at room temperature (77° F.). Don't use a microwave oven or warm water bath.

Solutions should be clear after thawing. If the solution remains cloudy or a precipitate forms at room temperature, do not use. Thawed solutions should not be refrozen; they are stable for 24 hours.

ADMINISTRATION

Direct injection: Temporarily discontinue medications being administered at the same site. Administer over 3 to 5 minutes.
Intermittent infusion: The reconstituted drug may be further diluted to concentrations of 1 to 20 mg/ml by adding it to 0.9% sodium chloride injection, dextrose 5% in water, or lactated Ringer's injection. Infuse diluted drug over 10 to 60 minutes.
Continuous infusion: not recommended.

INCOMPATIBILITY

Incompatible with aminoglycoside antibiotics.

ADVERSE REACTIONS

Life-threatening: anaphylaxis, hypotension, shock.
Other: altered color perception, candidiasis, diarrhea, dyspnea, epigastric pain, epistaxis, fever, generalized itching, hot flashes, hypersensitivity, nausea, pain at injection site, phlebitis, pleural effusion, pruritus, pseudomembranous colitis, respiratory distress, rash, superinfection, vaginitis, vomiting.

INTERACTIONS

Alcohol: disulfiram-like reaction. Alcohol should be avoided within 24 hours of administration.
Aminoglycosides: increased risk of nephrotoxicity.
Probenecid: increases both half-life and duration of measurable plasma concentrations of the drug.

EFFECTS ON DIAGNOSTIC TESTS

May cause false-positive results for urine glucose with copper sulfate tests (Clinitest). Glucose enzymatic tests (Clinistix, Tes-Tape) are unaffected.

SPECIAL CONSIDERATIONS

• Ask the patient if he's had any reaction to previous cephalosporin or

---

penicillin therapy before administering first dose. Expect to treat life-threatening hypersensitivity reactions with epinephrine, I.V. corticosteroids or antihistamines, pressor agents, or I.V. fluids.
• Advise patients to avoid alcohol during therapy and for 48 to 72 hours after end of treatment.
• Obtain specimen for culture and sensitivity before first dose. Therapy may begin pending test results.
• Prolonged use may result in overgrowth of nonsusceptible organisms. Monitor patient for superinfection.
• Drug may influence bleeding disorders. Monitor prothrombin time and administer vitamin K as ordered. Advise patient to report unusual bleeding or bruising.
• Advise patient to report diarrhea. Culture stool to rule out overgrowth of *Clostridium difficile*.
• Monitor patients with renal impairment frequently for signs of toxicity. Dosage may be reduced.

cefonicid sodium
Monocid

Pregnancy Risk Category: B

PHARMACOKINETICS
Distribution: widely distributed into body tissues and fluids, including myocardium, gallbladder, bile, bone, adipose tissue, prostate, uterus, sputum, and pleural fluid. Low concentrations appear in cerebrospinal fluid, GI tract, and aqueous humor. Drug crosses the placenta. Up to 98% is bound to plasma proteins.
Metabolism: not metabolized.
Excretion: in urine by tubular secretion, with 88% to 99% removed unchanged in 48 hours. Drug appears in breast milk. Serum half-life ranges from 3½ to 6 hours.

Action: peak serum level, immediately after administration.

MECHANISM OF ACTION
A semisynthetic second-generation cephalosporin, cefonicid achieves its bactericidal effects by inhibiting mucopeptide synthesis in the bacterial cell wall, thus promoting osmotic instability. Its broad spectrum of activity includes most gram-positive aerobic cocci, including *Staphylococcus aureus, Staphylococcus epidermidis, Streptococcus pneumoniae,* group A beta-hemolytic streptococci, and group B streptococci.

Susceptible gram-negative aerobic bacteria include most strains of *Neisseria meningitidis, N. gonorrhoeae,* and *Haemophilus influenzae;* many strains of *Citrobacter diversus, Escherichia coli, Klebsiella pneumoniae,* and *Proteus mirabilis;* and some strains of *Citrobacter freundii, Enterobacter aerogenes,* and *Providencia rettgeri.*

Susceptible anaerobic bacteria include *Clostridium, Fusobacterium, Peptostreptococcus, Propionibacterium acnes,* and *Veillonella.*

INDICATIONS & DOSAGE
• Septicemia and infections of the lower respiratory and urinary tracts, skin and skin structure, and bone and joints caused by susceptible organisms. *Adults:* 1 g q 24 hours; in uncomplicated infection, 0.5 g q 24 hours; in life-threatening infections, 2 g q 24 hours.
• Surgical prophylaxis. *Adults:* 1 g 60 minutes before surgery; may give 1 g q 24 hours for 2 days. *Cesarean section:* 1 g after umbilical cord is clamped.
Note: Adjust dosage in renal failure. In adults, adjust dosage if creatinine clearance falls below 60 ml/min.

CONTRAINDICATIONS & CAUTIONS

• Contraindicated in hypersensitivity to cephalosporins, penicillin, or penicillin-like drugs.
• In children, administer cautiously because safe use in this age-group hasn't been established.
• Use cautiously in patients with a history of GI disease (especially colitis) because of a heightened risk of pseudomembranous colitis.
• Give cautiously to the elderly and to patients with renal impairment because of possible toxicity.

PREPARATION & STORAGE

Reconstitute 500 mg vial with 2 ml of sterile water for injection (yields a concentration of 220 mg/ml) and 1 g vial with 2.5 ml of sterile water for injection (yields a concentration of 325 mg/ml). Shake well. Reconstitute piggyback vials with 50 to 100 ml of sterile water for injection, bacteriostatic water for injection, or 0.9% sodium chloride.

Compatible solutions include dextrose 5% and 0.15% potassium chloride; dextrose 5% in 0.2%, 0.45%, or 0.9% sodium chloride; dextrose 5% in Ringer's lactate; dextrose 5% or 10% in water; Ringer's injection; Ringer's lactate; 0.9% sodium chloride; and ⅙ M sodium lactate.

Solution remains stable for 24 hours at room temperature and for 72 hours if refrigerated.

ADMINISTRATION

Direct injection: Using a 21G or 23G needle, inject 2 ml of reconstituted drug into vein over 3 to 5 minutes. Or inject reconstituted drug into I.V. tubing containing a free-flowing, compatible solution.
Intermittent infusion: Infuse 50 to 100 ml of diluted drug over 20 to 30 minutes into the tubing of a free-flowing, compatible solution.

Continuous infusion: not recommended.

INCOMPATIBILITY

No incompatibilities reported.

ADVERSE REACTIONS

Life-threatening: anaphylaxis.
Other: anal and genital pruritus; bacterial and fungal superinfection; burning sensation, abscess, sloughing at injection site; diarrhea; dizziness; fatigue; headache; leukopenia; malaise; nausea; neutropenia; phlebitis; pseudomembranous colitis; thrombophlebitis; urticaria; vertigo; vomiting.

INTERACTIONS

Aminoglycosides, carmustine, loop diuretics, streptozocin: heightened risk of nephrotoxicity.
Probenecid: decreased cefonicid excretion.

EFFECTS ON DIAGNOSTIC TESTS

Coombs' test: positive findings.
Eosinophil and platelet counts: elevated.
Serum alkaline phosphatase, LDH, SGOT, SGPT: increased levels.
Urine glucose: false-positive results when tested with cupric sulfate (Benedict's solution, Clinitest).

SPECIAL CONSIDERATIONS

• Treat overdose or anaphylaxis symptomatically.
• Check for previous penicillin or cephalosporin hypersensitivity. Negative history doesn't rule out future allergic reaction.
• Obtain specimens for culture and sensitivity testing before first dose. Therapy may start before results are available.
• If diarrhea persists during therapy, collect stool specimens to rule out pseudomembranous colitis.

• Monitor BUN and serum creatinine levels to assess renal function. Adjust dosage accordingly.
• Cefonicid is useful for managing infections requiring prolonged outpatient therapy.
• Use Clinistix or Tes-Tape for urine glucose determinations to prevent spurious results.
• If the patient is undergoing dialysis, maintain the prescribed dosage. Only small amounts of drug are removed by dialysis.
• Observe patient for fungal and bacterial superinfection with prolonged use.

cefoperazone sodium
Cefobid♦

Pregnancy Risk Category: B

PHARMACOKINETICS
Distribution: throughout body tissues and fluids, including ascitic and pleural fluid, middle ear fluid, aqueous humor, bile, sputum, tonsils, sinus membranes, endometrium, myometrium, lungs, prostate, and bone. Slight amounts appear in cerebrospinal fluid with uninflamed meninges, higher amounts with inflammation. Drug crosses the placenta; it's 93% bound to plasma protein.
Metabolism: not metabolized.
Excretion: primarily in bile, with 15% to 30% excreted unchanged in urine within 24 hours. In severe hepatic disease or biliary obstruction, 90% is excreted in urine. Small amounts of drug appear in breast milk. Mean serum half-life is approximately 2 hours.
Action: peak serum level, upon completion of infusion.

MECHANISM OF ACTION
A semisynthetic third-generation cephalosporin, cefoperazone achieves its bactericidal effects by inhibiting mucopeptide synthesis in the bacterial cell wall, promoting osmotic instability. Its broad spectrum of activity includes gram-positive aerobic cocci, such as most strains of *Staphylococcus aureus, Staphylococcus epidermidis,* groups A and B streptococci, *Streptococcus viridans, S. pneumoniae, S. faecalis, S. faecium,* and *S. durans* and some strains of *Listeria monocytogenes.*

Susceptible gram-negative aerobic bacteria include *Citrobacter diversus, C. freundii, Enterobacter aerogenes, E. cloacae, Escherichia coli, Klebsiella oxytoca, Morganella morganii, Proteus mirabilis, P. vulgaris, Providencia, Salmonella, Shigella, Yersinia enterocolitica, Pseudomonas, Haemophilus influenzae, H. parainfluenzae, Neisseria gonorrhoeae,* and *N. meningitidis.*

Susceptible anaerobes include *Bifidobacterium, Eubacterium, Fusobacterium, Peptococcus, Peptostreptococcus, Propionibacterium, Veillonella,* and *Clostridium* (including some strains of *C. difficile*).

INDICATIONS & DOSAGE
• Septicemia, peritonitis, and gynecologic, skin, and urinary and respiratory tract infections caused by susceptible organisms. *Adults:* 1 to 2 g q 12 hours for 2 to 3 days. Daily dosage of 16 g has been given without complications.
Note: Adjust dosage in renal failure. For adults, no adjustment usually necessary; however, dosages of 4 g per day may be given cautiously to patients with hepatic impairment. Patients with both hepatic and renal impairment should not receive more than 1 g (base) daily without serum level determinations.

CONTRAINDICATIONS & CAUTIONS

• Contraindicated in cephalosporin or penicillin hypersensitivity.
• Use cautiously in hypoprothrombinemia and in bleeding disorders because of possible exacerbation; and in ulcerative colitis, regional enteritis, or antibiotic-associated colitis because of an increased risk of pseudomembranous colitis.
• Also use cautiously during prolonged parenteral or enteral nutrition and in patients with poor nutritional status, malabsorption, or alcohol dependence because of an increased risk of vitamin K deficiency.
• Safe use hasn't been established for children.

PREPARATION & STORAGE

Reconstitute 1 g of cefoperazone with 5 ml of compatible diluent. Shake vial vigorously until drug dissolves. Let vial stand to allow foam to dissipate before drawing up.

After reconstitution, dilute further by adding 20 to 40 ml of compatible diluent for intermittent infusion and enough diluent to make a solution of 2 to 25 mg/ml for a continuous infusion. Compatible solutions include bacteriostatic water for injection, dextrose 5% or 10% in water, Ringer's lactate, dextrose 5% in Ringer's lactate, dextrose 5% in 0.2% or 0.9% sodium chloride, Normosol-R, dextrose 5% and Normosol-M, 0.9% sodium chloride, and sterile water for injection. Solutions remain stable for 24 hours at room temperature and for 5 days if refrigerated.

ADMINISTRATION

Direct injection: not recommended. If employed, though, use a 21G or 23G needle to inject reconstituted drug into vein over 3 to 5 minutes. Alternatively, inject into I.V. tubing containing a free-flowing, compatible solution.
Intermittent infusion: Infuse solution over 15 to 30 minutes into I.V. tubing containing a compatible solution.
Continuous infusion: Infuse solution containing 2 to 25 mg/ml at ordered rate.

INCOMPATIBILITY

Incompatible with aminoglycosides.

ADVERSE REACTIONS

Life-threatening: anaphylaxis.
Other: abdominal cramps, anal and genital pruritus, bacterial and fungal superinfection, bleeding, chills, diarrhea, dizziness, eosinophilia, glossitis, headache, hypoprothrombinemia, local pain, nausea, neutropenia, phlebitis, pseudomembranous colitis, rash, tremors, urticaria, vitamin K deficiency, vomiting.

INTERACTIONS

Alcohol: disulfiram-like reaction if taken within 72 hours of drug.
Aminoglycosides: heightened risk of nephrotoxicity and possible synergistic effect against some gram-negative organisms.
Anticoagulants, platelet aggregation inhibitors: possible bleeding.
Clavulanic acid: possible synergistic effect against many Enterobacteriaceae, *Pseudomonas aeruginosa*, *Staphylococcus aureus,* and *Bacteroides fragilis.*

EFFECTS ON DIAGNOSTIC TESTS

BUN, serum creatinine: elevated levels.
Coombs' test: positive findings.
Hematocrit, hemoglobin, neutrophils: reduced levels.
Serum alkaline phosphatase, SGOT, SGPT: increased levels.

Urine glucose: false-positive results when tested with cupric sulfate (Benedict's solution, Clinitest).

SPECIAL CONSIDERATIONS
• Treat overdose symptomatically. Hemodialysis enhances drug removal.
• Check for cephalosporin or penicillin hypersensitivity before first dose. Negative history doesn't rule out future allergic reaction.
• Obtain specimens for culture and sensitivity testing before first dose. Therapy may start before results are available.
• Monitor BUN and serum creatinine levels to assess renal function.
• Monitor patients with hepatic disease or biliary obstruction frequently for signs of toxicity.
• Monitor CBC and prothrombin time to assess bleeding disturbances.
• Vitamin K may be given to patients receiving high drug doses, to debilitated patients, to those with hepatic or renal impairment.
• Give prescribed dosage after hemodialysis treatment.
• Use glucose oxidase methods (Clinistix, Tes-Tape) for urine glucose determinations to avoid spurious results.
• Observe patient for fungal and bacterial superinfection with prolonged use.
• Advise the patient to avoid alcohol during therapy and for 48 to 72 hours after treatment ends.

---

ceforanide
Precef

Pregnancy Risk Category: B

PHARMACOKINETICS
Distribution: throughout body tissues and fluids, including pericardial and synovial fluid, bile, gallbladder, bone, skeletal muscle, vaginal and uterine tissue, jejunum, and myocardium. Drug isn't readily distributed into cerebrospinal fluid even with inflamed meninges. Not known if drug crosses the placenta. It's 76% to 83% bound to plasma proteins.
Metabolism: not metabolized.
Excretion: in the urine by glomerular filtration and renal tubular secretion, with 78% to 95% removed in 12 hours. Not known if drug appears in breast milk. Serum half-life averages 3 hours.
Action: peak serum level, immediately after infusion.

MECHANISM OF ACTION
A semisynthetic second-generation cephalosporin, ceforanide achieves its bactericidal effects by inhibiting mucopeptide synthesis in the bacterial cell wall, promoting osmotic instability. Its broad spectrum of activity includes most gram-positive aerobic cocci, including *Staphylococcus aureus, Staphylococcus epidermidis, Streptococcus pneumoniae, Streptococcus viridans*, group A beta-hemolytic streptococci, and group B streptococci.

Susceptible gram-negative aerobic bacteria include most strains of *Neisseria gonorrhoeae* and *N. meningitidis* and many strains of *Haemophilus influenzae, H. parainfluenzae, Citrobacter diversus, C. freundii, Eikenella corrodens, Escherichia coli, Klebsiella, Proteus mirabilis, Salmonella,* and *Shigella.* Susceptible anaerobic bacteria include *Fusobacterium, Peptococcus, Peptostreptococcus,* and strains of *Clostridium.*

INDICATIONS & DOSAGE
• Infection caused by susceptible organisms. *Adults:* 0.5 to 1 g q 12 hours. Can increase to 2 to 4 g q 12 hours in severe infection. *Children*

---

age 1 and older: 10 to 20 mg/kg q 12 hours.
• Surgical prophylaxis. *Adults:* 0.5 to 1 g 1 hour before surgery; after surgery, 0.5 to 1 g q 12 hours for 48 hours, as needed.
Note: Adjust dosage in renal failure. A reduced dosage may be needed for adults with a creatinine clearance below 20 ml/min. After initial loading dose of 750 mg, adjust dosage as follows: If clearance is less than 5 ml/min, dosage is 250 mg q 12 hours; if 5 to 20 ml/min, 250 mg q 6 hours; if more than 20 ml/min, 500 mg q 6 hours.

CONTRAINDICATIONS & CAUTIONS
• Contraindicated in hypersensitivity to cephalosporins, penicillin, or penicillin-like products.
• Use cautiously in patients with a history of GI disease (especially colitis) because of a magnified risk of pseudomembranous colitis.
• Give cautiously in impaired renal function because of an increased risk of toxicity.

PREPARATION & STORAGE
Dilute contents of 500 mg or 1 g vial or piggyback unit with 5 to 10 ml, respectively, of compatible solution; shake container immediately. Compatible solutions include dextrose 5% or 10% in water, dextrose 5% in Ringer's lactate, dextrose 5% in 0.2% or 0.45% sodium chloride solution, Ringer's lactate, 0.9% sodium chloride, and sterile water for injection.
  Dilute further for infusion. Solution remains stable for 48 hours at room temperature, 14 days when refrigerated, and 90 days when frozen.

ADMINISTRATION
Direct injection: Using a 21G or 23G needle, inject 5 to 10 ml into vein over 3 to 5 minutes. Alternatively, inject into I.V. tubing containing a compatible solution.
Intermittent infusion: Dilute reconstituted drug in 50 to 100 ml of compatible solution. Use secondary I.V. tubing or volume-control set, and discontinue administration of solution in primary I.V. With a 21G or 23G needle, infuse solution over 30 minutes.
Continuous infusion: not recommended.

INCOMPATIBILITY
No incompatibilities reported.

ADVERSE REACTIONS
Life-threatening: anaphylaxis.
Other: bacterial and fungal superinfection, confusion, diarrhea, eosinophilia, headache, hypotension, lethargy, light-headedness, nausea, neutropenia, pain and swelling at injection site, phlebitis, pruritus, pseudomembranous colitis, rash, transient thrombocytopenia, urticaria, vomiting.

INTERACTIONS
Aminoglycosides, loop diuretics: increased risk of nephrotoxicity.

EFFECTS ON DIAGNOSTIC TESTS
BUN: elevated levels.
Coombs' test: positive findings.
Serum alkaline phosphatase, SGOT, SGPT: increased levels.
Serum creatinine: falsely elevated values when Jaffé reaction is used.
Urine glucose: false-positive results when tested with cupric sulfate (Benedict's solution, Clinitest).

SPECIAL CONSIDERATIONS
• Treat overdose symptomatically. Hemodialysis removes drug.
• Check for cephalosporin or penicillin hypersensitivity before giving

first dose. Negative history doesn't rule out future allergic reaction.
• Obtain specimens for culture and sensitivity testing before first dose. Therapy may start before results are available.
• If diarrhea persists during therapy, collect stool specimens to rule out possible pseudomembranous colitis.
• Assess renal function. May be necessary to reduce dosage in renal impairment.
• Monitor hepatic function periodically during therapy.
• Use glucose oxidase methods (Clinistix, Tes-Tape) for urine glucose determinations to avoid spurious results.

cefotaxime sodium
Claforan♦

Pregnancy Risk Category: B

PHARMACOKINETICS
Distribution: throughout most body tissues and fluids. Therapeutic concentrations reach middle ear and cerebrospinal fluid, especially if meninges are inflamed. Drug readily crosses the placenta; it's 13% to 38% bound to plasma proteins.
Metabolism: partly metabolized in liver and kidneys.
Excretion: excreted rapidly by glomerular filtration and renal tubular secretion. Serum half-life is about 60 to 90 minutes. Drug appears in breast milk.
Action: peak serum level at end of infusion.

MECHANISM OF ACTION
Inhibits mucopeptide synthesis in the bacterial cell wall, promoting osmotic instability. Its broad spectrum of activity includes most gram-negative aerobic bacteria, such as *Citro-*

bacter freundii, C. diversus, Enterobacter aerogenes, E. cloacae, Escherichia coli, Klebsiella pneumoniae, K. oxytoca, Morganella morganii, Proteus mirabilis, P. vulgaris, Providencia rettgeri, Salmonella, Serratia marcescens, Shigella, and *Haemophilus influenzae;* some strains of *Pseudomonas;* and ampicillin-resistant, penicillinase-resistant, and non-penicillinase-resistant strains of *Neisseria gonorrhoeae* and *N. meningitidis.*

Drug is effective against some gram-positive aerobic bacteria, including most strains of *Staphylococcus aureus,* group A and group B streptococci, and *Streptococcus pneumoniae* and some strains of *Streptococcus viridans.*

Susceptible anaerobic bacteria include *Bacteroides, Eubacterium, Fusobacterium, Peptococcus, Peptostreptococcus, Propionibacterium, Veillonella,* and some strains of *Clostridium.*

INDICATIONS & DOSAGE
• Severe life-threatening infections caused by susceptible organisms. *Adults:* 2 g q 4 hours. Maximum dosage, 12 g daily.
• Moderate to severe infections caused by susceptible organisms. *Adults and children weighing 50 kg or more:* 1 to 2 g q 6 hours. *Children age 1 month to 12 years (weighing less than 50 kg):* 50 to 180 mg/kg daily in 4 to 6 equally divided doses. *Neonates age 1 to 4 weeks:* 25 to 50 mg/kg q 8 hours. *Neonates under age 1 week:* 25 to 50 mg/kg q 12 hours.
• Uncomplicated infections caused by susceptible organisms. *Adults:* 1 g q 12 hours.
• Disseminated gonorrhea. *Adults:* 500 mg q.i.d. for 7 days. *Children*

---

weighing less than 45 kg: 50 mg/kg daily in divided doses for 7 days. *Neonates:* 25 to 50 mg/kg b.i.d. or t.i.d. for 10 to 14 days.
• Gonococcal ophthalmia. *Adults:* 500 mg q.i.d. for 5 days.
• Gonococcal meningitis. *Children weighing less than 45 kg:* 200 mg/kg daily in divided doses for at least 10 days. *Neonates:* 50 mg/kg b.i.d. or t.i.d. for 10 to 14 days.
• Surgical prophylaxis. *Adults:* 1 g 30 to 90 minutes before surgery. *Cesarean section:* 1 g once umbilical cord is clamped, then 1 g 6 to 12 hours later.
Note: Adjust dosage in renal failure. Adult patients with creatinine clearance less than 20 ml/min should receive half the usual dose.

CONTRAINDICATIONS & CAUTIONS
• Contraindicated in cephalosporin hypersensitivity. Use cautiously in penicillin hypersensitivity because of possible allergic reaction.
• In patients with a history of GI disease (especially colitis), administer carefully because of an increased risk of pseudomembranous colitis.
• Give drug cautiously in renal impairment because of prolonged excretion.

PREPARATION & STORAGE
Available in vials containing 500 mg, 1 g, or 2 g and in infusion bottles containing 1 or 2 g. Reconstitute vials with 10 ml of sterile water for injection. Shake well to dissolve. I.V. infusion bottles can be further diluted in 50 to 100 ml of dextrose 5% in water or 0.9% sodium chloride.

Reconstituted drug can be diluted in 500 to 1,000 ml of compatible solution for continuous infusion. These solutions include dextrose 5% or 10% in water; 0.9% sodium chlo-

ride; dextrose 5% in 0.2%, 0.45%, or 0.9% sodium chloride; invert sugar 10% in water; Ringer's lactate; and ⅙ M sodium lactate.

Reconstituted solutions remain stable for 24 hours at 77° F. (25° C.) and for 10 days at less than 41° F. (5° C.).

ADMINISTRATION
Direct injection: Give over 3 to 5 minutes directly into an intermittent infusion device or through an I.V. line containing a free-flowing, compatible solution.
Intermittent infusion: Infuse diluted solution over 20 to 30 minutes into a butterfly or scalp vein needle or through an I.V. line containing a compatible solution. Interrupt flow of primary I.V. if piggyback method is used.
Continuous infusion: Give ordered infusion over 24 hours.

INCOMPATIBILITY
Incompatible with aminoglycosides, aminophylline, and sodium bicarbonate injection.

ADVERSE REACTIONS
Life-threatening: anaphylaxis.
Other: abdominal pain, agitation, anorexia, bacterial and fungal superinfection, colitis, confusion, diarrhea, eosinophilia, fatigue, fever, granulocytopenia, headache, leukopenia, nausea, neutropenia, nocturnal perspiration, phlebitis, pruritus, pseudomembranous colitis, rash, thrombophlebitis, vomiting.

INTERACTIONS
Aminoglycosides: increased risk of nephrotoxicity.

EFFECTS ON DIAGNOSTIC TESTS
BUN, serum creatinine: elevated levels.

Coombs' test: positive findings.
Serum alkaline phosphatase,
SGOT, SGPT: increased levels.
Urine alanine aminopeptidase: transient rise.

SPECIAL CONSIDERATIONS
• Treat overdose symptomatically. Hemodialysis or peritoneal dialysis removes drug.
• Check for previous penicillin or cephalosporin hypersensitivity. Negative history doesn't rule out future allergic reaction.
• Obtain specimens for culture and sensitivity testing before first dose. Therapy may start before test results are available.
• If diarrhea persists during therapy, collect stool specimens to rule out possible pseudomembranous colitis.
• Observe patient for fungal and bacterial superinfection with prolonged use.
• Monitor patients with renal impairment frequently for signs of drug toxicity. Dosage may be reduced.

cefotetan disodium
Cefotan

Pregnancy Risk Category: B

PHARMACOKINETICS
Distribution: throughout body tissues and fluids, but with limited distribution into cerebrospinal fluid. Drug crosses the placenta; it's 76% to 91% bound to plasma proteins.
Metabolism: not metabolized.
Excretion: unchanged by kidneys, primarily by glomerular filtration, with 50% to 80% removed in 24 hours. About 20% is excreted in bile. Serum half-life averages about 4 hours. Drug appears in breast milk.
Action: peak level, 30 minutes.

MECHANISM OF ACTION
A semisynthetic cephamycin antibiotic, cefotetan achieves its bactericidal effects by inhibiting mucopeptide synthesis in the bacterial cell wall, promoting osmotic instability. Its spectrum of activity includes gram-positive aerobic bacteria, including *Staphylococcus aureus*; most strains of group A beta-hemolytic streptococci and groups B, C, and G streptococci; and some strains of *Streptococcus pneumoniae* and *Staphylococcus epidermidis*.

Susceptible gram-negative aerobic bacteria include *Neisseria meningitidis;* most strains of *Neisseria gonorrhoeae, Haemophilus influenzae, Citrobacter diversus, C. freundii, Enterobacter aerogenes, E. agglomerans, E. cloacae, Escherichia coli, Hafnia alvei, Klebsiella oxytoca, K. ozaenae, K. pneumoniae, Morganella morganii, Proteus mirabilis, P. vulgaris, Providencia rettgeri, P. stuartii, Serratia marcescens, Salmonella, Shigella,* and *Yersinia enterocolitica;* and some strains of *Alcaligenes odorans* and *Moraxella.*

Susceptible gram-positive anaerobic bacteria include *Actinomyces, Clostridium, Peptococcus, Peptostreptococcus,* and *Propionibacterium.* Susceptible gram-negative anaerobic bacteria include *Bacteroides, Fusobacterium,* and *Veillonella.*

INDICATIONS & DOSAGE
• Infections (except for urinary tract) caused by susceptible organisms. *Adults:* 1 to 2 g q 12 hours; 3 g q 12 hours in life-threatening infections.
• Urinary tract infection. *Adults:* 500 mg q 12 hours or 1 to 2 g once daily or b.i.d.
• Surgical prophylaxis. *Adults:* 1 to 2 g 30 to 60 minutes before surgery. For cesarean section, give dose as

soon as umbilical cord is clamped. Maximum daily dosage, 6 g.

Note: Adjust dosage in renal failure. Doses or frequency of administration must be modified according to the degree of renal impairment, severity of infection, and susceptibility of organisms. Adult dosage reflects creatinine clearance. If creatinine clearance is less than 10 ml/min, dosage is usual adult dose q 48 hours, or one-fourth the usual dose q 12 hours; if 10 to 30 ml/min, usual dose q 24 hours or one-half usual dose q 12 hours; if 30 ml/min or greater, give usual adult dose.

Hemodialysis patients should be given one-fourth the usual adult dose q 24 hours on days between treatments, and one-half the usual dose on the day of hemodialysis.

CONTRAINDICATIONS & CAUTIONS

• Contraindicated in cephalosporin hypersensitivity.
• Use cautiously in penicillin hypersensitivity and in patients with a history of GI disease (especially colitis) because of an increased risk of pseudomembranous colitis.
• Also use cautiously in renal impairment because of prolonged excretion, and in bleeding disorders because drug may cause hypoprothrombinemia and hemorrhage.
• Safe use in children hasn't been established.

PREPARATION & STORAGE

Available as a white to pale yellow powder in 1 g and 2 g vials and infusion vials. Reconstitute vials with 10 to 20 ml of sterile water for injection. Reconstitute infusion vials with 50 to 100 ml of dextrose 5% in water or 0.9% sodium chloride. After reconstitution, solution remains stable for 24 hours at room temperature, for 96 hours if refrigerated, and for 1 week if frozen.

ADMINISTRATION

Direct injection: Inject reconstituted drug directly into vein over 3 to 5 minutes.

Intermittent infusion: Over 20 to 30 minutes, infuse solution through a butterfly or scalp vein needle or into the tubing of a free-flowing, compatible solution. Interrupt flow of primary I.V. solution during cefotetan administration.

Continuous infusion: not recommended.

INCOMPATIBILITY

Incompatible with aminoglycosides.

ADVERSE REACTIONS

Life-threatening: anaphylaxis.
Other: abdominal pain; chills; diarrhea; eosinophilia; fever; leukopenia; nausea; neutropenia; pain, inflammation, and swelling at infusion site; phlebitis; pruritus; pseudomembranous colitis; rash; thrombocytopenia; thrombocytosis; vomiting.

INTERACTIONS

Alcohol: disulfiram-like reaction if used within 72 hours of cefotetan.
Aminoglycosides: additive effects against certain organisms and increased risk of nephrotoxicity.
Beta-lactam antibiotics: additive effects against certain organisms.

EFFECTS ON DIAGNOSTIC TESTS

Coombs' test: positive findings.
Prothrombin time: possibly prolonged.
Serum alkaline phosphatase, LDH, SGOT, SGPT: increased levels.
Serum or urine creatinine: false-positive results when Jaffé reaction is used.

Urine glucose: false-positive results when tested with cupric sulfate (Benedict's solution, Clinitest).
Urine protein: false-positive results.

SPECIAL CONSIDERATIONS
• Treat overdose symptomatically. Hemodialysis or peritoneal dialysis may promote drug removal.
• Check for previous penicillin or cephalosporin hypersensitivity. Negative history doesn't rule out future allergic reaction.
• Obtain specimens for culture and sensitivity testing before first dose. Therapy may start before results are available.
• If diarrhea persists during therapy, collect stool specimens to rule out possible pseudomembranous colitis.
• Use Clinistix or Tes-Tape for urine glucose determinations to avoid spurious results.
• Observe patient for superinfection with prolonged use.

cefoxitin sodium
Mefoxin♦

Pregnancy Risk Category: B

PHARMACOKINETICS
Distribution: widely distributed into most body tissues and fluids, including ascitic, pleural, and synovial fluid. Present in bile in absence of obstruction. Poor diffusion into cerebrospinal fluid even with inflamed meninges. Drug readily crosses the placenta.
Metabolism: about 2% metabolized in liver.
Excretion: about 85% removed in urine by glomerular filtration and tubular secretion within 6 hours. Small amounts appear in breast milk. Serum half-life after I.V. dose is 41 to 59 minutes.

Action: peak level, 3 to 5 minutes after infusion.

MECHANISM OF ACTION
Classified as a second-generation cephalosporin, cefoxitin achieves its bactericidal effects by inhibiting mucopeptide synthesis in the bacterial cell wall. Its spectrum of activity includes gram-positive aerobic bacteria, including most strains of alpha- and beta-hemolytic streptococci, *Streptococcus pneumoniae*, and staphylococci (especially most strains of penicillin G–resistant *Staphylococcus aureus*).
   Susceptible gram-negative aerobic bacteria include *Escherichia coli*, *Klebsiella*, *Morganella morganii*, *Proteus mirabilis*, *P. vulgaris*, *Providencia rettgeri*, *Salmonella*, *Shigella*, *Neisseria gonorrhoeae*, and most strains of *Haemophilus influenzae*. Susceptible anaerobic bacteria include *Bacteroides*, *Fusobacterium*, *Peptococcus*, *Peptostreptococcus*, and *Clostridium*.

INDICATIONS & DOSAGE
• Severe infections caused by susceptible organisms. *Adults:* 1 to 2 g t.i.d. or q.i.d; in life-threatening infections, up to 12 g divided t.i.d. or q.i.d. *Children age 3 months and older:* 80 to 160 mg/kg divided into four to six equal doses.
• Disseminated gonorrhea caused by penicillinase-producing strains of *Neisseria gonorrhoeae. Adults:* 1 g q.i.d. for 7 days.
• Gonococcal ophthalmia. *Adults:* 1 g q.i.d. for 5 days.
• Surgical prophylaxis. *Adults:* 2 g 30 to 60 minutes before surgery, then 2 g q 6 hours for 1 day after surgery. *Children age 3 months and older:* 30 to 40 mg/kg 30 to 60 minutes before surgery, then 30 to 40 mg/kg q 6 hours for up to 24 hours after surgery.

Note: Adjust dosage in renal failure. Doses or frequency of administration must be modified according to the degree of renal impairment, severity of infection, and susceptibility of organism. Adult dosage reflects creatinine clearance. If creatinine clearance is less than 5 ml/min, dose is 500 mg to 1 g q 24 to 48 hours; if 5 to 9 ml/min, 500 mg to 1 g q 12 to 24 hours; if 10 to 29 ml/min, 1 to 2 g q 12 to 24 hours; if 30 to 50 ml/min, 1 to 2 g q 8 to 12 hours; if greater than 50 ml/min, give usual adult dose.

CONTRAINDICATIONS & CAUTIONS

• Contraindicated in cephalosporin hypersensitivity. Use cautiously in patients with a history of penicillin or other allergies.
• Administer carefully in renal impairment because of a heightened risk of toxicity.
• In patients with a history of GI disease (especially colitis), use cautiously because of an increased risk of pseudomembranous colitis.

PREPARATION & STORAGE

Available in 1 g and 2 g vials, PVC bags, and infusion bottles. Store vials at 86° F. (30° C.).

Reconstitute 1 g and 2 g vials with 10 ml of sterile water for injection. For intermittent infusion, reconstitute 1 g and 2 g infusion bags or bottles with 50 to 100 ml of a compatible solution. For continuous infusion, reconstitute and add up to 1 liter of a compatible solution, such as dextrose 5% or 10% in water; dextrose 5% in 0.2%, 0.45%, or 0.9% sodium chloride; Ringer's injection; Ringer's lactate; 0.9% sodium chloride; 1⁄6 M sodium lactate; invert sugar 5% or 10% in water; and dextrose 5% and Ionosol B.

Solutions remain stable for 24 hours at room temperature. Both powder and solutions may turn amber, but this doesn't indicate significant change in potency.

ADMINISTRATION

Direct injection: Inject diluted drug over 3 to 5 minutes directly into vein, through an intermittent infusion device, or into an I.V. line containing a free-flowing, compatible solution.

Intermittent infusion: Give 50 to 100 ml solution through a butterfly or scalp vein needle, an intermittent infusion device, or a patent I.V. line at the ordered flow rate. Interrupt primary solution during cefoxitin infusion. Administer over 15 to 30 minutes.

Continuous infusion: Infuse up to 1 liter of solution over the prescribed duration.

INCOMPATIBILITY

Possibly incompatible with aminoglycosides.

ADVERSE REACTIONS

Life-threatening: anaphylaxis.
Other: bacterial and fungal superinfection, bone marrow depression, diarrhea, eosinophilia, exfoliative dermatitis, fever, granulocytopenia, hypotension, leukopenia, nausea, neutropenia, oliguria, pruritus, pseudomembranous colitis, rash, renal toxicity, thrombocytopenia, thrombophlebitis, urticaria, vomiting.

INTERACTIONS

Aminoglycosides, colistin, polymyxin B, vancomycin: heightened risk of nephrotoxicity.
Probenecid: reduced cefoxitin excretion.

EFFECTS ON DIAGNOSTIC TESTS

BUN, serum alkaline phosphatase, creatinine, LDH, SGOT, SGPT: increased levels.

Coombs' test: positive findings.

Serum or urine creatinine: false-positive findings when Jaffé method is used.

Urine glucose: false-positive results when tested with cupric sulfate (Benedict's solution, Clinitest).

SPECIAL CONSIDERATIONS

• Treat overdose symptomatically. Hemodialysis helps remove drug.

• Check for previous penicillin or cephalosporin hypersensitivity. Negative history doesn't rule out future allergic reaction.

• Obtain specimens for culture and sensitivity testing before first dose. Therapy may start before test results are available.

• If diarrhea persists during therapy, collect stool specimens to rule out possible pseudomembranous colitis.

• Monitor intake and output and serum creatinine and BUN levels to help detect nephrotoxicity.

• Incidence of thrombophlebitis decreases when butterfly or scalp vein needle is used.

• Drug can be removed by hemodialysis. Loading dose of 1 to 2 g should be given after hemodialysis session. Maintenance doses should reflect patient's creatinine clearance.

• Use Clinistix or Tes-Tape for urine glucose determinations to avoid spurious results.

• Observe patient for fungal and bacterial superinfection with prolonged use.

ceftazidime
Fortaz♦, Magnacef♦♦, Tazicef, Tazidime

Pregnancy Risk Category: B

PHARMACOKINETICS

Distribution: widespread; therapeutic levels appear in bone, heart, skin, skeletal muscle, gallbladder, sputum, bile, urine (especially), aqueous humor, and synovial, peritoneal, lymphatic, and cerebrospinal fluid. Distribution half-life averages 20 minutes. Drug is 5% to 24% bound to serum protein. It crosses the placenta and appears in amniotic fluid.

Metabolism: not metabolized.

Excretion: in the urine by glomerular filtration as unchanged drug; about half is removed in 2 hours and all in 24 hours. Elimination half-life is 85 to 120 minutes. Drug appears in breast milk.

Action: onset, immediate; peak level, 15 to 30 minutes.

MECHANISM OF ACTION

A semisynthetic third-generation cephalosporin, ceftazidime achieves its bactericidal effects by inhibiting mucopeptide synthesis in the bacterial cell wall, promoting osmotic instability. Its broad spectrum of activity includes most gram-positive aerobic cocci, including *Staphylococcus aureus, Staphylococcus epidermidis, Streptococcus pneumoniae,* group A beta-hemolytic streptococci, group B streptococci, and *Streptococcus viridans.*

Susceptible gram-negative aerobic bacteria include *Acinetobacter, Branhamella catarrhalis, Citrobacter diversus, C. freundii, Enterobacter aerogenes, E. agglomerans, E. cloacae, Eikenella corrodens, Esche-*

richia coli, Klebsiella oxytoca, K. pneumoniae, Morganella morganii, Pasteurella multocida, Proteus mirabilis, Proteus vulgaris, Providencia rettgeri, Providencia stuartii, Serratia marcescens, Salmonella, Shigella, Yersinia enterocolitica, many Pseudomonas species, Haemophilus influenzae, H. parainfluenzae, H. ducreyi, Neisseria gonorrhoeae, and N. meningitidis.

Susceptible anaerobic organisms include Bifidobacterium, Eubacterium, Lactobacillus, Peptococcus, Peptostreptococcus, Propionibacterium, Clostridium, and some strains of C. difficile.

INDICATIONS & DOSAGE

• Uncomplicated infections (except for urinary tract) caused by susceptible organisms. Adults and children over age 12: 1 g q 8 to 12 hours; maximum daily dosage, 6 g. Dosage depends on susceptibility of organism and severity of infection. Children age 1 month to 12 years: 30 to 50 mg/kg q 8 hours; maximum daily dosage, 6 g. Neonates: 30 mg/kg q 12 hours (or 50 mg/kg q 8 hours in immunosuppression).

• Urinary tract infection. Adults and children over age 12: in uncomplicated infection, 250 mg q 12 hours; in severe infection, 500 mg q 8 to 12 hours.

• Bone and joint infection. Adults and children over age 12: 2 g q 12 hours.

• Uncomplicated pneumonia, mild skin and skin structure infections. Adults and children over age 12: 500 mg to 1 g q 8 hours.

• Peritonitis, meningitis, severe gynecologic infections, other life-threatening infections. Adults and children over age 12: 2 g q 8 hours.

• Pseudomonal lung infection in cystic fibrosis patients with normal renal function. Adults and children

over age 12: 30 to 50 mg/kg q 8 hours; maximum daily dosage, 6 g. Note: Adjust dosage in renal failure. For adults, give 1 g loading dose. Maintenance dosage reflects creatinine clearance: 1 g q 12 hours for clearance of 31 to 50 ml/min; 1 g q 24 hours for 16 to 30 ml/min; 500 mg q 24 hours for 5 to 15 ml/min; and 500 mg q 48 hours for less than 5 ml/min.

For hemodialysis patients, give a loading dose of 1 g, then 1 g after each session. For peritoneal dialysis patients, give a loading dose of 1 g, then 500 mg q 24 hours.

CONTRAINDICATIONS & CAUTIONS

• Contraindicated in cephalosporin hypersensitivity. Use cautiously in patients with penicillin hypersensitivity or a history of allergies.

• In patients with a history of GI disease (especially colitis), give cautiously because of an increased risk of pseudomembranous colitis.

• Give cautiously in renal impairment because of higher and more prolonged serum concentrations.

PREPARATION & STORAGE

Available as a white to off-white sterile powder in 500 mg, 1 g, and 2 g vials; also available in 1 g and 2 g piggyback vials for infusion. Powder and solution may darken, but potency isn't generally changed. Store powder at 59° to 86° F. (15° to 30° C.). Protect from light.

Piggyback vials are supplied under reduced pressure because carbon dioxide is released and positive pressure develops when the drug is reconstituted. Venting may be necessary. Follow each brand's reconstitution instructions.

To reconstitute a 500 mg vial, add 5 ml of sterile water for injection, yielding a concentration of 100 mg/

ml. To reconstitute a 1 g vial, add 3 ml of sterile water for injection to yield a concentration of 280 mg/ml, or 10 ml to yield 95 to 100 mg/ml. To reconstitute a 2 g vial, add 10 ml of sterile water for injection to yield a concentration of 180 mg/ml.

If you're using the 1 or 2 g piggyback vial, reconstitute with 10 ml of sterile water for injection and dilute with 90 ml of a compatible I.V. solution. The resultant solution will contain 10 mg/ml for the 1 g vial and 20 mg/ml for the 2 g vial.

Solutions usually remain potent for 17 to 24 hours at room temperature and for 7 days when refrigerated. If stored at $-4°$ F. ($-20°$ C.) immediately after reconstitution, they usually remain potent for 3 to 6 months. Avoid heating after thawing or refreezing. Thawed solutions usually retain potency for 8 to 24 hours at room temperature and for 4 to 7 days if refrigerated. Don't use if solution is cloudy or contains a precipitate.

For infusions at concentrations between 1 and 40 mg/ml, use these solutions: 0.9% sodium chloride injection; ⅙ M sodium lactate injection; dextrose 5% in 0.2%, 0.45%, or 0.9% sodium chloride; or dextrose 5% or 10% in water. For concentrations between 1 and 20 mg/ml, use Ringer's injection, Ringer's lactate injection, invert sugar 10% in sterile water for injection, or dextrose 5% and Normosol-M. These solutions may be stored for 24 hours at room temperature or for 7 days if refrigerated. Solutions in dextrose 5% or 0.9% sodium chloride remain stable for at least 6 hours at room temperature in plastic tubing, drip chambers, or volume-control devices of infusion sets.

ADMINISTRATION
Direct injection: First remove any carbon dioxide bubbles. Then inject reconstituted drug directly into vein over 3 to 5 minutes. Alternatively, give through an I.V. line containing a free-flowing, compatible solution.
Intermittent infusion: Using a Y-type administration set, infuse solution over 15 to 30 minutes. Discontinue primary solution during ceftazidime infusion.
Continuous infusion: Infuse prescribed volume over 24 hours. Don't use thawed solutions.

INCOMPATIBILITY
Incompatible with aminoglycosides and sodium bicarbonate solutions.

ADVERSE REACTIONS
Life-threatening: anaphylaxis.
Other: abdominal cramps, bacterial and fungal superinfection, diarrhea, dizziness, dysgeusia, dyspnea, eosinophilia, fever, headache, injection site reaction (inflammation, pain), leukopenia, nausea, paresthesias, pruritus, pseudomembranous colitis, rash, sore mouth or tongue, thrombocytosis, urticaria, vomiting.

INTERACTIONS
Aminoglycosides: increased risk of nephrotoxicity and synergistic effect against *Pseudomonas aeruginosa* and Enterobacteriaceae.
Azlocillin, carbenicillin, cefsulodin, mezlocillin, piperacillin: synergistic effect against *P. aeruginosa.*
Clavulanic acid: synergistic effect against *Bacteroides fragilis* resistant to ceftazidime alone.
Metronidazole: partial synergistic effect against *Clostridium.*
Probenecid: prolonged and increased serum concentrations of ceftazidime.

EFFECTS ON DIAGNOSTIC TESTS

BUN: elevated levels.

Coombs' test: positive findings (may also occur in neonates whose mothers received drug before delivery).

Serum creatinine: transiently elevated levels.

Serum alkaline phosphatase, LDH, SGOT, SGPT: increased levels.

Urine glucose: false-positive results when tested with cupric sulfate (Benedict's solution, Clinitest).

SPECIAL CONSIDERATIONS

• Treat overdose and anaphylactic reaction symptomatically.

• Check for previous penicillin or cephalosporin hypersensitivity before giving first dose. Negative history doesn't rule out future allergic reaction.

• Obtain specimens for culture and sensitivity testing before first dose. Therapy may start before results are available.

• If diarrhea persists during therapy, collect stool specimens to rule out possible pseudomembranous colitis.

• Closely monitor renal function if patient has renal impairment or is receiving aminoglycoside antibiotics or potent diuretics because of potential for nephrotoxicity.

• If patient must restrict sodium intake, include 54 mg sodium per gram of ceftazidime in daily count.

• Observe patient for superinfection with prolonged use.

---

ceftizoxime sodium
Cefizox

Pregnancy Risk Category: B

PHARMACOKINETICS

Distribution: widespread, appearing in gallbladder, bone, heart, prostate, uterus, saliva, aqueous humor, bile, surgical wounds, and pleural, ascitic, and peritoneal fluids. Drug crosses the placenta. Also appears in cerebrospinal fluid when meninges are inflamed.

Metabolism: not metabolized.

Excretion: primarily in urine; mostly unchanged in 8 hours, with complete elimination in 24 hours. Serum half-life ranges from 85 to 115 minutes. Drug also appears in breast milk.

Action: onset, immediately after administration; peak level, after 30 minutes.

MECHANISM OF ACTION

Inhibits mucopeptide synthesis in the bacterial cell wall, promoting osmotic instability. Drug's spectrum of activity includes such gram-positive aerobic bacteria as *Staphylococcus aureus,* many strains of *S. epidermidis,* group A and group B streptococci, *Streptococcus pneumoniae,* and *Corynebacterium diphtheriae.*

Susceptible gram-negative aerobic bacteria include *Citrobacter freundii, Enterobacter aerogenes, E. cloacae, Escherichia coli, Klebsiella pneumoniae, Morganella morganii, Proteus mirabilis, P. vulgaris, Providencia, Salmonella, Shigella, Serratia marcescens, Haemophilus influenzae* (including ampicillin-resistant strains), *Neisseria gonorrhoeae* (including penicillin-resistant strains), *N. meningitidis* and some strains of *Acinetobacter, Aeromonas hydrophila, Moraxella, Pseudomonas aeruginosa, Yersinia enterocolitica,* and *Pasteurella multocida.*

Susceptible anaerobic bacteria include *Actinomyces, Bacteroides, Bifidobacterium, Eubacterium, Fusobacterium, Peptococcus, Peptostreptococcus, Propionibacterium, Veillonella,* and strains of *Clostridium.*

INDICATIONS & DOSAGE

• Life-threatening infections caused by susceptible organisms. *Adults:* 3 to 4 g q 8 hours. In renal impairment, a loading dose of 500 mg to 1 g may be given. Maintenance dose is determined by creatinine clearance. If clearance exceeds 80 ml/minute, give usual adult dosage; if it ranges from 50 to 79 ml/minute, give 750 mg to 1.5 g q 8 hours; if it ranges from 5 to 49 ml/minute, give 500 mg to 1 g q 12 hours; below 5 ml/minute, give 500 mg to 1 g q 48 hours, or 500 mg q 24 hours. *Children over age 6 months:* 200 mg/kg daily in divided doses. Maximum dosage, 12 g daily.

• Uncomplicated infections (except those of the urinary tract) to severe infections caused by susceptible organisms. *Adults:* 1 to 2 g q 8 to 12 hours. Maximum dosage, 12 g daily. In renal impairment, maintenance dosage determined by creatinine clearance. If clearance exceeds 80 ml/minute, give usual adult dosage; if it ranges from 50 to 79 ml/minute, give 500 mg q 8 hours; if it ranges from 5 to 49 ml/minute, give 250 to 500 mg q 12 hours; below 5 ml/minute, give 500 mg q 48 hours or 250 mg q 24 hours. *Children over age 6 months:* 50 mg/kg q 6 to 8 hours.

• Uncomplicated urinary tract infection caused by susceptible organisms. *Adults:* 500 mg q 12 hours. Give higher dosage in *P. aeruginosa* infection.

CONTRAINDICATIONS & CAUTIONS

• Contraindicated in cephalosporin hypersensitivity. Use cautiously in patients with penicillin hypersensitivity or a history of allergies.

• Use cautiously in patients with a history of GI disease (especially colitis) because of an increased risk of pseudomembranous colitis.

• Use cautiously in patients with renal impairment because of risk of toxicity from prolonged serum clearance.

PREPARATION & STORAGE

Available as a white to pale yellow crystalline powder in 1 and 2 g vials; protect from light and store at 59° to 86° F. (15° to 30° C.). Drug is also supplied as a frozen solution in 50 ml single-dose plastic containers, equivalent to 1 or 2 g in dextrose 5% in water; store frozen but not below −4° F. (−20° C.).

When reconstituting powder, add 10 ml of sterile water to the 1 g vial and 20 ml to the 2 g vial. This yields a concentration of 95 mg/ml.

Reconstitute piggyback vials with 50 to 100 ml of 0.9% sodium chloride injection. Alternatively, use dextrose 5% or 10% in water; dextrose 5% in 0.2%, 0.45%, or 0.9% sodium chloride; Ringer's injection; Ringer's lactate; invert sugar 10% in sterile water for injection; or 5% sodium bicarbonate in sterile water for injection. Shake well. For continuous infusion, add to compatible solution an amount appropriate for the patient's condition. Solutions remain stable for 24 hours at room temperature or for 96 hours if refrigerated. They may turn yellow to amber, but this color change doesn't affect potency. However, don't use if solution is cloudy or contains precipitate.

Thaw frozen solution at room temperature. Discard if you detect leaks, cloudiness, precipitation, or a broken seal. After thawing, the solution remains stable for 24 hours at room temperature or for 10 days if refrigerated. Don't refreeze.

ADMINISTRATION

Direct injection: Inject reconstituted drug over 3 to 5 minutes directly into a vein or an I.V. line containing a com-

patible solution. Don't inject commercially available frozen solutions intended for infusion.
Intermittent infusion: Infuse 50 to 100 ml of diluted drug into established I.V. line over 15 to 30 minutes.
Continuous infusion: Using an infusion pump, give solution over 24 hours.

INCOMPATIBILITY
Incompatible with aminoglycosides.

ADVERSE REACTIONS
Life-threatening: anaphylaxis.
Other: anemia, bacterial and fungal superinfection, chills, diarrhea, dizziness, edema, eosinophilia, fatigue, fever, headache, injection site reaction (burning, cellulitis, induration, pain, phlebitis, pseudomembranous colitis, sterile abscess, thrombophlebitis, tissue sloughing), leukopenia, malaise, nausea, neutropenia, paresthesias, pruritus, rash, thrombocytopenia, thrombocytosis, urticaria, vertigo, vomiting.

INTERACTIONS
Aminoglycosides: heightened risk of nephrotoxicity and synergistic effect against *P. aeruginosa, S. marcescens,* and Enterobacteriaceae.
Probenecid: prolonged elimination half-life of ceftizoxime.

EFFECTS ON DIAGNOSTIC TESTS
BUN, serum creatinine: elevated levels.
Coombs' test: positive findings (may also occur in neonates whose mothers received drug before delivery).
Serum alkaline phosphatase, LDH, SGOT, SGPT: increased levels.

SPECIAL CONSIDERATIONS
• Treat overdose and anaphylactic reaction symptomatically and supportively. Hemodialysis may help to remove drug.
• Check for previous penicillin or cephalosporin hypersensitivity before giving first dose. Negative history doesn't rule out future allergic reaction.
• Obtain specimens for culture and sensitivity testing before first dose. Therapy may start before results are available.
• If diarrhea persists during therapy, collect stool specimens to rule out possible pseudomembranous colitis.
• If patient receives high doses, takes other antibiotics (especially aminoglycosides), or has renal impairment, monitor renal function and intake and output because of the risk of nephrotoxicity.
• If the patient has sodium restrictions, be sure to account for 60 mg of sodium in each gram of drug.
• Frozen solution contains dextrose 5%.
• If the patient is undergoing hemodialysis, give dose after dialysis session. Supplemental doses aren't required.
• Observe patient for superinfection with prolonged use.

ceftriaxone sodium
Rocephin

Pregnancy Risk Category: B

PHARMACOKINETICS
Distribution: widespread, with therapeutic levels found in myometrium, gallbladder, bone, lungs, prostate, bile, sputum, and peritoneal, ascitic, synovial, pleural, and blister fluids. Higher concentrations appear in cerebrospinal fluid when meninges are inflamed. Drug is 58% to 96% bound to plasma proteins; it readily crosses the placenta.

Metabolism: partly in liver, and partly in intestine after biliary excretion.

Excretion: by renal and biliary routes; 40% to 60% excreted unchanged in urine by glomerular filtration, the remainder removed in feces unchanged or as metabolites. Low levels appear in breast milk. Elimination half-life is 6 to 9 hours.

Action: peak level, 30 minutes.

MECHANISM OF ACTION

A semisynthetic third-generation cephalosporin, ceftriaxone achieves its bactericidal effects by inhibiting mucopeptide synthesis in the bacterial cell wall, promoting osmotic instability. Its broad spectrum of activity includes gram-positive bacteria, including *Staphylococcus aureus, Staphylococcus epidermidis, Streptococcus pneumoniae,* group A beta-hemolytic streptococci, and groups B and D streptococci.

Susceptible gram-negative bacteria include *Neisseria gonorrhoeae, N. meningitidis, Escherichia coli, Klebsiella pneumoniae, Morganella morganii, Haemophilus influenzae* (including ampicillin-resistant strains), *H. parainfluenzae, Enterobacter aerogenes, E. cloacae, Citrobacter, Proteus mirabilis, P. vulgaris, Providencia rettgeri, P. stuartii, Pseudomonas, Serratia marcescens, Salmonella, Shigella, Yersinia enterocolitica, Acinetobacter, Moraxella,* and *Eikenella corrodens.*

Susceptible anaerobic bacteria include *Actinomyces, Borrelia burgdorferi, Fusobacterium, Lactobacillus, Peptococcus, Peptostreptococcus, Propionibacterium,* and *Veillonella.*

INDICATIONS & DOSAGE

• Severe infections caused by susceptible organisms. *Adults:* 1 to 2 g once daily or in divided doses q 12 hours. Maximum of 4 g daily. Dosage depends on infection type and severity. *Children under age 12:* 50 to 75 mg/kg daily in divided doses q 12 hours. Maximum of 2 g daily.

• Meningitis. *Adults and children:* 100 mg/kg daily in divided doses q 12 hours. May give 75 mg/kg loading dose. Maximum of 4 g daily.

• Disseminated gonococcal infections. *Adults:* 1 g daily for 7 days.

• Surgical prophylaxis. *Adults:* 1 g 30 minutes to 2 hours before surgery, then 750 mg q 8 to 12 hours. Discontinue within 24 hours.

• Acute pelvic inflammatory disease. *Prepubertal children:* 100 mg/kg daily with other antibiotics.

• Lyme disease. *Adults:* 1 to 2 g q 12 to 24 hours.

CONTRAINDICATIONS & CAUTIONS

• Contraindicated in cephalosporin hypersensitivity.

• Use cautiously in patients with penicillin hypersensitivity, a history of allergies, or renal or hepatic impairment. In renal or hepatic impairment, dosage adjustment not usually necessary. However, dose should not exceed 2 g per day while monitoring serum levels.

• In patients with a history of GI disease (especially colitis), administer carefully because of a magnified risk of pseudomembranous colitis.

PREPARATION & STORAGE

Available as a white to yellowish orange crystalline powder in vials containing 250 mg, 500 mg, 1 g, or 2 g. Also available in 1 g and 2 g piggyback vials. When reconstituted, solution turns light yellow to amber, depending on the diluent, drug concentration, and storage duration.

Reconstitute with sterile water for injection, 0.9% sodium chloride injection, dextrose 5% or 10% injection, or a combination of sodium chloride and dextrose injection and other compatible solutions. These include sodium lactate, invert sugar 10%, sodium bicarbonate 5%, Freamine III, dextrose 5% and Normosol-M, dextrose 5% and Ionosol B, and mannitol 5% or 10%.

Reconstitute by adding 2.4 ml diluent to the 250 mg vial, 4.8 ml to the 500 mg vial, 9.6 ml to the 1 g vial, and 19.2 ml to the 2 g vial. Reconstitute the 1 g piggyback vial with 10 ml diluent and the 2 g vial with 20 ml diluent. All reconstituted solutions yield a concentration that averages 100 mg/ml.

After reconstitution, dilute further for intermittent infusion to desired concentration. Concentrations of 10 to 40 mg/ml are recommended, but lesser ones can be used.

I.V. dilutions are stable for 24 hours at room temperature.

ADMINISTRATION
Direct injection: Inject reconstituted drug over 2 to 4 minutes directly into a vein, through an intermittent infusion device, or into an I.V. line containing a compatible solution.
Intermittent infusion: Give diluted drug over 15 to 30 minutes, using an intermittent infusion device or an I.V. line containing a compatible solution. Administer over 10 to 30 minutes in neonates or children.
Continuous infusion: not recommended.

INCOMPATIBILITY
Incompatible with aminoglycosides.

ADVERSE REACTIONS
Life-threatening: anaphylaxis.
Other: abdominal cramps, anemia, bacterial and fungal superinfection, diaphoresis, diarrhea, dizziness, dysgeusia, dyspepsia, dyspnea, eosinophilia, flushing, genital pruritus, headache, hypersensitivity reaction (chills, fever, pruritus, rash), hypoprothrombinemia (rare), injection site reaction (pain, phlebitis), leukopenia, nausea, neutropenia, pseudomembranous colitis, sore mouth or tongue, thrombocytopenia, thrombocytosis, vomiting.

INTERACTIONS
Aminoglycosides: increased risk of nephrotoxicity and synergistic effect against *P. aeruginosa, S. marcescens,* and Enterobacteriaceae.
Probenecid: decreased ceftriaxone excretion.

EFFECTS ON DIAGNOSTIC TESTS
BUN, serum creatinine: elevated levels.
Prothrombin time: prolonged.
Serum alkaline phosphatase, bilirubin, SGOT, SGPT: increased levels.
Urinalysis: casts possible.
Urine glucose: false-positive findings if using cupric sulfate (Clinitest, Benedict's solution).

SPECIAL CONSIDERATIONS
• Treat overdose symptomatically.
• Check for previous penicillin or cephalosporin allergy before giving first dose. Negative history doesn't rule out future allergic reaction.
• Obtain specimens for culture and sensitivity testing before first dose. Therapy may start before results are available.
• If diarrhea persists during therapy, collect stool specimens to rule out possible pseudomembranous colitis.
• If patient receives high doses (more than 2 g daily), takes other antibiotics (especially aminoglycosides), or has renal impairment, monitor renal function and intake and output because of the risk of nephrotoxicity.

• If the patient has sodium restrictions, include 83 mg of sodium per gram of ceftriaxone in daily count.
• Treatment should continue for at least 2 days after symptoms of infection disappear. Usual duration of 4 to 14 days may be prolonged in severe infection.
• Use glucose oxidase methods (Clinistix, Tes-Tape) for urine glucose determinations to avoid spurious results.
• Drug isn't removed by hemodialysis or peritoneal dialysis.
• Observe patient for superinfection with prolonged use.
• High doses and rapid infusion rates increase risk of cholelithiasis.

---

cefuroxime sodium
Kefurox, Zinacef♦

Pregnancy Risk Category: B

PHARMACOKINETICS
Distribution: throughout fluids and tissues, with therapeutic levels found in pleural and synovial fluid, cerebrospinal fluid (in meningeal inflammation), bile, sputum, bone, and aqueous humor. Drug is 33% to 50% bound to plasma proteins. It crosses the placenta.
Metabolism: not metabolized.
Excretion: in urine by glomerular filtration and tubular secretion as unchanged drug; most removed within 6 hours, 90% to 100% within 24 hours. Serum half-life is 1 to 2 hours. Drug appears in breast milk.
Action: peak serum level, 15 minutes.

MECHANISM OF ACTION
A semisynthetic second-generation cephalosporin, cefuroxime achieves its bactericidal effects by inhibiting mucopeptide synthesis in the bacterial cell wall, promoting osmotic instability. Drug's spectrum of activity includes most gram-positive aerobic cocci, such as *Staphylococcus aureus, Staphylococcus epidermidis, Streptococcus pneumoniae,* group A beta-hemolytic streptococci, and group B streptococci. Drug is also effective against many gram-negative aerobic bacteria, including *Neisseria gonorrhoeae, Escherichia coli, Klebsiella pneumoniae, Proteus mirabilis, P. inconstans, Salmonella, Shigella, Enterobacter aerogenes, Morganella morganii, Providencia rettgeri, Haemophilus parainfluenzae,* ampicillin-resistant strains of *Haemophilus influenzae,* most strains of *Neisseria meningitidis,* many strains of *Citrobacter diversus,* and some strains of *C. freundii.*

Susceptible anaerobic bacteria include *Actinomyces, Clostridium, Eubacterium, Fusobacterium, Lactobacillus, Peptococcus, Peptostreptococcus, Propionibacterium acnes,* and *Veillonella.*

INDICATIONS & DOSAGE
• Uncomplicated urinary tract infections, skin and skin structure infections, disseminated gonococcal infections, and uncomplicated pneumonia caused by susceptible organisms. *Adults:* 750 mg q 8 hours. *Children over age 3 months:* 50 to 100 mg/kg daily in divided doses q 6 to 8 hours.
• Severe or complicated infections caused by susceptible organisms. *Adults:* 1.5 g q 8 hours.
• Bacterial meningitis. *Adults:* up to 3 g q 8 hours.
• Life-threatening infections or infections caused by less susceptible organisms. *Adults:* 1.5 g q 6 hours. *Note:* Dosage in renal failure reflects creatinine clearance. For adults with a creatinine clearance above 20 ml/min, give 750 mg to 1.5 g q 8 hours. If it

---

ranges from 10 to 20 ml/min, give 750 mg q 12 hours; below 10 ml/min, 750 mg q 24 hours.

If the patient's undergoing hemodialysis, give dose at end of session.
• Preoperative prophylaxis for clean-contaminated or potentially contaminated surgery. *Adults:* 1.5 g 30 to 60 minutes before surgery and during prolonged procedures, then 750 mg q 8 hours for at least 24 hours afterward. Open-heart surgery patients should receive 1.5 g initially and q 12 hours, to total of 6 g.

CONTRAINDICATIONS & CAUTIONS
• Contraindicated in hypersensitivity to cephalosporins.
• Use cautiously in known hypersensitivity to penicillin and in ulcerative colitis, regional enteritis, and antibiotic-associated colitis because of a heightened risk of pseudomembranous colitis.
• Also use cautiously in renal dysfunction because of the risk of toxicity.

PREPARATION & STORAGE
Available as a sterile powder in 750 mg and 1.5 g vials. Store vials between 59° and 86° F. (15° and 30° C.) and protect from light.

Reconstitute 750 mg vial with 9 ml of sterile water for injection, withdrawing 8 ml for 750 mg dose. For the 1.5 g vial, reconstitute with 16 ml of sterile water for injection, withdrawing the entire volume for a 1.5 g dose. After reconstitution, the solutions maintain potency for 24 hours at room temperature and for 48 hours if refrigerated. Properly frozen solutions can be stored for up to 6 months.

For infusion, dilute 750 mg or 1.5 g in 50 to 100 ml of dextrose 5% in water for injection. Solution will maintain potency for 24 hours at room temperature and for 7 days if refrigerated. Other compatible solutions include dextrose 5% in 0.2%, 0.45%, or 0.9% sodium chloride; dextrose 10% in water; invert sugar 10%; Ringer's injection; Ringer's lactate; 0.9% sodium chloride; and ⅙ M sodium lactate.

ADD-Vantage vials should be reconstituted according to the manufacturer's directions.

ADMINISTRATION
Direct injection: Give directly into vein over 3 to 5 minutes, or inject into an I.V. line containing a free-flowing, compatible solution.
Intermittent infusion: Infuse solution over 15 to 60 minutes. Discontinue primary infusion during cefuroxime administration.
Continuous infusion: Using an established I.V. line, infuse the solution at the ordered rate.

INCOMPATIBILITY
Incompatible with aminoglycosides.

ADVERSE REACTIONS
Life-threatening: anaphylaxis.
Other: bacterial and fungal superinfection, diarrhea, nausea, nephrotoxicity, pseudomembranous colitis, thrombophlebitis.

INTERACTIONS
Aminoglycosides: synergistic effect against some susceptible organisms.
Diuretics: increased risk of renal impairment.
Probenecid: increased or prolonged cefuroxime serum concentration.

EFFECTS ON DIAGNOSTIC TESTS
Coombs' test: positive findings.
Hematocrit, hemoglobin level: reduced.
Serum alkaline phosphatase, LDH, SGOT, SGPT: increased levels.

Serum bilirubin: elevated levels.
Serum glucose: false-negative reaction using ferricyanide tests.
Urine glucose: false-positive results when tested with cupric sulfate (Benedict's solution, Clinitest).
WBC count: eosinophilia, neutropenia, leukopenia.

SPECIAL CONSIDERATIONS

• Treat overdose or anaphylaxis symptomatically. Hemodialysis and peritoneal dialysis can remove drug.
• Check for previous penicillin or cephalosporin hypersensitivity. Negative history doesn't rule out future allergic reaction.
• Obtain specimens for culture and sensitivity testing before giving first dose. Therapy may start before results are available.
• If diarrhea persists during therapy, collect stool specimens to rule out possible pseudomembranous colitis.
• If patient has sodium restrictions, include 54.2 mg of sodium for each gram of cefuroxime in daily count.
• Monitor intake and output and serum creatinine and BUN levels to avoid risk of nephrotoxicity.
• Use Clinistix or Tes-Tape for urine glucose determinations to prevent spurious results.

cephalothin sodium
Keflin♦♦, Keflin Neutral

Pregnancy Risk Category: B

PHARMACOKINETICS
Distribution: throughout most body tissues and fluids. Drug readily crosses the placenta.
Metabolism: 10% to 40% metabolized in liver and kidneys.
Excretion: 60% to 95% in urine as unchanged drug and metabolite by tubular secretion. Serum half-life ranges from 30 to 60 minutes. Low levels appear in breast milk.
Action: peak serum levels, 15 to 30 minutes; duration, 4 to 5 hours.

MECHANISM OF ACTION
A semisynthetic first-generation cephalosporin, cephalothin achieves its bactericidal effects by inhibiting mucopeptide synthesis of the bacterial cell wall, promoting osmotic instability. Its spectrum of activity includes most gram-positive aerobic cocci, including *Staphylococcus aureus, Staphylococcus epidermidis,* group A beta-hemolytic streptococci, group B streptococci, and *Streptococcus pneumoniae.* The drug may have limited effects against such gram-negative aerobic cocci as *Escherichia coli, Klebsiella pneumoniae, Proteus mirabilis,* and *Shigella.*

INDICATIONS & DOSAGE
• Severe infection caused by susceptible organisms. *Adults:* 2 g q 4 hours, if needed.
• Uncomplicated infection caused by susceptible organisms. *Adults:* 500 mg to 1 g q 4 to 6 hours. *Children:* 20 to 40 mg/kg q 4 to 6 hours.
• Surgical prophylaxis. *Adults:* 1 to 2 g 30 to 60 minutes before surgery; 1 to 2 g q 6 hours for 24 hours after it, then single dose of 20 to 30 mg/kg. For lengthy surgery, give 1 to 2 g intraoperatively. *Children:* 20 to 30 mg/kg 30 to 60 minutes before surgery, then q 6 hours for 24 hours. *Note:* Adjust dosage in renal failure. For adults, give loading dose of 1 to 2 g. Maintenance dosage reflects creatinine clearance. Maximum dosage is 2 g q 6 hours for clearance of 50 to 80 ml/min, 1.5 g q 6 hours for 25 to 50 ml/min, 1 g q 6 hours for 10 to 25 ml/min, 0.5 g q 6 hours for

2 to 10 ml/min, and 0.5 g q 8 hours for lower levels.

CONTRAINDICATIONS & CAUTIONS
• Contraindicated in cephalosporin hypersensitivity.
• Use with caution in hypersensitivity to penicillins or other drugs.
• In GI disease (especially colitis), give cautiously because of an increased risk of pseudomembranous colitis.
• Also give cautiously in renal impairment because of the drug's prolonged elimination half-life.

PREPARATION & STORAGE
Available as a white crystalline powder in 1, 2, and 4 g vials. Also available as a solution containing 1 or 2 g of cephalothin in dextrose 5% injection. Store powder between 59° and 86° F. (15° and 30° C.).

Reconstitute powder with sterile water for injection, 0.9% sodium chloride, dextrose 5% in water, Ringer's lactate, or other solutions with a pH of less than 5. For direct injection or intermittent infusion, add 10 ml of a compatible solution for each gram; for continuous infusion, add 20 ml solution for each 4 g. Solution may be diluted further for infusion. Compatible solutions include dextrose 5% in Ringer's lactate, dextrose 5% in 0.9% sodium chloride, dextrose 5% or 10% in water, dextrose 5% in Isolyte M, dextrose 5% in Isolyte P, Ringer's lactate, and 0.9% sodium chloride.

After reconstitution, solutions remain potent for 96 hours when refrigerated and for 12 weeks when frozen at −4° F. (−20° C.). Warm slowly at room temperature before use. Don't refreeze after thawing. Concentrated solutions may darken at room temperature; this doesn't affect potency.

ADMINISTRATION
Direct injection: Give directly into vein over 3 to 5 minutes, or give slowly through an I.V. line containing a free-flowing, compatible solution.
Intermittent infusion: Using a Y-type administration set, infuse solution over prescribed duration. Discontinue primary infusion during cephalothin administration.
Continuous infusion: Give ordered volume over 24 hours.

INCOMPATIBILITY
Incompatible with aminoglycosides, aminophylline, bleomycin sulfate, calcium chloride, calcium gluceptate, calcium gluconate, cimetidine, colistimethate sodium, dopamine, doxorubicin, erythromycin lactobionate, methylprednisolone sodium succinate, norepinephrine injection, oxytetracycline, penicillin G, potassium, phenobarbital sodium, polymyxin B, prochlorperazine edisylate, and tetracycline hydrochloride.

ADVERSE REACTIONS
Life-threatening: anaphylaxis.
Other: bacterial and fungal superinfection, chills, diarrhea, dizziness, edema, fever, headache, leukopenia, malaise, nausea, nephrotoxicity, neutropenia, paresthesias, pruritus, pseudomembranous colitis, rash, severe phlebitis and thrombophlebitis, thrombocytopenia, thrombocytosis, toxic paranoid reaction, urticaria, vertigo, vomiting.

INTERACTIONS
Aminoglycosides: increased risk of nephrotoxicity; also possible synergistic effect against some organisms.
Probenecid: elevated cephalothin blood levels.

EFFECTS ON DIAGNOSTIC TESTS

BUN, serum alkaline phosphatase, SGOT, SGPT: increased levels.
Coombs' test: positive results.
Prothrombin time: prolonged.
Urine glucose: false-positive results when tested with cupric sulfate (Benedict's solution, Clinitest).
Urine and serum creatinine: false-positive results when using Jaffé method.

SPECIAL CONSIDERATIONS

• Treat overdose symptomatically. Hemodialysis or peritoneal dialysis removes drug.
• Check for previous penicillin or cephalosporin hypersensitivity before first dose. Negative history doesn't rule out future allergic reaction.
• Obtain specimens for culture and sensitivity testing before first dose. Therapy may start before results are available.
• If diarrhea persists during therapy, collect stool specimens to rule out possible pseudomembranous colitis.
• Check I.V. site frequently for signs of phlebitis. Severe phlebitis occurs most commonly when patient receives more than 6 g daily for longer than 3 days.
• If patient must restrict sodium, include 63 mg of sodium per gram of cephalothin in daily count.
• Monitor renal function because of risk of nephrotoxicity from reduced serum clearance. Dose may be reduced.
• Use Clinistix or Tes-Tape for urine glucose determinations to prevent spurious results.
• Observe patient for fungal and bacterial superinfection with prolonged use.

cephapirin sodium
Cefadyl♦

Pregnancy Risk Category: B

PHARMACOKINETICS

Distribution: throughout body tissues, fluids (including pleural and synovial fluid), and bone. Only small amounts penetrate the blood-brain barrier, even if meninges are inflamed. Drug crosses the placenta, with fetal levels exceeding maternal ones by about 10%. Drug is 44% to 50% bound to plasma proteins.
Metabolism: partly in plasma, liver, and kidneys to desacetylcephapirin. About half the antibacterial activity comes from the parent compound and 20% from desacetylcephapirin.
Excretion: in urine by glomerular filtration and tubular secretion and reabsorption; 70% to 94% is removed unchanged in 6 hours and the rest is excreted as metabolite. Drug appears in breast milk. Serum half-life averages 35 minutes.
Action: peak serum levels, immediately after administration.

MECHANISM OF ACTION

A semisynthetic first-generation cephalosporin, cephapirin achieves its bactericidal effects by inhibiting mucopeptide synthesis in the bacterial cell wall, promoting osmotic instability. It is active against most gram-positive aerobic cocci, including *Staphylococcus aureus, Staphylococcus epidermidis,* group A beta-hemolytic streptococci, group B streptococci, and *Streptococcus pneumoniae.* The drug may have limited effects against such gram-negative aerobic cocci as *Escherichia coli, Klebsiella pneumoniae, Proteus mirabilis,* and *Shigella.*

Unmarked trade names available in the United States only.
♦Also available in Canada.   ♦♦Available in Canada only.

INDICATIONS & DOSAGE

• Severe infection caused by susceptible organisms or infection caused by less susceptible organisms. *Adults:* 1 to 3 g q 4 to 6 hours. Maximum of 12 g daily.

• Mild to moderate infection caused by susceptible organisms. *Adults:* 0.5 to 1 g q 4 to 6 hours. *Children age 3 months and older:* 10 to 20 mg/kg q 6 hours.

• Surgical prophylaxis. *Adults:* 1 to 2 g 30 to 60 minutes before surgery, repeated intraoperatively, then q 6 hours for 24 hours after surgery. Prophylaxis may continue for up to 5 days if severe complications loom. *Note:* Adjust dosage in renal failure. For adults, give lower dose of 7.5 to 15 mg/kg q 12 hours.

CONTRAINDICATIONS & CAUTIONS

• Contraindicated in cephalosporin hypersensitivity.

• Use with caution in hypersensitivity to penicillins or other drugs and in renal impairment.

• In GI disease (especially colitis), use cautiously because of a heightened risk of pseudomembranous colitis.

• Safe use in infants under age 3 months hasn't been established.

PREPARATION & STORAGE

Available as a white powder in 500 mg and 1, 2, and 4 g vials; store at 59° to 86° F. (15° to 30° C.). For direct injection, reconstitute with 10 ml of sterile water for injection, 0.9% sodium chloride, or dextrose 5% in water. For infusion, add 40 to 50 ml of dextrose 5% in Ringer's injection; dextrose 5% in Ringer's lactate; dextrose 5% in 0.2%, 0.45%, or 0.9% sodium chloride; dextrose 5%, 10%, or 20% in water; invert sugar 20% and 0.9% sodium chloride; Ringer's injection or Ringer's lactate injection; 0.9% sodium chloride; ⅙ M sodium lactate; dextrose 10% in Ionosol G; Ionosol D-CM; Normosol-R; or dextrose 5% in Normosol-R.

Solution concentrations of 50 to 400 mg/ml remain stable for 12 hours at room temperature. A concentration of 5 mg/ml stays stable for 10 days if refrigerated. All solutions may be frozen in the original vial immediately after reconstitution. Thawed slowly to room temperature, they remain stable for at least 12 hours. Solutions may turn yellow, but this doesn't affect potency.

Cephapirin is also available in 20 g I.V. packs. Add 67 ml of 0.9% sodium chloride, dextrose 5% in water, or sterile water to yield a concentration of 250 mg/ml.

ADMINISTRATION

Direct injection: Give directly into vein over 3 to 5 minutes.

Intermittent infusion: Using a Y-type administration set, infuse into an I.V. line containing a free-flowing, compatible solution. If you're using a 4 g piggyback vial, discontinue primary infusion while giving cephapirin.

Continuous infusion: Give solution over 24 hours.

INCOMPATIBILITY

Incompatible with aminoglycosides, aminophylline, ascorbic acid injection, epinephrine hydrochloride, oxytetracycline, phenytoin sodium, tetracycline hydrochloride, and thiopental sodium.

ADVERSE REACTIONS

Life-threatening: anaphylaxis.
Other: bacterial and fungal superinfection, chills, diarrhea, dizziness, eosinophilia, fever, leukopenia, malaise, nausea, neutropenia, phlebitis, pruritus, pseudomembranous colitis,

rash, thrombocytopenia, thrombocytosis, thrombophlebitis, urticaria, vertigo, vomiting.

INTERACTIONS
Aminoglycosides: synergistic antibacterial effects against some organisms and increased risk of nephrotoxicity.
Nephrotoxic drugs: heightened risk of nephrotoxicity.
Probenecid: increased and prolonged cephapirin serum concentrations.

EFFECTS ON DIAGNOSTIC TESTS
BUN: elevated levels.
Coombs' test: positive results.
Serum alkaline phosphatase, bilirubin, LDH, SGOT, SGPT: increased levels.
Urine glucose: false-positive results when tested with cupric sulfate (Benedict's solution, Clinitest).

SPECIAL CONSIDERATIONS
• Treat overdose symptomatically.
• Check for previous penicillin or cephalosporin hypersensitivity before first dose. Negative history doesn't rule out future allergic reaction.
• Obtain specimens for culture and sensitivity testing before first dose. Therapy may start before results are available.
• If diarrhea persists during therapy, collect stool specimens to rule out possible pseudomembranous colitis.
• If patient has sodium restrictions, keep in mind that each gram of drug contains 54 mg of sodium.
• Monitor renal function because of risk of nephrotoxicity from reduced clearance. Dose may be reduced.
• Give hemodialysis patient 7.5 to 15 mg/kg before dialysis and every 12 hours thereafter.
• Use Clinistix or Tes-Tape for urine glucose determinations to prevent spurious results.

• Observe patient for superinfection with prolonged use.

cephradine
Velosef♦

Pregnancy Risk Category: B

PHARMACOKINETICS
Distribution: well dispersed to bone, tissue, pleural and synovial fluids, kidneys, and middle ear but barely distributed to cerebrospinal fluid even with meningeal inflammation. Drug is 6% to 20% bound to plasma protein. It crosses the placenta.
Metabolism: not metabolized.
Excretion: in urine by glomerular filtration and tubular secretion as unchanged drug, with 60% to 90% removed within 6 hours. Serum half-life ranges from 40 to 120 minutes. Drug appears in breast milk.
Action: peak serum levels, 5 minutes.

MECHANISM OF ACTION
A semisynthetic first-generation cephalosporin, cephradine achieves its bactericidal effects by inhibiting mucopeptide synthesis in the bacterial cell wall, promoting osmotic instability. Its spectrum of activity includes most gram-positive aerobic cocci, including *Staphylococcus aureus, Staphylococcus epidermidis,* group A beta-hemolytic streptococci, group B streptococci, and *Streptococcus pneumoniae*. The drug may have limited effects against such gram-negative aerobic cocci as *Escherichia coli, Klebsiella pneumoniae, Proteus mirabilis,* and *Shigella*.

INDICATIONS & DOSAGE
• Severe infections caused by susceptible organisms. *Adults:* 500 mg

---

to 1 g b.i.d. to q.i.d., not to exceed 8 g daily.
• Infections caused by susceptible organisms. *Adults:* 250 to 500 mg q 6 hours or 500 mg q 12 hours. *Children age 9 months and older:* 12 to 25 mg q 6 to 12 hours. Maximum dosage is 8 g daily.
• Surgical prophylaxis. *Adults:* 1 g 30 to 90 minutes before surgery, then q 4 to 6 hours for up to 24 hours after it. In cesarean surgery, give first dose when umbilical cord is clamped, then give q 6 or 12 hours for two doses.
Note: Adjust dosage in renal failure according to degree of renal impairment, severity of infection, and susceptibility of organism. For adults, dosage reflects creatinine clearance. If clearance is less than 5 ml/min, dosage is 500 mg to 1 g q 48 to 72 hours; if 5 to 19 ml/min, 500 mg to 1 g q 48 hours; if 20 to 59 ml/min, 500 mg to 1 g q 24 hours; if more than 60 ml/min, give usual adult dose.

CONTRAINDICATIONS & CAUTIONS
• Contraindicated in cephalosporin hypersensitivity.
• Use with caution in hypersensitivity to penicillins or other drugs.
• In GI disease (especially colitis), give cautiously because of an increased risk of pseudomembranous colitis.
• Also give cautiously in renal impairment because of prolonged elimination half-life.

PREPARATION & STORAGE
Available as a white crystalline powder in 250 mg, 500 mg, and 1 g vials; as a sodium-free powder; and as 100 ml infusion bottles containing 2 or 4 g of cephradine. Protect powder from light and store at room temperature; don't use if discolored.

Bottles remain stable at room temperature for 10 hours.
Reconstitute vials with sterile water for injection or dextrose 5% in water. For direct injection, dissolve 250 or 500 mg of powder in 5 ml, 1 g of powder in 10 ml. For intermittent infusion, dilute reconstituted powder with 150 to 200 ml of a compatible solution. For continuous infusion, dilute with a larger volume to a concentration of 5 mg/ml or less. Compatible solutions include dextrose 5% or 10% in water, ⅙ M sodium lactate, invert sugar 10% and water, and dextrose 5% and Ionosol B. Ringer's lactate may be used to reconstitute and dilute sodium-free cephadrine powder.
Solutions with a concentration of 50 mg/ml or less remain stable for 10 hours at room temperature; those with a concentration of 50 to 100 mg/ml may be frozen at −4° F. (−20° C.) in their original containers immediately after reconstitution, remaining stable for 6 weeks.

ADMINISTRATION
Direct injection: Inject into vein over 3 to 5 minutes.
Intermittent infusion: Slowly infuse 150 to 200 ml solution using an established I.V. line. Alternatively, hang the 100 ml infusion bottle from an I.V. pole and infuse directly over 20 to 30 minutes.
Continuous infusion: Infuse solution over the prescribed duration.

INCOMPATIBILITY
Incompatible with calcium salts, Ringer's injection or Ringer's lactate, dextrose 5% in Ringer's lactate injection, and Normosol-R and 0.9% sodium chloride. Cephradine shouldn't be mixed with penicillins, aminoglycosides, or other cephalosporins.

ADVERSE REACTIONS
Life-threatening: anaphylaxis.
Other: bacterial and fungal superinfection, chest tightness, chills, diarrhea, dizziness, edema, eosinophilia, fever, headache, hepatomegaly, leukopenia, malaise, nausea, neutropenia, paresthesias, pruritus, pseudomembranous colitis, rash, thrombocytopenia, thrombocytosis, thrombophlebitis, urticaria, vertigo, vomiting.

INTERACTIONS
Aminoglycosides: additive or synergistic effects against certain organisms and increased risk of nephrotoxicity.
Nephrotoxic drugs: heightened risk of nephrotoxicity.
Probenecid: prolonged cephradine serum concentrations.

EFFECTS ON DIAGNOSTIC TESTS
Coombs' test: positive results.
Urine glucose: false-positive results when tested with cupric sulfate (Benedict's solution, Clinitest).

SPECIAL CONSIDERATIONS
• Check for previous penicillin or cephalosporin hypersensitivity before first dose. Negative history doesn't rule out future allergic reaction.
• Obtain specimens for culture and sensitivity testing before first dose. Therapy may start before results are available.
• If diarrhea persists during therapy, collect stool specimens to rule out possible pseudomembranous colitis.
• If patient has sodium restrictions, keep in mind that each gram of drug contains 6 mg of sodium.
• Monitor BUN and serum creatinine levels regularly. Reduced dosage may be necessary.
• Check infusion site for signs of phlebitis.
• Use Clinistix or Tes-Tape for urine glucose determinations to prevent spurious results.
• Observe patient for superinfection with prolonged use.

chloramphenicol sodium succinate
Chloromycetin Sodium Succinate♦, Mychel-S, Pentamycetin♦♦

Pregnancy Risk Category: C

PHARMACOKINETICS
Distribution: throughout most body tissues and fluids. Highest concentrations occur in the liver and kidneys, lowest ones in the brain and cerebrospinal fluid. Drug crosses the placenta, but cord levels remain lower than maternal ones. It's about 60% bound to plasma proteins.
Metabolism: hydrolyzed in plasma to free chloramphenicol and inactivated in the liver by glucuronyl transferase.
Excretion: 68% to 99% removed in urine over 3 days, mostly as metabolites. Small amounts appear in bile, feces, and breast milk. Elimination half-life ranges from 90 minutes to 4 hours. In neonates ages 1 to 2 days, half-life is 24 hours or more. In neonates ages 10 to 16 days, half-life is 10 hours.
Action: peak serum level, 1 hour.

MECHANISM OF ACTION
Usually bacteriostatic, chloramphenicol may also act bactericidally in high concentrations. Drug binds to 50S ribosomal subunit, inhibiting peptide bond formation. It's effective against many gram-positive aerobic bacteria, including *Streptococcus pneumoniae* and other streptococci; many gram-negative aerobic bacteria, including *Haemophilus influen-*

zae, Neisseria meningitidis, Salmonella, and *Shigella;* and many anaerobic bacteria, including *Bacteroides melaninogenicus, B. fragilis, Clostridium, Fusobacterium,* and *Veillonella.* Other susceptible organisms include *Rickettsia, Chlamydia,* and *Mycoplasma.*

INDICATIONS & DOSAGE
• Severe infections caused by susceptible organisms. *Adults and children:* 12.5 to 25 mg/kg q 6 hours. Reduce high doses as soon as possible. *Neonates:* 6.25 mg/kg q 6 hours. Full-term neonates over age 2 weeks may receive up to 12.5 mg/kg q 4 hours.

High doses should be used only to maintain effective serum levels. Adjust dosage based on patient response and therapeutic serum level (peak of 10 to 20 mcg/ml, trough of 5 to 10 mcg/ml).

CONTRAINDICATIONS & CAUTIONS
• Contraindicated in chloramphenicol hypersensitivity.
• Use cautiously in hepatic or renal impairment and with other myelosuppressive drugs because of a heightened risk of toxicity.
• During pregnancy, use only for life-threatening infections.
• Administer cautiously and in reduced dosage in infants to avoid cardiovascular collapse (gray baby syndrome).

PREPARATION & STORAGE
Available as a white or yellow powder in 1 g and 10 g vials. Reconstitute with 10 ml of dextrose 5% in water or bacteriostatic water for injection. Shake well.

For intermittent infusion, dilute required dose in 50 ml of a compatible solution. (Most solutions are compatible.) Preparation remains stable for 30 days if refrigerated. Avoid freezing. Don't use cloudy solutions.

ADMINISTRATION
Direct injection: Don't give any concentration exceeding 100 mg/ml. Inject reconstituted drug over 1 to 3 minutes directly into a vein or into an I.V. line containing a free-flowing, compatible solution.
Intermittent infusion: Give over 15 to 20 minutes through an established I.V. line containing a free-flowing compatible solution.
Continuous infusion: not recommended.

INCOMPATIBILITY
Incompatible with carbenicillin disodium, chlorpromazine, glycopyrrolate, hydroxyzine hydrochloride, oxytetracycline, prochlorperazine edisylate, promethazine, and tetracycline hydrochloride.

ADVERSE REACTIONS
Life-threatening: anaphylaxis, aplastic anemia, bone marrow depression, cardiovascular collapse (in neonates), granulocytopenia, gray baby syndrome, hypoplastic anemia, thrombocytopenia.
Other: bacterial and fungal superinfection, confusion, delirium, depression, diarrhea, headache, nausea, optic and peripheral neuritis, vomiting, weakness in hands and feet.

INTERACTIONS
Acetaminophen: possible reduced chloramphenicol excretion.
Alfentanil: decreased plasma clearance and prolonged duration.
Bactericidal antibiotics: reduced effectiveness.
Bone marrow depressants: heightened risk of myelosuppression.
Hydantoins: decreased chloramphenicol metabolism.

Iron preparations, vitamin B₁₂: delayed hematopoietic response.
Oral antidiabetics: enhanced hypoglycemic effect.
Pyridoxine: decreased effectiveness, requiring a dosage increase.

EFFECTS ON DIAGNOSTIC TESTS
Bentiromide test: invalid results.
Urine glucose: false-positive results with cupric sulfate (Benedict's solution, Clinitest).

SPECIAL CONSIDERATIONS
• Treat overdose symptomatically. Charcoal hemoperfusion (but not hemodialysis) effectively removes drug.
• Chloramphenicol should be used only for severe infections that fail to respond to other drugs because of the risk of serious toxicity. Change to oral dose as soon as possible.
• Herxheimer-like reactions have occurred when treating patients with typhoid fever, probably resulting from release of bacterial endotoxins.
• In children under age 2 years, watch for signs of gray syndrome (failure to feed, vomiting, abdominal distention, pallor, cyanosis, irregular respirations). Discontinue drug and notify doctor immediately if these signs appear.
• Monitor CBC, platelet count, serum iron level, and reticulocyte count before and every 2 days during therapy. Stop drug immediately if anemias develop.
• Check injection site daily for phlebitis.
• Carefully monitor serum levels in patient with renal or hepatic impairment because of slight difference between therapeutic and toxic levels. Dosage may be reduced.
• If patient has sodium restrictions, keep in mind that solution contains 52 mg of sodium per gram.

• Use glucose oxidase methods (Clinistix, Tes-Tape) for urine glucose determinations to avoid spurious results.
• Observe patient for fungal and bacterial superinfection with prolonged use.

chlordiazepoxide hydrochloride
Librium♦

Controlled Substance Schedule IV
Pregnancy Risk Category: D

PHARMACOKINETICS
Distribution: throughout body tissues and across the blood-brain barrier and the placenta.
Metabolism: in liver to active metabolites.
Excretion: in urine as active and inactive metabolites, with small amounts removed in feces. Serum half-life is 5 to 30 hours. Drug and metabolites appear in breast milk.
Action: onset, 1 to 5 minutes; duration, 15 to 60 minutes.

MECHANISM OF ACTION
May suppress the limbic subcortical levels of the CNS, resulting in CNS depression ranging from mild sedation to coma. The drug also possesses skeletal muscle relaxant and anticonvulsant properties.

INDICATIONS & DOSAGE
• Short-term management of acute or severe anxiety. *Adults:* 50 to 100 mg initially, then 25 to 50 mg t.i.d. or q.i.d., as needed. *Children over age 12:* 25 to 50 mg t.i.d. or q.i.d.
• Acute alcohol withdrawal and management of associated agitation. *Adults:* 50 to 100 mg initially, then repeated q 2 to 4 hours, as needed, up to a maximum of 300 mg daily.

CONTRAINDICATIONS & CAUTIONS

• Contraindicated in chlordiazepoxide hypersensitivity; in shock or unstable blood pressure because of the drug's hypotensive effects; in coma because of further sedation; and in acute alcohol intoxication with depressed vital signs because of possible deepened CNS depression.
• Contraindicated in patients with psychosis and hyperkinesis because of possible paradoxical reaction.
• Also contraindicated in patients with a history of drug dependence or emotional instability; in glaucoma; in hypoalbuminemia; in severe depression and myasthenia gravis; and in severe chronic obstructive pulmonary disease.
• Give cautiously in hepatic or renal impairment and in elderly or debilitated patients because of slowed drug metabolism and excretion.

PREPARATION & STORAGE

Available as a dry powder in an amber ampule containing 100 mg of drug. Don't use the I.M. diluent provided by the manufacturer for I.V. reconstitution because air bubbles will form. Instead, dilute powder with 5 ml of sterile 0.9% sodium chloride or sterile water for injection to yield a concentration of 20 mg/ml. Gently rotate ampule until powder dissolves. Protect from light. Administer immediately and discard any unused solution.

ADMINISTRATION

Direct injection: Inject reconstituted drug into vein over at least 1 minute. Alternatively, inject drug into I.V. tubing at a site directly above needle or cannula insertion site. After injection, flush tubing with 0.9% sodium chloride.
Intermittent infusion: not recommended.
Continuous infusion: not recommended.

INCOMPATIBILITY

Incompatible with benzquinamide. However, manufacturer recommends that chlordiazepoxide not be mixed with any other drug.

ADVERSE REACTIONS

Life-threatening: anaphylaxis, apnea, bradycardia, cardiac arrest, hypotension.
Other: agranulocytosis, anorexia, ataxia, bitter or metallic taste, blurred vision, confusion, constipation, diplopia, dizziness, drowsiness, dry mouth, edema, fatigue, headache, hiccups, increased salivation and bronchial secretions, jaundice, nausea, nystagmus, paradoxical CNS excitation (especially in children and psychiatric patients), photosensitivity, pruritus, rash, status epilepticus, swollen tongue, syncope, thrombophlebitis, urticaria, vertigo, vivid dreams, weakness.

INTERACTIONS

Alcohol, barbiturates, MAO inhibitors, parenteral magnesium sulfate, phenothiazines, psychotropics, tricyclic antidepressants, valproic acid, other CNS depressants: deepened CNS depression.
Antihypertensives: potentiated hypotension.
Carbamazepine: possible reduced serum levels of either drug.
Cimetidine, disulfiram: elevated serum levels.
Ketamine: increased risk of hypotension and respiratory depression.
Levodopa: reduced control of parkinsonian symptoms.
Oral contraceptives: possible impaired metabolism.

EFFECTS ON DIAGNOSTIC TESTS

EEG: altered wave patterns of low-voltage, fast activity.

Gravindex® pregnancy test: false-positive results.

Serum alkaline phosphatase, bilirubin, LDH, SGOT, SGPT: increased levels.

Urine 17-ketosteroids: elevated or reduced levels.

SPECIAL CONSIDERATIONS

• *Treatment of overdose:* Provide supportive care. Maintain airway patency and give I.V. fluids. Administer norepinephrine or metaraminol for hypotension. Use of caffeine and sodium benzoate is controversial and of short-term benefit in reversing CNS depression.

• Take vital signs before therapy, and monitor them carefully during and after injection. Be especially alert for hypotension, respiratory depression, and bradycardia. Report them to doctor immediately. Keep resuscitation equipment readily available.

• Maintain bed rest for at least 3 hours after injection.

• Institute safety measures to prevent falls and injuries caused by hypotension, confusion, or oversedation.

• Monitor CBC and liver function studies during prolonged therapy.

• Be alert for signs of drug dependency.

• Drug isn't appreciably removed by hemodialysis.

• May contain benzyl alcohol.

---

chlorothiazide sodium
Diuril Intravenous Sodium

Pregnancy Risk Category: D

PHARMACOKINETICS

Distribution: into extracellular space and across the placenta. Variable protein binding.

Metabolism: apparently not metabolized.

Excretion: in urine by glomerular filtration and proximal tubular secretion within 5 hours; 95% excreted unchanged. Drug appears in breast milk.

Action: onset, 15 minutes; peak effect, 30 minutes; duration, 2 hours.

MECHANISM OF ACTION

Although chlorothiazide's precise mechanism of action isn't known, the drug apparently alters tubular cell metabolism in the cortical diluting segment of the nephron. It increases excretion of sodium, chloride, and water. Natriuresis is accompanied by some loss of potassium and bicarbonate.

Direct arteriolar dilation may contribute to the drug's antihypertensive effect.

INDICATIONS & DOSAGE

• Treatment of edema in an emergency or in NPO patient. *Adults:* initially, 0.5 to 2 g daily in divided doses given b.i.d.; subsequent dosages reflect patient response.

CONTRAINDICATIONS & CAUTIONS

• Contraindicated in anuria and hypersensitivity to thiazides, sulfonamides, or thimerosal, a preservative.

• Use cautiously in hepatic impairment and progressive hepatic disease because electrolyte imbalance may

---

precipitate hepatic coma; in electrolyte imbalance because of possible exacerbation; and in renal impairment because azotemia can occur.
• Also use cautiously in lupus erythematosus because drug may exacerbate the disorder, and in sympathectomy because of enhanced antihypertensive effects.
• Drug isn't recommended for pediatric use.

PREPARATION & STORAGE
Available as a dry white powder in 500 mg vials. Reconstitute with at least 18 ml of sterile water for injection. For infusion, further dilute with 0.2%, 0.45%, or 0.9% sodium chloride solution; dextrose 5% in 0.2%, 0.45%, or 0.9% sodium chloride; Ringer's lactate; Dextran 6% in 0.9% sodium chloride; Dextran 6% in dextrose 5%; ⅙ M sodium lactate; and invert sugar 5% or 10% in water. Solutions remain stable for 24 hours at room temperature.

ADMINISTRATION
Direct injection: Inject reconstituted drug directly into vein, through an I.V. line containing a free-flowing, compatible solution, or through an intermittent infusion device.
Intermittent infusion: Give diluted solution using an intermittent infusion device or an I.V. line containing a free-flowing, compatible solution over the prescribed duration.
Continuous infusion: not recommended.

INCOMPATIBILITY
Incompatible with whole blood, its derivatives, and these solutions: Ionosol B, D, or G and invert sugar 10%; Ionosol B or D-CM and dextrose 5%; Ionosol PSL; Normosol-M (900 calories); Normosol-M in dextrose 5%; and Normosol-R in dextrose 5%.

Also incompatible with amikacin, chlorpromazine, codeine, hydralazine, insulin, levorphanol, methadone, morphine, norepinephrine bitartrate, polymyxin B, procaine, prochlorperazine edisylate, prochlorperazine mesylate, promazine, promethazine hydrochloride, streptomycin, tetracycline hydrochloride, triflupromazine, and vancomycin.

ADVERSE REACTIONS
Life-threatening: anaphylaxis, CNS depression, coma, hepatic encephalopathy secondary to electrolyte imbalance.
Other (mostly dose-related): agranulocytosis, aplastic anemia, dilutional hyponatremia, dizziness, fever, headache, hypercalcemia, hyperglycemia and glycosuria in diabetes, hypokalemia, hypomagnesemia, muscle spasms, nausea, orthostatic hypotension, paresthesias, photosensitivity, polyarteritis nodosa, purpura, rash, respiratory distress, restlessness, thrombocytopenic purpura, urticaria, vertigo, yellow vision.

INTERACTIONS
ACTH, adrenocorticoids, amphotericin B (parenteral), glucocorticoids: worsened electrolyte imbalance.
Alcohol, barbiturates, opiates: worsened orthostatic hypotension.
Allopurinol, colchicine, probenecid, sulfinpyrazone: elevated serum uric acid level and renal impairment.
Amiodarone: increased risk of dysrhythmias associated with hypokalemia.
Antihypertensives: potentiated hypotension.
Anti-inflammatory analgesics, estrogens, sympathomimetics: decreased antihypertensive effects.

Calcium-containing drugs: hypercalcemia resulting from reduced calcium excretion.
Carbonic anhydrase inhibitors: increased diuresis.
Cardiac glycosides: heightened risk of toxicity.
Dopamine: enhanced diuresis.
Insulin, oral antidiabetics: elevated serum glucose levels.
Lithium: toxicity caused by reduced renal clearance.
Methenamine: reduced effectiveness.
Neuromuscular blocking agents: prolonged effects.
Sodium bicarbonate: increased risk of alkalosis.

EFFECTS ON DIAGNOSTIC TESTS

Bentiromide test: unreliable findings. Discontinue drug at least 3 days before test.
Glucose tolerance test: unreliable findings.
Histamine, phentolamine, and tyramine tests for pheochromocytoma: false-negative results.
Serum bilirubin, cholesterol, glucose, triglycerides, uric acid: increased levels.
Serum calcium, magnesium, potassium, protein-bound iodine, sodium: decreased levels.
Urine hydroxycorticosteroids: reduced levels.

SPECIAL CONSIDERATIONS

• *Treatment of overdose:* Signaled by lethargy progressing to coma without evidence of electrolyte imbalance or dehydration, an overdose should be treated supportively. Monitor serum electrolyte levels and renal function, and replace fluid and electrolytes as needed. Provide measures to support respiratory, cardiovascular, and renal function, if necessary.

• Carefully monitor intake and output and serum electrolyte levels.
• Provide potassium replacements.
• If dilutional hyponatremia occurs, restrict fluids to 500 ml daily and withdraw drug. This complication occurs most commonly in hot weather and in patients with congestive heart failure or hepatic disease.
• Because chlorothiazide raises serum glucose and uric acid levels, patients taking antidiabetic or antigout drugs may require a dosage adjustment.
• Patients with preexisting hepatic disease are most susceptible to hypokalemic hypochloremic alkalosis.
• Elderly patients may be more sensitive to the drug's effects.

chlorpheniramine maleate
Chlor-Pro, Chlor-Trimeton, Phenetron

Pregnancy Risk Category: B

PHARMACOKINETICS

Distribution: rapidly and extensively distributed throughout the body and CNS, with 69% to 72% of drug bound to plasma proteins. Highest concentrations occur in the lungs, heart, kidneys, brain, spleen, and small intestine. Drug probably crosses the placenta.
Metabolism: in the liver.
Excretion: apparently almost completely in urine; small amounts (under 1%) appear in feces and breast milk. Excretion rate falls as urine pH rises. About 35% is excreted within 48 hours, primarily as metabolites. Serum half-life ranges from 12 to 43 hours for adults and from 10 to 13 hours for children. In patients with chronic renal failure, serum half-life may increase to 330 hours.

Action: peak level, at end of infusion; duration, 4 to 25 hours.

MECHANISM OF ACTION
Chlorpheniramine competes with H_1-receptors on effector cells to prevent, but not reverse, the histamine-mediated response.

INDICATIONS & DOSAGE
• Allergic transfusion reaction. *Adults and children over age 11:* 10 to 20 mg as a single dose. Maximum dosage, 40 mg in 24 hours.
• Adjunctive treatment of anaphylaxis. *Adults and children over age 11:* 15 to 20 mg as a single dose after acute symptoms have been controlled by epinephrine administration and other measures.
• Uncomplicated allergic conditions in NPO patient. *Adults and children over age 11:* 5 to 20 mg as a single dose.

CONTRAINDICATIONS & CAUTIONS
• Contraindicated in patients with antihistamine hypersensitivity, in neonates, and in premature infants.
• Give cautiously in narrow-angle glaucoma, stenotic peptic ulcer, pyloroduodenal obstruction, symptomatic prostatic hypertrophy, and bladder neck obstruction. Severity of symptoms may increase.
• Because of an atropine-like effect, use drug cautiously in increased intraocular pressure, hyperthyroidism, cardiovascular disease, and asthma.
• Use cautiously in patients with renal dysfunction because of increased risk of toxicity.

PREPARATION & STORAGE
Available in 1 ml ampules (concentration of 10 mg/ml). For intermittent infusion, dilute drug with 50 to 100 ml of a compatible solution (most solutions are compatible).

Protect solution from light to prevent discoloration; discard if discolored. Store at room temperature or refrigerate.

ADMINISTRATION
Direct injection: Slowly inject reconstituted drug into an I.V. line containing a free-flowing, compatible solution.
Intermittent infusion: Infuse slowly using an established I.V. line.
Continuous infusion: not recommended.

INCOMPATIBILITY
Incompatible with calcium chloride, iodipamide meglumine, kanamycin sulfate, norepinephrine bitartrate, and phenobarbital sodium.

ADVERSE REACTIONS
Life-threatening: anaphylaxis.
Other: acute labyrinthitis; blurred vision; chest tightness; chills; confusion; constipation; diaphoresis; diarrhea; diplopia; disturbed coordination; dizziness; dry mouth, nose, and throat; epigastric distress; euphoria; excitation; extrasystole; fatigue; headache; hypotension; hysteria; insomnia; irritability; nasal congestion; nausea; nervousness; neuritis; palpitations; paresthesias; photosensitivity; rash; restlessness; sedation; seizures; tachycardia; thickened bronchial secretions; tinnitus; tremors; urinary frequency and difficulty; urticaria; vertigo; vomiting; wheezing.

INTERACTIONS
Alcohol, other CNS depressants: deepened CNS depression.
Antimuscarinics: potentiated effects.
MAO inhibitors: prolonged and intensified anticholinergic effects.
Ototoxic drugs: possible masked symptoms of ototoxicity.

Phenytoin: possible increased effects.

EFFECTS ON DIAGNOSTIC TESTS
Skin tests for allergy: spurious results.

SPECIAL CONSIDERATIONS
• *Treatment of overdose:* Signs and symptoms of overdose include fixed, dilated pupils, flushed face, dry mouth, fever, excitation, hallucinations, ataxia, incoordination, athetosis, tonic-clonic seizures, and postictal depression that potentially may lead to coma, cardiorespiratory collapse, and death.

Treatment is symptomatic and supportive. If a vasopressor is needed, use norepinephrine or phenylephrine, not epinephrine. Physostigmine can help counteract CNS anticholinergic effects. If seizures continue, diazepam I.V. can be used. Treat fever with cold packs or tepid water sponging. Alcohol sponging should not be used.

• Young children are much more susceptible to toxic effects than adults.
• If patient is drowsy, give coffee or tea. If dry mouth occurs, give sugarless gum, sour hard candy, or ice chips.
• Withdraw drug 4 days before skin tests for allergy.
• Chlor-Pro may contain benzyl alcohol.

chlorpromazine hydrochloride
Largactil♦♦, Ormazine, Promaz

Pregnancy Risk Category: C

PHARMACOKINETICS
Distribution: widely distributed to most body fluids, with high concentrations in the brain, lungs, liver, kidneys, and spleen. Drug readily crosses the placenta and blood-brain barrier and is 92% to 97% bound to plasma proteins.
Metabolism: extensively metabolized in the liver, primarily to inactive metabolites, via hydroxylation, oxidation, demethylation, sulfoxide formation, and conjugation with gluconic acid.
Excretion: mainly as metabolites, primarily in the urine, but also in feces. Drug appears in breast milk.
Action: onset, unknown; duration, unknown.

MECHANISM OF ACTION
The drug achieves an antiemetic effect by blocking the vagus nerve in the GI tract. It also inhibits or blocks dopamine receptors in the chemoreceptor trigger zone of the medulla.

INDICATIONS AND DOSAGE
• Severe hiccoughs. *Adults:* 25 to 50 mg infused at rate of 1 mg/min.
• Adjunctive treatment for tetanus. *Adults:* 25 to 50 mg. *Children age 6 months or older:* 0.55 mg/kg q 6 to 8 hours. Maximum dose: 40 mg for children weighing less than 22.7 kg and 75 mg for children weighing 22.7 to 45.5 kg.
• Vomiting during surgery. *Adults:* 2 mg q 2 minutes. Total dose: 25 mg. *Children:* 1 mg q 2 minutes. Total dose: 0.275 mg/kg. May repeat dose

in 30 minutes if hypotension does not occur.

CONTRAINDICATIONS & CAUTIONS
• Contraindicated in hypersensitivity to phenothiazines and sulfites.
• Also contraindicated in severe toxic CNS depression, subcortical brain damage, bone marrow depression, and severe cardiovascular disorders because drug may worsen these conditions.
• Avoid use in such neurologic disorders as Reye's syndrome, meningitis, encephalopathy, and encephalitis because drug may mask symptoms or confuse diagnosis.
• Use carefully in patients with hypocalcemia to avoid possible dystonic reactions. Use cautiously in alcoholism because of possible deepened CNS depression.
• Also use cautiously in debilitated patients because of the increased risk of toxicity, and in elderly patients because of the increased risk of severe adverse effects.
• Because chlorpromazine may precipitate glaucoma, give cautiously to patients with glaucoma or a predisposition to this disorder.
• Administer cautiously to patients with hepatic or renal disease because they metabolize and excrete drug more slowly and therefore face a greater risk of toxicity. Also administer cautiously in Parkinson's disease because of possible potentiation of extrapyramidal effects.
• Use cautiously in peptic ulcer disease or urine retention because drug may exacerbate these conditions; in respiratory disease because of CNS depression and suppression of cough reflex; in seizure disorders because drug may lower seizure threshold; and in symptomatic prostatic hypertrophy because of increased risk of urine retention.

• Give carefully to patients who show severe reactions to insulin or electroconvulsive therapy.

PREPARATION AND STORAGE
Available in 1 and 2 ml ampuls and 10 ml multiple dose vials containing 25 mg/ml concentration. Store below 104° F. (40° C.), preferably between 59° and 86° F. (15° and 30° C.). Protect from light and freezing. Discard if darker than light amber or if precipitate forms.
   For direct injection, dilute with 0.9% sodium chloride to a 1 mg/ml concentration.
   For infusion, add ordered dose to 500 to 1,000 ml of 0.9% sodium chloride.

ADMINISTRATION
Direct injection: Slowly inject ordered amount of diluted drug (1 mg/ml concentration) into the tubing of a patent I.V. line. Direct injection is generally used for adjunctive treatment of tetanus and vomiting during surgery.
Intermittent infusion: not recommended.
Continuous infusion: Slowly infuse ordered dose diluted in 500 to 1,000 ml. Used for treatment of severe hiccoughs.

INCOMPATIBILITY
Incompatible with aminophylline, amphotericin B, ampicillin, atropine, chloramphenicol sodium succinate, chlorothiazide, cimetidine, dimenhydrinate, heparin, methicillin, methohexital, penicillin, pentobarbital, phenobarbital, thiopental, and solutions having a pH of 4 to 5.

ADVERSE REACTIONS
Life-threatening: anaphylaxis, angioedema, bronchospasm, cardiac arrest, laryngeal edema, laryngospasm, neuroleptic malignant syn-

drome (hyperthermia, altered mental status, altered blood pressure, tachycardia), severe hypotension.

Other: anorexia, anxiety, cerebral edema, contact dermatitis, constipation, dizziness, drowsiness, dyspepsia, dystonia, EKG changes, erythema, headache, hypotension, increased appetite, paralytic ileus, photosensitivity, restlessness, seizures, syncope, tachycardia, urticaria.

INTERACTIONS

Alcohol, CNS depressants, magnesium sulfate (parenteral): deepened CNS and respiratory depression.

Amantadine, antidyskinetics, antihistamines, antimuscarinics (especially atropine and related compounds): possible intensified antimuscarinic effects.

Amphetamines: reduced stimulant effects.

Anticonvulsants (including barbiturates): possible lowered seizure threshold, requiring dosage adjustment of these drugs.

Apomorphine: deepened CNS depression, possible decreased emetic response to this drug.

Appetite suppressants: possible antagonized anorectic effects.

Beta-adrenergic blockers: elevated serum levels of each drug.

Bone marrow depressants: possible increased leukopenia or thrombocytopenia.

Bromocriptine: possible inhibited effects.

Dopamine: possible antagonized peripheral vasoconstriction with high doses of dopamine.

Ephedrine, metaraminol: possible reduced pressor response.

Epinephrine: severe hypotension and tachycardia, resulting from blocked alpha-adrenergic effects.

Guanadrel, guanethidine: possible diminished hypotensive effects.

Hypotension-producing drugs: increased risk of severe hypotension.

Levodopa: inhibited antiparkinson effects.

Lithium: extrapyramidal symptoms and possible accelerated excretion.

MAO inhibitors, tricyclic antidepressants: possible intensified sedative and antimuscarinic effects of these drugs or chlorpromazine. Also increased risk of neuroleptic malignant syndrome.

Mephentermine: antagonized pressor effects.

Methoxamine, phenylephrine: possible decreased pressor effects and reduced duration of action of these drugs.

Metrizamide: possible lowered seizure threshold.

Other photosensitizing drugs: possible additive photosensitivity.

Ototoxic drugs (especially antibiotics): possible masked symptoms of ototoxicity.

Phenytoin: increased risk of phenytoin toxicity because of inhibited phenytoin metabolism.

Quinidine: possible additive cardiac effects.

Riboflavin: possible increased requirements.

Systemic methoxsalen, trioxsalen, tetracyclines: possible potentiated intraocular photochemical damage.

EFFECTS ON DIAGNOSTIC TESTS

EKG: possible changes in Q and T waves.

Gonadorelin test: blunted response because of increased serum prolactin levels.

Metapyrone test: possible reduced secretion of corticotropin.

Serum phenylalanine screening: possible false-positive results.

Urine pregnancy tests: possible false-positive or false-negative results, depending on test.

WBC and differential counts: possible decrease.

SPECIAL CONSIDERATIONS
• *Treatment of overdose:* No specific treatment as such; however, anticholinergic drugs may help control extrapyramidal symptoms. Treat severe hypotension with vasopressors, such as norepinephrine or phenylephrine (but not epinephrine).
• Because of possible hypotension, give I.V. only to patients on bed rest or to acute ambulatory patients who can be closely monitored. Monitor elderly patients carefully because they are especially vulnerable to hypotension and extrapyramidal symptoms. Usually, elderly or debilitated patients require a lowered dose.
• Establish baseline blood pressure and heart rate and monitor for tachycardia and hypotension. Keep patient lying down for at least 1 hour after injection, and advise him to change position slowly.
• After drug discontinuation, notify doctor if patient experiences dizziness, nausea and vomiting; GI upset, pain, trembling of hands and fingers; or controlled, repetitive movements of the mouth, tongue, and jaw.
• Keep in mind that chlorpromazine's antiemetic effect can obscure diagnosis of a condition with nausea as a primary symptom. Also remember that this drug prolongs sleep in postoperative patients.
• Give sugarless gum, sour hard candy, or mouthwash as needed to relieve dry mouth.
• Monitor intake and output for urine retention and constipation.
• To prevent dermatitis, avoid skin contact with drug.
• Advise women against breast-feeding during therapy.
• Elderly and pediatric patients are at greater risk of hypotensive and extrapyramidal reactions.

cimetidine hydrochloride
Tagamet♦

Pregnancy Risk Category: B

PHARMACOKINETICS
Distribution: throughout body tissues and across the placenta. Drug is 15% to 20% bound to plasma proteins.
Metabolism: in liver to sulfoxide and 5-hydroxymethyl derivatives.
Excretion: in urine, primarily unchanged, with remainder removed as two metabolites; 80% to 90% of drug is excreted in urine in 24 hours. Remainder excreted in feces. Serum half-life is 2 to 3 hours. Drug appears in breast milk.
Action: onset, immediately after I.V. injection; duration, 4 to 5 hours.

MECHANISM OF ACTION
Drug reduces gastric acid output and concentration by competitively inhibiting histamine's action on the H_2-receptors of gastric parietal cells, thereby raising gastric pH to 5 or higher. It reduces both basal and stimulated gastric acid production and helps reduce pepsin secretion by decreasing gastric juice volume.

INDICATIONS & DOSAGE
• Active gastric or duodenal ulcer. *Adults:* 300 mg q 6 to 8 hours (q 12 hours if creatinine clearance is less than 30 ml/minute). Maximum of 2,400 mg daily. Adjust dosage to maintain a gastric pH of greater than 5. *Children:* 5 to 10 mg/kg every 6 to 8 hours.
• Stress ulcers, peptic esophagitis, upper GI bleeding (when not caused by major vessel erosion). *Adults:* 300 to 400 mg q.i.d.
• Prophylaxis of aspiration pneumonitis. *Adults:* 300 mg I.M. before in-

duction of anesthesia followed by 300 mg I.V. q 4 hours until patient responds to verbal commands.
• Pathologic hypersecretory conditions or intractable ulcers. *Adults:* loading dose of 300 mg, then adjust dosage to patient's requirements.
Note: Reduced dosage may be necessary for adult patients with hepatic or renal failure.

CONTRAINDICATIONS & CAUTIONS
• Use cautiously in elderly patients and in patients with renal or hepatic insufficiency because of an increased risk of toxicity. Also use cautiously in patients under age 16 because of limited dosage data.

PREPARATION & STORAGE
Available in 2 ml single-dose disposable syringes containing 300 mg cimetidine; in 8 ml multidose vials containing 300 mg/2 ml; and in PVC bags containing 300 mg/50 ml.

For direct injection, dilute dose (including the single-dose form) with 20 ml of 0.9% sodium chloride for injection. For infusion, dilute with 50 to 100 ml of a compatible solution, such as amino acid solution, dextrose 5% in water, Ringer's injection, Ringer's lactate, invert sugar 5% in water, 0.9% sodium chloride, or dextrose 5% in 0.2%, 0.45%, or 0.9% sodium chloride.

Use reconstituted solutions within 48 hours. Check expiration dates. Protect from light and store at room temperature. Solution becomes cloudy if refrigerated. Discard solutions if discolored or if precipitate appears.

ADMINISTRATION
Direct injection: Inject diluted drug over at least 2 minutes directly into vein or through an I.V. line containing a free-flowing, compatible solu-

tion. Rapid injection may increase the risk of dysrhythmias and hypotension.
Intermittent infusion: Give 50 to 100 ml of diluted drug over 15 to 20 minutes, using an intermittent infusion device or infused into an I.V. line containing a free-flowing, compatible solution.
Continuous infusion: Dilute 900 mg of drug in 100 to 1,000 ml of compatible solution. Using an infusion pump, give no more than 37.5 mg/ hour. Total dosage not to exceed 900 mg daily.

INCOMPATIBILITY
Incompatible with aminophylline, amphotericin B, barbiturates, cefamandole, cefazolin, cephalothin, pentobarbital sodium, and a combination of pentobarbital sodium and atropine sulfate.

ADVERSE REACTIONS
Life-threatening: cardiac arrest; dysrhythmias, including sinus bradycardia, unifocal and multifocal premature ventricular contractions, ventricular fibrillation, and ventricular tachycardia; hypotension.
Other: agitation, agranulocytosis, anxiety, aplastic anemia, arthralgia, atrial fibrillation, bradycardia, confusion, diarrhea, disorientation, dizziness, fever, hallucinations, headache, hepatotoxicity, maculopapular or acnelike rash, myalgia, nephrotoxicity, neutropenia, palpitations, premature atrial contractions, psychosis, somnolence, urticaria.

INTERACTIONS
Alprazolam, chlordiazepoxide, diazepam, flurazepam, triazolam, tricyclic antidepressants: impaired metabolism.
Caffeine, ethanol: increased CNS effects.

Unmarked trade names available in the United States only.
♦ Also available in Canada.   ♦ ♦ Available in Canada only.

Calcium channel blockers, labe-talol, lidocaine, metoprolol, pro-pranolol, quinidine: decreased metabolism.
Disulfiram, estrogen-containing oral contraceptives, isoniazid: altered metabolism resulting from inhibition of hepatic microsomal enzymes.
Ketoconazole: reduced absorption possible because of increased gastric pH. Give at least 2 hours apart.
Metronidazole, phenytoin, sulfonyl-ureas, theophylline: impaired metabolism.
Myelosuppressive drugs (alkylating agents, antimetabolites): possible potentiated toxicity.
Procainamide: reduced excretion.
Triamterene: decreased metabolism and excretion.
Warfarin and similar anticoagu-lants: elevated serum levels.

EFFECTS ON DIAGNOSTIC TESTS
Gastric acid stimulation test (using pentagastrin): depressed gastric acid levels.
Serum alkaline phosphatase, creati-nine, prolactin, SGOT, SGPT: possible elevated levels.
Skin test for allergies: false-negative results because of inhibited cutaneous histamine response.

SPECIAL CONSIDERATIONS
• Treat overdose symptomatically. Treat tachycardia with a beta blocker. Hemodialysis promotes drug clearance.
• If cimetidine and coumarin antico-agulants must be given together, closely monitor prothrombin times and adjust dosage as necessary.
• Renal or hepatic failure requires dosage adjustment.
• If the patient's undergoing hemo-dialysis, give drug after dialysis session and every 12 hours during the interdialysis period.

• Malignant gastric ulcers have been shown to heal transiently on cimeti-dine therapy and must be closely monitored.
• Raised gastric pH may permit can-didal overgrowth in stomach.
• Elderly patients may be subject to cimetidine-induced confusion.
• Because cimetidine alters gastric pH, it may affect the bioavailability of many oral drugs.
• Cimetidine inhibits hepatic micro-somal enzymes and may decrease the metabolism of many drugs.
• Advise women taking cimetidine to avoid becoming pregnant. Also advise against breast-feeding during therapy.

ciprofloxacin
Cipro I.V.

Pregnancy Risk Category: C

PHARMACOKINETICS
Distribution: throughout body tissues; tissue concentration commonly exceeds serum concentrations. Crosses the placenta.
Metabolism: chiefly in liver.
Excretion: in normal renal function, 40% to 50% excreted in urine within 24 hours. Small amounts excreted in bile. Drug appears in breast milk.
Action: peak level, immediately after infusion.

MECHANISM OF ACTION
A broad spectrum quinolone antibi-otic, drug's exact mechanism un-known, but its bactericidal effects may result from inhibition of bacte-rial DNA replication in susceptible organisms.

INDICATIONS & DOSAGE
• Mild to moderate urinary tract in-fections. *Adults:* 200 mg q 12 hours.

• Severe to complicated urinary tract infections. *Adults:* 400 mg q 12 hours.

• Mild to moderate infections of lower respiratory tract, skin and skin structure, bone and joint infections. *Adults:* 400 mg q 12 hours.

Note: Dosage in renal failure reflects creatinine clearance. For adults with a clearance less than 29 ml/min, dosage is 200 to 400 mg q 18 to 24 hours.

Duration of treatment depends on severity of infection, but usually 7 to 14 days. Bone and joint infections may require treatment for 4 to 6 weeks or more.

CONTRAINDICATIONS & CAUTIONS

• Contraindicated in hypersensitivity to quinolone antimicrobial agents, in pregnant or breast-feeding women, and in patients under age 18.

• Contraindicated in concurrent I.V. therapy with theophylline.

• Use cautiously in elderly patients and in patients with renal impairment. Also use cautiously in patients with central nervous system disorders.

PREPARATION & STORAGE

Available as a clear, colorless to slightly yellow solution in 200 mg and 400 mg vials (injection concentrate). Dilute vials before use.

Reconstitute with 0.9% sodium chloride injection or 5% dextrose injection to concentrations of 1 to 2 mg/ml.

I.V. dilutions are stable for up to 14 days at room temperature or when refrigerated.

Premixed solution is also available in flexible containers of 200 mg in 100 ml 5% dextrose, and 400 mg in 200 ml 5% dextrose.

ADMINISTRATION

Continuous infusion: Infuse diluted solution over 60 minutes.

Intermittent infusion: Discontinue flow of any concurrent I.V. solutions temporarily while infusing drug.

INCOMPATIBILITY

None reported.

ADVERSE REACTIONS

Life-threatening: anaphylaxis, cardiovascular collapse, cardiopulmonary arrest, renal failure.

Other: abdominal pain or discomfort, arthralgia, confusion, crystalluria, diarrhea, eosinophilia, erythema, hallucinations, headache, light-headedness, local burning, nausea, oral candidiasis, paresthesia, photosensitivity, pruritus, rash, restlessness, seizures, swelling, thrombophlebitis, tremor.

INTERACTIONS

Antacids containing magnesium, aluminum, or calcium: decreased absorption of ciprofloxacin.

Alkalizers (urine): reduced solubility of ciprofloxacin.

Caffeine: increased half-life of caffeine and risk of CNS stimulation with concurrent use.

Probenecid: possible elevated ciprofloxacin level.

Theophylline: increased plasma theophylline concentrations; prolonged theophylline half-life.

EFFECTS ON DIAGNOSTIC TESTS

Alkaline phosphatase, SGPT, SGOT, LDH, serum bilirubin: hepatic elevations.

Blood glucose, triglycerides: elevated levels.

BUN, serum creatinine, uric acid: elevated levels.

Eosinophil: elevated levels.

Hemoglobin, hematocrit: decreased levels.

SPECIAL CONSIDERATIONS

• *Treatment of overdose:* Treat symptomatically and maintain adequate hydration.
• Carefully monitor SGPT, SGOT, LDH, CPK, serum bilirubin, eosinophil and platelet counts, and serum creatinine, BUN, uric acid, blood glucose, and triglyceride levels.
• Obtain specimen for culture and sensitivity tests before giving first dose.
• Observe patient for superinfection with prolonged use.
• Make sure patient has adequate hydration to avoid crystalluria.
• If patient is ambulatory, warn him of risk of dizziness.
• If patient is breast-feeding, give alternate drug or stop breast-feeding during therapy.
• Advise patient to avoid caffeine.
• Advise home care patient that hypersensitivity is common even after first dose. If skin rash or other allergic reaction occurs, have patient stop drug and notify his doctor.
• Warn home care patient of possible photosensitivity reaction.

---

cisplatin
(cis-platinum)
Platinol♦, Platinol-AQ

Pregnancy Risk Category: C

PHARMACOKINETICS
Distribution: throughout body fluids and tissues; highest levels in the liver, kidneys, intestines, and prostate. Cerebrospinal fluid concentrations are low. Readily crosses the blood-brain barrier and apparently crosses the placenta. It's extensively bound to plasma proteins.

Metabolism: rapid nonenzymatic conversion to inactive metabolites.
Excretion: in urine, predominantly by glomerular filtration, with 15% to 50% excreted within 48 hours. Drug's extensive binding prolongs excretion; 27% to 45% isn't eliminated for 3 to 10 days. Not known if drug appears in breast milk. Initial half-life averages about 35 minutes; terminal half-life, about 75 hours.
Action: peak level, at end of infusion; duration, several days.

MECHANISM OF ACTION
Precise mechanism of action unknown. Apparently, the drug crosslinks strands of DNA material, inhibiting DNA synthesis and leading to cell death.

INDICATIONS & DOSAGE
• Metastatic testicular tumors.
Adults: 20 mg/m² daily for 5 days q 3 weeks for three or four cycles, or 120 mg/m² single dose q 3 to 4 weeks for three cycles.
• Metastatic ovarian tumors. *Adults:* as part of combination therapy, 50 mg/m² q 3 to 4 weeks; as a single agent, 100 mg/m² q 4 weeks. Alternative dosages, 30 to 120 mg/m² q 4 to 5 weeks.
• Advanced bladder cancer when surgery or radiotherapy is no longer possible. *Adults:* 50 to 70 mg/m² q 3 to 4 weeks.
• Head and neck tumors. *Adults:* as part of combination therapy, 50 to 120 mg/m² according to hospital protocol; as a single agent, 80 to 120 mg/m² q 3 weeks or 50 mg/m² on 1st and 8th day of every 4-week cycle. *Children:* 60 mg/m² daily for 2 days q 3 to 4 weeks.
• Cervical carcinoma. *Adults:* 50 to 100 mg/m² q 3 weeks.
• Non-small-cell lung carcinoma. *Adults:* as part of combination therapy, 40 to 120 mg/m² q 3 to 6 weeks

as directed; as a single agent, 75 to 120 mg/m² q 3 to 6 weeks or 50 mg/m² on 1st and 8th day of every 4-week cycle.
• Osteogenic sarcoma, neuroblastoma. *Children:* 90 mg/m² q 3 weeks or 30 mg/m² q week.

CONTRAINDICATIONS & CAUTIONS
• Contraindicated in hypersensitivity to platinum-containing compounds.
• Also contraindicated in renal disease because of the risk of nephrotoxicity. Renal impairment usually occurs during the 2nd week after infusion but may occur within several days with high-dose regimens.
• Avoid use in existing or recent chicken pox or herpes zoster. Immunosuppressive properties increase the risk of generalized disease.
• To lessen the risk of cumulative immunosuppression, use cautiously in patients with preexisting myelosuppression or who have had cytotoxic drug or radiation therapy.
• Give cautiously to patients with hearing impairment because of an increased risk of cumulative ototoxicity; with existing or recent infection to avoid severe infection; and with gout or urate calculi because of possible hyperuricemia.

PREPARATION & STORAGE
Use extreme caution when preparing or giving cisplatin to avoid mutagenic, teratogenic, and carcinogenic risks. Use a biological containment cabinet and avoid contact with skin. Wear mask and gloves. If solution comes in contact with skin or mucosa, immediately wash thoroughly with soap and water. Dispose of needles, syringes, vials, and any unused drug carefully.

Available as a white powder in 10 and 50 mg vials. Protect unopened vials from bright sunlight; however, exposure to fluorescent light causes no problems. Store for up to 2 years at room temperature.

Reconstitute 10 mg vial with 10 ml of sterile water, 50 mg vial with 50 ml of sterile water (drug is also available as an aqueous solution of 50 mg/50 ml and 100 mg/100 ml). For intermittent infusion, dilute reconstituted drug in 2 liters of 0.33% or 0.45% sodium chloride along with 37.5 g of mannitol.

Precipitation may cause loss of potency. To avoid this, don't use needles, syringes, or I.V. kits containing aluminum parts and don't refrigerate reconstituted solutions.

Reconstituted solutions remain stable for 20 hours at room temperature. Solutions prepared with bacteriostatic water for injection with benzyl alcohol or parabens are stable for 72 hours.

ADMINISTRATION
Hydrate patient using 0.9% sodium chloride before giving drug. Maintain urine output of 150 to 400 ml/hour at onset of administration and for 4 to 6 hours thereafter.
Direct injection: not recommended.
Intermittent infusion: Give diluted solution through a separate I.V. line, using a 21G or 23G needle. Infuse over 6 to 8 hours or follow hospital protocol.
Continuous infusion: Infuse diluted solution over 24 hours or 5 days, according to hospital protocol.

INCOMPATIBILITY
Incompatible with aluminum, sodium bicarbonate, dextrose 5% in water, 0.1% sodium chloride, and solutions with a chloride content under 2%.

ADVERSE REACTIONS

Life-threatening: anaphylaxis, myelosuppression (anemia, thrombocytopenia, leukopenia).
Other: blindness, cardiac abnormalities, electrolyte disturbances (hypomagnesemia, hypocalcemia, hypokalemia, hypophosphatemia), hyperuricemia, nausea and vomiting, nephrotoxicity, neurotoxicity (peripheral neuropathy, seizures, loss of taste), optic neuritis, ototoxicity (tinnitus, high-frequency hearing loss, vestibular effects), papilledema, phlebitis.

INTERACTIONS

Aminoglycosides: heightened risk of nephrotoxicity and ototoxicity if given within 2 weeks after infusion.
Amphotericin B: increased risk of nephrotoxicity.
Bleomycin, methotrexate: altered elimination.
Etoposide: impaired elimination.
Live vaccine: possible potentiation of virus replication.
Myelosuppressive agents: additive bone marrow suppression.
Nephrotoxic or ototoxic drugs: magnified risk of toxicity.

EFFECTS ON DIAGNOSTIC TESTS

BUN, serum creatinine, uric acid: increased levels.
Creatinine clearance: reduced rate possible (sign of nephrotoxicity).
Serum calcium, magnesium, phosphate, potassium: possible decreased levels.
SGOT, SGPT: elevated levels.

SPECIAL CONSIDERATIONS

• *Treatment of overdose:* No specific antidote for overdose exists. Treat hepatic and hematologic toxicity symptomatically. Monitor vital signs during infusion.

• If anaphylaxis occurs, treat symptomatically.
• Determine serum magnesium, potassium, calcium, and creatinine levels, BUN levels, and creatinine clearance before first infusion and each course.
• Maintain urine output of 100 to 200 ml/hour for 18 to 24 hours after therapy.
• Nausea and vomiting may be severe enough to discontinue treatment. Nausea usually begins 1 to 6 hours after administration and may last for 24 hours or more. For an antiemetic, administer high doses of metoclopramide, diphenhydramine, or dexamethasone before and after each dose.
• Regularly perform neurologic examinations. Discontinue drug if neurotoxicity occurs.
• Monitor CBC and platelet count weekly; myelosuppression may be cumulative. Leukocyte and platelet nadirs generally occur 18 to 23 days after a single dose. Levels usually return to baseline within 13 to 62 days. Don't repeat dose unless platelet count exceeds 100,000/mm^3, WBC count is over 4,000/mm^3, creatinine level is under 1.5 mg/dl, or BUN level is under 25 mg/dl.
• Monitor liver and kidney function. Renal insufficiency, usually reversible, may occur within 4 weeks of administration. Patients with mild to moderate renal impairment may receive 50% to 75% of recommended dose. Regimens of I.V. hydration and diuresis and 6- to 8-hour infusions reduce the incidence and severity of nephrotoxicity.
• Perform audiometric tests before each course to detect high-frequency hearing loss. Up to one-third of patients show signs of ototoxicity after a single dose. Ototoxicity may be cumulative and severer in children.

• Cisplatin raises serum uric acid levels. Patients taking antigout drugs may need a dosage adjustment.

• Adequate hydration, allopurinol administration, and alkalinization of urine may prevent or minimize uric acid nephropathy from elevated serum uric acid levels.

• Cisplatin can be removed by hemodialysis for 3 hours after administration.

• Advise women of childbearing age to avoid becoming pregnant during therapy. Suggest consulting with doctor before making the decision to become pregnant.

---

clindamycin phosphate
Cleocin Phosphate, Dalacin C♦♦

Pregnancy Risk Category: B

PHARMACOKINETICS
Distribution: throughout body tissues and fluids, including saliva, bone, bile, and ascitic, pleural, and synovial fluid, with about 93% bound to plasma proteins. Drug readily crosses the placenta, but even with inflamed meninges, only small amounts reach cerebrospinal fluid.
Metabolism: partly changed in liver to active and inactive metabolites. Metabolic rate increases in children.
Excretion: in urine, bile, and feces as metabolites. Drug appears in breast milk. Its half-life is 2 to 3 hours.
Action: peak serum level, at end of infusion.

MECHANISM OF ACTION
Clindamycin is bactericidal or bacteriostatic, depending on its concentration and the susceptibility of the organism. Drug inhibits protein synthesis of susceptible bacteria.

Its spectrum of activity includes staphylococci, *Streptococcus pneumoniae,* and most other gram-positive cocci. Susceptible gram-negative and gram-positive anaerobic organisms include *Actinomyces, Bacteroides, Eubacterium, Fusobacterium, Propionibacterium, Peptococcus, Peptostreptococcus, Veillonella, Clostridium perfringens, Clostridium tetani, Corynebacterium diphtheriae,* and *Mycoplasma.*

INDICATIONS & DOSAGE
• Severe infections caused by susceptible organisms. *Adults:* 600 mg to 2.7 g equally divided q 6, 8, or 12 hours or by continuous infusion to maintain serum levels of 4 to 6 mcg/ml. May increase to 4.8 g daily for life-threatening infections. *Children over age 1 month:* 15 to 40 mg/ kg equally divided q 6 to 8 hours. *Children age 1 month or under:* 15 to 20 mg/kg equally divided q 6 to 8 hours. Maximum dosage, 300 mg daily.

CONTRAINDICATIONS & CAUTIONS
• Contraindicated in clindamycin or lincomycin hypersensitivity.
• Use cautiously in patients with GI disorders because of increased risk of pseudomembranous colitis, and in patients with renal or hepatic impairment because it may exacerbate these conditions. Also use cautiously in neonates because the drug contains benzyl alcohol, which in large doses can cause toxicity.

PREPARATION & STORAGE
Available in a concentration of 150 mg/ml in 2 and 4 ml ampules and 6 ml vials. Store below 104° F. (40° C.), preferably between 59° and 86° F. (15° and 30° C.). Protect from freezing.

For a concentration of 6 mg/ml or less, add 25 ml of compatible solution to each 150 mg of clindamycin (300 mg/50 ml). Compatible solutions include dextrose 5% or 10% in water, Isolyte H, Isolyte M and dextrose 5%, Isolyte P and dextrose 5%, Normosol-R, Ringer's lactate, and 0.9% sodium chloride.

Solutions should be used within 24 hours.

ADMINISTRATION
Direct injection: not recommended.
Intermittent infusion: Infuse drug diluted to a concentration of 6 mg/ml or less through an intermittent infusion device or into an I.V. line containing a free-flowing, compatible solution. Infuse 300 mg/50 ml over 10 minutes, 600 mg/100 ml over 20 minutes, or 900 mg/150 ml over 30 minutes. Don't infuse more than 1,200 mg over 1 hour.
Continuous infusion: Administer as a single, rapid infusion, then follow with a continuous infusion, using a diluted concentration of 6 mg/ml.

For serum levels above 4 mcg/ml, rapidly infuse 10 mg/minute for 30 minutes, then give maintenance dose of 0.75 mg/minute. For serum levels above 5 mcg/ml, rapidly infuse 15 mg/minute for 30 minutes, then give maintenance dose of 1 mg/minute. For serum levels above 6 mcg/ml, rapidly infuse 20 mg/minute for 30 minutes, then give maintenance dose of 1.25 mg/minute.

Bear in mind that overly rapid infusion can cause cardiac arrest.

INCOMPATIBILITY
Incompatible with aminophylline, ampicillin, barbiturates, calcium gluconate, magnesium sulfate, phenytoin sodium, and theophylline. Drug is also incompatible with rubber closures, such as those on I.V. tubing.

ADVERSE REACTIONS
Life-threatening: anaphylaxis.
Other: abdominal pain; anorexia; bacterial and fungal superinfection; bloating; diarrhea; eosinophilia; erythema; pain, pruritus, and swelling at infusion site; esophagitis; fever; flatulence; hypotension; leukopenia; maculopapular or morbilliform rash; nausea; neutropenia; nonspecific colitis; pseudomembranous colitis; tenesmus; thrombocytopenia; thrombophlebitis; unpleasant or metallic taste; urticaria; vomiting; weight loss.

INTERACTIONS
Antimyasthenics: possible antagonistic antimyasthenic effect.
Chloramphenicol, erythromycin: possible diminished clindamycin effect.
Hydrocarbon inhalation anesthetics, neuromuscular blocking agents: enhanced muscle relaxant action.
Neurotoxic drugs: increased risk of neurotoxicity.
Opioid analgesics: additive respiratory depression.

EFFECTS ON DIAGNOSTIC TESTS
Serum alkaline phosphatase, SGOT, SGPT: possible increased levels.

SPECIAL CONSIDERATIONS
• Obtain specimens for culture and sensitivity tests. Therapy may begin before test results are available.
• During long-term therapy, monitor kidney and liver function tests and blood cell counts. As ordered, adjust dosage accordingly.
• Keep in mind that colitis may not develop for several weeks after the drug has been discontinued.
• If severe, persistent diarrhea occurs, discontinue drug and obtain a stool specimen for culture.

Unmarked trade names available in the United States only.
♦ Also available in Canada.   ♦ ♦ Available in Canada only.

• To prevent toxin retention, avoid opiates or diphenoxylate when treating clindamycin-induced colitis.
• Not significantly removed by hemodialysis or peritoneal dialysis.
• May contain benzyl alcohol.
• Observe patient for superinfection with prolonged use.

codeine phosphate♦

Controlled Substance Schedule II
Pregnancy Risk Category: C

PHARMACOKINETICS
Distribution: rapidly distributed to kidneys, liver, spleen, and lungs. Minimal protein binding.
Metabolism: in the liver.
Excretion: excreted mainly in the urine as norcodeine and conjugated morphine. Small amounts are excreted in the feces and the drug appears in breast milk. Elimination half-life is 2 to 3 hours.
Action: peak effect, 20 to 30 minutes; duration, 4 to 5 hours.

MECHANISM OF ACTION
Codeine binds with stereospecific receptors in the CNS, altering the perception of pain and the emotional response to it.

INDICATIONS & DOSAGE
• Mild to moderate pain. *Adults:* 15 to 60 mg q 4 to 6 hours.

CONTRAINDICATIONS & CAUTIONS
• Contraindicated in hypersensitivity to codeine or sulfites; in acute respiratory depression because the drug may exacerbate the condition; and in premature neonates.
• Because it may slow elimination of toxins, codeine is contraindicated in diarrhea associated with pseudomembranous colitis or poisoning.
• Contraindicated in pulmonary edema caused by a chemical respiratory irritant. Codeine causes vasodilation, which may produce adverse hemodynamic effects.
• Use with caution in altered respiratory function because of an increased risk of respiratory depression; in dysrhythmias because drug can increase response through a vagolytic action; and in seizure disorders because drug may induce or exacerbate seizures.
• Because of the potential for abuse, use cautiously in patients experiencing drug dependency, emotional instability, or suicidal ideation.
• Administer carefully in acute abdominal conditions because codeine may mask symptoms; in gallbladder disease because drug may increase biliary contractions; in inflammatory bowel disease because toxic megacolon may develop; and after recent GI surgery because drug may alter GI motility.
• Because of the increased risk of respiratory depression and prolonged CNS depression, use cautiously in hypothyroidism. Also use cautiously in head injury and increased intracranial pressure (from intracranial lesions) because codeine may mask clinical changes and elevate cerebrospinal fluid (CSF) pressure.
• In hepatic and renal impairment, administer cautiously because of an increased risk of toxicity.
• Because codeine can cause urine retention, give cautiously in prostatic hypertrophy, urethral stricture, or recent urinary tract surgery.
• Note that elderly and pediatric patients are more likely to suffer respiratory depression.

PREPARATION AND STORAGE

Available in concentrations of 15, 30, and 60 mg/ml in 1 ml vials and 2 ml disposable units.

Store below 104° F. (40° C.), preferably between 59° and 86° F. (15° and 30° C.). Protect from light and freezing. Do not use solution if it becomes more than slightly discolored or contains a precipitate.

ADMINISTRATION

Direct injection: Inject diluted drug over 4 to 5 minutes through I.V. tubing containing a free-flowing, compatible solution.

Intermittent infusion: Infuse diluted drug slowly at ordered rate.

Continuous infusion: Infuse diluted drug slowly at ordered rate.

INCOMPATIBILITY

Incompatible with aminophylline, ammonium chloride, amobarbital, bromides, chlorothiazide sodium, heparin, iodides, methicillin, pentobarbital, phenobarbital, phenytoin, salts of heavy metals, secobarbital, sodium bicarbonate, sodium iodide, and thiopental.

ADVERSE REACTIONS

Life-threatening: anaphylaxis, respiratory depression (particularly in elderly patients).

Other: cold, clammy skin; confusion, severe dizziness, severe drowsiness, low blood pressure, restlessness, pinpoint pupils, bradycardia, severe weakness, troubled breathing, diarrhea, tachycardia, nausea and vomiting, shivering, and stomach cramps.

INTERACTIONS

Antidiarrheals, antiperistaltics: enhanced risk of constipation and CNS depression.

Antihypertensives, diuretics: increased risk of hypotension.

Antimuscarinics: increased risk of paralytic ileus.

Buprenorphine: possible reduced therapeutic effects of codeine.

Hydroxyzine: possible increased analgesia and CNS depression.

MAO inhibitors: severe, unpredictable adverse reactions when given within 21 days of codeine. Reduce codeine dose, as ordered.

Metoclopramide: antagonistic effect on GI motility.

Naloxone: antagonistic effects on the analgesic and the CNS and respiratory depressant action of codeine.

Naltrexone: blocked therapeutic effect of codeine and possible precipitation of withdrawal symptoms in drug-dependent patients.

Neuromuscular blocking agents: possible additive respiratory depression.

Opioid-agonist analgesics: possible additive respiratory and CNS depression and hypotension.

Other CNS depressants: deepened CNS depression and risk of addiction.

EFFECTS ON DIAGNOSTIC TESTS

Gastric emptying studies: possible delayed emptying.

Hepatobiliary imaging with technetium 99m disofenin: delayed visualization, falsely resembling obstruction of common bile duct.

Lumbar puncture: elevated CSF pressure caused by carbon dioxide retention induced by respiratory depression.

Serum amylase, lipase: possible increased levels.

SPECIAL CONSIDERATIONS

• *Treatment of overdose:* To reverse respiratory depression, administer naloxone, as ordered.

• Rapid infusion can cause life-threatening adverse reactions.

• If administering by direct injection, monitor vital signs and respiratory status during injection and every 15 minutes for at least 1 hour after injection. Also monitor vital signs and respiratory status during continuous and intermittent infusion.
• Keep emergency resuscitation equipment available.
• To minimize hypotension, administer drug with patient lying down. Tell him to get up slowly to lessen dizziness and faintness.
• Codeine stimulates vasopressin release and may heighten the risk of water intoxication.
• Assess bowel function and obtain order for stool softener if indicated.
• Available in United States and Canada by generic name. Preparations manufactured in the United States contain sulfites, but Canadian preparations do not.

corticotropin (ACTH)
ACTHAR♦

Pregnancy Risk Category: C

PHARMACOKINETICS
Distribution: unknown. Drug is transported with Cohn protein fractions II and III and rapidly removed from plasma by many tissues. It doesn't cross the placenta.
Metabolism: enzymatically cleaved by the plasmin-plasminogen system.
Excretion: unknown.
Action: peak level, 1 hour after infusion; duration, 2 to 4 hours.

MECHANISM OF ACTION
Corticotropin stimulates the adrenal cortex to secrete cortisol, corticosterone, several weakly androgenic substances, and small amounts of aldosterone.

INDICATIONS & DOSAGE
• Diagnosis of adrenocortical insufficiency in otherwise normal patients and in those with complete primary adrenal insufficiency. *Adults:* 10 to 25 units over 8 hours.
• Evaluation of adrenocortical reserve in secondary adrenocortical insufficiency or hypopituitarism. *Adults:* 10 to 25 units over 8 hours daily on 4 to 5 successive days.
• Rapid screening of adrenocortical insufficiency. *Adults:* 25 units by rapid injection.

CONTRAINDICATIONS & CAUTIONS
• Contraindicated in hypersensitivity to corticotropin or pork proteins.
• Keep antihistamines and emergency resuscitation equipment nearby when giving corticotropin because of the risk of anaphylaxis. Remain with patient for entire infusion, especially during home care.
• Use cautiously in Cushing's syndrome because of the risk of acute adrenal hemorrhage. If administration is necessary, avoid repeat doses.
• Also use cautiously in cardiac disease, hypertension, or renal impairment because of an increased risk of fluid retention.
• Because the drug can exacerbate or mask symptoms of certain disorders, give cautiously in diabetes mellitus, ulcerative colitis, diverticulitis, gastritis, and esophagitis.
• Because corticotropin can blunt the immune response, give cautiously in systemic fungal infections, ocular herpes simplex, uncontrolled bacterial or viral infections, osteoporosis, scleroderma, or active or latent tuberculosis, or in a patient with a history of tuberculosis, or a positive tuberculin skin test.
• Administer cautiously in open-angle glaucoma because of the risk of increased intraocular pressure; in

myasthenia gravis because the drug can worsen weakness, possibly leading to respiratory distress; in hyperlipidemia because glucocorticoids can further raise serum fatty acid or cholesterol levels; and in hypoalbuminemia, hepatic cirrhosis, or nephrotic syndrome because of the heightened risk of toxicity from reduced availability of albumin for glucocorticoid binding.
• In hyperthyroidism, give corticotropin cautiously because of impaired glucocorticoid effect from accelerated metabolism.
• In hypothyroidism, give cautiously because of a magnified glucocorticoid effect.

PREPARATION & STORAGE
Available as a lyophilized white or near-white, water-soluble solid in 25 or 40 unit vials. Reconstitute with sterile water for injection or 0.9% sodium chloride for injection so that required dose is contained in 1 to 2 ml of solution. For continuous infusion, further dilute in 500 ml of a compatible solution, such as Ringer's lactate, 0.9% sodium chloride, dextrose 5% in water, or dextrose 5% in 0.9% sodium chloride. Reconstituted solutions remain stable for 1 to 7 days when stored at 36° to 46° F. (2° to 8° C.).

ADMINISTRATION
Direct injection: Inject reconstituted drug directly into vein or through an I.V. line containing a free-flowing, compatible solution.
Intermittent infusion: not recommended.
Continuous infusion: Infuse diluted solution over 8 hours.

INCOMPATIBILITY
Incompatible with aminophylline and sodium bicarbonate.

ADVERSE REACTIONS
Life-threatening: anaphylaxis.
Other: depression, emotional instability, euphoria, headache, hirsutism, hypertension, hypokalemic acidosis, hypothalamic-pituitary insufficiency, impaired wound healing, insomnia, mood swings, nausea, peptic ulcer, potassium loss, psychosis, seizures, sensitivity reactions, sodium retention with edema, vertebral compression fractures, vertigo, vomiting, weakness.

INTERACTIONS
Aminoglutethimide, mitotane: diminished adrenal response to corticotropin.
Amphotericin B: possible decreased adrenal response to corticotropin. May cause hypokalemia.
Anticoagulants, thrombolytics: reduced effects.
Cortisone, hydrocortisone: if given on test day, possible abnormally high baseline plasma cortisol levels, followed by a paradoxical decline in plasma cortisol levels.
Digitalis glycosides: increased risk of arrhythmias or digitalis toxicity associated with hypokalemia.
Estrogens: elevated plasma cortisol levels if given before and after corticotropin.
Hepatic enzyme-inducing drugs: possible increased glucocorticoid metabolism.
Indomethacin, salicylates: possible increased risk of GI ulcers.
^{131}I: reduced uptake.
Mexiletine: accelerated metabolism.
Nondepolarizing neuromuscular blockers: possible enhanced blockade.
Potassium-depleting drugs: magnified potassium-wasting effects of corticotropin.
Potassium-sparing diuretics, potassium supplements: diminished effects.

Sodium-containing drugs: possible edema and hypertension.
Somatrem, somatropin: inhibited growth response.
Spironolactone: if given on test day, possible falsely elevated plasma cortisol levels if fluorometric methods are used.

EFFECTS ON DIAGNOSTIC TESTS

^{123}I uptake: possible reduced uptake.
Serum and urine glucose, serum sodium: possible increased levels.
Serum potassium: possible decreased levels.
Skin tests: possible suppressed response.
Urine estradiol: possible falsely decreased levels if Brown's method is used.
Urine estrogen: possible altered results if colorimetric-fluorometric procedures are used.

SPECIAL CONSIDERATIONS

• Increasing the dosage prolongs corticotropin's duration of action.
• Repeated infusions on successive days heighten adrenocortical response to further stimulation.
• Drug raises blood glucose level; patients with diabetes may require increased insulin dosage.
• Prolonged therapy may require calorie or sodium restriction, or potassium supplementation.
• Monitor patient's weight and intake and output.

---

cosyntropin
Cortrosyn♦

Pregnancy Risk Category: C

PHARMACOKINETICS
Distribution: unknown. Drug doesn't cross the placenta.
Metabolism: not known.
Excretion: not known. Also not known if drug appears in breast milk. Drug's half-life is about 15 minutes.
Action: peak serum level, 1 hour; duration, 2 to 3 hours.

MECHANISM OF ACTION
A synthetic peptide corresponding to amino acids 1 to 24 of human adrenocorticotropic hormone (ACTH), cosyntropin combines with receptors in the adrenal cell plasma membrane to stimulate secretion of cortisol, corticosterone, weak androgenic substances, and a small amount of aldosterone. A cosyntropin dose of 0.25 mg is pharmacologically equal to 25 units of natural ACTH.

INDICATIONS & DOSAGE
• Rapid screening test of adrenal function. *Adults and children age 2 and over:* 0.25 mg. *Children under age 2:* 0.125 mg.
• Adrenal stimulus. *Adults:* 0.25 to 0.75 mg.

CONTRAINDICATIONS & CAUTIONS
• Use cautiously in patients with corticotropin hypersensitivity or allergic disorders.

PREPARATION AND STORAGE
Available in two-vial packets. To reconstitute, add 1 ml of 0.9% sodium chloride injection to vial containing 0.25 mg of cosyntropin to yield a concentration of 250 mcg/ml. For infusion, dilute cosyntropin with dextrose 5% in water or 0.9% sodium chloride.

Before reconstitution, store at 59° to 86° F. (15° to 30° C.), unless manufacturer specifies otherwise. After reconstitution, solution remains stable for 24 hours at room temperature and for 3 weeks if re-

---

Unmarked trade names available in the United States only.
♦Also available in Canada.   ♦♦Available in Canada only.

frigerated at 36° to 46° F. (2° to 8° C.). Solutions diluted further remain stable for 12 hours at room temperature.

ADMINISTRATION
Direct injection: Inject reconstituted drug into vein through an intermittent infusion device over 2 minutes. Alternatively, inject drug through an I.V. line containing a free-flowing, compatible solution, but interrupt primary infusion during injection. *Intermittent infusion:* not recommended.
Continuous infusion: Infuse diluted solution at 0.04 mg/hour over 4 to 8 hours.

INCOMPATIBILITY
Incompatible with blood or plasma because enzymes inactivate drug.

ADVERSE REACTIONS
Life-threatening: anaphylaxis.
Other: flushing, pruritus.

INTERACTIONS
Adrenocorticoids, glucocorticoids (except betamethasone, dexamethasone, prednisone), especially cortisone and hydrocortisone: if taken on test day, abnormally high baseline plasma cortisol levels, followed by a paradoxical decline in levels after cosyntropin administration.

EFFECTS ON DIAGNOSTIC TESTS
Free hemoglobin, serum bilirubin: elevated levels.
Plasma cortisol: falsely elevated levels if fluorometric methods used.

SPECIAL CONSIDERATIONS
• Keep emergency resuscitation equipment nearby when giving drug because of the risk of anaphylaxis.

• Highest plasma cortisol levels occur about 45 to 60 minutes after cosyntropin administration.

co-trimoxazole (sulfamethoxazole-trimethoprim)
Bactrim I.V. Infusion, Septra I.V. Infusion♦

Pregnancy Risk Category: C (D if near term)

PHARMACOKINETICS
Distribution: throughout body tissues and fluids, such as aqueous humor, middle ear fluid, prostatic fluid, bile, and cerebrospinal fluid. Trimethoprim is 44% bound to plasma proteins; sulfamethoxazole, 70% bound. Drug crosses the placenta.
Metabolism: in the liver. Trimethoprim is metabolized to hydroxylated metabolites; sulfamethoxazole is acetylated and conjugated with glucuronic acid.
Excretion: in urine, through glomerular filtration and renal tubular secretion, and in small amounts in feces. From 50% to 60% of trimethoprim is excreted primarily unchanged in 24 hours; 45% to 70% of sulfamethoxazole is excreted within 24 hours. Co-trimoxazole appears in breast milk.

In adults with normal renal function, trimethoprim has a serum half-life of 8 to 11 hours; sulfamethoxazole, 10 to 13 hours. Half-life may triple in chronic renal failure. In children under age 10, serum half-life averages almost 7 hours.
Action: peak serum level, 1 hour; duration, 11 to 18 hours.

MECHANISM OF ACTION

Containing trimethoprim (bactericidal) and sulfamethoxazole (bacteriostatic), co-trimoxazole sequentially inhibits enzymes of folic acid pathways and bacterial thymidine synthesis. The drug's spectrum of activity includes many gram-positive aerobic bacteria, including most strains of *Streptococcus pneumoniae,* many strains of *Staphylococcus aureus,* group A and beta-hemolytic streptococci, and *Nocardia.* Susceptible gram-negative aerobic bacteria include *Acinetobacter, Enterobacter, Escherichia coli, Klebsiella pneumoniae, Proteus mirabilis, Salmonella, Shigella, Haemophilus influenzae* (including ampicillin-resistant strains), *Haemophilus ducreyi, Neisseria gonorrhoeae, Providencia, Serratia,* and many indole-positive strains of *Proteus.* Co-trimoxazole is also active against the protozoa *Pneumocystis carinii.*

INDICATIONS & DOSAGE

• Systemic bacterial infections caused by susceptible organisms. *Adults and children age 2 months and over:* 10 to 12.5 mg/kg of sulfamethoxazole and 2 to 2.5 mg/kg of trimethoprim q 6 hours; 13.3 to 16.7 mg/kg of sulfamethoxazole and 2.7 to 3.3 mg/kg of trimethoprim q 8 hours; or 20 to 25 mg/kg of sulfamethoxazole and 4 to 5 mg/kg of trimethoprim q 12 hours.
• *Pneumocystis carinii* pneumonitis. *Adults and children:* 100 mg/kg of sulfamethoxazole and 20 mg/kg of trimethoprim in equally divided doses q 6 hours for 14 days.
Note: Dosage in renal failure reflects creatinine clearance. If clearance is less than 15 ml/min in adults, use is not recommended; if 15 to 30 ml/min, give half usual adult dose; if more than 30 ml/min, give usual adult dose. Contraindicated in children if clearance is less than 20 ml/min; if 20 to 30 ml/min, give half usual pediatric dose; if more than 30 ml/min, give usual pediatric dose.

CONTRAINDICATIONS & CAUTIONS

• Contraindicated in neonates because sulfonamides cause kernicterus.
• Contraindicated in hypersensitivity to sulfonamides or trimethoprim.
• Use cautiously in patients with hypersensitivity to furosemide, thiazide diuretics, sulfonylureas, or carbonic anhydrase inhibitors because they may also be hypersensitive to sulfonamides.
• Also use cautiously in patients with renal or hepatic impairment, bronchial asthma, G6PD deficiency, folic acid deficiency, or AIDS because of the increased incidence of adverse reactions.
• Administer carefully to the elderly because of risk of toxicity.
• Also administer carefully to patients receiving chemotherapy because of an increased risk of myelosuppression; to mentally retarded children because reduced folate levels can worsen psychomotor regression; and to patients with streptococcal pharyngitis because of the risk of organism resistance.

PREPARATION & STORAGE

Available in 5 ml ampules and 5, 10, and 30 ml vials. Before infusion, add 125 ml of dextrose 5% in water to dilute a 5 ml vial. New concentration contains 0.64 mg of trimethoprim and 3.2 mg of sulfamethoxazole. Diluted 1:25 solution is stable for 6 hours at room temperature. Solutions containing 0.64 to 0.83 mg of trimethoprim and 3.2 to 4 mg of sulfamethoxazole stay stable for 4 hours; those containing 0.8 to 1.1 mg of trimethoprim and 4 to 5.3 mg of sulfamethoxazole remain stable for 2 hours.

Don't refrigerate drug or solutions. Discard cloudy solutions or those that contain precipitates.

ADMINISTRATION

Direct injection: not recommended.
Intermittent infusion: Using a 21G to 23G needle, infuse appropriate dose of diluted drug into an I.V. line of free-flowing dextrose 5% in water over 60 to 90 minutes. Or infuse drug into a flushed and patent intermittent infusion device. If the only available site is tubing that contains incompatible solutions, flush tubing with 10 ml of sterile water for injection before and after infusion and turn off primary I.V. solution during co-trimoxazole administration.
Continuous infusion: not recommended.

INCOMPATIBILITY

Incompatible with verapamil. Manufacturer recommends mixing no other drugs with co-trimoxazole.

Avoid diluting with any solution but dextrose 5% in water because drug components lose potency.

ADVERSE REACTIONS

Life-threatening: anaphylaxis, erythema multiforme (Stevens-Johnson syndrome), hepatic necrosis.
Other: abdominal pain, agranulocytosis, allergic myocarditis, apathy, aplastic anemia, arthralgia, aseptic meningitis, chills, conjunctivitis, depression, diuresis, drug fever, eosinophilia, exfoliative dermatitis, fatigue, glossitis, goiter, hallucinations, headache, hepatitis, hypoglycemia, hypoprothrombinemia, infusion site reaction (pain, irritation, inflammation, phlebitis), insomnia, jaundice, leukopenia, megaloblastic or hemolytic anemia, meningitis, methemoglobinemia, nervousness, neutropenia, pancreatitis, periorbital edema, peripheral neuritis, photosensitivity, pruritus, pseudomembranous enterocolitis, renal failure, seizures, serum sickness, stomatitis, thrombocytopenia, tinnitus, toxic nephrosis with oliguria and anuria, urticaria, weakness.

INTERACTIONS

Aminobenzoic acid (PABA): possible reduced antibacterial effects.
Diuretics (especially thiazides): heightened risk of thrombocytopenic purpura in the elderly.
Hemolytics: increased risk of toxic effects.
Methenamine: enhanced risk of crystalluria and formation of insoluble precipitates with sulfonamides.
Methotrexate, phenylbutazone, sulfinpyrazone: increased risk of toxicity.
Other bone-marrow depressants: magnified risk of leukopenia or thrombocytopenia.
Other hepatotoxic drugs: heightened risk of hepatotoxicity.
Penicillins: antagonized bactericidal effects.
Phenytoin: increased incidence of folate deficiency; decreased vitamin K metabolism.
Probenecid: heightened and prolonged sulfonamide levels.
Warfarin: prolonged clearance.

EFFECTS ON DIAGNOSTIC TESTS

BUN, serum bilirubin, creatinine, SGOT, SGPT: increased levels.
Partial thromboplastin time, prothrombin time: prolonged.

SPECIAL CONSIDERATIONS

• Obtain specimens for culture and sensitivity tests before giving first dose. Therapy may begin before receiving results. Monitor BUN, serum creatinine, CBC and platelet count,

partial thromboplastin time, prothrombin time, electrolyte levels, and urinalysis. Also monitor intake and output, and give enough fluids to maintain a urine output of at least 1,200 ml daily in adults.
• Closely monitor patients with AIDS because they're susceptible to severe adverse effects.
• Leucovorin can be given for bone marrow depression and folic acid supplements for hematologic side effects.
• Trimethoprim and active sulfamethoxazole are partially removed by dialysis.
• Observe patient for superinfection with prolonged use.

---

crotaline antivenin, polyvalent (North and South American anti-snakebite serum, pit viper antivenin)
Antivenin (Crotalidae) Polyvalent (Equine)

Pregnancy Risk Category: C

PHARMACOKINETICS
Distribution: not known.
Metabolism: not known.
Excretion: not known.
Action: peak plasma level, immediately on injection.

MECHANISM OF ACTION
Antivenin contains globulins that neutralize toxic effects of bites from crotalid snakes, including the rattlesnake, copperhead and cottonmouth moccasins, fer-de-lance and other species of *Bothrops,* cantil, and bushmaster of Central and South America. Drug isn't effective against coral snake venoms.

INDICATIONS & DOSAGE
• Severe crotalid snake bites. *Adults and children:* Initial dosage reflects severity of envenomation. For minimal envenomation, give 20 to 40 ml (2 to 4 vials); for moderate envenomation, 50 to 90 ml (5 to 9 vials); for severe envenomation, 100 to 150 ml or more (10 to 15 vials). Base additional doses on patient response. If swelling and systemic signs continue, give another 10 to 50 ml.

CONTRAINDICATIONS & CAUTIONS
• Use cautiously in patients with asthma, hay fever, or allergies to horses or horse serums.

PREPARATION & STORAGE
Available in a two-vial pack containing one vial of lyophilized powder and one vial of 10 ml bacteriostatic water for injection. Reconstitute with diluent provided. Gently roll vial between hands to hasten dissolution. Don't shake vigorously. For infusion, further dilute with 0.9% sodium chloride or dextrose 5% in water in concentrations of 1:1 to 1:10, and mix gently.
    Store reconstituted solution at room temperature. Avoid freezing. Use reconstituted solution within 48 hours, diluted solution within 12 hours.

ADMINISTRATION
Give doses within 4 hours after bite. Drug's effectiveness is questionable if given more than 12 hours after envenomation.
Direct injection: not recommended.
Intermittent infusion: Give initial 5 to 10 ml of reconstituted solution over 3 to 5 minutes while carefully observing patient. If no adverse reactions occur, infuse at rate based on severity of envenomation and patient's tolerance.

Continuous infusion: not recommended.

INCOMPATIBILITY
No incompatibilities reported.

ADVERSE REACTIONS
Life-threatening: anaphylaxis.
Other: serum sickness 5 to 24 days after administration.

INTERACTIONS
None reported.

EFFECTS ON DIAGNOSTIC TESTS
None reported.

SPECIAL CONSIDERATIONS
• If you're unfamiliar with snake-bite management, obtain advice from a poison control center or an expert, such as a herpetologist at a large zoo. Crotalid bites can cause severe tissue damage or even death.
• Always perform a skin test before giving antivenin, to determine patient sensitivity. To perform test, give intradermal injection of 0.02 to 0.03 ml of a 1:10 dilution of normal equine serum or antivenin in 0.9% sodium chloride. Urticarial wheal indicates a positive result. The shorter the time between injection and onset of reaction, the greater the patient's sensitivity.
• Use desensitization for hypersensitive patients or those with allergies.
• Keep emergency airway equipment and anaphylaxis kit nearby in case of severe systemic reactions to antivenin (usually within 30 minutes of administration). If hypersensitivity reaction occurs, slow infusion rate and treat symptomatically.
• Never inject antivenin into a finger or toe.
• Give corticosteroids, as ordered, for serum sickness. Be alert for arthralgia, edema, fever, lymphade-

nopathy, malaise, nausea, pain, weakness (possibly leading to permanent atrophy), peripheral neuritis, urticaria, and vomiting.
• Some clinicians suggest that epinephrine solution be infused along with antivenin in patients at risk for systemic reaction to antivenin. Antihistamines can mask severity of envenomation symptoms.

cryoprecipitated antihemophilic factor

Pregnancy Risk Category: C

COMPOSITION
Derived from whole blood, cryoprecipitate contains about 80 to 120 units of Factor VIII:C (antihemophilic factor), 250 mg of fibrinogen, and 40% to 70% of Factor VIII:vWF (von Willebrand's factor) and 20% to 30% of the Factor XIII present in the initial unit of blood. These proteins are suspended in 10 to 15 ml of plasma.

MECHANISM OF ACTION
Replaces missing clotting factor.

INDICATIONS & DOSAGE
• Deficiences of Factor VIII (hemophilia A and von Willebrand's disease), Factor XIII, or fibrinogen.
Adults and children: Dosage is determined by severity of deficiency and bleeding, patient's age and weight, and presence of Factor VIII inhibitors. Usually, a Factor VIII level of 30% of normal provides effective hemostasis. However, for bleeding or surgical preparation, a level of 50% is desirable. Repeat dose q 8 to 12 hours to maintain desired level.
    To calculate the number of units of cryoprecipitate needed to achieve

the desired Factor VIII level, use these calculations:

—Multiply the patient's weight (kg) by 40 ml/kg to obtain the approximate plasma volume (PV).

—Multiply PV by the desired increase in Factor VIII. Then divide the product by 100 to obtain the number of Factor VIII units to be transfused.

—Divide Factor VIII units by 80 (approximate number of Factor VIII units per unit of cryoprecipitate) to obtain the number of cryoprecipitate units to be transfused.

For instance, suppose the patient weighs 50 kg, his Factor VIII level is 10%, and the desired Factor VIII level is 50%. Start by multiplying 50 kg by 40 ml/kg to obtain the plasma volume (2,000). Now multiply 2,000 by 40 (the difference between the desired and actual Factor VIII level) and divide by 100. The result: 800 Factor VIII units needed. Finally, divide 800 by 80 to obtain the number of cryoprecipitated units (10) to be transfused.

CONTRAINDICATIONS & CAUTIONS

• Contraindicated in patients with coagulation deficiencies other than those caused by low levels of Factor VIII, Factor XIII, or fibrinogen.

• Use cautiously in patients with type A, B, or AB blood because cryoprecipitate may contain A and B isohemagglutinins, which can cause intravascular hemolysis.

PREPARATION & STORAGE

In cryoprecipitate preparation, 1 unit of plasma is separated from 1 unit of whole blood and frozen within 6 hours. Later the plasma is slowly thawed at 39° F. (4° C.), and a white precipitate forms. The supernatant plasma is removed, leaving the coagulation proteins in 10 to 15 ml of plasma. The cryoprecipitate is immediately refrozen and can be stored for up to 1 year.

Allow 30 to 60 minutes for the blood bank to thaw and label cryoprecipitate. Refrigerate after thawing to prevent reformation of cold precipitates. Transfuse within 6 hours.

The total number of units prescribed may be pooled into a single container in the blood bank or issued in individual bags. Rinse single bags with 10 to 20 ml of 0.9% sodium chloride to flush all cryoprecipitate from the container.

ADMINISTRATION

Direct injection: Withdraw solution through a filtered needle into a 20 ml syringe. Inject as rapidly as possible through a 21G to 23G needle. Observe closely for signs of infiltration (swelling, pain). This technique is typically used only for neonates.

Intermittent infusion: not recommended.

Continuous infusion: Using a standard blood filter, infuse rapidly through a 19G to 21G needle.

INCOMPATIBILITY

Incompatible with all drugs and solutions, except 0.9% sodium chloride.

ADVERSE REACTIONS

Life-threatening: anaphylaxis.
Other: breathing difficulty, flushing, hypotension, lethargy, nausea, paresthesias, pruritus, tachycardia, urticaria, visual disturbances, vomiting.

INTERACTIONS

None reported.

EFFECTS ON DIAGNOSTIC TESTS

Coombs' test: possible antibody attachment to RBCs if enough incompatible plasma is given.

Unmarked trade names available in the United States only.
♦ Also available in Canada.   ♦ ♦ Available in Canada only.

Factors VIII, XIII: increased levels.
Fibrinogen: elevated levels.

SPECIAL CONSIDERATIONS
• *Treatment of anaphylaxis:* Onset is acute; signs include anxiety, urticaria, and wheezing, progressing to cyanosis, shock, and cardiac arrest. Stop infusion immediately and keep vein open with 0.9% sodium chloride. Treat hypotension and other complications symptomatically.
• Before requesting cryoprecipitate from the blood bank, record the patient's vital signs and ensure venous catheter patency.
• Because cryoprecipitate contains no RBCs, red cell cross matching isn't necessary. Cryoprecipitate-rich plasma should be ABO-compatible.
• Monitor vital signs during administration. If adverse reactions occur, reduce the rate. Give antihistamines, as ordered, to prevent or treat reactions such as anaphylaxis.
• Monitor fibrinogen levels when giving large amounts of drug.
• Keep in mind that cryoprecipitate carries the risk of transmitting viral diseases, such as hepatitis, cytomegalovirus infection, and AIDS.

cyclophosphamide
Cytoxan♦, Neosar

Pregnancy Risk Category: C

PHARMACOKINETICS
Distribution: throughout body tissues, with 10% to 50% of alkylating metabolites (but not parent drug) bound to plasma proteins. Drug crosses the blood-brain barrier (appearing in cerebrospinal fluid in subtherapeutic concentrations) and probably the placenta.
Metabolism: primarily in liver to active metabolites.

Excretion: in urine, with 15% to 30% excreted unchanged and the rest removed as metabolites; 36% to 99% is excreted in 48 hours. Drug appears in breast milk.
Action: peak serum level, 1 hour; duration, 72 hours.

MECHANISM OF ACTION
An alkylating agent, cyclophosphamide prevents cell division by crosslinking DNA strands or by breaking the DNA molecule itself, thereby interfering with DNA replication and RNA transcription. It also inhibits protein synthesis and acts as a potent immunosuppressive.

INDICATIONS & DOSAGE
• Lymphomas; acute leukemia (in adults); cancers of the lung, brain, breast, and reproductive organs; autoimmune diseases (such as rheumatoid arthritis); and prevention of graft-versus-host disease in organ transplants. Dosage reflects patient's disease, condition, and response as well as use of other treatments.
Adults: initially, 40 to 50 mg/kg in divided doses over 2 to 5 days. Maintenance dosage is 10 to 15 mg/kg q 7 to 10 days or 3 to 5 mg/kg twice weekly. *Children:* initially, 2 to 8 mg/kg or 60 to 250 mg/m^2 once weekly for 6 weeks, depending on susceptibility of neoplasm. Maintenance dosage depends on patient tolerance and presence of a WBC count of 2,500 to 4,000/mm^3. Recommended maintenance dosage is 10 to 15 mg/kg q 7 to 10 days, or 30 mg/kg q 3 to 4 weeks or when bone marrow recovers.

CONTRAINDICATIONS & CAUTIONS
• Contraindicated in existing or recent chicken pox or herpes zoster because of an increased risk of generalized infection.

• Use cautiously in patients with bone marrow depression, tumor infiltration of bone marrow, previous therapy with radiation or other cytotoxic agents, or impaired hepatic or renal function because of an increased risk of toxicity. Also use cautiously in patients with a history of gout or urate renal stones because of the risk of hyperuricemia.

PREPARATION & STORAGE

To avoid mutagenic, teratogenic, and carcinogenic risks, use a biological containment cabinet, wear gloves and mask, and use syringes with tight fittings (Luer-lok) to prevent leakage. Dispose of needles, syringes, vials, and unused drug correctly.

Available in 100 mg, 200 mg, 500 mg, 1 g, and 2 g vials. Reconstitute with sterile water for injection or bacteriostatic water for injection (paraben preserved only) to a concentration of 20 mg/ml. The powder contains enough sodium chloride to produce an isotonic solution. Shake vigorously. Unreconstituted drug stays stable at room temperature; reconstituted drug remains stable for 24 hours at room temperature and for 6 days if refrigerated. Discard any unused drug after 24 hours.

Other compatible solutions include dextrose 5% in Ringer's lactate, dextrose 5% in 0.9% sodium chloride, Ringer's lactate, 0.45% or 0.9% sodium chloride, and ⅙ M sodium lactate.

ADMINISTRATION

Use a new site for each injection or infusion. Heparin locks aren't recommended.
Direct injection: Using a 23G to 25G winged-tip needle, inject reconstituted drug directly into vein over 2 to 3 minutes.

Intermittent infusion: Using a 23G to 25G winged-tip needle, infuse diluted drug over 15 to 20 minutes.
Continuous infusion: not recommended.

INCOMPATIBILITY

No incompatibilities reported.

ADVERSE REACTIONS

Life-threatening: cardiotoxicity (with high doses), interstitial pulmonary fibrosis (with high doses over prolonged period).
Other: alopecia, amenorrhea, anorexia, bladder carcinomas, bladder fibrosis, colitis (possibly hemorrhagic), diaphoresis, diarrhea, dizziness, facial flushing, faintness, headache, hemorrhagic cystitis, hepatotoxicity, hyperkalemia, hypernatremia (including seizures), hyperuricemia, hypotension, mucosal irritation, myelosuppression, nausea, nephrotoxicity, oropharyngeal sensation, syndrome of inappropriate antidiuretic hormone secretion (SIADH), testicular atrophy, tongue burning, urticaria, vomiting.

INTERACTIONS

Allopurinol: increased bone marrow depression.
Anticoagulants (oral): enhanced activity.
Barbiturates, other hepatic enzyme inducers: increased cyclophosphamide toxicity.
Bone marrow depressants: worsened bone marrow depression.
Cardiotoxic drugs: possible potentiated effects.
Immunosuppressants: increased risk of infection and neoplasms.
Succinylcholine: prolonged effects with high cyclophosphamide doses.
Vincristine, VM-26: enhanced cyclophosphamide effects.

EFFECTS ON DIAGNOSTIC TESTS

Papanicolaou test: possible false-positive results.

Serum pseudocholinesterase: rarely, decreased levels.

Serum and urine uric acid: elevated levels.

Skin tests: possible suppression of positive reaction.

SPECIAL CONSIDERATIONS

• Treat overdose supportively.
• Encourage patient to drink plenty of fluids before, during, and for 72 hours after treatment, to avoid hemorrhagic cystitis. If symptoms (hematuria, painful urination) occur, discontinue drug immediately. Monitor urine for hematuria and specific gravity.
• Infuse slowly to prevent facial flushing.
• Monitor CBC, kidney and liver function, and uric acid levels.
• High I.V. dosage may cause SIADH leading to hyponatremia.
• Alkalinizing urine, providing good hydration, and possibly giving allopurinol may prevent or minimize hyperuricemia.
• Inform patient that reversible alopecia is common.
• Drug can be removed by dialysis.
• Monitor for infection in patients with leukopenia. If infection occurs, give antibiotics, if ordered.

---

cyclosporine
Sandimmune

Pregnancy Risk Category: C

PHARMACOKINETICS

Distribution: throughout fluids and tissues, with about 90% bound to plasma proteins. Distribution in blood depends on dose; with high drug concentrations, WBCs and RBCs become saturated. Drug crosses the placenta.

Metabolism: extensively changed in liver, to at least 17 metabolites.

Excretion: eliminated primarily in bile, 6% in urine; only 0.1% excreted unchanged. Drug appears in breast milk. It has a biphasic half-life: initial phase, about 70 minutes; terminal phase, 19 to 27 hours.

Action: peak levels, at end of infusion.

MECHANISM OF ACTION

Cyclosporine inhibits interleukin-2, which plays a major role in cell-mediated and humoral immunity.

INDICATIONS & DOSAGE

• Prophylaxis and treatment of organ tissue rejection. *Adults and children:* 2 to 6 mg/kg daily, beginning 4 to 12 hours before surgery and continuing after surgery until patient can tolerate oral form. Adjust dose to maintain plasma trough levels of 50 to 300 ng/ml.

CONTRAINDICATIONS & CAUTIONS

• Contraindicated in hypersensitivity to drug or diluent (polyoxyl 35 castor oil).
• Also contraindicated in existing or recent chicken pox or herpes zoster because of an increased risk of generalized disease.
• Use cautiously in patients with hyperkalemia or infection because drug may worsen these conditions, and in hepatic or renal impairment because of an increased risk of toxicity.

PREPARATION & STORAGE

Available in 5 ml ampules containing a concentration of 50 mg/ml. For infusion, dilute each milliliter of drug in 20 to 100 ml of 0.9% sodium chloride or dextrose 5% in water.

Unmarked trade names available in the United States only.
♦ Also available in Canada.   ♦ ♦ Available in Canada only.

Reconstituted solutions remain stable for up to 24 hours in dextrose 5% in water injection and for 6 to 12 hours in 0.9% sodium chloride injection (6 hours in PVC containers and 12 hours in glass containers). Store below 104 F. (40° C.), preferably at 59° to 86° F. (15° to 30° C.) Don't freeze or expose to light.

ADMINISTRATION
Direct injection: not recommended.
Intermittent infusion: not recommended.
Continuous infusion: Infuse diluted drug slowly over 2 to 6 hours or up to 24 hours. Bear in mind that significant amounts of drug are lost when given through PVC tubing.

INCOMPATIBILITY
No incompatibilities reported.

ADVERSE REACTIONS
Life-threatening: anaphylaxis.
Other: acne, anxiety, bacterial or fungal infections, chills, confusion, conjunctivitis, diarrhea, dyspnea, dysrhythmias, edema, facial or neck flushing, fatigue, fever, gingival hyperplasia, gynecomastia, hand tremors, headache, hearing loss, hematuria, hemolytic-uremic syndrome, hirsutism, hyperkalemia, hypertension, lymphoproliferative disorders (including lymphomas), nausea, paresthesias, seizures, sinusitis, tinnitus, vomiting, weakness, wheezing.

INTERACTIONS
Androgens, cimetidine, danazol, diltiazem, erythromycin, ketoconazole, miconazole: possible increased cyclosporine levels and risk of nephrotoxicity.
Banked blood, low-salt milk, potassium-containing products, potassium-sparing diuretics: possible heightened risk of hyperkalemia.

Immunosuppressants (except corticosteroids): possible risk of lymphomas and secondary infection.
I.V. sulfmethazine, phenobarbital, phenytoin, rifampin, trimethoprim: possible diminished cyclosporine levels.
Nephrotoxic drugs: enhanced risk of nephrotoxicity.

EFFECTS ON DIAGNOSTIC TESTS
BUN, serum creatinine, potassium, uric acid: possible increased levels.
Serum alkaline phosphatase, amylase, bilirubin, SGOT, SGPT: possible elevated levels.
Serum magnesium: possible reduced levels.

SPECIAL CONSIDERATIONS
• Treat overdose symptomatically.
• Because I.V. administration may cause anaphylaxis, give only to patients who can't tolerate oral dose.
• Monitor the patient continuously for the first 30 minutes and then at frequent intervals because of the risk of anaphylaxis. Keep resuscitation equipment nearby.
• Treat infection promptly, then reduce dosage or discontinue drug, as ordered.
• Parenteral dose of cyclosporine is one-third of oral dose.
• If infusing drug during home care, protect solution from light.
• Drug can't be removed by hemodialysis.

cytarabine
(arabinoside, ARA-C,
cytarabine arabinoside)
Cytosar-U

Pregnancy Risk Category: C

PHARMACOKINETICS
Distribution: rapidly and widely dispersed throughout body tissues, with high concentrations in GI mucosa and liver. Drug crosses the blood-brain barrier and the placenta. Protein binding is low.
Metabolism: rapidly and extensively changed in liver; also metabolized in kidneys, GI mucosa, granulocytes, and other tissues.
Excretion: 50% to 80% of dose excreted in urine within 24 hours, with about 90% removed as inactive metabolites and 10% as unchanged drug. Not known if drug or its metabolites appear in breast milk. Drug's biphasic half-life has an initial phase of 10 minutes and a terminal phase of 1 to 3 hours.
Action: peak serum level, immediately after infusion.

MECHANISM OF ACTION
As an antineoplastic antimetabolite, cytarabine interferes with DNA synthesis by blocking conversion of cytidine to deoxycytidine. It affects rapidly dividing cells in S phase. It also suppresses humoral or cell-mediated immune responses. The drug may have antiviral properties.

INDICATIONS & DOSAGE
• Induction of remission in acute myelogenous or lymphocytic leukemia. *Adults and children:* 200 mg/m² daily for 5 days by continuous infusion, then 2 weeks off the drug; maintenance dosage is 70 to 200 mg/m² daily for 2 to 5 days at monthly intervals. Dosage varies, depending on regimen.
• Refractory leukemia or non-Hodgkin's lymphoma. *Adults and children:* 3 g/m² q 12 hours for up to 12 days.

CONTRAINDICATIONS & CAUTIONS
• Contraindicated in hypersensitivity to drug.
• Also contraindicated in existing or recent chicken pox or herpes zoster infection because of an increased risk of generalized disease.
• Use cautiously in preexisting myelosuppression because cytarabine exacerbates this condition. Also use cautiously in hepatic impairment because the liver detoxifies much of the dose, and in renal impairment because of reduced drug excretion.
• Because of an increased risk of hyperuricemia, give carefully in patients with a history of gout or urate renal calculi.

PREPARATION & STORAGE
To avoid mutagenic, teratogenic, and carcinogenic risks, use a biological containment cabinet, wear gloves and mask, and use syringes with tight fittings (Luer Lock) to prevent drug leakage. Dispose of needles, syringes, vials, and unused drug correctly.
Drug is available in 100 and 500 mg vials. Reconstitute 100 mg vial with 5 ml of bacteriostatic water for injection (with benzyl alcohol), for a concentration of 20 mg/ml. Reconstitute 500 mg vial with 10 ml of bacteriostatic water for injection (with benzyl alcohol), for a concentration of 50 mg/ml. However, avoid using benzyl alcohol as a diluent when preparing high-dose cytarabine. Reconstituted solution remains stable for 48 hours at room temperature. Discard if cloudy.

Unmarked trade names available in the United States only.
♦Also available in Canada.   ♦♦Available in Canada only.

For infusion, dilute with dextrose 5% in water or with 0.9% sodium chloride; solution stays stable for 8 days at room temperature. Other compatible solutions include dextrose 5% in 0.9% sodium chloride and dextrose 5% in Ringer's lactate.

ADMINISTRATION
Direct injection: Give directly into vein or through a winged-tip needle, an intermittent infusion device, or an I.V. line containing a free-flowing, compatible solution.
Intermittent infusion: Infuse diluted solution over 1 hour or as ordered.
Continuous infusion: Infuse diluted solution over ordered duration, usually 5 days.

INCOMPATIBILITY
Incompatible with carbenicillin, cephalothin, fluorouracil, heparin sodium, methylprednisolone sodium succinate, nafcillin, oxacillin, and penicillin.

ADVERSE REACTIONS
Life-threatening: anaphylaxis; with high doses, severe cardiac, CNS, GI, and pulmonary toxicity.
Other: abdominal or chest pain, acute aseptic meningitis (with high dose therapy), alopecia, anorexia, cerebral and cerebellar dysfunction (with high dose therapy), conjunctivitis, decubitus or esophageal ulcers, diarrhea, diffuse interstitial pneumonitis (with high dose therapy), dizziness, drowsiness, esophagitis, fever, freckles, GI bleeding, hemorrhagic conjunctivitis and keratitis (with high dose therapy), hyperuricemia, jaundice, myelosuppression, nausea, neuritis, oral and anal ulcers, pancreatitis (with high dose therapy), peripheral neuropathy (with high dose therapy), rash, renal or hepatic dysfunction, sore throat, thrombophlebitis or cellulitis at infusion site, urine retention, vomiting.

INTERACTIONS
Bone marrow depressants: worsened myelosuppression.
Digoxin: decreased oral absorption of digoxin in patients receiving combination chemotherapy including cytarabine.
Methotrexate: possible enhanced cytotoxic effects.

EFFECTS ON DIAGNOSTIC TESTS
Serum alkaline phosphatase, bilirubin, SGOT, SGPT: elevated levels.

SPECIAL CONSIDERATIONS
• When giving high-dose cytarabine, perform a thorough neurologic assessment before every dose. Check for nystagmus, ataxia, dysarthria, memory loss, weakness, and vertigo. Note whether patient has an abnormal gait or a weak grasp. Afterward, observe for signs of toxicity, and ask family members to help.
• If toxicity occurs, don't give next dose of cytarabine. Notify doctor. He may withhold drug for 24 hours if just one sign is present; with multiple signs, he may discontinue drug because high doses can cause permanent brain damage.
• Many doctors order prophylactic ophthalmic steroid solutions and pyridoxine (100 mg daily) for patients receiving high dose therapy.
• Monitor kidney and liver function.
• Check for signs of infection and give antibiotics, as ordered.
• Treat skin reactions resulting from high-dose cytarabine with agents used in burn therapy. Reactions most commonly affect the palms, soles, and extensor surfaces.
• If patient develops diarrhea, give meticulous skin care to avoid or

treat perirectal abscess. Be alert for electrolyte imbalance, malabsorption, and pressure ulcers.
• Treat nausea and vomiting with antiemetics.
• Prevent or minimize uric acid nephropathy by providing good hydration, alkalinizing urine, or administering allopurinol.
• Initial WBC nadir occurs at 7 to 9 days, with level briefly rising at about 12 days; second nadir occurs at 15 to 24 days, with level rapidly rising above baseline in next 10 days. Platelet count declines at 5 days, with a nadir at 12 to 15 days; levels rise above baseline in the next 10 days.

dacarbazine
DTIC♦♦, DTIC-Dome

Pregnancy Risk Category: C

PHARMACOKINETICS
Distribution: localized in some body tissues, probably liver, and slightly bound to plasma proteins. Drug enters cerebrospinal fluid, reaching concentrations of about 14% of serum levels. Not known if drug crosses the placenta.
Metabolism: extensively metabolized in liver.
Excretion: in urine by renal tubular secretion, with 30% to 50% of drug and metabolites excreted in 6 hours. Not known if drug appears in breast milk. Biphasic half-life lasts 19 minutes for initial phase and about 5 hours for terminal phase.
Action: peak level, immediately after administration.

MECHANISM OF ACTION
Not fully understood. Drug apparently acts as an alkylating agent, is probably not cell cycle–specific, and causes slight immunosuppression.

INDICATIONS & DOSAGE
• Malignant melanoma. *Adults:* 2 to 4.5 mg/kg daily for 10 days, repeated q 4 weeks; or 250 mg/m² daily for 5 days, repeated q 3 weeks.
• Hodgkin's disease. *Adults:* 150 mg/m² daily for 5 days (in combination with other drugs), repeated q 4 weeks; or 375 mg/m² on day 1 (in combination with other drugs), repeated q 15 days.

CONTRAINDICATIONS & CAUTIONS
• Contraindicated in recent or existing chicken pox or herpes zoster infection because of an increased risk of generalized disease dacarbazine hypersensitivity.
• Give with caution to myelosuppressed patients and to those with hepatic or renal impairment.

PREPARATION & STORAGE
Use caution when preparing drug to avoid mutagenic, teratogenic, and carcinogenic risks. Use a biological containment cabinet and wear gloves and mask. Use syringes with tight fittings (Luer-lok) to prevent drug leakage and dispose of needles, syringes, vials, and unused drug correctly. Avoid contaminating work surfaces.
Drug comes as a powder in 100 and 200 mg vials that require refrigeration at 36° to 46° F. (2° to 8° C.) and protection from light. Reconstitute by adding 9.9 ml of sterile water to 100 mg vial or 19.7 ml of sterile water to 200 mg vial. Dilute further for infusion by mixing reconstituted solution with 250 ml of either dextrose 5% in water or 0.9% sodium chloride for infusion. Reconstituted drug remains stable for 8 hours at room temperature and for

up to 72 hours if refrigerated. Diluted solutions remain stable for 8 hours at room temperature and for up to 24 hours if refrigerated. If solution changes to pink it indicates decomposition.

ADMINISTRATION

When possible, give by infusion; injection can be painful.
Direct injection: Using a 21G or 23G needle, inject drug directly into vein or through an intermittent infusion device over 1 minute. Apply hot packs to injection site to alleviate pain or burning.
Intermittent infusion: Using a 21G or 23G needle, infuse diluted drug over 15 to 30 minutes.
Continuous infusion: not recommended.

INCOMPATIBILITY

Incompatible with hydrocortisone sodium succinate.

ADVERSE REACTIONS

Life-threatening: anaphylaxis, hepatotoxicity; leukopenia and thrombocytopenia, usually 2 to 4 weeks after dose.
Other: alopecia, anorexia, blurred vision, confusion, facial flushing, fever, headache, malaise, myalgia, nausea, pain and burning at injection site, paresthesias, photosensitivity, seizures, tissue damage and pain with extravasation, vomiting.

INTERACTIONS

Allopurinol: possible worsened hypouricemia.
Bone marrow depressants: worsened myelosuppression.
Hepatic enzyme inducers (such as barbiturates): possible enhanced dacarbazine effects.

EFFECTS ON DIAGNOSTIC TESTS

BUN, serum alkaline phosphatase, SGOT, SGPT: possible increased levels.

SPECIAL CONSIDERATIONS

• Restrict food and fluids 4 to 6 hours before giving drug to help reduce nausea and vomiting. Some clinicians recommend that patients be well hydrated 1 hour before receiving drug. Give antiemetics, if necessary.
• Monitor hematologic status carefully. WBC nadir is 21 to 25 days; platelet nadir, 16 days. Recovery usually occurs in 3 to 5 days.
• Also monitor kidney and liver function carefully; dysfunction can delay drug excretion.
• Avoid extravasation. If it occurs, stop drug and give at another site.
• If infection occurs when patient is leukopenic, give antibiotics, if ordered.
• Drug is often used in combination therapy with other antineoplastics.
• Advise ambulatory patient to avoid sunlight and sunlamps for first two days of therapy.
• Tell home care patient to avoid contact with people with infections.

dactinomycin (actinomycin D)
Cosmegen♦

Pregnancy Risk Category: C

PHARMACOKINETICS

Distribution: rapidly distributed into tissues, with high concentrations in bone marrow and nucleated cells. Drug penetrates cerebrospinal fluid poorly but apparently crosses placenta. Tissue binding is extensive.
Metabolism: minimal.

Excretion: in bile and urine as unchanged drug. Half-life is 36 hours. Not known if drug appears in breast milk.
Action: peak serum levels, immediately after infusion.

MECHANISM OF ACTION
An antineoplastic antibiotic with cytotoxic action, dactinomycin forms a complex with DNA to inhibit RNA synthesis. Greatest activity apparently occurs in phase G_1. The drug may also have immunosuppressive and hypocalcemic properties.

INDICATIONS & DOSAGE
Dosage varies, depending on patient tolerance, size and location of tumor, and use of other treatments.
• Choriocarcinoma, Ewing's sarcoma, rhabdomyosarcoma, testicular cancer, uterine cancer, Wilms' tumor. *Adults:* 500 mcg daily for maximum of 5 days. *Children over age 6 months:* 15 mcg/kg daily for 5 days or total dose of 2.5 mg/m² over 1 week. Both adults and children may have a second course after 3 weeks if toxic effects have subsided.

CONTRAINDICATIONS & CAUTIONS
• Contraindicated in recent or active chicken pox or herpes zoster infection because of the risk of generalized disease and in children age 6 months and under because of an increased risk of toxicity.
• Use cautiously in patients with gout or a history of urate renal calculi because of the risk of hyperuricemia; and in myelosuppressed patients.

PREPARATION & STORAGE
Because of mutagenic, teratogenic, and carcinogenic risks, use a biological containment cabinet during drug preparation. Wear gloves and mask, use syringes with tight fittings (Luer-lok) to prevent drug leakage, and contamination of work surface. Properly dispose of needles, syringes, vials, and unused drug.

To prepare drug, reconstitute each 500 mcg vial with 1.1 ml of sterile water without preservative to yield 0.5 mg/ml; use 2.2 ml to yield 0.25 mg/ml. For infusion, dilute the clear, gold-colored reconstituted drug with dextrose 5% in water or with 0.9% sodium chloride. Refrigerate reconstituted drug for up to 72 hours. Store intact vials at 59° to 86° F. (15° to 30° C.).

ADMINISTRATION
Direct injection: Inject 500 mcg over a few minutes, preferably through a side port in an I.V. line containing freely flowing dextrose 5% in water or 0.9% sodium chloride. Assess vein patency frequently. After injection, run the I.V. solution for 2 to 5 minutes or inject 5 to 10 ml of I.V. solution through tubing to remove residual drug.
Intermittent infusion: Infuse diluted dose over 10 to 15 minutes into tubing of a free-flowing I.V. solution.
Continuous infusion: not recommended.

INCOMPATIBILITY
Incompatible with diluents containing preservatives.

ADVERSE REACTIONS
Life-threatening: anaphylaxis, pancytopenia.
Other: abdominal pain, acne, alopecia, anorexia, cheilosis, diarrhea, dysphagia, esophagitis, fatigue, fever, GI ulcers, glossitis, hyperpigmentation of previously irradiated skin, hypocalcemia, maculopapular rash, myalgia, nausea, pain and erythema at injection site, proctitis,

---

pruritus, ulcerative stomatitis, vomiting.

INTERACTIONS
Bone marrow depressants: worsened myelosuppression.
Doxorubicin: increased risk of cardiotoxicity.
Vitamin K: possible reduced effects.

EFFECTS ON DIAGNOSTIC TESTS
Bioassays for determining antibacterial drug levels: altered results.
Serum and urine uric acid: possible increased levels.
SGOT: rarely, elevated levels.

SPECIAL CONSIDERATIONS
• Monitor for extravasation, which can produce necrosis, cellulitis, phlebitis, and possible muscle contracture. The drug is a vesicant, and the extravasation risk rises as the duration of infusion lengthens.
• If extravasation occurs, discontinue infusion and aspirate as much drug as possible. Infiltrate area with 4 ml of isotonic sodium thiosulfate (1 g/10 ml) diluted with 6 ml of sterile water for injection, with 50 to 100 mg of hydrocortisone sodium succinate, or with ascorbic acid injection, or treat according to institution policy. Cover with sterile gauze and apply cold compresses.
• Monitor CBC and platelet count. Keep doctor informed; he may withhold drug until recovery occurs. Severe hematologic toxicity may require supportive measures, antibiotics for secondary infections, and blood transfusions.
• Identify and monitor previously irradiated skin for radiation recall—a flare-up of skin irritation or even necrosis may appear.
• Give antiemetics before administering drug.

• Doctor may discontinue dactinomycin if stomatitis or diarrhea occurs in a patient also receiving another antineoplastic drug.
• Providing adequate hydration, alkalinizing urine, or administering allopurinol may prevent or minimize uric acid nephropathy.
• Monitor renal and hepatic functions.

---

dantrolene sodium
Dantrium Intravenous♦

Pregnancy Risk Category: C

PHARMACOKINETICS
Distribution: throughout tissues, with substantial amounts reversibly bound to plasma proteins, especially albumin.
Metabolism: in liver to 5-hydroxy derivative, which is less active than parent compound, and to its amino derivative by reproductive pathways.
Excretion: in urine, mainly as metabolites. Drug probably appears in breast milk. Its half-life is 5 hours.
Action: peak plasma level, immediately after administration.

MECHANISM OF ACTION
Drug interferes with calcium ion release from sarcoplasmic reticulum, reducing myoplasmic concentration of calcium ions, thus helping to inactivate the catabolic processes associated with malignant hyperthermia crisis.

INDICATIONS & DOSAGE
• Adjunctive treatment of malignant hyperthermia crisis. *Adults and children:* 1 mg/kg; may repeat to a total of 10 mg/kg. To prevent recurrence, may change to oral form.

CONTRAINDICATIONS & CAUTIONS

• Contraindicated in patients with active hepatic disease, upper motor neuron disorders, and in whom spasticity helps maintain upright posture and balance.

• Use cautiously in COPD and in patients with cardiac impairment because of the increased risk of pleural effusion or pericarditis.

PREPARATION & STORAGE

Supplied in 20 mg vials. Reconstitute drug with 60 ml of sterile water (without a bacteriostatic agent) for a concentration of 0.333 mg/ml. Solution remains stable for 6 hours when stored at 59° to 86° F. (15° to 30° C.). Protect from light.

ADMINISTRATION

Direct injection: Rapidly inject drug directly into vein or through an I.V. line containing a free-flowing compatible solution.
Intermittent infusion: not recommended.
Continuous infusion: not recommended.

INCOMPATIBILITY

Not compatible with 5% dextrose or 0.9% sodium chloride. Drug shouldn't be mixed with any other drugs in a syringe.

ADVERSE REACTIONS

Life-threatening: none reported.
Other: chills; confusion; constipation; depression; diarrhea; dizziness; drowsiness; fatigue; fever; hallucinations; headache; hepatotoxicity, especially with long-term oral use; light-headedness; myalgia; nausea; nervousness; phlebitis; photosensitivity reactions; pruritus; rash; sweating; tachycardia; thrombophlebitis; urinary difficulty, frequency, incontinence, or retention; visual disturbances; weakness.

INTERACTIONS

Calcium channel blockers: ventricular fibrillation and cardiovascular collapse associated with severe hypokalemia.
CNS depressants: excessive depression.

EFFECTS ON DIAGNOSTIC TESTS

Serum alkaline phosphatase, BUN, LDH, total bilirubin: increased levels.
SGOT, SGPT: elevated levels.

SPECIAL CONSIDERATIONS

• As ordered, while administering dantrolene, also provide oxygen, treatments for metabolic acidosis, and cooling measures. Maintain urine output and monitor serum electrolyte levels.

• Because of solution's high pH, avoid extravasation.

• Obtain baseline neuromuscular functions for later functions comparisons.

• Monitor liver and renal function tests as well as blood cell count, especially if therapy is prolonged.

---

daunorubicin hydrochloride (daunomycin hydrochloride, rubidomycin hydrochloride)
Cerubidine♦

Pregnancy Risk Category: D

PHARMACOKINETICS

Distribution: rapid and throughout body tissues. Highest concentrations in spleen, kidneys, liver, lungs, and heart. Crosses placenta but probably not the blood-brain barrier.

Metabolism: slow and extensive in liver.

Excretion: primarily in bile, with 14% to 23% removed in urine. Not known if drug appears in breast milk. Its biphasic half-life consists of an initial phase of 40 minutes and a terminal phase of 2 days.

MECHANISM OF ACTION

This antineoplastic antibiotic binds with the DNA molecule, interfering with DNA and DNA-dependent RNA synthesis. Although most cytotoxic in the S phase, the drug isn't cell cycle–specific. It has immunosuppressive and antibacterial properties.

INDICATIONS & DOSAGE

• Acute myelogenous and acute lymphocytic leukemia; in children, various lymphomas and solid tumors. *Adults:* 30 to 60 mg/m² daily for 3 to 5 days or 0.8 to 1 mg/kg daily for 3 to 6 days. *Children:* 25 mg/m² weekly in combination with other chemotherapeutic drugs.

• Induction of remission in acute myelogenous leukemia. *Adults:* 60 mg/m² daily for 3 days, repeated q 3 to 4 weeks. Maximum total lifetime dosage is 550 mg/m². Previous chest irradiation requires a limit of 450 mg/m².

Note: Reduce dose in hepatic impairment.

CONTRAINDICATIONS & CAUTIONS

• Contraindicated in existing or recent chicken pox or herpes zoster infection because of an increased risk of generalized disease.

• Give cautiously to patients with preexisting myelosuppression and patients with cardiac disease or to those who've had previous therapy with doxorubicin, cyclophosphamide, dacarbazine, dactinomycin, or mitomycin because of an increased risk of cardiomyopathy.

• In patients with a history of gout or urate renal calculi, give drug carefully because of a heightened risk of hyperuricemia.

• Use with caution in hepatic or renal impairment because of a magnified risk of toxicity. Adjust dose as needed.

PREPARATION & STORAGE

Because of mutagenic, teratogenic, and carcinogenic risks, use a biological containment cabinet and wear gloves and mask. Use syringes with tight fittings (Luer-lok) to prevent drug leakage and dispose of needles, syringes, vials, and unused drug correctly. Avoid contaminating work surfaces.

Drug is available in 20 mg glass vials. Reconstitute with 4 ml sterile water for injection, then withdraw desired dose into syringe containing 10 to 15 ml of dextrose 5% in water or 0.9% sodium chloride. Unreconstituted drug remains stable for 2 years at room temperature if protected from direct sunlight, although decompensation causes it to become bluish purple. Reconstituted solution remains stable for 36 hours if refrigerated and for 24 hours at room temperature if protected from direct sunlight.

ADMINISTRATION

Direct injection: Give drug through the side port of a newly started I.V. line, preferably using a 23G or 25G winged-tip needle. Infuse a 10 to 15 ml solution over 2 to 3 minutes, a 50 ml solution over 10 to 15 minutes, or a 100 ml solution over 30 to 45 minutes. Throughout administration, periodically flush vein with primary I.V. solution.

Closely monitor for signs of infiltration, and instruct the patient to promptly report any changes in sensation, such as burning at the I.V. site. Extravasation can cause slow, progressive necrosis of skin and painful ulcers. If it occurs, stop injection and aspirate as much of drug as possible. Then immediately infiltrate the area with 50 to 100 ml of hydrocortisone sodium succinate or sodium bicarbonate, and apply cold compresses.

Intermittent infusion: not recommended.

Continuous infusion: not recommended.

INCOMPATIBILITY

Incompatible with heparin and dexamethasone. Best not to mix with *any* other drugs.

ADVERSE REACTIONS

Life-threatening: cardiotoxicity.
Other: abdominal pain, alopecia, contact dermatitis, diarrhea, esophagitis, hyperuricemia, myelosuppression, nausea, oral ulcers, pigmentation of fingernails and toenails, rash, red urine, stomatitis, urticaria, vomiting.

INTERACTIONS

Doxorubicin: increased risk of cardiotoxicity.
Other hepatotoxic drugs: increased risk of hepatotoxicity.

EFFECTS ON DIAGNOSTIC TESTS

Serum alkaline phosphatase, bilirubin, SGOT: temporarily increased levels.

SPECIAL CONSIDERATIONS

• Daunorubicin can reactivate radiation-induced skin lesions. If this occurs, reduce dosage as ordered.
• Keeping patient well hydrated, alkalinizing urine, and possibly administering allopurinol can prevent or minimize uric acid nephropathy.
• As ordered, give antibiotics for infections that develop during myelosuppression.
• Using a scalp tourniquet to prevent or minimize alopecia increases risk of micrometastatic scalp lesions.
• Monitor EKG (before treatment and monthly during therapy), CBC, and hepatic function.
• Tell home care patient to avoid exposure to people with infections.
• Give antiemetic to prevent nausea and vomiting, as ordered.

deferoxamine mesylate
Desferal Mesylate♦

Pregnancy Risk Category: C

PHARMACOKINETICS

Distribution: throughout body tissues. Drug crosses the placenta.
Metabolism: in tissues and plasma enzymes by an unknown mechanism.
Excretion: in urine, as the iron chelate ferrioxamine, giving urine a red tint; some removed through bile in feces. Not known if drug appears in breast milk. Serum half-life is about 1 hour.
Action: onset, immediate; peak levels, immediately after infusion.

MECHANISM OF ACTION

Deferoxamine chelates iron, forming ferrioxamine, a stable water-soluble compound easily excreted by the kidneys. It can remove iron from ferritin and hemosiderin in the body. Theoretically, 100 parts by weight can bind 8.5 parts of ferric iron. Drug also chelates aluminum.

INDICATIONS & DOSAGE

• Acute iron intoxication. *Adults:* 1 g initially, followed by 0.5 g q 4

hours for 2 doses, then 0.5 g q 4 to 12 hours, depending on patient's condition. Total daily dosage shouldn't exceed 6 g. *Children over age 3:* 20 mg/kg or 600 mg/m² initially, followed by 10 mg/kg or 300 mg/m² q 4 hours for 2 doses. Total dosage shouldn't exceed 6 g daily.
• Chronic iron intoxication. *Adults:* 2 g/unit of blood infused into a separate vein over 12 hours in addition to I.M. dose.

CONTRAINDICATIONS & CAUTIONS
• Contraindicated in severe renal disease or anuria because ferrioxamine and deferoxamine are excreted by the kidneys, and in primary hemochromatosis because phlebotomy is more effective.
• Use cautiously in pyelonephritis to avoid exacerbating this disorder.

PREPARATION & STORAGE
Available in 500 mg vials. Reconstitute by adding 2 ml of sterile water for injection to each vial. Further dilute for I.V. infusion by adding 0.9% sodium chloride, dextrose 5% in water, or Ringer's lactate. Reconstituted solutions remain stable for 1 week. Store below 104° F. (40° C.), preferably between 59° and 86° F. (15° and 30° C.), and protect from light.

ADMINISTRATION
Direct injection: not recommended.
Intermittent infusion: Infuse diluted solution directly into vein or through an I.V. line containing a free-flowing compatible solution at an hourly rate not exceeding 15 mg/kg.
Continuous infusion: not recommended.

INCOMPATIBILITY
Incompatible with all drugs in a solution or in a syringe.

ADVERSE REACTIONS
Life-threatening: anaphylaxis.
Other: fever, pain, and induration at injection site; red urine; tachycardia.
With overly rapid administration: erythema, flushing, hypotension, seizures, shock, urticaria.

INTERACTIONS
Ascorbic acid: with small doses, possible enhanced chelating action of deferoxamine.

EFFECTS ON DIAGNOSTIC TESTS
Colorimetric serum iron test: falsely lowered level.

SPECIAL CONSIDERATIONS
• Most effective when given early in treatment of iron intoxication. Not intended as a substitute for standard measures used in iron intoxication, drug is used only in potentially fatal intoxication (serum iron greater than 400 mcg/dl) or when patient has severe symptoms—coma, seizures, or cardiovascular collapse.
• Monitor intake and output.
• Ferrioxamine can be removed by dialysis.

---

deslanoside
Cedilanid♦♦, Cedilanid-D

Pregnancy Risk Category: C

PHARMACOKINETICS
Distribution: throughout body tissues, with high concentrations in skeletal muscle, liver, brain, kidneys, and heart. Cardiac concentrations are 15 to 30 times higher than plasma concentrations and twice that of skeletal muscle. Deslanoside is about 25% bound to plasma proteins. It crosses the placenta.
Metabolism: minimal.

Excretion: mainly in urine as unchanged drug, with about 20% excreted in 24 hours. Not known if drug appears in breast milk. Its half-life is 33 to 36 hours—longer in renal dysfunction.

Action: onset, 10 to 30 minutes; peak level, 1 to 3 hours.

MECHANISM OF ACTION

A digitalis glycoside, deslanoside depresses the SA node and increases the refractory period of the AV node through a direct action and by increasing vagal output from CNS. It also indirectly increases intracellular calcium by inhibiting sodium, potassium, and adenosine triphosphatase (ATPase), resulting in an inotropic action.

INDICATIONS & DOSAGE

Deslanoside has a low therapeutic index, requiring an individualized dosage carefully based on the patient's response, cardiovascular status, and renal function.

• Rapid digitalization in congestive heart failure, paroxysmal atrial tachycardia, atrial fibrillation and flutter. *Adults:* 1.2 to 1.6 mg as a single dose or 0.8 mg initially, repeated in 4 hours. *Children over age 3:* 0.0075 to 0.0112 mg/kg q 3 to 4 hours for 2 or 3 doses, as needed. *Children age 2 weeks to 3 years:* 0.008 to 0.012 mg/kg q 3 to 4 hours for 2 or 3 doses, as needed. *Premature and full-term neonates with reduced renal function or myocarditis:* 0.007 to 0.011 mg/kg q 3 to 4 hours for 2 or 3 doses, as needed.

CONTRAINDICATIONS & CAUTIONS

• Contraindicated in deslanoside hypersensitivity and in digitalis-induced toxicity, ventricular fibrillation, and ventricular tachycardia (unless caused by congestive

heart failure) because of the risk of exacerbating dysrhythmias.

• Use with extreme caution in acute glomerulonephritis and congestive heart failure because of the increased risk of toxicity.

• Because of an increased risk of digitalis-induced dysrhythmias, use cautiously in hypothyroidism, acute myocardial infarction, incomplete arteriovenous block, severe heart failure, chronic constrictive pericarditis, acute myocarditis, renal insufficiency, hypoxia, sick sinus syndrome, myxedema, and Wolff-Parkinson-White syndrome with atrial fibrillation.

• In the elderly and in patients who've received digitalis within the past 3 weeks, also use cautiously because of risk of dysrhythmias.

• Give cautiously in hypokalemia, hypomagnesemia, or hypercalcemia because drug can cause digitalis toxicity; in renal impairment because of increased risk of toxicity; in idiopathic hypertrophic subaortic stenosis because of risk of left ventricular outflow obstruction; and in heightened carotid sinus sensitivity because drug increases vagal tone.

PREPARATION & STORAGE

Available in 2 ml ampules (0.2 mg/ml). Store between 59° and 86° F. (15° and 30° C.). Drug is compatible with most solutions, including dextrose 5% in water, dextrose 5% in Ringer's lactate, and 0.9% sodium chloride in Ringer's lactate solution.

ADMINISTRATION

Direct injection: Inject drug directly into a vein or an established I.V. line over at least 5 minutes.

Intermittent infusion: not recommended.

Continuous infusion: not recommended.

INCOMPATIBILITY
No incompatibilities reported.

ADVERSE REACTIONS
Life-threatening: anaphylaxis, atrioventricular block, profound sinus bradycardia, ventricular tachycardia.
Other: agitation, anorexia, atrial and junctional tachycardia, blurred vision, diarrhea, diplopia, dizziness, fatigue, generalized weakness, gynecomastia, hallucinations, headache, hypotension, light flashes, malaise, nausea, paresthesias, photophobia, premature ventricular contractions, rash, stupor, urticaria, vertigo, vomiting, yellow-green halos around visual images.

INTERACTIONS
Amphotericin B, carbenicillin, corticosteroids, diuretics, ticarcillin: possible digitalis toxicity associated with hypokalemia.
Calcium channel blockers: increased serum deslanoside levels.
Calcium salts: possible dysrhythmias resulting from effects on cardiac contractility and excitability.
Edrophonium: possible excessive bradycardia.
Heparin: possible antagonistic anticoagulant effect.
Other cardiac glycosides, pancuronium, succinylcholine, sympathomimetics: heightened risk of dysrhythmias.
Thyroid hormones: possible decreased deslanoside effects.

EFFECTS ON DIAGNOSTIC TESTS
None reported.

SPECIAL CONSIDERATIONS
• *Treatment of overdose:* If signs of toxicity (bradycardia, nausea, vomiting, anorexia) occur, discontinue drug and treat symptomatically. Monitor electrolyte levels and EKG.

Correct hypoxia and acid-base, fluid, and electrolyte imbalances, as needed. As ordered, give I.V. phenytoin or lidocaine for dysrhythmias and atropine for symptomatic bradycardia. Deslanoside is excreted rapidly, so its toxic effects dissipate faster than those of other glycosides.
• Before first dose, obtain baseline heart rate and rhythm, blood pressure, and serum electrolyte levels. Ask patient if he's taken a cardiac glycoside in the past 3 weeks.
• Take patient's apical-radial pulse for a full minute. A pulse rate of 60 beats/minute or less can signal toxicity. If this occurs, stop the infusion and notify doctor. Also report any sudden rise in heart rate, irregular beats, and especially regularization of a previously irregular rhythm. If any of these occur, check blood pressure and obtain a 12-lead EKG.
• During therapy, monitor serum potassium level. Take corrective action before hypokalemia occurs.
• Deslanoside isn't appreciably removed by dialysis.

desmopressin acetate
DDAVP Injection♦, Stimate

Pregnancy Risk Category: B

PHARMACOKINETICS
Distribution: not fully understood. Not known if drug crosses the placenta or the blood-brain barrier.
Metabolism: possibly in kidneys.
Excretion: exact mechanism unknown. Drug appears in breast milk. Plasma levels decline biphasically, with half-lives of 8 and 76 minutes.
Action: peak levels, 90 minutes to 3 hours.

MECHANISM OF ACTION
As an antidiuretic, desmopressin promotes reabsorption of water by renal collecting ducts, resulting in increased urine osmolality and diminished urine flow. As an antihemorrhagic, it temporarily raises concentrations of Factor VIII:C, Factor VIII:R (von Willebrand's factor), and other components of Factor VIII complex.

INDICATIONS & DOSAGE
• Nonnephrogenic diabetes insipidus, temporary polyuria and polydipsia associated with pituitary trauma. *Adults and children age 12 and over:* 1 to 2 mcg q 12 hours. Dosage depends on changes in urine volume and osmolality and on control of nocturia.
• Hemophilia A and von Willebrand's disease. *Adults and children age 3 months and older:* 0.3 mcg/kg.

CONTRAINDICATIONS & CAUTIONS
• Contraindicated in hypersensitivity to desmopressin, in children under age 3 months because safety hasn't been established, and in patients with the Type IIB form of von Willebrand's disease because the drug can cause platelet aggregation.
• Use cautiously in patients with coronary artery insufficiency or hypertension because high doses can raise blood pressure.
• As an antidiuretic, the drug's safety hasn't been established for children under age 12.

PREPARATION & STORAGE
Available in 10 ml multidose vials and 1 ml ampules, with concentrations of 4 mcg/ml. For infusion, dilute the appropriate dose in 50 ml of 0.9% sodium chloride (for adults and children who weigh over 10 kg) or in 10 ml of 0.9% sodium chloride (for children who weigh 10 kg or less). Store at 39° F. (4° C.) unless manufacturer specifies otherwise; protect from freezing.

ADMINISTRATION
Direct injection: not recommended.
Intermittent infusion: Infuse diluted drug over 15 to 30 minutes. Rapid administration may produce hypotension.
Continuous infusion: not recommended.

INCOMPATIBILITY
No incompatibilities reported.

ADVERSE REACTIONS
Life-threatening: anaphylaxis.
Other: facial flushing, hyponatremia, hypotension, local erythema, mild abdominal cramps, nausea, slight rise in blood pressure, swelling and burning at injection site, tachycardia, transient headache, vulval pain, water intoxication (drowsiness, headache, vomiting).

INTERACTIONS
Alcohol, demeclocycline, epinephrine (large doses), heparin, lithium: possible reduced antidiuretic effect.
Chlorpropamide, fludrocortisone, urea: possible potentiated antidiuretic effect.
Clofibrate: potentiated and prolonged antidiuretic effect.

EFFECTS ON DIAGNOSTIC TESTS
None reported.

SPECIAL CONSIDERATIONS
• *Treatment of overdose:* Reduce desmopressin dosage. If fluid overload is severe, give furosemide.
• During infusion, monitor patient's blood pressure and pulse. After infusion, monitor his intake and output and serum sodium level.

• If patient has a hemorrhagic disorder, monitor Factor VIII, Factor VIII:R co-factor, Factor VIII antigen levels, and activated partial thromboplastin time.
• If patient has diabetes insipidus, monitor urine volume and osmolality. Also periodically monitor serum osmolality.
• Measure response to antidiuretic therapy by volume and frequency of urination and by duration of sleep.
• If patient doesn't need the drug for its antidiuretic effect, tell him to drink only enough to satisfy his thirst, to reduce the risk of water intoxication and hyponatremia.
• I.V. desmopressin has 10 times the antidiuretic effect of the same dose administered intranasally.
• Giving drug more than every 48 hours may cause tachyphylaxis.
• Drug has been successfully used to reduce blood loss during cardiac surgery.

---

dexamethasone sodium phosphate
Dalalone, Decadrol, Decadron Phosphate♦, Decaject, Dekasol, Dexacen-4, Dexameth, Dexasone, Dexon, Dexone, Hexadrol Phosphate, Solurex

Pregnancy Risk Category: C

PHARMACOKINETICS
Distribution: throughout muscles, liver, skin, intestines, and kidneys. Drug crosses the placenta and the blood-brain barrier.
Metabolism: primarily in the liver and, to a lesser degree, in the kidneys and other tissues to inactive compounds.
Excretion: in urine as inactive metabolites, primarily glucuronides and sulfates but also as unconjugated

products. Small amounts of unchanged drug are excreted in urine, negligible amounts in bile. Drug also appears in breast milk. Its half-life averages about 4 hours.
Action: rapid onset and varied duration, depending on dose, frequency of administration, and length of therapy.

MECHANISM OF ACTION
A synthetic glucocorticoid, dexamethasone decreases inflammation by stabilizing leukocyte lysosomal membranes. It also suppresses pituitary release of corticotropin (ACTH), thereby halting adrenocortical secretion of corticosteroids and stifling the immune response. The drug also influences protein, fat, and carbohydrate metabolism.

INDICATIONS & DOSAGE
• Adjunctive treatment of shock. *Adults:* 1 to 6 mg/kg in a single dose, 40 mg q 2 to 6 hours, or 20 mg in a single dose followed by 3 mg/kg over 24 hours in a continuous infusion.
• Adjunctive treatment of cerebral edema. *Adults:* 10 mg initially, then doses given I.M. For inoperable or recurrent brain tumors, 2 mg I.V. maintenance dose may be given b.i.d. or t.i.d.
• Inflammatory conditions or allergic reactions. *Adults:* usually, 0.5 to 9 mg daily. Maximum dosage is 80 mg daily. *Children:* 6 to 40 mcg/kg once or twice daily.

CONTRAINDICATIONS & CAUTIONS
• Contraindicated in sensitivity to any component of drug, including sulfites. Sodium bisulfites can cause severe allergic reactions.
• Also contraindicated in peptic ulcers (except if life-threatening) be-

cause of the increased risk of GI bleeding.

• Use cautiously in diverticulitis and nonspecific ulcerative colitis if any risk of perforation, abscess, or other pyogenic infection exists; in recent intestinal anastomoses because drug may exacerbate the condition or mask its signs; and in seizure disorders, diabetes mellitus, osteoporosis, and bacterial, viral, or fungal infections because drug can exacerbate these disorders.

• Also use cautiously in hypothyroidism or cirrhosis because of the risk of an exaggerated drug response; in cardiac disease, congestive heart failure, renal insufficiency, or hypertension because of the risk of fluid retention; and in thromboembolic disease because the drug increases blood coagulability and the risk of intravascular thrombosis.

• Administer carefully in ocular herpes simplex because of the risk of corneal perforation; in patients with a history of tuberculosis or with positive skin tests because the drug may reactivate disease; in glaucoma because the drug can raise intraocular pressure; in hepatic impairment or hypoalbuminemia because of an increased risk of toxicity; and in hyperlipidemia because drug can raise serum cholesterol or fatty acid levels.

• In hyperthyroidism, use cautiously because accelerated metabolism may reduce drug effect; in hypothyroidism, slowed metabolism may enhance drug effect.

PREPARATION & STORAGE

Available in concentrations of 4, 10, 20, and 24 mg/ml in vials and syringes in a range of sizes. The solution is clear but may appear yellow at higher concentrations. Dilute dexamethasone in dextrose 5% in water or 0.9% sodium chloride for intermittent or continuous infusion. Protect solutions from light and freezing.

ADMINISTRATION

Direct injection: Give undiluted drug over at least 1 minute.
Intermittent infusion: Give diluted drug as ordered.
Continuous infusion: Infuse diluted drug over 24 hours.

INCOMPATIBILITY

Incompatible with daunorubicin, doxorubicin, and vancomycin.

ADVERSE REACTIONS

Most reactions are dose- or duration-dependent.
Life-threatening: anaphylaxis.
Other: acne, cataracts, congestive heart failure, delayed wound healing, edema, euphoria, GI irritation, glaucoma, growth suppression in children, hyperglycemia, hypertension, hypokalemia, increased appetite, increased susceptibility to infection, insomnia, pancreatitis and pancreatic destruction (with high doses), peptic ulcer, psychotic behavior, weakness. *In children:* Increased intracranial pressure can cause abducens or oculomotor nerve paralysis, headache, papilledema, or vision loss.

INTERACTIONS

Anticholinesterase drugs: severe weakness in patients with myasthenia gravis. Use cautiously.
Cardiac glycosides: increased risk of dysrhythmias.
Estrogen: enhanced dexamethasone effects.
Hepatic enzyme inhibitors: increased glucocorticoid metabolism.
Indomethacin, other ulcerogenic drugs: heightened risk of GI ulcers.

Insulin: elevated serum levels, requiring dexamethasone dosage adjustment.
131I: reduced uptake.
Mexiletine: accelerated metabolism.
Mitotane: suppressed adrenocortical function, requiring higher doses of dexamethasone.
Potassium-depleting diuretics, other potassium-depleting drugs: possible enhanced potassium loss.
Salicylates: enhanced salicylate clearance, requiring dosage increase.
Toxoids and live or inactivated vaccines: diminished response.

EFFECTS ON DIAGNOSTIC TESTS

ACTH stimulation, plasma cortisol: decreased levels.
Basophil, eosinophil, lymphocyte, monocyte counts: reduced.
Gonadorelin tests: altered results because of modified pituitary secretion of gonadatropins.
123I uptake, protein-bound iodine, serum T_4: reduced levels.
Nitroblue tetrazolium test for systemic bacterial infections: possible false-negative results.
Platelet count: increased or decreased.
Radionuclide brain and skeletal imaging: altered results when pertechnetate Tc 99m or technetium 99m medronate is used.
Serum and urine glucose; polymorphonuclear leukocytes; serum cholesterol, fatty acid, sodium, uric acid: elevated levels.
Serum calcium, potassium: decreased levels.
Skin tests: suppressed reactions.
Urine 14-ketosteroids and 17-hydroxycorticosteroids: reduced levels.

SPECIAL CONSIDERATIONS
● Because of the risk of hypersensitivity reactions, keep emergency resuscitation equipment nearby before starting therapy.
● Monitor patient for injury or signs of infection during therapy.
● As ordered, titrate drug to lowest effective dose.
● I.V. administration is usually followed by use of I.M. or P.O. route.
● Short-term administration is unlikely to cause adverse reactions, even with massive doses. Long-term therapy may retard bone growth in infants and children and should be closely monitored.
● Dexamethasone is used effectively to treat nausea and vomiting from chemotherapy.
● Dalalone, Decadron Phosphate, Decaject, Dekasol, Dexacen-4, Dexone, and Solurex may contain sulfites. Hexadol Phosphate contains benzyl alcohol.

---

dexpanthenol (D-pantothenyl alcohol injection)
Ilopan

Pregnancy Risk Category: C

PHARMACOKINETICS
Distribution: throughout body tissues after conversion to pantothenic acid, a precursor of coenzyme A. Highest concentrations occur in the liver, adrenal glands, heart, and kidneys. Not known if drug crosses the placenta.
Metabolism: not fully understood.
Excretion: 70% in urine, 30% in feces. Not known if drug appears in breast milk.
Action: not known.

MECHANISM OF ACTION
The alcohol analogue of D-pantothenic acid, dexpanthenol helps to transfer acetyl groups to form ace-

tylcholine, which stimulates and tones intestinal smooth muscles.

INDICATIONS & DOSAGE
• Prophylaxis immediately after major abdominal surgery to stimulate intestinal peristalsis and avoid abdominal distention, flatus retention, and delayed return of normal intestinal motility. *Adults:* 500 mg. If prompt relief isn't obtained, consider other methods of stimulating peristalsis.

CONTRAINDICATIONS & CAUTIONS
• Contraindicated in dexpanthenol hypersensitivity; in mechanical obstruction because therapy requires correcting the obstruction (not relieving symptoms); and in hemophilia because of the risk of prolonged bleeding time.
• Safety and effectiveness in children haven't been established.

PREPARATION & STORAGE
A viscous liquid available in 2, 10, and 30 ml vials as well as in 2 ml disposable syringes containing 250 mg/ml. Dilute in dextrose 5% in water or in Ringer's lactate. Don't expose drug to excessive heat or cold.

ADMINISTRATION
Direct injection: not recommended.
Intermittent infusion: Piggyback into an established I.V. line. Infuse slowly.
Continuous infusion: not recommended.

INCOMPATIBILITY
Incompatible with alkalies and strong acids.

ADVERSE REACTIONS
Life-threatening: anaphylaxis.

Other: agitation (in elderly patients), diarrhea, dyspnea, generalized dermatitis, intestinal colic, patchy erythema, pruritus, slight drop in blood pressure, tingling, urticaria, vomiting.

INTERACTIONS
Antibiotics, barbiturates, narcotics: possible increased risk of allergic reaction.
Succinylcholine: possible prolonged effect if given within 1 hour of dexpanthenol.

EFFECTS ON DIAGNOSTIC TESTS
None reported.

SPECIAL CONSIDERATIONS
• Use of dexpanthenol to stimulate intestinal peristalsis remains controversial; its benefit hasn't been proved.
• Because drug effect may be diminished in hypokalemia, give potassium supplements and, if needed, increase dexpanthenol dosage.

dextran

Low molecular weight: Dextran 40
10% Dextran 40 in 5% Dextrose Injection; 10% Dextran 40 in 0.9% Sodium Chloride Injection; 10% Gentran 40 in 5% Dextrose Injection; 10% Gentran 40 in 0.9% Sodium Chloride Injection; 10% LMD in 5% Dextrose Injection; 10% LMD in 0.9% Sodium Chloride Injection; 10% Rheomacrodex in 5% Dextrose Injection; 10% Rheomacrodex in 0.9% Sodium Chloride Injection

High molecular weight: Dextran 70 and 75
6% Dextran 70 in 5% Dextrose Injection; 6% Dextran 70 in 0.9% Sodium Chloride Injection; 6% Dextran 75 in 5% Dextrose Injection; 6% Dextran 75 in 0.9% Sodium Chloride Injection; 6% Gentran 70 in 0.9% Sodium Chloride Injection; Macrodex in 0.9% Sodium Chloride Injection

Pregnancy Risk Category: C

COMPOSITION
Dextran is available in both low- and high-molecular-weight forms that contain dextrose or sodium chloride.

MECHANISM OF ACTION
A short-acting plasma volume expander, low-molecular-weight dextran increases plasma volume by twice its own volume. It helps to restore normal circulatory dynamics, increasing arterial and pulse pressure, central venous pressure, and cardiac output. It also improves microcirculatory flow to prevent venous stasis and mobilizes water from body tissues to increase urine output.

High-molecular-weight dextran has colloidal properties similar to those of human albumin. It expands plasma volume by slightly more than its own volume; then the volume decreases over 24 hours. It improves hemodynamic status for at least 24 hours. A glucose polymer, it's degraded to glucose and excreted in urine.

INDICATIONS & DOSAGE
• Adjunctive treatment of shock from hemorrhage, burns, surgery, or other trauma. *Adults and children:* Dosage reflects fluid loss and resultant hemoconcentration. Total dosage of 10% low-molecular-weight solution shouldn't exceed 2 g/kg (20 ml/kg) for first 24 hours, then 1 g/kg (10 ml/kg) daily for 4 days. Total dosage of 6% high-molecular-weight solution shouldn't exceed 1.2 g/kg (20 ml/kg) for first 24 hours, then 0.6 g/kg (10 ml/kg) daily, as needed.
• Prophylaxis of venous thrombosis and pulmonary embolism. *Adults:* 50 to 100 g (500 to 1,000 ml) of 10% low-molecular-weight solution during surgery, then 50 g daily for 2 to 3 days, followed by 50 g q 2 or 3 days for up to 2 weeks.

CONTRAINDICATIONS & CAUTIONS
• Contraindicated in hypersensitivity to dextran.
• Also contraindicated in pulmonary edema because of exacerbation of the condition; in marked thrombocytopenia, coagulation defects, and bleeding disorders because of the increased risk of prolonged bleeding time; and in renal disease with severe oliguria or anuria because of the heightened risk of circulatory overload.

• In extreme dehydration, avoid using low-molecular-weight dextran because renal failure can occur.
• Give cautiously (especially sodium chloride solutions) in heart failure and cardiac decompensation because of the increased risk of pulmonary edema.
• Also give cautiously in hemorrhage because increased perfusion pressure and improved microvascular flow can cause additional blood loss.

PREPARATION & STORAGE
Low-molecular-weight dextran is available in 500 ml bottles as a 10% solution diluted in 0.9% sodium chloride or dextrose 5% in water. High-molecular-weight dextran comes in 500 ml bottles as a 6% solution diluted in 0.9% sodium chloride or dextrose 5% in water. Store solutions at a constant temperature, preferably 77° F. (25° C.). Crystals may form at low temperatures. If this occurs, submerge bottle in warm water to dissolve crystals before infusing. Don't administer cloudy solutions.

ADMINISTRATION
Direct injection: not recommended.
Intermittent infusion: Rapidly infuse first 500 ml of low-molecular-weight dextran over 15 to 30 minutes. Slowly infuse remainder based on patient response. In an emergency, infuse high-molecular-weight dextran at 1.2 to 2.4 g (20 to 40 ml)/minute. In normovolemic patients, don't exceed 0.24 g (4 ml)/minute.
Continuous infusion: Infuse over 24 hours based on patient's condition and response.

INCOMPATIBILITY
Incompatible with ascorbic acid, chlortetracycline, phytonadione, promethazine, and protein hydrolysate.

Don't add any drug to a bottle of dextran solution.

ADVERSE REACTIONS
Life-threatening: anaphylaxis.
Other: arthralgia, chest tightness, extravasation, fever, hypervolemia, nausea, urticaria, vomiting, wheezing.

INTERACTIONS
None reported.

EFFECTS ON DIAGNOSTIC TESTS
Blood cross matching, typing, Rh determinations: with high-molecular-weight dextran, altered results stemming from rouleaux formation in RBCs. Draw blood for type and cross matching before giving dextran.
Hematocrit: possible reduced levels.
Serum glucose: increased levels when test uses sulfuric or acetic acid hydrolysis or turbidimeter measurements.
Serum or urine bilirubin: with low-molecular-weight dextran, altered levels in tests using alcohol.
SGOT, SGPT: with low-molecular-weight dextran, increased levels.
Total protein: with low-molecular-weight dextran, altered results in tests using biuret reagents.

SPECIAL CONSIDERATIONS
• Monitor pulse, blood pressure, central venous pressure, and urine output every 5 to 15 minutes for the first hour and then hourly. Watch for signs of fluid overload or hypersensitivity.
• Discontinue the infusion at the first sign of allergic reaction, but maintain I.V. access. Give antihistamines, ephedrine, or epinephrine, as needed. Keep resuscitation equipment available.

• Maintain hydration with additional I.V. fluids. Dextran is a colloid hypertonic solution that attracts water from the extravascular space and causes tissue dehydration.

• Slow or discontinue the infusion if central venous pressure rises rapidly (normal pressure is 7 to 14 mm H_2O) or if the patient is anuric or oliguric after receiving 500 ml of dextran. Give mannitol to help increase urine flow.

• Change I.V. tubing or flush well with 0.9% sodium chloride before transfusing blood. Dextran may cause blood coagulation in the tubing.

• Dextran can impair coagulation, possibly leading to additional blood loss. Notify doctor if bleeding increases or if hematocrit drops below 30%.

• Use high-molecular-weight dextran only when whole blood or blood products aren't available. It isn't a substitute for whole blood or plasma proteins because it has no oxygen-carrying ability.

dextrose in sodium chloride solutions

Pregnancy Risk Category: C

COMPOSITION
These solutions contain combinations of hypotonic or isotonic concentrations of dextrose and sodium chloride. Solutions of dextrose 2.5% or 5% and 0.45% sodium chloride are hypotonic. Others are isotonic.

INDICATIONS & CONCENTRATION
• Temporary treatment of circulatory insufficiency and shock when plasma volume expander isn't available, and as fluid replacement in burned, de-

hydrated, and other patients. *Adults and children:* Concentration and infusion rate reflect patient's age, weight, condition, and fluid, electrolyte, and acid-base balance.

CONTRAINDICATIONS & CAUTIONS
• Contraindicated in diabetic coma or allergy to corn or corn products.

• Avoid use or give with extreme caution during concurrent corticosteroid therapy and in congestive heart failure, severe renal insufficiency, and edema with sodium retention because of the increased risk of circulatory overload.

• Use cautiously in renal impairment because of the increased risk of sodium retention; in urinary obstruction because of the risk of circulatory overload; and in diabetes mellitus or carbohydrate intolerance because of exacerbated hyperglycemia.

PREPARATION & STORAGE
Available in 250, 500, and 1,000 ml bottles and PVC bags. Dextrose 5% in 0.2% sodium chloride also comes in 150 ml containers. Concentrations include dextrose 2.5% in 0.45% sodium chloride; dextrose 5% in 0.11%, 0.2%, 0.225%, 0.3%, 0.45%, or 0.9% sodium chloride; and dextrose 10% in 0.2% or 0.9% sodium chloride. Store solutions in a cool, dry place, and protect from freezing or extreme heat. Don't administer cloudy solutions.

ADMINISTRATION
Direct injection: not recommended.
Intermittent infusion: not recommended.
Continuous infusion: Infuse through a peripheral or central vein at ordered rate.

INCOMPATIBILITY
Incompatible with amphotericin B, ampicillin sodium, amsacrine, diazepam, erythromycin lactobionate, mannitol, phenytoin, and warfarin.

ADVERSE REACTIONS
Life-threatening: none.
Other: extravasation, fever, fluid overload, hypernatremia, hypervolemia, hypokalemia, hypovitaminosis, metabolic acidosis or alkalosis, phlebitis, thrombosis.

INTERACTIONS
None reported.

EFFECTS ON DIAGNOSTIC TESTS
BUN: possible increased levels.

SPECIAL CONSIDERATIONS
• Monitor changes in fluid balance, electrolyte levels, and acid-base balance during prolonged parenteral therapy. Give electrolyte supplements as needed.
• Watch closely for fluid overload (exacerbated hypertension, signs of congestive heart failure or pulmonary edema), especially in the elderly or in patients with renal or cardiac disease.

dextrose in water solutions (glucose solutions)

Pregnancy Risk Category: C

COMPOSITION
Containing glucose and water, these solutions vary in tonicity and concentration. Solutions of 2.5% are hypotonic, solutions of 5% are isotonic, and solutions over 10% are hypertonic.

INDICATIONS & CONCENTRATION
• Provision of calories and water to meet metabolic and hydration needs. *Adults and children:* 2.5%, 5%, or 10% solution.
• Hyperkalemia and conditions that require adequate calories but little water. *Adults and children:* 20% solution.
• Promotion of diuresis. *Adults and children:* 20% to 50% solution.
• Base solution for I.V. hyperalimentation. *Adults and children:* 10% to 70% solution.
• Adjunctive treatment of shock. *Adults and children:* 40% to 70% solution.
• Cerebral edema, pregnancy-induced hypertension, renal disease, acute hypoglycemia, and as a sclerosing agent. *Adults and children:* 50% solution.
• Acute symptomatic hypoglycemia. *Infants and neonates:* 10% to 25% solution.

CONTRAINDICATIONS & CAUTIONS
• Hypertonic solutions are contraindicated in neurosurgical procedures, delirium tremens with dehydration, and intracranial or intraspinal hemorrhage because they may cause hyperosmolar syndrome, and in anuria because of the risk of circulatory overload.
• All dextrose solutions are contraindicated in diabetic coma because of the risk of exacerbation, and in allergies to corn or corn products because solution is made from corn sugar.
• Use dextrose solutions cautiously in patients with renal disease, cardiac disease, and hypertension because of the risk of circulatory overload; in overt or subclinical diabetes mellitus because solution may exacerbate hyperglycemia; in urinary

obstruction because of excretion difficulty; and in carbohydrate intolerance because solution may cause hyperosmolar syndrome.

PREPARATION & STORAGE
Available in 50, 100, 150, 250, 500, and 1,000 ml bottles or PVC bags in the following concentrations: 2.5%, 5%, 7.7%, 10%, 11.5%, 20%, 25%, 30%, 38%, 38.5%, 40%, 50%, 60%, and 70%. Because dextrose is an excellent medium for bacterial growth, store solutions in a cool, dry place. Protect from freezing and extreme heat. Don't administer cloudy solutions.

ADMINISTRATION
Avoid extravasation because tissue sloughing and necrosis can occur. Never infuse hypertonic solutions rapidly because this can cause hyperglycemia and fluid shift.
Direct injection: Give 50 ml of 50% solution at 3 ml/minute.
Intermittent infusion: not recommended.
Continuous infusion: Give isotonic solutions through a peripheral vein, hypertonic solutions through a central venous line. Rate depends on the solution's concentration and the patient's age and condition. An hourly rate above 0.5 g/kg may cause glycosuria in healthy people. Maximum rate shouldn't exceed 0.8 g/kg/hour.

INCOMPATIBILITY
Incompatible with ampicillin sodium, cisplatin, diazepam, erythromycin lactobionate, fat emulsions (10% and 25% solutions), phenytoin, procainamide, thiopental (solutions of 10% and above), warfarin, and whole blood.

ADVERSE REACTIONS
Life-threatening: none reported.

Other: extravasation, fever (from contaminated solution), glycosuria or hyperglycemia (from prolonged infusion, hypertonic solution, or metabolic insufficiency), hyperosmolar syndrome (confusion, unconsciousness caused by rapid administration of hypertonic solution), hypervolemia, hypokalemia, hypovitaminosis, infusion site reaction (local pain, phlebitis, or sclerosed veins with prolonged infusion of hypertonic solution), metabolic acidosis or alkalosis, thrombosis, water intoxication (from prolonged infusion of hypotonic or isotonic solution).

INTERACTIONS
None reported.

EFFECTS ON DIAGNOSTIC TESTS
Serum glucose: increased levels with prolonged infusion of hypertonic solution.
Urine glucose: positive results with prolonged infusion of hypertonic solution.

SPECIAL CONSIDERATIONS
● Monitor serum glucose levels—hypertonic solutions especially can alter insulin requirements, and prolonged infusion of nutrients can diminish insulin production and secretion. Watch for signs of hyperglycemia. If they occur, reduce infusion rate and give insulin.
● To avoid rebound hypoglycemia, substitute dextrose 5% or 10% after discontinuing hypertonic solutions.
● Monitor intake and output and weight, and watch for signs of fluid overload (exacerbated hypertension, signs of congestive heart failure or pulmonary edema), especially in the elderly or in patients with renal or cardiac disease.
● Expect osmotic diuresis when giving hypertonic solutions.

• Monitor serum electrolyte and acid-base balance during prolonged administration. Give electrolyte supplements, as needed.

dezocine
Dalgan

Pregnancy Risk Category: C

PHARMACOKINETICS
Distribution: widely distributed; effective plasma levels are 5 ng/ml.
Metabolism: in liver.
Excretion: in urine, mostly as metabolites. Not known if the drug appears in breast milk.
Action: onset, within 15 minutes; duration, 2 to 4 hours; half-life, 2.4 hours.

MECHANISM OF ACTION
A synthetic opioid agonist-antagonist, dezocine produces postoperative analgesia qualitatively similar to postoperative analgesia produced by morphine.

INDICATIONS & DOSAGE
• Moderate to severe pain when use of an opioid analgesic is inappropriate. *Adults:* initially, 5 mg I.V., then 2.5 to 10 mg I.V. q 2 to 4 hours.

CONTRAINDICATIONS & CAUTIONS
• Contraindicated in hypersensitivity to the drug.
• Contraindicated in patients who are opioid-dependent because it may precipitate a withdrawal syndrome and in patients with chronic pain because it can precipitate an abstinence syndrome if the patient has a substantial tolerance to opiates.
• Because dezocine produces a dose-dependent respiratory depression similar to that of morphine (usually peaking within 15 minutes of administration), use only in clinical settings where adequate respiratory support and an opiate antagonist (naloxone hydrochloride) are available.
• Injection contains sulfite preservatives, which may cause allergic reactions in hypersensitive patients.
• Use cautiously and in lower doses in patients with renal dysfunction and in those with chronic respiratory disease.
• Like other narcotic agonist-antagonists, dezocine abuse is a potential risk in patients with a history of opiate use or dependence.
• Use with extreme caution in patients with head injury because clinical signs may be obscured by the CNS depressant effects of the drug. Related drugs have caused elevations of CSF pressure in head injury patients.
• Use cautiously in patients undergoing biliary surgery. Related drugs have caused significant increases in pressure within the common bile duct.
• As with other potent analgesics, administer dezocine cautiously to elderly patients.

PREPARATION & STORAGE
Available in 2 ml single dose vials and 2 ml prefilled syringes containing 5 mg/ml, 10 mg/ml, or 15 mg/ml. Also available in a 10 ml, 10 mg/ml multiple dose container. Store at room temperature and protect from light.

ADMINISTRATION
Direct injection: Infuse ordered dose over at least 5 minutes.
Intermittent infusion: not recommended.
Continuous infusion: not recommended.

INCOMPATIBILITY
None reported. Studies are limited. Do not mix with other drugs until more data are available. Call pharmacy for more information.

ADVERSE REACTIONS
Life-threatening: none reported.
Other: abdominal distress, anxiety, chest pain, chills, constipation, diarrhea, dizziness, dry mouth, edema, flushing, headache, hypertension, hypotension, irregular heartbeat, local irritation at the injection site, mood disorders, nausea, pallor, pruritus, rash, sleep disturbances, slurred speech, sweating, thrombophlebitis, vertigo, vomiting.

INTERACTIONS
Alcohol or other CNS depressants: increased risk of CNS depression.
Opiates: increased risk of precipitating acute abstinence syndrome in patients who are dependent upon opiates.

EFFECTS ON DIAGNOSTIC TESTS
None reported

SPECIAL CONSIDERATIONS
• *Treatment of overdose:* Treatment is supportive. Maintain the airway and administer oxygen as ordered. Administer naloxone hydrochloride (Narcan) to reverse respiratory depressant effects.
• Warn the patient to move about cautiously because the drug may cause dizziness.
• Breast feeding is not recommended during dezocine therapy because of the risk of adverse effects to the infant.
• Plasma concentrations higher than 45 ng/ml are associated with an increased incidence of adverse effects.
• Maximum dosage for I.V. use has not been determined. Maximum recommended single I.M. dose is 20 mg, with a maximum daily I.M. dosage of 120 mg.

diazepam
Valium♦, Zetran

Controlled Substance Schedule IV
Pregnancy Risk Category: D

PHARMACOKINETICS
Distribution: throughout body tissues, with 80% to 99% bound to plasma proteins.
Metabolism: in the liver.
Excretion: in urine as metabolites; small amounts in feces. Drug appears in breast milk. Its half-life is 20 to 50 hours.
Action: onset, 1 to 5 minutes; duration, 15 to 60 minutes.

MECHANISM OF ACTION
The sites and mechanism of action of diazepam aren't completely understood. However, the drug is thought to enhance or facilitate the action of the neurotransmitter gamma-aminobutyric acid, which depresses the CNS at the limbic and subcortical levels, producing an antianxiety effect.

As an anticonvulsant, diazepam suppresses the spread of impulses from irritable foci in the cortex, thalamus, and limbic structures. As a skeletal muscle relaxant, it purportedly inhibits polysynaptic afferent pathways. As an amnesic, its mechanism of action isn't known.

INDICATIONS & DOSAGE

• Short-term, symptomatic relief of anxiety or as a skeletal muscle relaxant in N.P.O. patient. *Adults and children over age 12:* 2 to 10 mg (0.4 to 2 ml) q 3 to 4 hours. May repeat in 1 hour, with maximum of 30 mg in 8 hours. Give 2 to 5 mg to elderly patient or when another sedative has been given.

• Cardioversion. *Adults:* 5 to 15 mg (1 to 3 ml) just before procedure as amnesic agent.

• Endoscopy. *Adults:* up to 20 mg before procedure, then titrated to desired effect. May produce anterograde amnesia.

• Tetanus. *Adults and children age 5 and older:* 5 to 10 mg. May repeat dose in 3 to 4 hours. *Infants over age 1 month:* 1 to 2 mg q 3 to 4 hours.

• Status epilepticus and recurrent seizures. *Adults:* 5 to 20 mg by slow I.V. push at 2 to 5 mg/minute. May repeat dose q 5 to 10 minutes up to maximum of 60 mg. Give 2 to 5 mg to elderly or debilitated patient; in recurrent seizures, dose may be repeated in 20 to 30 minutes. *Children age 5 and older:* 0.5 to 1 mg q 2 to 5 minutes up to a total dose of 10 mg. May be repeated in 2 to 4 hours. *Infants over age 1 month:* 0.2 to 0.5 mg q 2 to 5 minutes up to a total dose of 5 mg. May be repeated in 2 to 4 hours.

CONTRAINDICATIONS & CAUTIONS

• Contraindicated in hypersensitivity to drug; in acute narrow-angle glaucoma or untreated chronic open-angle glaucoma because of drug's possible anticholinergic effect; in shock or coma because drug's hypotensive or hypnotic effects may be prolonged or worsened; and in acute alcohol intoxication because drug deepens CNS depression.

• Also contraindicated in pregnant women because of possible fetal malformations and in infants younger than 30 days because of slow drug metabolism.

• Give with extreme caution to patients with limited pulmonary reserve because of the risk of apnea and cardiac arrest. Also give with extreme caution for endoscopy, keeping emergency resuscitation equipment readily available in case of laryngospasm.

• Give diazepam cautiously to psychotic patients because of possible paradoxical reaction; to depressed patients because of possible worsened depression; and to patients with myasthenia gravis or porphyria because of possible exacerbation.

• Also administer cautiously to patients with renal or hepatic impairment because of delayed drug elimination; to patients with hypoalbuminemia because of higher incidence of adverse effects; to elderly or debilitated patients because of increased CNS effects; and to addiction-prone patients.

PREPARATION & STORAGE

Available in 10 ml bottles (5 mg/ml), prefilled syringes, and 2 ml ampules. Protect vials from light. Don't mix with I.V. solutions. Also don't store in plastic syringes or in administration sets because diazepam interacts with plastic.

ADMINISTRATION

Direct injection: Slowly inject undiluted drug into large vein or cannula at a rate of less than 5 mg/minute for adults and 0.25 mg/kg of body weight over 3 minutes for children. Avoid extravasation. If you inject drug into tubing, choose a site directly above the needle or cannula insertion site. Afterward, flush with 0.9% sodium chloride.

Intermittent infusion: not used. Drug precipitates in any solution.
Continuous infusion: not used. Drug precipitates in any solution.

INCOMPATIBILITY
Incompatible with *all* other drugs and I.V. solutions.

ADVERSE REACTIONS
Life-threatening: bradycardia, cardiovascular collapse, hypotension, respiratory depression.
Other: ataxia, blurred or double vision, confusion, depression, desquamation, dizziness, drowsiness, dysarthria, fatigue, hangover, headache, lethargy, nausea, nightmares, nystagmus, pain and phlebitis at injection site, rash, slurred speech, syncope, tremors, urinary incontinence or retention, urticaria, vertigo, vomiting.

INTERACTIONS
Alcohol, barbiturates, general anesthetics, narcotics, phenothiazines: intensified CNS depression.
Antihypertensives: potentiated effects.
Cimetidine: elevated diazepam levels resulting from diminished hepatic metabolism.
Isoniazid, rifampin: possible increased serum diazepam levels.
Ketamine: heightened risk of hypotension or respiratory depression.
Levodopa: diminished therapeutic effects.
Magnesium sulfate: potentiated CNS effects.
MAO inhibitors, other antidepressants: deepened CNS depression.
Neuromuscular blocking drugs: deepened respiratory depression. Monitor respirations closely.

EFFECTS ON DIAGNOSTIC TESTS
EEG: minor changes in wave patterns, usually low-voltage fast activity, during and after therapy.
Liver function tests and serum bilirubin: altered levels.

SPECIAL CONSIDERATIONS
• *Treatment of overdose:* Give dopamine, norepinephrine, or metaraminol for hypotension.
• Always keep emergency resuscitation equipment nearby when giving I.V. diazepam. Obtain baseline respiratory rate before administration, and notify doctor if rate falls below 12 breaths/minute. Also obtain baseline blood pressure, and monitor carefully during and after administration.
• Monitor respiratory rate for 1 hour after administration. If rate falls below 8 breaths/minute, arouse patient and encourage him to breathe at rate of 10 to 12 breaths/minute. If you can't arouse patient, maintain airway patency and use a hand-held respirator to maintain rate of 10 to 12 breaths/minute. Notify doctor; he may decide to intubate patient.
• If patient's receiving a narcotic, reduce its dosage by at least a third.
• Keep patient in bed for 3 hours after parenteral administration.
• Observe infusion site for signs of phlebitis.
• Discontinue drug if paradoxical reaction occurs, typified by anxiety, acute excitation, hallucinations, increased muscle spasticity, insomnia, or rage.
• Keep in mind that abrupt withdrawal after high doses or extended use can cause seizures and delirium.
• Drug isn't appreciably removed by hemodialysis.
• May contain benzyl alcohol.

diazoxide
Hyperstat

Pregnancy Risk Category: C

PHARMACOKINETICS
Distribution: highest concentrations found in kidneys, liver, and adrenal glands, with about 90% bound to plasma proteins. Drug crosses the placenta and blood-brain barrier.
Metabolism: in the liver by oxidation and conjugation.
Excretion: in urine by glomerular filtration, with about 50% excreted unchanged. Not known if drug appears in breast milk. Its half-life is 21 to 45 hours—longer in patients with renal impairment and possibly shorter in children.
Action: onset, 1 minute; duration, 30 minutes to 72 hours.

MECHANISM OF ACTION
The drug's hypotensive effect isn't entirely understood. However, diazoxide does act directly on arterial smooth muscle, causing vasodilation. It also reduces peripheral resistance by inhibiting alpha-adrenergic receptors.

INDICATIONS & DOSAGE
• Emergency treatment of malignant hypertension or hypertensive crisis.
Adults: 1 to 3 mg/kg up to 150 mg, repeated q 5 to 15 minutes as needed. Maintenance dosages given q 4 to 24 hours up to 1.2 g daily.
Children: 1 to 3 mg/kg q 5 to 15 minutes as needed. Maintenance dosages given q 4 to 24 hours.

CONTRAINDICATIONS & CAUTIONS
• Contraindicated in patients with hypersensitivity to thiazide diuretics or sulfonamide-type agents; they may be sensitive to diazoxide, too.
• Also contraindicated in hypertension associated with aortic coarctation or arteriovenous shunt because therapy should treat underlying condition.
• Use cautiously during labor because drug can stop uterine contractions; in impaired cerebral or cardiac function because drug can cause transient myocardial or cerebral ischemia; in uremia because of potentiated hypotensive effect; and in diabetes because drug can aggravate hyperglycemia, requiring a dosage adjustment in insulin or oral agents.
• Also give cautiously to patients who could be harmed by fluid and sodium retention, rapid blood pressure reduction, tachycardia, decreased perfusion, or renal impairment.

PREPARATION & STORAGE
Available in 20 ml ampules of 300 mg. Store between 59° and 86° F. (15° and 30° C.), and protect from freezing, heat, and light.

ADMINISTRATION
Direct injection: Inject undiluted drug directly into peripheral vein or peripheral I.V. line over 10 to 30 seconds. Avoid extravasation because the drug is extremely alkaline. If extravasation occurs, infiltrate the area with sodium chloride solution, then apply warm compresses. Relieve pain by infiltrating a local anesthetic.
Intermittent infusion: not recommended.
Continuous infusion: not recommended.

INCOMPATIBILITY
No incompatibilities reported.

ADVERSE REACTIONS

Life-threatening: anaphylaxis, congestive heart failure, excessive hypotension (overdose).

Other: abdominal discomfort, altered taste, angina, anorexia, anxiety, back pain, burning, chest pain, confusion, constipation, diabetic ketoacidosis (in renal impairment), diarrhea, dizziness, drowsiness, dry mouth, dysrhythmias, edema, facial flushing or redness, generalized or localized warmth, headache, hyperglycemia, ileus, light-headedness, nausea, orthostatic hypotension, pain at injection site, paralysis, paresthesias, pruritus, retention of nitrogenous wastes, salivation, seizures, severe muscle cramps, sweating, tachycardia, tinnitus, unconsciousness, urinary retention, vomiting, weakness, weight gain.

INTERACTIONS

Allopurinol, colchicine, probenecid, sulfinpyrazone: possible decreased effectiveness resulting from elevated serum uric acid levels.
Anticoagulants (coumarin or indanedione derivatives): possible enhanced effect.
Antihypertensives: possible intensified hypotensive effect if given within 6 hours of diazoxide.
Anti-inflammatory analgesics, NSAIDs(especially indomethacin): antagonized hypotensive effects of diazoxide.
Beta blockers: potentiated hypotensive effects and avoidance of diazoxide-induced tachycardia.
Insulin, oral antidiabetic drugs: reversed hyperglycemic effects of diazoxide.
Phenytoin: subtherapeutic levels or toxicity and risk of hyperglycemia, resulting from altered metabolism or plasma protein binding.
Thiazide and loop diuretics: possible increased antihypertensive, hyperglycemic, and hyperuricemic effects of diazoxide.

EFFECTS ON DIAGNOSTIC TESTS

BUN, serum alkaline phosphatase, free fatty acids, glucose, sodium, uric acid, SGOT: elevated levels.
Creatinine clearance: reduced.
Hematocrit, hemoglobin, immunoglobulin G: decreased.
Insulin response to glucagon: false-negative results.
Urine bicarbonate, chloride, potassium: reduced levels.

SPECIAL CONSIDERATIONS

• *Treatment of overdose:* For excessive hypotension, give vasopressors (norepinephrine or metaraminol) and place patient in Trendelenburg's position. Treat acute hyperglycemia or ketoacidosis with insulin, and restore fluid and electrolyte balance.
• Keep patient supine during infusion and for 15 to 30 minutes afterward. If he becomes hypotensive, keep him supine for at least 1 hour. If he receives furosemide along with diazoxide, keep him supine for 8 to 10 hours.
• Record blood pressure during and after rapid infusion to monitor rapid fall. Closely monitor until blood pressure is stable, then hourly.
• Also monitor intake and output for fluid retention. Weigh patient daily.
• Watch diabetic patient for signs of severe hyperglycemia or hyperosmolar nonketotic coma. Give insulin, as needed.
• I.V. diazoxide therapy usually lasts no longer than 5 days and is followed by oral antihypertensive therapy. Don't give drug for more than 10 days.
• Long-term monitoring is necessary because drug has a long half-life.
• Diazoxide is used investigationally for chronic hypertension.

- Administer drug rapidly; slow injection causes a reduced response because of the drug's extensive protein binding.
- Diazoxide and its metabolites are removed by hemodialysis and peritoneal dialysis.

diethylstilbestrol diphosphate (DES)
Honvol♦♦, Stilphostrol

Pregnancy Risk Category: X

PHARMACOKINETICS
Distribution: throughout body tissues, with highest concentrations in fat deposits. About 50% to 80% is bound to plasma proteins. Drug crosses the placenta.
Metabolism: in the liver, inactivated primarily by conjugation.
Excretion: mainly eliminated in urine as a glucuronide, with small amounts in feces. Drug appears in breast milk.
Action: peak serum level, immediately after administration.

MECHANISM OF ACTION
This estrogen's exact mechanism of action isn't known. The drug is thought to bind with intracellular receptor proteins, increasing synthesis of DNA, RNA, and protein in responsive tissues. It reduces pituitary release of follicle-stimulating hormone and luteinizing hormone.

INDICATIONS & DOSAGE
- Palliative treatment of postmenopausal breast cancer and prostatic cancer. *Adults:* 0.5 to 1 g daily for 5 or more consecutive days, as needed. Maintenance dosage is 0.25 to 0.5 g once or twice weekly.

CONTRAINDICATIONS & CAUTIONS
- Contraindicated in gallbladder disease because of an increased risk of recurrence; in thromboembolic disease or thrombophlebitis because of an increased risk of myocardial infarction and pulmonary embolism in men; and in metastatic bone disease because of an increased risk of severe hypercalcemia.
- Also contraindicated in abnormal or undiagnosed vaginal bleeding, because the underlying disorder should be identified and treated, and in pregnancy.
- Use cautiously in patients with porphyria, a history of uterine fibroids, hypertension, cardiac disease, hepatic or renal dysfunction, depression, migraine headaches, or benign cystic breast disease because drug can worsen these conditions.
- In congestive heart failure, give carefully because sodium retention can aggravate this condition.

PREPARATION & STORAGE
Available in 250 mg/5 ml vials. Dilute colorless to straw-colored drug with 300 ml of dextrose 5% in water or 0.9% sodium chloride. Store at 59° to 86° F. (15° to 30° C.); avoid freezing.

ADMINISTRATION
Direct injection: not recommended.
Intermittent infusion: Inject diluted drug into an I.V. line containing a free-flowing compatible solution, and infuse at 1 to 2 ml/minute for 10 to 15 minutes. Adjust rate so that remaining solution infuses within 1 hour. Infuse drug slowly—rapid infusion can cause perineal or vaginal burning.
Continuous infusion: not recommended.

ADVERSE REACTIONS

Life-threatening: none reported.
Other: alopecia, anorexia, breast
tenderness, dizziness, folic acid deficiency, gynecomastia, headache, hirsutism, hypercalcemia, hypertension,
impotence, increased nipple pigmentation, lethargy, nausea, sodium retention, thrombophlebitis, uterine
bleeding, vomiting.

INTERACTIONS

Anticoagulants: decreased effects.
Antidiabetic drugs: reduced glucose
tolerance.
Barbiturates, hydantoins: reduced
diethylstilbestrol effect.
Corticosteroids: potentiated hydrocortisone effects.

EFFECTS ON DIAGNOSTIC TESTS

Factors VII, VIII, IX, X: possible
elevated levels.
*Glucose tolerance test, T_3 resin up-
take:* possible reduced levels.
Metyrapone test: reduced response.
*Norepinephrine-induced platelet
test:* possible increased platelet aggregation.
Prothrombin time: possibly prolonged.
Serum cholesterol: possible reduced
levels.
Serum lipoproteins, triglycerides:
possible increased levels.
*Serum T_4, thyroxine-binding globu-
lin:* possible elevated levels.
Sulfobromophthalein test: increased
response.

SPECIAL CONSIDERATIONS

• Monitor patient closely for signs
of hypercalcemia (polyuria, polydipsia, weakness, constipation, and
changes in mental status). Instruct
him to report any such signs immediately. If untreated, hypercalcemia
can rapidly progress to coma and
death.

• High-dose therapy causes an increased risk of thrombophlebitis and
other thromboembolic complications
(pulmonary embolism, myocardial
infarction, and cerebrovascular accident).
• If specimens must be analyzed by
a pathologist, indicate that the patient is receiving estrogen therapy.

---

digoxin
Lanoxin♦

Pregnancy Risk Category: C

PHARMACOKINETICS

Distribution: throughout body tissues, with high concentrations in
skeletal muscle, liver, heart, brain,
and kidneys. About 20% to 30%
binds to plasma proteins. Drug
doesn't accumulate in adipose tissue,
but it does cross the placenta.
Metabolism: in the liver and the biliary tract, although variable among
patients.
Excretion: in urine by glomerular
filtration and active renal tubular secretion, with 50% to 70% excreted
unchanged and the remainder excreted as metabolites. Small amounts
of drug and metabolites are also excreted in bile. Drug appears in
breast milk. Its half-life is 34 to 44
hours in normal renal function, longer in renal impairment.
Action: onset, 5 to 30 minutes; peak
level, 1 to 5 hours.

MECHANISM OF ACTION

A digitalis glycoside that depresses
the SA node and increases the refractory period of the AV node. It
also indirectly increases intracellular
calcium by inhibiting adenosine triphosphatase (ATPase).

INDICATIONS & DOSAGE

• Congestive heart failure, atrial flutter and fibrillation, atrial tachycardias (including paroxysmal atrial tachycardia). *Adults and children over age 10:* loading dose, 0.5 to 1 mg (alternatively, .008 to .012 mg/kg); maintenance dose, 0.125 to 0.5 mg daily (usual dose is 0.25 mg). *Children age 5 to 10:* loading dose, 0.015 to 0.03 mg/kg; maintenance dose, 25% to 35% of loading dose. *Children age 2 to 5:* loading dose, 0.025 to 0.035 mg/kg; maintenance dose, 25% to 35% of loading dose. *Children age 1 month to 2 years:* loading dose, 0.03 to 0.05 mg/kg; maintenance dose, 25% to 35% of loading dose. *Full-term neonates under age 1 month:* loading dose, 0.02 to 0.03 mg/kg; maintenance dose, 25% to 35% of loading dose. *Premature infants:* loading dose, 0.015 to 0.025 mg/kg; maintenance dose, 20% to 30% of loading dose.

CONTRAINDICATIONS & CAUTIONS

• Contraindicated in patients with digitalis-induced toxicity because of the risk of additive toxicity and in patients with ventricular fibrillation or ventricular tachycardia (except when caused by congestive heart failure) because of the risk of exacerbating dysrhythmias.
• Use with extreme caution in acute glomerulonephritis and congestive heart failure because of the increased risk of toxicity.
• Because of the increased risk of *digitalis-induced* dysrhythmias, use cautiously in the elderly and in patients with acute myocardial infarction, incomplete atrioventricular block, severe heart failure, hypothyroidism, or chronic constrictive pericarditis.
• Because of the heightened risk of dysrhythmias, use cautiously in patients who've received any digitalis preparation within the past 3 weeks and in patients with acute myocarditis, renal insufficiency, severe pulmonary disease, hypoxia, sick sinus syndrome, myxedema, or Wolff-Parkinson-White syndrome with atrial fibrillation.
• In idiopathic hypertrophic subaortic stenosis, administer carefully because of possible increased left ventricular outflow obstruction.
• Also administer cautiously in hypokalemia, hypomagnesemia, or hypercalcemia because of the risk of digitalis toxicity; in heightened carotid sinus sensitivity because digoxin increases vagal tone; and in renal impairment because of the magnified risk of toxicity.

PREPARATION & STORAGE

Available in 1 and 2 ml ampules (0.25 mg/ml) for adults and in 1 ml ampules (0.1 mg/ml) for children. Store drug at room temperature.

Dilute with 10 ml of dextrose 5% in water, 0.9% sodium chloride, or sterile water, or give undiluted. Drug can precipitate if less than a fourfold dilution is used. Give diluted drug immediately.

ADMINISTRATION

Direct injection: Inject undiluted drug over at least 5 minutes as close to I.V. insertion site as possible.
Intermittent infusion: not recommended.
Continuous infusion: not recommended.

INCOMPATIBILITY

Incompatible with dobutamine. However, the manufacturer recommends *not* mixing digoxin with any other drug or administering in the same I.V. line with any other drugs.

ADVERSE REACTIONS

Life-threatening: anaphylaxis, atrioventricular block, profound sinus bradycardia, ventricular tachycardia.
Other: agitation, anorexia, atrial and junctional tachycardia, blurred vision, diarrhea, diplopia, dizziness, fatigue, generalized weakness, gynecomastia, hallucinations, headache, hypotension, light flashes, malaise, nausea, paresthesias, photophobia, premature ventricular contractions, rash, stupor, urticaria, vertigo, vomiting, yellow-green halos around visual images.

INTERACTIONS

Amiodarone, captopril, diltiazem, nifedipine, quinidine, verapamil: increased digoxin levels.
Amphotericin B, carbenicillin, corticosteroids, diuretics, ticarcillin: possible digitalis toxicity associated with hypokalemia.
Bretylium tosylate: aggravated dysrhythmias associated with digitalis toxicity.
Calcium salts: severe dysrhythmias caused by effects on cardiac contractility and excitability.
Edrophonium: possible excessive slowing of heart rate.
Heparin: partially counteracted anticoagulant effect.
Pancuronium, rauwolfia alkaloids, succinylcholine, sympathomimetics: possible heightened risk of dysrhythmias.

EFFECTS ON DIAGNOSTIC TESTS

None reported.

SPECIAL CONSIDERATIONS

• *Treatment of overdose:* Discontinue drug at the first sign of toxicity (in adults, anorexia, diarrhea, nausea, and vomiting; in children, most common sign is cardiac dysrhythmias). Monitor EKG continuously and maintain patient's serum potassium level between 3.5 and 5 mEq/liter. Treat bradycardia with 0.5 to 1 mg of I.V. atropine; treat ventricular dysrhythmias with phenytoin (drug of choice) or with lidocaine and procainamide. If symptomatic bradycardia or atrioventricular block occurs, anticipate temporary transvenous pacing. Digoxin-immune FAB can be used to bind with digoxin and reduce toxicity in life-threatening overdose.
• Check patient's apical pulse for a full minute before each dose. Report any significant changes (pulse rate less than 60 or more than 100 beats/minute, or irregular beats). A pulse rate below 60 may indicate toxicity. Also report blood pressure changes, and anticipate an order for a 12-lead EKG.
• Digoxin has a low therapeutic index, requiring an individualized dosage based on patient's ideal body weight and response to drug.
• Divide the loading dose over 24 hours. The first dose is 50% of the total loading dose; the next two doses, given 4 to 8 hours apart, are 25% of the loading dose. The loading dose may be omitted in patients with congestive heart failure and reduced in patients with renal failure.
• Use a continuous EKG to monitor patients on I.V. digoxin for development or improvement of dysrhythmias. If dysrhythmias (a symptom of toxicity) develop, notify the doctor immediately. Then treat toxicity.
• Elderly patients occasionally suffer hallucinations, delusions, and anxiety from digoxin toxicity. Notify the doctor immediately if these symptoms occur. Protect the patient by raising the bed side rails, helping him walk, using restraints if necessary, and reorienting, reassuring, and observing him frequently.

Unmarked trade names available in the United States only.
♦ Also available in Canada.   ♦ ♦ Available in Canada only.

digoxin-immune FAB
Digibind

Pregnancy Risk Category: C

PHARMACOKINETICS
Distribution: not fully understood, but drug appears to be rapidly distributed throughout extracellular space.
Metabolism: not metabolized.
Excretion: in urine by glomerular filtration, principally as cardiac glycoside–FAB fragment complex. Elimination half-life is 14 to 20 hours.
Action: peaks at end of infusion.

MECHANISM OF ACTION
Drug prevents or reverses toxic effects of cardiac glycosides. Specific antigen-binding fragments bind with free digoxin or digitoxin intravascularly or in extracellular spaces, making them unavailable for binding at site of action.

INDICATIONS & DOSAGE
• Potentially life-threatening cardiac glycoside toxicity. *Adults and children:* dosage based on ingested amount or serum level of digoxin or digitoxin.

For digoxin tablets, solution, or I.M. injection, find the antidote dose (in mg) by multiplying the ingested amount (in mg) by 0.8; divide answer by 0.6 and multiply by 40. For digitoxin tablets, digoxin capsules, or I.V. digoxin or digitoxin, find the antidote dose (in mg) by dividing the ingested dose (in mg) by 0.6 and multiplying by 40.

If the serum digoxin or digitoxin level is known, determine dosage as follows: Multiply the serum *digoxin* level (in ng/ml) by the patient's weight (kg), divide by 100, and multiply by 40. Or multiply the serum *digitoxin* level (in ng/ml) by the patient's weight (in kg), divide by 1,000, and multiply by 40.

In acute toxicity or if an estimated ingested amount or serum drug level isn't known, administer 20 vials (800 mg) of digoxin-immune FAB. This dosage should be effective in most life-threatening ingestions in adults and children, but it may cause volume overload in young children.

CONTRAINDICATIONS & CAUTIONS
• Experience with this drug is limited. Recommended only for life-threatening situations. Use cautiously in congestive heart failure; digitalis glycoside levels may fall below effective inotropic concentrations.
• If hypokalemia occurs, administer potassium supplements cautiously to avoid hyperkalemia. Allergic reactions, though rare, can occur.

PREPARATION & STORAGE
Available in 40 mg vials. Reconstitute with 4 ml of sterile water for injection. For infusion, further dilute solution with 0.9% sodium chloride. For children and other patients who need small doses, reconstitute 40 mg vial with 36 ml of 0.9% sodium chloride for a 1 mg/ml concentration. Use reconstituted solution promptly. If not used immediately, refrigerate for up to 4 hours.

ADMINISTRATION
Direct injection: If cardiac arrest is imminent, rapidly inject directly into vein or I.V. line containing a free-flowing compatible solution, using a 0.22-micron filter needle.
Intermittent infusion: not recommended.
Continuous infusion: Infuse diluted solution over 15 to 30 minutes through a 0.22-micron filter needle.

INCOMPATIBILITY
No incompatibilities reported.

ADVERSE REACTIONS
Life-threatening: exacerbation of low cardiac output states or congestive heart failure.
Other: hypokalemia, rapid ventricular response in patients with atrial fibrillation.

INTERACTIONS
Cardiac glycosides: reversed effects.

EFFECTS ON DIAGNOSTIC TESTS
Serum digitoxin, digoxin: increased levels of inactive drug.
Serum potassium: elevated in cardiac glycoside toxicity; diminished levels when toxicity is reversed.

SPECIAL CONSIDERATIONS
• Obtain serum digoxin or digitoxin levels before giving digoxin-immune FAB because serum studies will be difficult to interpret afterward.
• Closely monitor vital signs, EKG, and serum potassium level during and after administration.
• Overly high doses can cause allergic reaction, febrile reaction, or delayed serum sickness. Don't attempt redigitalization until the elimination of Digibind is complete—which can take up to 1 week.
• Digoxin doses above 10 mg in healthy adults (4 mg in healthy children) can cause cardiac arrest.
• If patient is allergic to sheep proteins or has previously reacted to digoxin-immune FAB and his condition is not life-threatening, consider skin testing. Dilute 0.1 ml of reconstituted drug in 10 ml of sterile saline solution. Inject 0.1 ml of this solution intradermally, and examine site after 20 minutes. Urticarial wheal surrounded by erythema indicates positive result.

dihydroergotamine mesylate
D.H.E. 45

Pregnancy Risk Category: X

PHARMACOKINETICS
Distribution: throughout body tissues, with 90% bound to plasma proteins. Dihydroergotamine crosses the blood-brain barrier and placenta.
Metabolism: in the liver.
Excretion: in urine and feces, primarily as metabolites.
Action: onset, less than 5 minutes; duration, 1 to 4 hours.

MECHANISM OF ACTION
Dihydroergotamine causes peripheral vasoconstriction by stimulating alpha-adrenergic receptors. It directly affects cranial vessels, causing vasoconstriction and reduction in amplitude of pulsations associated with vascular headaches. It also causes vasodilation in hypertonic vessels and may reduce catecholamine and serotonin levels.

INDICATIONS & DOSAGE
• Rapid control of vascular headaches (including migraine and cluster headaches). *Adults:* 1 mg at start of attack, then 1 mg in 1 hour, as needed; not to exceed 2 mg daily or 6 mg weekly.

CONTRAINDICATIONS & CAUTIONS
• Contraindicated in patients with a history of hypersensitivity to ergot alkaloids.
• Also contraindicated in children because safety and efficacy haven't been proved; in peripheral vascular

disease, coronary artery disease, and severe hypertension because drug can increase vasoconstriction and induce vasospasm; in hepatic or renal impairment because impaired drug metabolism can lead to ergot poisoning; and in patients with infection or sepsis because these conditions may enhance drug's vasoconstrictive effects.

• Use cautiously in the elderly. They may be predisposed to peripheral vascular disease and have slowed drug clearance.

PREPARATION & STORAGE
Available as a colorless solution in 1 mg/ml vials. Drug doesn't need dilution for I.V. use. Protect from light, freezing, and heat. Store at 59° to 86° F. (15° to 30° C.). Don't administer discolored solutions.

ADMINISTRATION
Direct injection: Inject directly into vein over 3 minutes.
Intermittent infusion: not recommended.
Continuous infusion: not recommended.

INCOMPATIBILITY
No incompatibilities reported.

ADVERSE REACTIONS
Life-threatening: anaphylaxis, coronary vasospasm.
Other: dizziness, headache, localized edema in legs and feet, muscle pain in extremities, nausea, pale and cold hands and feet, paresthesias, peripheral ischemia, precordial distress and pain, tachycardia or bradycardia, vomiting, weakness in legs.

INTERACTIONS
Other ergot alkaloids and vasoconstrictors: increased vasoconstrictive effects. Adjust dosage, if ordered.

Tobacco: in heavy smokers, additional vasoconstriction and peripheral ischemia related to nicotine's effects.

EFFECTS ON DIAGNOSTIC TESTS
None reported.

SPECIAL CONSIDERATIONS
• *Treatment of overdose:* Provide symptomatic care. Support respirations as needed. For severe vasospasm, apply warmth to ischemic extremities to prevent tissue damage. Carefully administer vasodilators, such as nitroprusside, prazosin, or tolazine, because they can cause hypotension.
• Give dihydroergotamine with prodromal signs or as soon as possible after headache begins. Dosage and speed of relief may be directly related to prompt administration.
• After the initial dose, advise patient to lie down and relax in a quiet, darkened room.
• Instruct him to avoid alcohol and tobacco, which can aggravate vasoconstriction and headache, and to avoid exposure to cold, which also increases vasoconstriction.
• Protect extremities from injury if paresthesias occur.

---

dimenhydrinate
Dinate, Dommanate, Dramamine, Dramanate, Dramocen, Dramoject, Dymenate, Gravol♦♦, Hydrate, Wehamine

Pregnancy Risk Category: B

PHARMACOKINETICS
Distribution: probably throughout body tissues. Drug crosses the placenta and blood-brain barrier.
Metabolism: in the liver.

Excretion: in urine, primarily as metabolites. Small amounts appear in breast milk.
Action: onset, immediate; duration, 3 to 6 hours.

MECHANISM OF ACTION
Although dimenhydrinate's action isn't completely understood, it competes with histamine at H_1-receptors to prevent, but not reverse, the actions of histamine. The drug also inhibits acetylcholine, which in turn inhibits the vestibular and reticular systems. It also depresses the CNS.

INDICATIONS & DOSAGE
• Prophylactic and symptomatic treatment of nausea and vomiting.
Adults: 50 mg q 4 hours, as needed. Or if drowsiness doesn't occur, 100 mg q 4 hours.

CONTRAINDICATIONS & CAUTIONS
• Contraindicated in hypersensitivity to dimenhydrinate and its components.
• Also contraindicated in children under age 2 because safety and efficacy haven't been proved.
• Use cautiously in prostatic hypertrophy, stenosing peptic ulcer, pyloroduodenal obstruction, bladder neck obstruction, narrow-angle glaucoma, bronchial asthma, seizures, or dysrhythmias because of exacerbation.

PREPARATION & STORAGE
Available in 5 and 10 ml ampules of 50 mg/ml. Dilute each 50 mg (1 ml) with 10 ml of 0.9% sodium chloride or dextrose 5% in water before injection. Store diluted solution for up to 10 days at 59° to 86° F. (15° to 30° C.); avoid freezing.

ADMINISTRATION
Direct injection: Inject diluted drug into vein or into a previously established I.V. line over 2 minutes.
Intermittent infusion: not recommended.
Continuous infusion: not recommended.

INCOMPATIBILITY
Incompatible with aminophylline, ammonium chloride, amobarbital sodium, chlorpromazine, glycopyrrolate, hydrocortisone sodium succinate, hydroxyzine hydrochloride, opium alkaloids, pentobarbital sodium, prochlorperazine edisylate, promazine, and thiopental.

ADVERSE REACTIONS
Life-threatening: anaphylaxis, respiratory depression (with massive overdose).
Other: anorexia; blurred vision; chest tightness; confusion; constipation; diarrhea; difficult or painful urination; diplopia; drowsiness; dry mouth, nose, and throat; epigastric distress; hallucinations; headache; hemolytic anemia; hypotension; insomnia (especially in children); malaise; nasal stuffiness; nausea; palpitations; photosensitivity; restlessness; tachycardia; thickened bronchial secretions; urticaria; wheezing.

INTERACTIONS
Antimuscarinics: enhanced effectiveness.
Apomorphine: decreased emetic effect.
Barbiturates, other CNS depressants: possible additive effects, precipitating overdose.
MAO inhibitors: deepened CNS depression.
Ototoxic drugs (such as cisplatin, vancomycin): masked ototoxic symptoms.

Tricyclic antidepressants: increased anticholinergic effect.

EFFECTS ON DIAGNOSTIC TESTS
Skin tests: false-positive results in tests using allergen extracts.

SPECIAL CONSIDERATIONS
• *Treatment of overdose:* In adults, 500 mg or more of dimenhydrinate may cause initial sedation followed by difficulty swallowing and speaking, psychosis, CNS excitation, seizures, and postictal depression. Signs in children include dilated pupils, flushed face, excitation, hallucinations, confusion, ataxia, intermittent clonic convulsions, coma, and cardiorespiratory collapse, which can lead to death. Treat symptomatically. For respiratory depression, provide mechanical ventilation and oxygen. Treat seizures with diazepam.
• Keep patient lying down during administration.
• CNS depression and hypotension are more common in the elderly.
• Dimenhydrinate can interfere with diagnosis of appendicitis.
• Most preparations (except Dommanate and Gravol) contain benzyl alcohol.

diphenhydramine hydrochloride
Benadryl♦, Benahist 10, Benahist 50, Benoject-10, Benoject-50, Diphenacen-10, Diphenacen-50, Hyrexin-50, Nordryl, Nordryl-50, Wehydryl-10, Wehydryl-50

Pregnancy Risk Category: C

PHARMACOKINETICS
Distribution: not fully understood. Highest concentrations appear in lungs, spleen, and brain; lower concentrations in heart, muscles, and liver. Drug crosses the placenta.
Metabolism: in the liver, where drug apparently undergoes first-pass metabolism to be biotransformed to dephenylmethoxyacetic acid and *N*-demethyl and *N,N*-didemethyl derivatives; 82% of drug is bound to plasma proteins.
Excretion: mainly in urine, primarily as metabolites, in 24 hours. Small amounts appear in breast milk. Half-life averages 5 hours.
Action: onset, 15 to 20 minutes; duration, 4 to 6 hours.

MECHANISM OF ACTION
Diphenhydramine competes with histamine for H_1-receptor sites on effector cells to prevent, but not reverse, the actions of histamine. The drug's anticholinergic properties are probably responsible for the antiemetic and sedative effects.

INDICATIONS & DOSAGE
• Allergic reactions. *Adults:* 10 to 50 mg q 4 to 6 hours or up to 100 mg/dose. Maximum 400 mg daily. *Children:* 1.25 mg/kg q 6 hours. Maximum dosage is 300 mg daily.
• Nausea and vertigo. *Adults:* 10 mg initially, increased to 20 to 50 mg q 2 to 3 hours, as needed. *Children:* 1 to 1.25 mg/kg q 6 hours. Maximum dosage is 300 mg daily.

CONTRAINDICATIONS & CAUTIONS
• Contraindicated in antihistamine hypersensitivity.
• Also contraindicated in neonates and premature infants because of the increased risk of antimuscarinic effects, such as CNS excitation, and the risk of seizures.
• Use cautiously in patients with lower respiratory tract symptoms, in-

cluding asthma, because drug thickens and dries secretions, making expectoration difficult.

• Use cautiously in narrow-angle glaucoma, stenosing peptic ulcer, pyloroduodenal obstruction, symptomatic prostatic hypertrophy, bladder neck obstruction, cardiovascular disease, or hypertension because the drug can worsen their symptoms.

PREPARATION & STORAGE
Available in 10 and 50 mg/ml vials. Store in light-resistant containers at 59° to 86° F. (15° to 30° C.), and avoid freezing. Further dilution isn't required for direct injection. Drug is compatible with most solutions.

ADMINISTRATION
Direct injection: Inject drug over 3 to 5 minutes directly into vein or into an I.V. line containing a free-flowing compatible solution.
Intermittent infusion: After diluting appropriate dosage, infuse slowly.
Continuous infusion: Infuse appropriate dosage slowly.

INCOMPATIBILITY
Incompatible with amobarbital sodium, amphotericin B, cephalothin, iodides, hydrocortisone sodium succinate, iodipamide, pentobarbital sodium, phenytoin sodium, secobarbital sodium, and thiopental sodium.

ADVERSE REACTIONS
Life-threatening: agranulocytosis, anaphylaxis, hemolytic anemia, thrombocytopenia.
Other: acute labyrinthitis; anorexia; blurred vision; chest tightness; chills; clumsiness; confusion; constipation; diaphoresis; diarrhea; diplopia; dizziness; dry mouth, nose, and throat; epigastric distress; euphoria; excitation; extrasystoles; fatigue; headache; hypotension; hysteria; insomnia; irritability; nasal congestion; nausea; neuritis; nightmares; palpitations; paresthesias; photosensitivity; rash; restlessness; sedation; seizures; tachycardia; thickened bronchial secretions; tinnitus; tremors; urinary difficulty or retention; urticaria; vertigo; vomiting; wheezing.

INTERACTIONS
Alcohol, hypnotics, sedatives, tranquilizers, other CNS depressants: deepened CNS depression.
Antimuscarinics: possible potentiated effects.
Apomorphine: decreased emetic effects.
MAO inhibitors: prolonged and intensified anticholinergic effects.
Ototoxic drugs (such as cisplatin, vancomycin): masked signs of ototoxicity.

EFFECTS ON DIAGNOSTIC TESTS
Skin tests: false-positive results in tests using allergen extracts.

SPECIAL CONSIDERATIONS
• *Treatment of overdose:* Reactions may vary from CNS depression in the elderly to CNS stimulation in children. Other reactions include dry mouth; fixed, dilated pupils; flushing; and GI symptoms. Treat symptomatically with oxygen and I.V. fluids. Give vasopressors for hypotension.
• Keep patient lying down, and monitor vital signs and level of consciousness during infusion.
• Avoid stimulants because they can cause seizures.
• Coffee and tea may reduce drowsiness; sugarless gum, sour hard candy, or ice chips may relieve dry mouth.
• Drug may interfere with diagnosis of appendicitis.
• Withdraw drug 4 days before skin tests.

diphtheria antitoxin, equine

Pregnancy Risk Category: D

PHARMACOKINETICS
Distribution: unknown.
Metabolism: unknown.
Excretion: unknown.
Action: peak level, immediately after administration.

MECHANISM OF ACTION
Neutralizes toxins produced by *Corynebacterium diphtheriae*.

INDICATIONS & DOSAGE
Dosage reflects site and size of diphtheria membrane, degree of toxicity, and duration of illness.
• Diphtheria. *Adults and children:* 20,000 to 40,000 units for pharyngeal or laryngeal disease lasting for 48 hours; 40,000 to 60,000 units for nasopharyngeal lesions; and 80,000 to 120,000 units for disease lasting for 3 or more days or for patients with brawny neck swelling.

CONTRAINDICATIONS & CAUTIONS
• Give with extreme caution to patients with allergic disorders or hypersensitivity to equine serum or horses.

PREPARATION & STORAGE
Diphtheria antitoxin is prepared from plasma or serum of healthy horses, which are hyperimmunized against diphtheria toxin. The antitoxin itself is a sterile, odorless, and colorless solution of refined and concentrated protein (mainly immunoglobulins) that's available in vials of 10,000 and 20,000 units with concentrations of at least 500 units/ml. Either cresol or m-cresol is added as a preservative.

Refrigerate the antitoxin at 36° to 46° F. (2° to 8° C.); freezing doesn't affect potency. Before infusion, warm the antitoxin to 90° to 93° F. (32° to 34° C.), never higher. Then dilute dose with 0.9% sodium chloride or dextrose 5% in water for a 1:20 concentration.

ADMINISTRATION
Direct injection: not used.
Intermittent infusion: not used.
Continuous infusion: Infuse diluted solution directly into vein at a rate of less than 1 ml/minute.

INCOMPATIBILITY
Incompatible with diphtheria toxoid, which may neutralize the vaccine.

ADVERSE REACTIONS
Life-threatening: anaphylaxis.
Other: serum sickness (arthralgia, fever, lymphadenopathy, malaise, pruritus, rash, urticaria), which may occur up to 12 days after administration.

INTERACTIONS
None reported.

EFFECTS ON DIAGNOSTIC TESTS
None reported.

SPECIAL CONSIDERATIONS
• Test for sensitivity in all patients, using both conjunctival and skin tests (intradermal or scratch) if possible. When results are positive or inconclusive, perform desensitization before giving antitoxin.
• Obtain specimens for culture and sensitivity testing before and after therapy. However, start therapy immediately, without waiting for test results.

• Give the entire dose at one time. Bear in mind that any delay in administration may raise dosage requirements or diminish the antitoxin's effectiveness.

• Systemic reactions are usually related to dose, sensitivity, or previous serum injections.

• As ordered, administer an anti-infective, such as erythromycin or penicillin G.

• Serum sickness occurs in 5% to 10% of adults receiving preventive antitoxin and may occur more commonly in adults receiving antitoxin for diphtheria. Treat serum sickness with salicylates, antihistamines, or corticosteroids. Accelerated serum sickness (incubation under 7 to 12 days) may occur in patients sensitized by previous equine serum therapy.

• Keep epinephrine and resuscitation equipment available for immediate treatment of anaphylaxis.

---

dobutamine hydrochloride
Dobutrex♦

Pregnancy Risk Category: C

PHARMACOKINETICS
Distribution: in plasma. Not known if drug crosses the placenta.
Metabolism: in the liver and other tissues to inactive compound 3-0-methyldobutamine. Drug also undergoes conjugation with glucuronic acid.
Excretion: primarily in urine as metabolites, with small amounts in feces. Half-life is about 2 minutes. Not known if drug appears in breast milk.
Action: onset, 1 to 2 minutes, or up to 10 minutes with slow infusion; duration, a few minutes.

MECHANISM OF ACTION
This direct-acting inotropic drug stimulates beta$_1$-receptors in the heart to increase myocardial contractility and stroke volume, thereby increasing cardiac output. Preload decreases because of reduced ventricular filling pressure; afterload declines because of reduced systemic vascular resistance. Dobutamine also produces mild chronotropic, hypertensive, arrhythmogenic, and vasodilative effects.

INDICATIONS & DOSAGE
• Short-term treatment of cardiac decompensation resulting from depressed contractility in heart disease or cardiac surgery. *Adults:* 2.5 to 15 mcg/kg/minute.

CONTRAINDICATIONS & CAUTIONS
• Contraindicated in dobutamine or sulfite hypersensitivity and in idiopathic hypertrophic subaortic stenosis because drug may exacerbate symptoms.

• Give cautiously in atrial fibrillation because drug facilitates atrioventricular conduction and rapid ventricular response; in hypertension because of the risk of an exaggerated pressor response; and after myocardial infarction because high doses may intensify oxygen demand, increasing ischemia.

• Also give cautiously in hypovolemia because therapy should aim to correct the condition and in premature ventricular contractions because the drug may worsen this dysrhythmia.

• Dobutamine shouldn't be used in children because its pediatric safety

---

and efficacy haven't been established.

PREPARATION & STORAGE

Supplied in 250 mg/20 ml vials. Before reconstitution, store at room temperature. Reconstitute with 10 ml of sterile water or dextrose 5% in water (25 mg/ml). Reconstituted solution remains potent for 6 hours at room temperature and for 48 hours if refrigerated.

Before administration, further dilute with at least 50 ml of dextrose 5% in water, dextrose 5% in 0.45% sodium chloride, 0.9% sodium chloride, or ⅙ M sodium lactate. For a concentration of 250 mcg/ml, mix 250 mg of drug in 1,000 ml solution; for 500 mcg/ml, mix 250 mg in 500 ml solution; for 1 mg/ml, mix 250 mg in 250 ml solution. Maximum concentration for infusion is 5 mg/ml.

Use diluted solution within 24 hours. Solution may turn pink from slight drug oxidation, but this doesn't significantly affect its potency. Avoid freezing; solution may crystallize.

ADMINISTRATION

Direct: not used.
Intermittent infusion: not used.
Continuous infusion: Administer via a central I.V. line, using an infusion pump for most accurate titration. Titrate appropriately diluted infusion, using the guidelines given in the following table.

Drug Delivery Rate (mcg/kg/minute)	Infusion Rate (ml/kg/minute)
	250 mcg/ml†
2.5	0.01
5.0	0.02
7.5	0.03
10.0	0.04
12.5	0.05
15.0	0.06
	500 mcg/ml†
2.5	0.005
5.0	0.01
7.5	0.015
10.0	0.02
12.5	0.025
15.0	0.03
	1,000 mcg/ml†
2.5	0.0025
5.0	0.005
7.5	0.0075
10.0	0.01
12.5	0.0125
15.0	0.015

†concentration

INCOMPATIBILITY

Incompatible with alkaline solutions, aminophylline, bretylium tosylate, bumetanide, calcium chloride, calcium gluconate, cefamandole, cefazolin, diazepam, digoxin, furosemide, heparin sodium, hydrocortisone, magnesium sulfate, neutral cephalothin, penicillin, phenytoin sodium, potassium chloride, potassium phosphate, regular insulin, sodium bicarbonate, sodium ethacrynate, and verapamil.

ADVERSE REACTIONS

Life-threatening: none reported.
Other: angina, dyspnea, headache, increased blood pressure, increased heart rate, mild leg cramps, nausea, palpitations, paresthesias, ventricular ectopy, vomiting.

INTERACTIONS
Anesthetics (cyclopropane and halothane): increased risk of ventricular dysrhythmias.
Beta-adrenergic blockers: antagonized beta₁ effects of dobutamine.
Guanadrel, guanethidine: elevated blood pressure and dysrhythmias, resulting from diminished hypotensive effects of these drugs and potentiated pressor effects of dobutamine.
Insulin: increased requirements in diabetics.
MAO inhibitors, tricyclic antidepressants: enhanced pressor effects of dobutamine.
Nitroprusside: additive effects, including higher cardiac output and lower pulmonary wedge pressure.
Rauwolfia alkaloids: prolonged effect of dobutamine because these drugs prevent its uptake into storage granules.

EFFECTS ON DIAGNOSTIC TESTS
None reported.

SPECIAL CONSIDERATIONS
• *Treatment of overdose:* Signs of overdose include tachycardia or excessive alteration in blood pressure. Reduce infusion rate or discontinue therapy until patient is stable. Because the drug has a short half-life, you needn't take other measures.
• Before treatment, correct hypovolemia with a volume expander and, as ordered, digitalize the patient who has a rapid ventricular response to atrial fibrillation.
• Monitor blood pressure and heart rate and rhythm continuously. Also monitor cardiac output and pulmonary wedge pressure.
• May contain sulfites.

dopamine hydrochloride
Dopastat, Intropin♦, Revimine♦♦

Pregnancy Risk Category: C

PHARMACOKINETICS
Distribution: throughout body but not across blood-brain barrier. Not known if drug crosses the placenta.
Metabolism: in the liver, kidneys, and plasma by monoamine oxidase and catechol-o-methyltransferase to inactive compounds. About 25% is metabolized to norepinephrine in adrenergic nerve terminals.
Excretion: primarily in urine, with about 80% removed in 24 hours as metabolites; small amount is excreted unchanged. Dopamine's half-life is about 2 minutes.
Action: onset, 5 minutes; duration, 3 to 10 minutes.

MECHANISM OF ACTION
I.V. doses of 0.5 to 2 mcg/kg/minute of dopamine stimulates dopaminergic receptors in the kidneys and mesenteric, coronary, and intracerebral vascular beds. Higher doses stimulate beta₁-adrenergic receptors and alpha-adrenergic receptors in the sympathetic nervous system.

INDICATIONS & DOSAGE
Dopamine infusion must be carefully adjusted to patient response.
• Adjunctive treatment of shock that persists after adequate fluid volume replacement or in which oliguria is refractory to other vasopressors. Used to increase cardiac output, blood pressure, and urine flow.
Adults: 1 to 5 mcg/kg/minute initially, increased by 1 to 4 mcg/kg/minute or less at 10- to 30-minute intervals until desired response is achieved. Maintenance dosage is usually under 20 mcg/kg/minute.

- Chronic refractory congestive heart failure. *Adults:* 0.5 to 2 mcg/kg/minute until desired response is achieved.
- Occlusive vascular disease. *Adults:* 1 mcg/kg/minute, increased by 5 to 10 mcg/kg/minute up to 50 mcg/kg/minute until desired response is achieved.
- Severe illness. *Adults:* 5 mcg/kg/minute initially, increased by 5 to 10 mcg/kg/minute up to 50 mcg/kg/minute until desired response is achieved.

CONTRAINDICATIONS & CAUTIONS
- Contraindicated in dopamine and sulfite hypersensitivity, and in pheochromocytoma because of the risk of severe hypertension.
- Also contraindicated in children because the drug's safety and efficacy haven't been proved.
- Use cautiously in tachydysrhythmias or ventricular dysrhythmias because the drug may worsen these conditions, and in occlusive disease (Raynaud's disease, arterial embolism) because the drug may impair circulation.

PREPARATION & STORAGE
Available in 5 ml vials, single-dose vials, and prefilled syringes of 200 mg (40 mg/ml), 400 mg (80 mg/ml), and 800 mg (160 mg/ml). Because the injectable solution is light-sensitive, it's available in protective vials. Dopamine also comes premixed with dextrose 5% in water for infusion in concentrations of 0.8, 1.6, and 3.2 mg/ml in 250 and 500 ml glass or PVC containers. Don't use discolored solutions or those darker than light yellow.

Dilute dopamine concentrate to 200 mg/250 ml or 200 mg/500 ml, using 0.9% sodium chloride, dextrose 5% in water, dextrose 5% in 0.9% sodium chloride, Ringer's lactate solution, dextrose 5% in Ringer's lactate solution, or 1/6 M sodium lactate. Dilution with 250 ml yields an 800 mcg/ml solution. Protect the diluted concentration from light. It's stable for 24 hours.

ADMINISTRATION
Direct injection: not used.
Intermittent infusion: not used.
Continuous infusion: Use an infusion control device to avoid inadvertent bolus administration of dopamine. Using an appropriately diluted concentration, administer dopamine through a long I.V. catheter in a large vein, such as the antecubital fossa, rather than in a hand or ankle vein because of the risk of extravasation. Continuously observe the infusion site for extravasation, which can lead to gangrene. If extravasation occurs, use a small-gauge needle to promptly infiltrate the area with 10 to 15 ml of 0.9% sodium chloride containing 5 to 10 mg of phentolamine.

INCOMPATIBILITY
Incompatible with amphotericin B, ampicillin sodium, cephalothin, gentamicin, iron salts, oxidizing agents, penicillin G potassium, and sodium bicarbonate or other alkaline solutions. Don't mix additives with a dopamine and dextrose solution because of the risk of incompatibility.

ADVERSE REACTIONS
Life-threatening: conduction abnormalities, hypotension, ventricular dysrhythmias (with high doses).
Other: allergic reactions (in preparations containing sulfites), angina, anxiety, azotemia, dyspnea, ectopic heartbeats, gangrene in extremities (with high doses in occlusive vascular disease), headache, hypertension,

nausea, piloerection, tachycardia, vomiting, widened QRS complex.

INTERACTIONS
Alpha-adrenergic blockers (such as phenoxybenzamine): decreased peripheral vasoconstriction with high dopamine doses.
Anesthetics (chloroform, cyclopropane, halothane, trichloroethylene): intensified risk of severe dysrhythmias or hypertension.
Antihypertensives: reduced antihypertensive effect if dopamine is given in sufficient amounts to produce alpha-adrenergic effects.
Beta-adrenergic blockers, sympathomimetics: decreased cardiac effects.
Cardiac glycosides, levodopa: possible heightened risk of dysrhythmias.
Diatrizoate, iothalamate, ioxaglate: if given after dopamine, increased neurologic effects during aortography.
Diuretics: enhanced diuresis.
Doxapram, oxytocin: increased vasopressor effects.
Ergonovine, methylergonovine, methysergide: increased vasopressor effects and possible enhanced vasconstriction.
Ergotamine: increased vasopressor effects and possible peripheral vascular ischemia and gangrene.
Guanadrel, guanethidine, mazindol, mecamylamine, methyldopa, methylphenidate, trimethaphan: possible increased vasopressor effects.
MAO inhibitors: prolonged and intensified dopamine effects.
Maprotiline, tricyclic antidepressants: possible potentiation of dopamine's cardiovascular effects.
Nitrates: possible reduced antianginal effects.
Phenytoin: possible hypotension and bradycardia.

Thyroid hormones: possible heightened effects of these hormones or of dopamine.

EFFECTS ON DIAGNOSTIC TESTS
None reported.

SPECIAL CONSIDERATIONS
• *Treatment of overdose:* Reduce infusion rate or temporarily discontinue. If this won't lower blood pressure (rare), give a short-acting alpha-adrenergic blocker, such as phentolamine.
• Correct hypovolemia before dopamine therapy.
• Before and during therapy, monitor heart rate, blood pressure, urine flow, peripheral perfusion, central venous pressure or pulmonary capillary wedge pressure, and cardiac output.
• When discontinuing drug, reduce infusion rate gradually to prevent severe hypotension.
• Infusion rates of 50 mcg/kg/minute have been used safely in advanced circulatory decompensation. Bear in mind that high doses of dopamine can increase renal vasoconstriction and peripheral resistance.
• May contain sulfites.

---

doxacurium chloride
Nuromax

Pregnancy Risk Category: C

PHARMACOKINETICS
Distribution: rapid; extent of protein binding unknown.
Metabolism: not metabolized.
Excretion: in urine and bile.
Action: onset, 3.5 to 9 minutes; duration, 55 to 160 minutes; half-life, 100 minutes.

MECHANISM OF ACTION

A nondepolarizing muscle relaxant, doxacurium competes with acetylcholine for receptor sites at the motor end plate.

INDICATIONS & DOSAGE

• To relax skeletal muscle during surgery as a adjunct to general anesthesia. *Adults:* Dosage is highly individualized. Considerable variation is normal. 0.05 mg/kg infused rapidly I.V. allows endotracheal intubation in 5 minutes in about 90% of patients when used as part of a thiopental/narcotic induction technique. Lower doses may require longer times before intubation is possible. Neuromuscular blockade at this dose will last for an average of 100 minutes. Higher doses (0.8 mg/kg) will produce intubating conditions more rapidly (within 4 minutes), but neuromuscular block will last for 160 minutes or more. If administered during anesthesia with enflurane, halothane, or isoflurane, consider reducing the dose by 33%. *Children over age 2:* Initially, 0.03 mg/kg administered during halothane anesthesia produces a block with an onset of 7 minutes and duration of 30 minutes; 0.05 mg/kg produces a block in 4 minutes lasting 45 minutes.
• Maintenance of skeletal muscle paralysis during general anesthesia. *Adults and children:* Follow initial dose (after 30 minutes) with 0.005 to 0.01 mg/kg every 30 minutes. In general, children require more frequent maintenance doses.

CONTRAINDICATIONS & CAUTIONS

• Contraindicated in patients hypersensitive to the drug; in patients requiring prolonged mechanical ventilation in the ICU; and patients who have received other nondepolarizing neuromuscular blockers.
• Contraindicated during caesarean section because safety to the neonate has not been established and the drug's long duration exceeds that of the procedure.
• Contraindicated in neonates because it contains benzyl alcohol which has been associated with fatalities in neonates.
• Give only under direct medical supervision and only if familiar with the use of neuromuscular blocking agents and techniques involved in maintaining a patent airway. Do not give unless facilities and equipment for artificial respiration, mechanical ventilation, oxygen therapy, intubation, and antagonist are available.
• Use cautiously and in reduced dosage in debilitated patients, obese patients, patients with metastatic cancer, severe electrolyte disturbances, neuromuscular diseases, and in patients in whom difficulty in reversal is anticipated.
• Use cautiously in nursing mothers, as it is not known whether doxacurium is excreted in breast milk.
• Use cautiously in patients with myasthenia gravis or myasthenic syndrome (Eaton-Lambert syndrome). These patients are particularly sensitive to the effects of nondepolarizing relaxants. Shorter-acting agents are recommended for such patients.

PREPARATION & STORAGE

Available in 5 ml vials containing 1 mg/ml. Reconstitute with dextrose 5% in water, 0.9% sodium chloride injection, dextrose 5% in 0.9% sodium chloride injection, lactated Ringer's injection, or dextrose 5% in lactated Ringer's injection. Diluted solutions are stable for 24 hours at room temperature; but because the preservative is diluted, there is a risk of contamination. Give immediately after reconstituting. Discard unused solution after 8 hours.

ADMINISTRATION

Direct injection: Inject ordered dose directly into a vein or tubing of a free-flowing I.V. solution.
Intermittent infusion: not recommended.
Continuous infusion: not recommended.

INCOMPATIBILITY

Incompatible with alkaline solutions (such as barbiturate solutions). Do not administer through the same I.V. line because a precipitate may form.

ADVERSE REACTIONS

Life-threatening: apnea, myocardial infarction, respiratory depression, and respiratory insufficiency.
Other: bronchospasm, diplopia, dyspnea, fever, flushing, hypotension, prolonged muscle weakness, urticaria, wheezing.

INTERACTIONS

Aminoglycosides (dihydrostreptomycin, gentamicin, kanamycin, neomycin, streptomycin); bacitracin; colistin; polymyxin B; sodium colistimethate; and tetracyclines: increased muscle weakness. Use together cautiously.
Inhalational anesthetics, magnesium salts, quinidine: may enhance activity (or increase duration of action) of nondepolarizing neuromuscular blocking agents.
Carbamazepine, phenytoin: may prolong the time to maximal block or shorten the duration of block.

EFFECTS ON DIAGNOSTIC TESTS

None reported.

SPECIAL CONSIDERATIONS

Treatment of overdose: Maintain patent airway and control ventilation. As ordered, give an anticholinester-ase agent in conjunction with an anticholinergic.
• Doxacurium has no effect on consciousness or pain threshold. Do not give drug until consciousness is obtunded by the general anesthetic.
• Because the drug has minimal vagolytic action, bradycardia during anesthesia may be common.
• Higher initial doses may be required in burn patients and in some patients with severe liver disease.
• Adjust dosage to ideal body weight in obese patients because prolonged neuromuscular block may occur.
• Adjust dosage as necessary for patients with renal or hepatic insufficiency who exhibit prolonged neuromuscular blockade.
• A nerve stimulator and train-of-four (T4) monitoring is recommended to assess recovery of muscle strength. Before attempting pharmacologic reversal with neostigmine, some evidence of spontaneous recovery should be apparent.
• Evidence suggests that acid-base or electrolyte imbalance may influence nondepolarizing neuromuscular blocking agents. Alkalosis may counteract the paralysis and acidosis may enhance it.
• When diluted as directed, doxacurium is compatible with alfentanil hydrochloride, fentanyl citrate, and sufentanil citrate.

---

doxapram hydrochloride
Dopram♦

Pregnancy Risk Category: B

PHARMACOKINETICS

Distribution: probably dispersed throughout body tissues. Not known if drug crosses the placenta.

Metabolism: probably metabolized rapidly.

Excretion: in urine and feces in 24 to 48 hours. Not known if drug appears in breast milk.

Action: onset, 20 to 40 seconds; duration, 5 to 12 minutes.

MECHANISM OF ACTION
Doxapram stimulates the entire CNS. It's thought to stimulate respiration through its effects on carotid chemoreceptors and the medullary respiratory center.

INDICATIONS & DOSAGE
• Postanesthesia respiratory depression or apnea unrelated to muscle relaxant drugs. *Adults and children over age 12:* 0.5 to 1 mg/kg, repeated, if necessary, q 5 minutes up to a total dose of 2 mg/kg.

When desired response is obtained or if adverse effects appear, reduce infusion rate to 1 to 3 mg/minute.
• Drug-induced CNS depression. *Adults and children over age 12:* 1 to 2 mg/kg initially, repeated in 5 minutes, then 1 to 2 mg/kg q 1 to 2 hours until patient awakens or up to maximum daily dosage of 3 grams.
• Chronic obstructive pulmonary disease (COPD) associated with acute hypercapnia. *Adults:* 1 to 2 mg/minute for up to 2 hours. Maximum infusion rate, 3 mg/minute.

CONTRAINDICATIONS & CAUTIONS
• Contraindicated in doxapram hypersensitivity; in seizure disorders because the drug may trigger seizures; and in neonates.
• Because doxapram won't improve ventilation, it's contraindicated in ventilatory incompetence caused by extreme dyspnea, airway obstruction, pneumothorax, muscle paresis, or flail chest.

• Also contraindicated in pulmonary embolism, acute asthma, restrictive respiratory disorders, and respiratory failure brought on by neuromuscular disorders.
• Avoid administering drug in severe hypertension, cerebrovascular accident, and head injury (may raise blood pressure and exacerbate these conditions); and in coronary artery disease and frank uncompensated heart failure (may increase cardiac work load and oxygen consumption).
• Give with extreme caution in cerebral edema, asthma, hyperthyroidism, severe tachycardia, cardiac disease, or pheochromocytoma because the drug's cardiac and pressor effects may worsen these conditions.

PREPARATION & STORAGE
Available in 20 ml multidose vials with a concentration of 20 mg/ml. Store between 59° and 86° F. (15° and 30° C.); avoid freezing.

Compatible with most I.V. fluids. For use in postanesthesia or drug-induced CNS depression, add 250 mg of drug to 250 ml dextrose 5% or 10% in water or 0.9% sodium chloride. In COPD, add 400 mg of drug to 180 ml of dextrose 5% or 10% in water or 0.9% sodium chloride.

ADMINISTRATION
Direct injection: Inject drug into a vein or into an I.V. line containing a free-flowing compatible solution.
Intermittent infusion: Give diluted solution at ordered rate (usually 1 to 2 mg/minute, but not exceeding 3 mg/minute) for up to 2 hours. If necessary, repeat in 30 minutes to 2 hours. Rapid infusion may cause hemolysis. Avoid extravasation or extended use of a single injection site; either may lead to thrombophlebitis or local skin irritation.
Continuous infusion: not used.

INCOMPATIBILITY
Incompatible with strongly alkaline drugs, such as aminophylline, sodium bicarbonate, or thiopental.

ADVERSE REACTIONS
Life-threatening: anaphylaxis.
Other: albuminuria, apprehension, bilateral Babinski's signs, bronchospasms, chest pain and tightness, cough, diarrhea, disorientation, dizziness, dyspnea, dysrhythmias, fever, flushing, headache, heart rate variations, hemolysis, hiccups, hyperactivity, hypertension, incontinence, increased deep tendon reflexes, involuntary movements, laryngospasm, lowered T waves, muscle spasticity, nausea, paresthesias (especially in genitalia and perineum), pruritus, pupillary dilation, rebound hypoventilation, seizures, sweating, tachypnea, thrombophlebitis at injection site, urine retention, vomiting, wheezing.

INTERACTIONS
CNS stimulants: possible additive effects.
General anesthetics: possible dysrhythmias.
MAO inhibitors, sympathomimetics: possible increased pressor effects.
Neuromuscular blockers: possible temporarily masked residual effects.

EFFECTS ON DIAGNOSTIC TESTS
BUN: elevated levels.
Hematocrit, hemoglobin, RBC count: decreased.
WBC count: further reduced in presence of leukopenia.

SPECIAL CONSIDERATIONS
• *Treatment of overdose:* Early signs include excessive pressor effects and skeletal muscle activity, tachycardia, and hyperactive deep tendon reflexes. Such signs may signal the need for an adjustment in dosage or infusion rate. Seizures, a more serious sign, don't usually occur at the recommended dosage; nevertheless, keep anticonvulsants, oxygen, and resuscitation equipment available.
• Establish an adequate airway before administering drug.
• Monitor blood pressure, pulse rate, and deep tendon reflexes.
• Discontinue doxapram if sudden hypotension or dyspnea develops.
• In COPD patients, draw samples for blood gas analysis before doxapram and oxygen administration, then at least every 30 minutes.
• Delay giving doxapram for at least 10 minutes after discontinuing general anesthetics, which are known to sensitize the myocardium.
• Doxapram has a narrow margin of safety. Do not use as an analeptic or with mechanical ventilation.

---

doxorubicin hydrochloride (hydroxydaunomycin hydrochloride)
Adriamycin RDF♦

Pregnancy Risk Category: D

PHARMACOKINETICS
Distribution: throughout plasma and tissues, especially in the heart, liver, kidneys, spleen, and lungs. Drug doesn't cross blood-brain barrier or concentrate in cerebrospinal fluid. It may cross the placenta.
Metabolism: rapidly metabolized in liver and other tissues (first-pass effect). The major metabolite, adriamycinol, has antineoplastic effects.
Excretion: primarily removed by liver as unchanged drug or metabolites. About 10% to 20% is excreted in feces in 24 hours and about 40% to 50% is eliminated in 7 days; 6% is removed in urine after 5 days.

Serum half-life is biphasic: initial phase, about 30 minutes; terminal phase, about 17 hours. Half-lives of metabolites are about 3 hours and 32 hours. Not known if drug appears in breast milk.

Action: peak level, after administration.

MECHANISM OF ACTION
Doxorubicin decreases DNA, RNA, and protein synthesis by binding to DNA through intercalation between base pairs. Drug acts in S phase of cell cycle.

INDICATIONS & DOSAGE
• Solid tumors, including carcinomas, soft tissue and osteogenic sarcomas, breast carcinoma, neuroblastoma, Wilms' tumor, malignant lymphomas, acute lymphocytic leukemia, acute myelocytic leukemia. *Adults:* 60 to 75 mg/m² as a single dose at 21-day intervals; 20 mg/m² weekly; or 25 to 30 mg/m² daily for 2 or 3 consecutive days q 3 to 4 weeks. Total lifetime dose shouldn't exceed 550 mg/m² because of risk of cumulative cardiotoxicity. *Children:* 30 mg/m² for 3 consecutive days q 4 weeks.
Note: Reduce dosage in hepatic impairment. If serum bilirubin level is 1.2 to 3 mg/dl, reduce dosage by 50%; if greater than 3 mg/dl, reduce dosage by 75%.

CONTRAINDICATIONS & CAUTIONS
• Contraindicated in myelosuppression and in patients who've received a total lifetime dose of 550 mg/m². Avoid giving a lifetime dose exceeding 400 mg/m² in patients who've received chest radiation therapy, a related tetracyclic chemotherapeutic drug (such as daunorubicin), or cyclophosphamide. Preliminary data suggest that cardiac toxicity may oc-

cur at doses lower than recommended cumulative limit.
• Also contraindicated in chicken pox or herpes zoster because of the risk of severe generalized disease.
• Use cautiously in gout or a history of urate stones (increased risk of hyperuricemia); in heart disease (heightened risk of cardiotoxicity); and in bone marrow infiltration (enhanced risk of myelosuppression).

PREPARATION & STORAGE
To avoid mutagenic, teratogenic, and carcinogenic risks when preparing doxorubicin, use a biological containment cabinet during preparation, wear a mask to avoid inhaling drug particles or solution, and put on gloves to avoid skin contact. If the drug comes in contact with skin or mucosa, immediately wash the area with soap and water.

Dispose of needles, vials, and unused drug correctly. Use syringes with tight (Luer-lok) fittings to prevent drug leakage. Avoid contamination of work surfaces.

Doxorubicin is supplied as a powder in 10, 20, and 50 mg vials. Store in a dry place, away from sunlight. Reconstitute with 0.9% sodium chloride, dextrose 5% in water, or sterile water for injection. Avoid using diluents containing preservatives or having a pH less than 3.0 or greater than 7.0.

To reconstitute drug, add 5 ml of diluent to 10 mg vial, 10 ml to 20 mg vial, or 25 ml to 50 mg vial. When using sterile water for injection, add 2 to 3 volumes of 0.9% sodium chloride to drug to make solution isotonic. Shake vial to help dissolve drug. Reconstituted drug remains stable for 24 hours at room temperature and for 48 hours at 39° to 50° F. (4° to 10° C.). For best results, use within 8 hours of reconstitution. Discard any unused drug.

ADMINISTRATION
Direct injection: Using a 21G or 23G winged-tip needle, inject drug into a large vein over 3 to 5 minutes. Or inject drug into tubing of free-flowing I.V. line containing 0.9% sodium chloride or dextrose 5% in water. Avoid injecting into veins over joints or extremities with compromised venous return or impaired lymphatic drainage. Flush administration set with 0.9% sodium chloride after use.

Avoid extravasation, which may be asymptomatic. If extravasation occurs, stop infusion, apply ice to area, notify doctor, and consider use of local corticosteroids. Restart infusion at another site.

Reduce administration rate if patient develops facial flushing or local erythema.
Intermittent infusion: not recommended.
Continuous infusion: not recommended.

INCOMPATIBILITY
Incompatible with aluminum, aminophylline, bacteriostatic diluents, cephalothin, dexamethasone sodium phosphate, diazepam, fluorouracil, furosemide, heparin sodium, and hydrocortisone sodium succinate.

ADVERSE REACTIONS
Life-threatening: acute cardiotoxicity, chronic congestive heart failure (dose-related).
Other: alopecia, anemia, chills, conjunctivitis, dyspnea, esophagitis, facial flushing, fever, hyperpigmented nail beds, hyperuricemia, joint pain, leukopenia (nadir 10 to 14 days after administration), nausea and vomiting, phlebosclerosis, radiation recall (darkened or reddened skin and severe dermatitis or mucositis in previously irradiated areas), severe soft tissue damage (from extravasation), sore throat, stomatitis, swollen feet and legs, tachycardia, thrombocytopenia, ulceration and necrosis of colon (in patients with acute myelocytic leukemia who are receiving cytarabine).

INTERACTIONS
Cyclophosphamide, dactinomycin, daunorubicin, mitomycin: increased risk of cardiotoxicity.
Hepatotoxic drugs: increased risk of toxicity.
Live virus vaccines: potentiated virus replication.
Myelosuppressant drugs, radiation therapy: heightened risk of bone marrow depression or, if chest has been irradiated, of cardiomyopathy.
Streptozocin: possible prolonged half-life of doxorubicin.

EFFECTS ON DIAGNOSTIC TESTS
Serum and urine uric acid: increased levels.

SPECIAL CONSIDERATIONS
• *Treatment of overdose:* Watch for increased toxic effects (mucositis, leukopenia, and thrombocytopenia). Give antibiotics, platelets, and granulocyte transfusions, as ordered. Treat mucositis symptomatically.
• Some degree of toxicity occurs with a therapeutic response.
• Regularly monitor EKG or echocardiogram in patients who've received 300 mg/m² or more of drug. Also monitor EKG, CBC, and liver function tests for signs of toxicity.
• Cardiotoxicity may be more common in children under age 2, in elderly patients, and in patients whose cumulative dose exceeds 550 mg/m².
• Watch for early signs of congestive heart failure (CHF); drug-induced condition often fails to respond to therapy. If CHF occurs, give cardiac glycosides,

diuretics, and peripheral vasodilators, as ordered.
• Prevent or minimize uric acid nephropathy through hydration, alkalinizing urine, or giving allopurinol.
• Administer antibiotics, as ordered, to patients with leukopenia or neutropenia who develop infection.
• Advise home care patient to avoid exposure to people with infections.
• Tell patient his urine and stools may be red for 1 to 2 days and that reversible alopecia may occur.

doxycycline hyclate
Doxy, Doxychel, Vibramycin♦

Pregnancy Risk Category: D

PHARMACOKINETICS
Distribution: widespread, to most body fluids, and highly protein-bound. Drug tends to localize in reticuloendothelial cells of the liver, spleen, and bone marrow. It crosses the blood-brain barrier, with cerebrospinal fluid levels about 25% of serum levels; prostatic levels are about 60% of serum levels. Therapeutic levels appear in eye. Drug crosses the placenta.
Metabolism: not metabolized but partly deactivated in the intestine by chelate formation.
Excretion: within 48 hours, 20% to 26% of drug is eliminated in urine via glomerular filtration and 20% to 40% is removed in feces. Drug also appears in breast milk. In normal renal function, half-life is 14 to 17 hours after a single dose and 22 to 24 hours after multiple doses.
Action: peak serum levels, immediately after infusion.

MECHANISM OF ACTION
Primarily bacteriostatic, doxycycline inhibits protein synthesis by preventing transfer RNA from binding to its messenger RNA complex. The drug's broad spectrum of activity includes many gram-positive bacteria, such as *Actinomyces israelii, Arachnia propionica, Bacillus anthracis, Clostridium perfringens, C. tetani, Listeria monocytogenes, Nocardia, Propionibacterium acnes*, and some strains of staphylococci and streptococci.

Drug proves effective against the gram-negative bacteria *Bartonella bacilliformis, Bordetella pertussis, Brucella, Calymmatobacterium granulomatis, Campylobacter fetus, Francisella tularensis, Haemophilus ducreyi, H. influenzae, Legionella pneumophila, Leptotrichia buccalis, Neisseria gonorrhoeae, N. meningitidis, Pasteurella multocida, Pseudomonas mallei, Pseudomonas pseudomallei, Shigella, Spirillum minor, Streptobacillus moniliformis, Vibrio cholerae, V. parahaemolyticus, Yersinia enterocolitica, Y. pestis*, and some strains of *Acinetobacter, Bacteroides, Enterobacter aerogenes, Escherichia coli*, and *Klebsiella*.

The drug is also effective against *Borrelia recurrentis, Chlamydia psittaci, C. trachomatis, Coxiella burnetii, Fusobacterium fusiforme, Leptospira, Mycobacterium fortuitum, Mycoplasma hominis, M. pneumoniae, Rickettsia akari, R. prowazekii, R. rickettsii, R. tsutsugamushi, R. typhi, Treponema pallidum, T. pertenue*, and *Ureaplasma urealyticum*.

INDICATIONS & DOSAGE
• Infections caused by susceptible organisms when P.O. use isn't feasible. *Adults and children over age 8 weighing more than 45 kg:* 200 mg q 12 hours on day 1, then 100 to 200 mg daily, depending on infection's severity. *Children over age 8 weighing 45 kg or less:* 4.4 mg/kg q 12 hours on day 1, then 2.2 to 4.4 mg/

kg q 12 hours, depending on infection's severity.
• Acute pelvic inflammatory disease (when *N. gonorrhoeae* or *C. trachomatis* is suspected). *Adults:* 100 mg q 12 hours (plus cefoxitin 2 g q 6 hours) daily for at least 4 days and then substitute oral doxycycline.
Note: Usual doses of doxycycline may be used in patients with impaired renal function. The usual antianabolic action of tetracyclines doesn't occur with doxycycline.

CONTRAINDICATIONS & CAUTIONS
• Contraindicated in hypersensitivity to any tetracycline. Contraindicated during bone and tooth development (last half of pregnancy and in children under age 8); may cause permanent tooth discoloration, enamel defects, and retarded bone growth.
• Use with caution in myasthenia gravis because of an increased risk of weakness; in patients with impaired renal function as serum half-life is prolonged; and in patients exposed to direct sunlight because of risk of photosensitivity.

PREPARATION & STORAGE
Available as a sterile powder in 100 and 200 mg vials. Before reconstitution, store at room temperature. Reconstitute 100 mg vial with 10 ml of sterile water for injection, 200 mg vial with 20 ml. Further dilute to a concentration of 0.1 to 1 mg/ml, using suitable diluent, such as 0.9% sodium chloride, dextrose 5% in water, Ringer's injection, invert sugar 10% in water, Ringer's lactate injection, dextrose 5% in Ringer's lactate, Normosol-M in dextrose 5%, Normosol-R in dextrose 5%, Plasma-Lyte 56 in dextrose 5%, or Plasma-Lyte 148 in dextrose 5%.

After reconstitution, dilutions using 0.9% sodium chloride or dextrose 5% in water remain stable for 48 hours at room temperature when protected from direct sunlight. Other appropriately diluted solutions retain potency for 12 hours at room temperature and for up to 72 hours if refrigerated and protected from light. To ensure stability, complete infusions within 6 hours.

When frozen immediately after reconstitution, solutions at concentrations of 10 mg/ml are stable for 8 weeks. Once thawed, don't refreeze.

ADMINISTRATION
Direct injection: not used.
Intermittent infusion: Infuse 100 mg (0.5 mg/ml) over 1 to 4 hours, depending on the dose. Avoid extravasation.
Continuous infusion: not used.

INCOMPATIBILITY
No incompatibilities reported.

ADVERSE REACTIONS
Life-threatening: exfoliative dermatitis.
Other: abdominal discomfort, anorexia, benign intracranial hypertension in adults (resolves when drug is discontinued), bulging fontanelles in infants, bulky and loose stools, darkened or discolored tongue, diarrhea, discolored nails, dizziness, dysphagia, eosinophilia, flatulence, glossitis, hemolytic anemia, itching and inflammatory anogenital lesions, Jarisch-Herxheimer reaction (in brucellosis or spirochetal infections), maculopapular and erythematous rash, nausea, neutropenia, photosensitivity, pseudomembranous colitis, superinfection, thrombocytopenia, thrombophlebitis, unusual thirst, urinary frequency.

Unmarked trade names available in the United States only.
♦ Also available in Canada.   ♦ ♦ Available in Canada only.

INTERACTIONS
Anticoagulants: depressed plasma prothrombin activity. Anticoagulant dosage may need to be adjusted.
Barbiturates, carbamazepine, phenytoin: decreased doxycycline levels.
Penicillins: impaired bactericidal action. Don't give with penicillins.
Oral contraceptives: decreased effectiveness with breakthrough bleeding.

EFFECTS ON DIAGNOSTIC TESTS
Urine catecholamines: falsely increased levels because of fluorescence interference in the Hingerty method.
Urine glucose: false-positive results using cupric sulfate methods (Clinitest, Benedict's solution) and false-negative results using oxidase methods (Clinistix, Tes-Tape).

SPECIAL CONSIDERATIONS
• Obtain specimens for culture and sensitivity before first dose. Therapy may begin before results are available.
• If syphilitic infection is suspected when treating other venereal diseases, a dark field examination should be performed before therapy. Blood serology should be repeated monthly for at least 4 months.
• If diarrhea persists during therapy, collect stool specimens to detect possible pseudomembranous colitis.
• Watch for signs of overgrowth. Check patient's tongue for signs of *Candida* infection, and stress good oral hygiene.
• Drug can't be removed by hemodialysis.
• Advise patient of possible photosensitivity reactions. Tell patient to avoid direct sunlight and ultraviolet light.
• If the patient is taking oral contraceptives, suggest that another form of contraceptive be used.

droperidol
Inapsine♦

Pregnancy Risk Category: C

PHARMACOKINETICS
Distribution: not fully understood. Drug crosses the blood-brain barrier and the placenta.
Metabolism: in the liver.
Excretion: in urine and feces.
Action: onset, 3 to 10 minutes; duration, 2 to 4 hours for sedation.

MECHANISM OF ACTION
Droperidol blocks central dopaminergic receptors, producing sedation and antiemetic effects. The drug also blocks alpha-adrenergic receptors.

INDICATIONS & DOSAGE
• Preoperative sedation and prevention or alleviation of nausea and vomiting. *Adults and children over age 12:* 2.5 to 10 mg given 30 to 60 minutes before surgery. *Children age 2 to 12:* 0.088 to 0.165 mg/kg given 30 to 60 minutes before surgery.
• Prevention or alleviation of postoperative nausea and vomiting, and of nausea and vomiting associated with cancer chemotherapy. *Adults:* 0.01 to 0.02 mg/kg.
• Adjunct to induction in general anesthesia. *Adults and children over age 12:* 0.22 to 0.275 mg/kg.
• Maintenance in general anesthesia. *Adults and children over age 12:* 1.25 to 2.5 mg. *Children age 2 to 12:* 0.088 to 0.165 mg/kg.
• Conscious sedation for diagnostic procedures. *Adults and children over age 12:* 1.25 to 2.5 mg I.V. titrated to patient response, after I.M. premedication.
• Adjunct in regional anesthesia. *Adults:* 2.5 to 5 mg.

CONTRAINDICATIONS & CAUTIONS
• Contraindicated in hypersensitivity to drug.
• Use cautiously in elderly, debilitated, and other poor-risk patients. As ordered, reduce the dosage, titrating slowly to patient response.
• Use cautiously in hepatic or renal impairment because of the heightened risk of toxicity and in hypotensive or hypovolemic patients to avoid exacerbating hypotension.

PREPARATION & STORAGE
Available in concentrations of 2.5 mg/ml in 1, 2, and 5 ml ampules and in 10 ml multidose vials. Protect from light and store at room temperature. Drug is compatible with all I.V. solutions.

ADMINISTRATION
When used as an anesthetic, drug should be given only by staff specially trained in giving I.V. anesthetics and managing their adverse reactions.
Direct injection: Inject directly into vein in small incremental boluses or into an established I.V. line containing a free-flowing solution.
Intermittent infusion: not recommended.
Continuous infusion: not recommended.

INCOMPATIBILITY
Incompatible with barbiturates.

ADVERSE REACTIONS
Life-threatening: with high doses, respiratory depression, severe hypotension.
Other: akathisia, anxiety, bronchospasm, chills, depression, dizziness, dystonia, emergence delirium, facial sweating, hallucinations, hyperactivity, laryngospasm, nightmares, oculogyric crisis (extended neck, flexed arms, fine tremors, upward rotation of eyes), postoperative drowsiness, respiratory depression, restlessness, tachycardia, transient hypotension (mild to moderate).

INTERACTIONS
CNS depressants: deepened CNS depression, possibly requiring dosage reduction.
Epinephrine: possible paradoxically lowered blood pressure because of droperidol's alpha-adrenergic blocking action.
Opiate analgesics: prolonged narcotic effect and respiratory depression.

EFFECTS ON DIAGNOSTIC TESTS
EEG: possible abnormal patterns for up to 12 hours.
Hemodynamic measurements: possible reduced pulmonary artery pressure.

SPECIAL CONSIDERATIONS
• *Treatment of overdose:* Provide supportive care. Maintain airway patency and administer vasopressors to correct hypotension. Observe the patient for 24 hours, keep him warm, and give fluids.
• Keep resuscitation equipment available during administration.
• Move and position patient slowly during anesthesia to avoid orthostatic hypotension.
• Watch for signs of an extrapyramidal reaction, such as akathisia or dystonia. Call doctor at once if any such signs occur.
• Frequently monitor patient's vital signs.
• When giving a narcotic analgesic with droperidol, reduce narcotic dosage by one quarter to one third for up to 12 hours or until patient becomes fully alert.

• Droperidol has been used experimentally to prevent or reduce nausea and vomiting caused by chemotherapeutic drugs, especially cisplatin.

edetate calcium disodium (calcium EDTA)
Calcium Disodium Versenate♦

Pregnancy Risk Category: C

PHARMACOKINETICS
Distribution: mainly in extracellular fluid. Drug doesn't penetrate erythrocytes or enter cerebrospinal fluid in appreciable amounts. Not known if drug crosses the placenta.
Metabolism: not metabolized.
Excretion: rapidly removed in urine by glomerular filtration. About 50% is eliminated in 1 hour; 95% in 24 hours. Drug is excreted unchanged or as metal chelates. Half-life ranges from 20 to 60 minutes. Not known if drug appears in breast milk.
Action: onset, 1 hour; duration, unknown.

MECHANISM OF ACTION
Divalent and trivalent metals (especially lead) displace calcium from edetate calcium disodium to form stable soluble complexes.

INDICATIONS & DOSAGE
• Diagnosis of lead poisoning (calcium mobilization test). *Adults and children:* 500 mg/m². Maximum dose, 1 g.
• Acute and chronic lead poisoning and lead encephalopathy. *Adults and children:* 1 g/m² daily for 3 to 5 days if serum lead levels are 25 to 100 mcg/dl; 1.5 g/m² daily for 3 to 5 days along with dimercaprol if serum lead levels exceed 100 mcg/dl. Children may require more than two courses of therapy.

CONTRAINDICATIONS & CAUTIONS
• Contraindicated in severe oliguria or anuria because of the drug's nephrotoxic effects.
• Don't use drug to diagnose lead poisoning if patient's serum lead level exceeds 55 mcg/dl.
• Administer with extreme caution in renal impairment because of the risk of nephrotoxicity. Reduce dosage, if ordered.
• Give cautiously in hypercalcemia because the drug may worsen the condition, and in lead encephalopathy because rapid administration may produce a sudden, lethal rise in intracranial pressure (ICP).

PREPARATION & STORAGE
Available in 5 ml ampules with a concentration of 200 mg/ml. For infusion, dilute with dextrose 5% in water or 0.9% sodium chloride to a concentration of 2 to 4 mg/ml. Store at room temperature.

ADMINISTRATION
Direct injection: not used.
Intermittent infusion: Infuse diluted drug into an established I.V. line at a rate guided by the patient's condition. In an *asymptomatic* patient, infuse half the daily dose over at least 1 hour every 12 hours. In a *symptomatic* patient, infuse half the daily dose over at least 2 hours, and give the second dose after 6 or more hours.
Continuous infusion: Infuse the single daily dose over 8 to 24 hours.

INCOMPATIBILITY
Incompatible with dextrose 10% in water, invert sugar 10% in water, invert sugar 10% in 0.9% sodium chloride, Ringer's lactate, Ringer's injection, protein hydrolysate, and ⅙ M sodium lactate. Also incompat-

ible with amphotericin B and hydralazine.

ADVERSE REACTIONS
Life-threatening: renal tubular necrosis leading to fatal nephrosis; suddenly increased ICP in cerebral edema.
Other: anorexia, dysrhythmias, headache, hematuria, hypercalcemia, hypertension, hypotension, myalgia, nausea, paresthesias, proteinuria, thrombophlebitis, urinary frequency and urgency, vomiting. *Within 8 hours after infusion:* excessive thirst, fatigue, nasal congestion, sneezing, sudden fever and chills. *With prolonged administration:* skin and mucous membrane lesions (subside with drug discontinuation), transient bone marrow depression.

INTERACTIONS
Adrenocorticosteroids: increased risk of nephrotoxicity.
Zinc-insulin preparations: shortened action resulting from zinc chelation.

EFFECTS ON DIAGNOSTIC TESTS
EKG: T-wave inversion.
Urine glucose: increased levels.

SPECIAL CONSIDERATIONS
• Strict adherence to dosage schedule is essential because of potentially fatal drug effects. Each course of therapy should last no more than 7 days, with a 2-week interval between courses.
• To avoid toxicity, use with dimercaprol.
• Before first dose, establish urine flow by giving I.V. dextrose 10%, with mannitol if necessary. If urine flow isn't established after 3 hours of fluid infusion, you can use edetate calcium disodium along with hemodialysis. Once urine flow is es-

tablished, maintain infusion rate to supply basal fluid and electrolyte requirements only. Stop drug when urine flow ceases.
• Monitor BUN level before and during therapy to detect renal impairment. Also monitor EKG during therapy to detect dysrhythmias.
• Perform urinalysis daily, checking especially for increased protein levels, erythrocytes, or large renal epithelial cells, to help determine if drug should be discontinued.
• Edetate calcium disodium has been used to treat magnesium intoxication.

edetate disodium (EDTA)
Chealamide, Disotate, Endrate

Pregnancy Risk Category: C

PHARMACOKINETICS
Distribution: not well understood. Drug doesn't enter cerebrospinal fluid in appreciable amounts.
Metabolism: not metabolized.
Excretion: rapidly excreted in urine. About 95% is excreted in 24 hours as calcium chelate. Serum half-life ranges from 20 to 60 minutes. Not known if drug appears in breast milk.
Action: peak serum level, immediately after administration.

MECHANISM OF ACTION
By forming chelates with calcium and divalent and trivalent metals, edetate disodium increases urinary excretion of calcium, magnesium, zinc, and other trace elements. Drug also exerts a negative inotropic effect on the heart.

INDICATIONS & DOSAGE
• Emergency treatment of hypercalcemia. *Adults:* 50 mg/kg daily up to

a maximum of 3 g daily. *Children:* 40 to 70 mg/kg daily or 50 mg/kg in a single dose.
• Digitalis-induced dysrhythmias. *Adults and children:* 15 mg/kg hourly, not to exceed 60 mg/kg daily.

CONTRAINDICATIONS & CAUTIONS
• Contraindicated in renal disease or reduced glomerular filtration because of the risk of nephrotoxicity.
• Also contraindicated in patients with seizures or intracranial lesions because drug-induced hypocalcemia may reduce seizure threshold.
• Avoid use in patients with active tuberculosis or healed calcified tubular lesions because drug may worsen these conditions.
• Because the drug affects myocardial contractility, use cautiously in cardiac disease.
• Administer cautiously in diabetes mellitus because drug may reduce serum glucose levels.
• Also administer cautiously in hypokalemia and hypocalcemia because the drug may exacerbate these conditions.

PREPARATION & STORAGE
Available in 20 ml ampules with a concentration of 150 mg/ml. Dilute in 500 ml of dextrose 5% in water or 0.9% sodium chloride. Store below 104° F. (40° C.), preferably between 59° and 86° F. (15° and 30° C.), and protect from freezing.

ADMINISTRATION
Direct injection: not recommended.
Intermittent infusion: not recommended.
Continuous infusion: Infuse diluted solution over 3 to 4 hours (preferably over 4 to 6 hours). Take care not to exceed the patient's cardiac reserve. Avoid extravasation because

drug is extremely irritating to tissues.

INCOMPATIBILITY
Incompatible with dextrose 5% and 5% alcohol.

ADVERSE REACTIONS
Life-threatening: nephrotoxicity, severe hypocalcemia.
Other: abdominal cramps, anemia, anorexia, back pain, calcium embolization, chills, diarrhea, erythematous skin eruptions, exfoliative dermatitis, fatigue, fever, glycosuria, headache, hyperuricemia, hypotension, malaise, muscle cramps, nausea, numbness, pain or burning at infusion site, transient circumoral paresthesias, transient drop in blood pressure, unusual thirst, vomiting, weakness.

INTERACTIONS
Zinc-insulin preparations: shortened duration resulting from zinc chelation.

EFFECTS ON DIAGNOSTIC TESTS
Serum alkaline phosphatase: decreased levels.
Serum calcium, glucose, magnesium, potassium: reduced levels.
Urine glucose: increased levels.

SPECIAL CONSIDERATIONS
• *Treatment of overdose:* Tetany, seizures, severe dysrhythmias, and respiratory arrest can result from overdose. Administer I.V. calcium.
• Before infusion, evaluate renal function. Monitor BUN levels periodically and urinalysis daily.
• Monitor EKG, especially when treating ventricular dysrhythmias associated with digitalis toxicity.
• After infusion, keep patient supine to avoid orthostatic hypotension.

- Monitor serum calcium levels after each dose. Be alert for a sudden drop.
- Monitor serum electrolyte levels in patients with hypokalemia or hypocalcemia.
- Drug isn't appropriate for treating atherosclerosis, arteriosclerosis, or coronary artery or peripheral vascular disease.

edrophonium chloride
Enlon, Reversol, Tensilon♦

Pregnancy Risk Category: C

PHARMACOKINETICS
Distribution: throughout body. Drug crosses the blood-brain barrier only with high doses. Probably crosses the placenta in limited amounts.
Metabolism: not well understood.
Excretion: in urine, but not well understood.
Action: onset, 30 to 60 seconds; duration, 5 to 10 minutes.

MECHANISM OF ACTION
Inhibits cholinesterase, allowing acetylcholine to accumulate at cholinergic synapses. Acetylcholine, in turn, causes bronchial constriction, bradycardia, miosis, and increased skeletal and intestinal muscle tone and salivary and sweat gland secretion.

INDICATIONS & DOSAGE
- Diagnosis of myasthenia gravis (MG). *Adults and children weighing over 34 kg:* 2 mg initially, then up to an additional 8 mg, depending on response. *Children weighing up to 34 kg:* 1 mg initially, then up to an additional 5 mg, depending on response.
- Evaluation of anticholinesterase therapy in MG. *Adults:* 1 to 2 mg

given 1 hour after last oral dose of anticholinesterase drug.
- Differentiation of myasthenic from cholinergic crisis. *Adults:* 1 mg initially. Dose may be repeated once if bradycardia or hypotension fails to occur. Total dose not to exceed 2 mg. Patients with myasthenic crisis show improved muscle strength.
- Antagonism of neuromuscular blocking agents (such as curare) after surgery. *Adults:* 10 mg initially. Dose may be repeated p.r.n. q 5 to 10 minutes. Maximum total dose, 40 mg.

CONTRAINDICATIONS & CAUTIONS
- Contraindicated in hypersensitivity to anticholinesterase drugs.
- Also contraindicated in patients with mechanical obstruction of the urinary or GI tract.
- Use cautiously in patients with dysrhythmias or bronchial asthma because drug may exacerbate these conditions.

PREPARATION & STORAGE
Available in 1 and 10 ml vials with a concentration of 10 mg/ml. Compatible with dextrose 5% in water, dextrose 5% in Ringer's lactate, Ringer's lactate, and 0.9% sodium chloride.

ADMINISTRATION
Drug should be given under close medical supervison.
Direct injection: To *diagnose MG,* draw 10 mg (1 ml) of drug into a tuberculin syringe with a 21G or 23G needle. Inject 2 mg (0.2 ml) directly into vein or into the tubing of a free-flowing I.V. line over 15 to 30 seconds. If patient shows no cholinergic effects after 45 seconds, give remaining 8 mg slowly in 2 mg increments. If cholinergic response oc-

curs, discontinue drug and give atropine.

To *evaluate anticholinesterase therapy in MG* or to *differentiate myasthenic from cholinergic crisis,* draw 2 mg (0.2 ml) into a tuberculin syringe and give slowly over 30 to 45 seconds in 1 mg increments.

To *antagonize neuromuscular blocking drugs,* inject drug over 30 to 45 seconds.

Intermittent infusion: not recommended.

Continuous infusion: not recommended.

INCOMPATIBILITY
No incompatibilities reported.

ADVERSE REACTIONS
Life-threatening: bronchospasm, cardiac arrest, respiratory paralysis. *Other:* bradycardia, cholinergic reactions (abdominal cramps, blurred or double vision, diaphoresis, diarrhea, excessive salivation, fasciculations, incoordination, increased bronchial secretions, lacrimation, nausea, pupillary constriction, urinary frequency, vomiting, weakness), hypotension.

INTERACTIONS
Cardiac glycosides: worsened bradycardia and atrioventricular block. *Depolarizing neuromuscular blocking agents (such as succinylcholine):* prolonged Phase I blockade. *Nondepolarizing neuromuscular blocking agents:* antagonized by edrophonium. *Other anticholinesterase drugs (such as ambenonium, neostigmine, pyridostigmine):* enhanced risk of cholinergic crisis (including paralysis) resulting from increased effects. *Quinidine:* possible blocked cholinergic effects of edrophonium.

EFFECTS ON DIAGNOSTIC TESTS
None reported.

SPECIAL CONSIDERATIONS
• *Treatment of overdose:* Weakness usually appears first in masticatory, swallowing, and neck muscles, then in shoulder and arm muscles. Subsequent weakness appears in pelvic, eye, and leg muscles. When cholinergic response occurs, give 0.4 to 0.5 mg atropine sulfate by direct I.V. injection to antagonize muscarinic effects of edrophonium.

• Before giving edrophonium, have 1 mg of atropine available for immediate injection. Keep suction, endotracheal intubation, and mechanical ventilation equipment readily available.

• Establish base line blood pressure, heart rate, and respiratory rate and quality. Keep patient on cardiac monitor during administration. Be alert for hypotension, bradycardia, and respiratory distress.

• If you're giving edrophonium to differentiate myasthenic from cholinergic crisis or to antagonize neuromuscular blocking drugs, initiate mechanical ventilation before administration.

• Evaluate vital capacity and muscle strength before and during administration.

• In patients over age 50, give 0.4 to 0.6 mg atropine sulfate, as ordered, along with edrophonium because of the heightened risk of bradycardia and hypotension.

• In patients sensitive to edrophonium, give small doses of drug along with atropine sulfate.

• Some MG patients experience effects lasting up to 30 minutes upon receiving drug for first time.

• Before giving drug to diagnose MG, stop all other anticholinesterase drugs for at least 8 hours. MG patients show a myasthenic response (marked but transient improvement in muscle strength). Non-MG patients show a cholinergic response (increased weakness, fasciculations, and other adverse muscarinic effects).

• When evaluating anticholinesterase therapy, keep in mind that a myasthenic response indicates an insufficient anticholinesterase dosage. A cholinergic response indicates an excessive anticholinesterase dosage.

• When differentiating myasthenic from cholinergic crisis, use the same guidelines as for evaluating anticholinesterase therapy. However, it may be difficult to distinguish myasthenic from cholinergic crisis in MG patients because muscarinic reactions and fasciculations may be diminished or absent.

• Edrophonium has also been used to treat paroxysmal atrial tachycardia.

• May contain sulfites.

enalaprilat
Vasotec I.V.

Pregnancy Risk Category: C

PHARMACOKINETICS
Distribution: Full distribution pattern is unknown. Drug crosses the placenta; it does not appear to cross the blood-brain barrier.
Metabolism: not metabolized.
Excretion: excreted in urine and feces.
Action: Peak antihypertensive effect occurs within 4 to 6 hours after a dose.

MECHANISM OF ACTION
Enalaprilat inhibits the angiotensin-converting enzyme (ACE) that catalyzes the conversion of angiotensin I to the vasoconstrictor substance angiotensin II. Reduced angiotensin II levels decrease peripheral arterial resistance, lowering blood pressure, and decrease aldosterone secretion, thus reducing sodium and water retention. (Enalapril maleate is an orally activated ACE inhibitor. Once administered, enalapril maleate is converted to enalaprilat.)

INDICATIONS & DOSAGE
• Mild to severe hypertension. *Adults:* 1.25 mg over a 5-minute period every 6 hours. The dose for patients being converted from the oral dose to the I.V. dose is the same.

• Diuretic therapy. *Adults:* 0.625 mg over a 5-minute period every 6 hours. If after 1 hour there is an inadequate clinical response, the dose may be repeated.
Note: Adjust dosage in renal impairment. For adults with a creatinine clearance below 30 ml/minute, the initial dose is 0.625 mg. Gradually titrate the dose according to response. Patients undergoing hemodialysis should receive a supplemental dose on dialysis days.

CONTRAINDICATIONS & CAUTIONS
• Contraindicated in hypersensitivity to the drug and in patients with history of angioedema related to previous treatment with an ACE inhibitor.

• Use with caution in patients with collagen vascular disease or immune system disorders and in patients taking drugs that may depress immune function or cause a decrease in WBC count.

• Use with caution in patients with renal dysfunction.

• Because of the risk of hyperkalemia, use with caution in patients taking potassium-sparing diuretics,

potassium supplements, and salt substitutes.
• Because of the risk of adverse effects associated with hypotension, use with caution in patients with vascular insufficiency, recent myocardial infarction, or cerebrovascular disease.
• Because trace amounts of enalaprilat are found in breast milk, exercise caution when administering the drug to nursing mothers.

PREPARATION & STORAGE

Available as a clear, colorless solution in 1 and 2 ml vials containing 1.25 mg per ml. May be diluted with up to 50 ml of the following compatible solutions: 5% dextrose injection, 0.9% sodium chloride injection, 0.9% sodium chloride injection in 5% dextrose, 5% dextrose in lactated Ringer's injection, or Isolyte E. Diluted solutions maintain full activity for 24 hours at room temperature. Store below 86° F. (30° C.).

ADMINISTRATION

Direct injection: may be administered as provided or diluted with up to 50 ml of a compatible diluent. Infuse slowly over at least 5 minutes.
Intermittent infusion: not recommended.
Continuous infusion: not recommended.

INCOMPATIBILITY

None reported.

ADVERSE REACTIONS

Life-threatening: agranulocytosis, cardiac arrest.
Other: angioedema, blurred vision, bone marrow depression, bronchospasm, cough, depression, diarrhea, dizziness, fatigue, headache, hypotension, ileus, insomnia, muscle cramps, nausea, neutropenia, or-

thostasis, rash, renal function impairment, syncope, thrombocytopenia.

INTERACTIONS

Aspirin and indomethacin: decreased enalaprilat effect.
Diuretics and other antihypertensives: increased hypotensive effect.
Lithium: decreased renal clearance of lithium.
Potassium-sparing diuretics, potassium supplements, and salt substitutes: increased risk of hyperkalemia.

EFFECTS ON DIAGNOSTIC TESTS

Bilirubin and liver enzyme: slightly elevated levels.
BUN and serum creatinine: elevated levels.
Hematocrit and hemoglobin: decreased levels.

SPECIAL CONSIDERATIONS

• *Treatment of overdose:* The most likely manifestation of overdosage is hypotension. The usual treatment is I.V. infusion of 0.9% sodium chloride. Enalaprilat may be removed from general circulation by hemodialysis. It has also been removed from neonatal circulation by peritoneal dialysis.
• Observe the patient for facial swelling and difficulty breathing, which may indicate angioedema. If angioedema of the face, extremities, lips, tongue, glottis, or larynx occurs, discontinue treatment with enalaprilat immediately. Institute appropriate therapy—epinephrine solution 1:1,000 (0.3 to 0.5 ml) S.C. and measures to ensure a patent airway. Monitor patient carefully until signs and symptoms disappear.
• Monitor WBC count and liver and kidney functions.

- Advise the patient that lightheadedness may occur and that sudden position changes may cause dizziness.
- If hypertension occurs, place the patient in a supine position and infuse 0.9% sodium chloride, as ordered.
- Because of the potential for decreased WBC count, observe the patient for signs of infection, such as sore throat, fever, and malaise.
- Because safe use of the drug during pregnancy has not been established, advise patients in the second or third trimesters of potential hazards to the fetus; recommend ultrasound examinations.
- Enalaprilat is usually used only when oral therapy with enalapril maleate is not feasible.
- Elderly patients may need lower doses because of impaired drug clearance.

---

ephedrine sulfate

Pregnancy Risk Category: C

PHARMACOKINETICS
Distribution: unknown. Drug presumably crosses the placenta.
Metabolism: slowly metabolized in liver. Small quantities are metabolized by oxidative deamination, demethylation, aromatic hydroxylation, and conjugation.
Excretion: in urine within 48 hours, mostly as unchanged drug and its metabolites. Rate of excretion depends on urine pH. Half-life ranges from 3 to 6 hours. Drug probably appears in breast milk.
Action: peak levels, immediately after administration; duration, 1 hour.

MECHANISM OF ACTION
Ephedrine stimulates alpha- and beta-adrenergic receptors, relaxing bronchial smooth muscle and increasing the automaticity of idioventricular and nodal pacemakers, producing a positive inotropic effect. The drug dilates coronary vessels and constricts renal arteries.

INDICATIONS & DOSAGE
- Bronchospasm. *Adults:* 12.5 to 25 mg. Subsequent doses based on patient response. Maximum dosage, 150 mg q 24 hours. *Children:* 0.5 to 0.75 mg/kg q 4 to 6 hours.
- Hypotension and temporary support of ventricular rate in bradycardia, atrioventricular block, carotid sinus syndrome, or Stokes-Adams syndrome. *Adults:* 5 to 25 mg, repeated in 5 to 10 minutes, if needed. Maximum dosage, 150 mg q 24 hours. *Children:* 0.5 to 0.75 mg/kg q 4 to 6 hours.

CONTRAINDICATIONS & CAUTIONS
- Contraindicated in hypersensitivity to the drug; in narrow-angle glaucoma because of the risk of increased ocular pressure; in psychoneurosis because of aggravating CNS effects; and in cardiac disease because drug increases oxygen consumption, stimulating the heart.
- Use with extreme caution in hypertension or hyperthyroidism because of the heightened risk of adverse reactions.
- Use ephedrine cautiously in elderly patients with prostatic hypertrophy because of the risk of urine retention; in diabetic patients because the drug raises serum glucose levels; and in patients with cardiovascular disease or pheochromocytoma because of pressor effects.

PREPARATION & STORAGE

Available in 1 ml vials with concentrations of 25 and 50 mg/ml. Store between 59° and 86° F. (15° and 30° C.) in light-resistant containers; drug gradually decomposes and darkens on exposure to light. Discard any unused, cloudy, or precipitated solutions. Drug is compatible with most common I.V. fluids.

ADMINISTRATION

Direct injection: Slowly inject drug directly into vein or into an I.V. line containing a free-flowing compatible solution.
Intermittent infusion: not recommended.
Continuous infusion: not recommended.

INCOMPATIBILITY

Incompatible with fructose; hydrocortisone sodium succinate; Ionosol B, D-CM, D, and G solutions; meperidine; pentobarbital sodium; secobarbital sodium; and thiopental.

ADVERSE REACTIONS

Life-threatening: anaphylaxis, extrasystoles, potentially fatal dysrhythmias (including ventricular fibrillation).
Other: acute urinary retention, agitation, anginal pain (in coronary insufficiency or ischemic heart disease), anorexia, anxiety, breathing difficulty, confusion, delirium, dizziness, dry nose and throat, mild epigastric distress, euphoria, fear, fever, hallucinations, headache, hyperactive reflexes, insomnia, irritability, light-headedness, nausea, painful urination, pallor, palpitations, precordial pain, restlessness, seizures, tachycardia, talkativeness, tremors, vomiting.

INTERACTIONS

Alpha-adrenergic blockers: possible decreased pressor response to ephedrine.
Antihypertensives: possible reduced effects.
Atropine: enhanced pressor response to ephedrine.
Beta-adrenergic blockers: possible reduced ephedrine effects, heightened risk of hypertension, and excessive bradycardia with heart block.
Cardiac glycosides: sensitization of myocardium to sympathomimetic effects.
CNS stimulants: possible excessive CNS stimulation.
Corticosteroids: possible increased metabolic clearance.
Diatrizoate, iothalamate, ioxaglate: possible enhanced CNS effects, such as paraplegia, if given after ephedrine because splanchnic vasoconstriction forces contrast media into vessels leading to spinal cord.
Doxapram, guanadrel, guanethidine: possible increased pressor effects.
Ergot alkaloids: possible enhanced vasodilation, peripheral vascular ischemia, and potentiated pressor effects, causing severe hypertension.
Furosemide, other diuretics: possible reduced arterial responsiveness to ephedrine.
General anesthetics (cyclopropane, halogenated hydrocarbons): possible increased cardiac irritability.
Levodopa: possible heightened risk of dysrhythmias.
MAO inhibitors: potentiated pressor effects of ephedrine.
Mazindol, methylphenidate: possible enhanced CNS stimulation and potentiated pressor effects.
Mecamylamine, methyldopa, trimethaphan: possible diminished hypotensive effects of these drugs and

---

enhanced pressor effects of ephedrine.

Nitrates: possible reduced effects.

Rauwolfia alkaloids: possible diminished hypotensive effects of these drugs and decreased pressor effects of ephedrine.

Sympathomimetics: possible additive effects and increased risk of toxicity.

Thyroid hormones: possible heightened thyroid hormone or ephedrine effects and enhanced risk of coronary insufficiency in coronary artery disease.

Urinary alkalizers (such as sodium bicarbonate, carbonic anhydrase inhibitors): prolonged ephedrine effects.

Xanthines: possible higher incidence of adverse reactions.

EFFECTS ON DIAGNOSTIC TESTS
None reported.

SPECIAL CONSIDERATIONS
• *Treatment of overdose:* Overdose may cause cardiovascular collapse. As ordered, give beta blockers for dysrhythmias; phentolamine mesylate for hypertension; diazepam or paraldehyde for seizures; and cold applications and I.V. dexamethasone for fever. Don't give vasopressors.
• Before giving ephedrine, correct hypovolemia.
• Monitor blood pressure and cardiac status before, during, and after therapy. Hypoxia, hypercapnia, and acidosis may reduce ephedrine's effectiveness.
• A sedative or tranquilizer may combat CNS stimulation.

epinephrine hydrochloride
Adrenalin Chloride Solution♦,
EpiPen Auto-Injector, EpiPen Jr.

Pregnancy Risk Category: C

PHARMACOKINETICS
Distribution: rapid and widespread. Crosses placenta but not the blood-brain barrier.

Metabolism: in sympathetic nerve endings, the liver, and other tissues to inactive metabolites.

Excretion: in urine, with about 40% as metabolites, mostly as sulfate conjugates, and small amounts unchanged. Appears in breast milk.

Action: onset, immediate; duration, brief.

MECHANISM OF ACTION
A sympathomimetic, epinephrine stimulates alpha- and beta-adrenergic receptors. Its major effects include relaxation of bronchial smooth muscle, cardiac stimulation, and dilation of skeletal muscle vasculature.

INDICATIONS & DOSAGE
• Bronchospasm and hypersensitivity reactions. *Adults:* 0.1 to 0.25 mg (1 ml to 2.5 ml of a 1:10,000 dilution) slowly over 5 to 10 minutes. May be followed by an infusion of 1 to 4 mcg/kg/minute. *Children:* 0.1 mg (10 ml of a 1:100,000 dilution) slowly over 5 to 10 minutes. May be followed by an infusion of 0.1 mcg/kg/minute, increased p.r.n. to a maximum of 1.5 mcg/kg/min.
• Cardiac arrest. *Adults:* 0.1 to 1 mg (1 to 10 ml of 1:10,000 dilution) repeated q 5 minutes p.r.n. May be followed by an infusion of 1 mcg/kg/minute, increased p.r.n. to 4 mcg/kg/minute. *Children:* 0.01 mg/kg (0.1 ml/kg of a 1:10,000 dilution) repeated q 5 minutes p.r.n. May be

followed by an infusion of 0.1 mcg/kg/minute, increased p.r.n. by 0.1 mcg/kg/minute to a maximum of 1 mcg/kg/minute. *Neonates:* 0.01 to 0.03 mg/kg (0.1 to 0.3 ml/kg of a 1:10,000 dilution) repeated q 5 minutes p.r.n.

CONTRAINDICATIONS & CAUTIONS
• Contraindicated in shock (except anaphylactic shock) because of increased myocardial oxygen demand; in organic brain damage, cerebral arteriosclerosis, organic heart disease, cardiac dilation, coronary insufficiency, and most dysrhythmias because the drug may worsen these conditions; and in narrow-angle glaucoma because of the risk of increased intraocular pressure.
• Give cautiously in hyperthyroidism, especially in elderly patients, because of the heightened risk of adverse reactions; in diabetes mellitus because the drug causes hyperglycemia, requiring an increased insulin dosage or a hypoglycemic drug; and in cardiovascular disorders, such as angina pectoris, tachycardia, congestive heart failure, coronary artery disease, and hypertension, because of possible exacerbation.
• Also use cautiously in sensitivity to sulfites or sympathomimetic amines because of an increased risk of hypersensitivity; in psychoneurosis because symptoms may worsen; and in Parkinson's disease because the drug temporarily increases rigidity or tremors.

PREPARATION & STORAGE
Available in 1 and 30 ml vials in concentrations of 0.1 mg/ml (1:10,000), 0.5 mg/ml (1:2,000), and 1 mg/ml (1:1,000). Also available in prefilled syringes containing 1 to 2 ml of 1 mg/ml concentration; 10 ml of 0.1 mg/ml; and 5 ml of 0.01 mg/ml. To obtain a solution of 4 mcg/ml, add 1 mg of drug to 250 ml of dextrose 5% in water or 0.9% sodium chloride. Compatible with most other I.V. solutions.

Protect epinephrine from light. (Keep ampules in carton until ready to use.) Discard brown solutions or solutions that contain a precipitate.

ADMINISTRATION
Direct injection: Slowly inject drug directly into vein or into an I.V. line containing a free-flowing compatible solution.
Intermittent infusion: Using an appropriately diluted concentration, piggyback drug into a compatible I.V. solution, and infuse at 1 to 4 mcg/minute.
Continuous infusion: not recommended.

INCOMPATIBILITY
Rapidly destroyed by alkalies or oxidizing agents, including halogens, nitrates, nitrites, permanganates, sodium bicarbonate, and salts of easily reducible metals (such as iron, copper, and zinc). Incompatible with aminophylline, cephapirin, mephentermine sulfate, warfarin, Ionosol D-CM, Ionosol PSL, and Ionosol T with dextrose 5%.

ADVERSE REACTIONS
Life-threatening: anaphylaxis, cerebral hemorrhage, ventricular dysrhythmias.
Other: agitation, anxiety, blurred vision, bradycardia, breathing difficulty, chest pain, chills, disorientation, dizziness, excitability, fever, hallucinations, headache, hypertension, impaired memory, insomnia, light-headedness, mood changes, muscle cramps, nausea, pallor, palpitations, restlessness, sweating, tachycardia, tremors, vomiting, weakness.

INTERACTIONS
Alpha-adrenergic blockers: reversed epinephrine effects.
Antihistamines, tricyclic antidepressants: potentiated epinephrine effects.
Beta-adrenergic blockers: antagonized cardiac and bronchodilatory effects of epinephrine.
Cardiac glycosides: anginal pain in coronary insufficiency.
Diatrizoate, iothalamate, ioxaglate: possible increased CNS effects, such as paraplegia, if given after epinephrine because splanchnic vasoconstriction forces contrast media into vessels leading to spinal cord.
Doxapram, guanadrel, guanethidine: possible increased pressor effects.
Ergot alkaloids: possible enhanced vasoconstriction, peripheral ischemia, and pressor effects, resulting in severe hypertension.
General anesthetics (cyclopropane, halogenated hydrocarbons): increased risk of ventricular dysrhythmias. Don't use together.
Levodopa: possible heightened risk of dysrhythmias.
Mazindol, methylphenidate: possible increased CNS stimulation and pressor effects of epinephrine.
Mecamylamine, methyldopa, trimethaphan: possible decreased antihypertensive effects and heightened pressor effects of epinephrine.
Other CNS stimulants and xanthines: additive CNS effects.
Sympathomimetics: additive effects and heightened risk of epinephrine or sympathomimetic toxicity.
Thyroid hormones: possible increased thyroid hormone or epinephrine effects and enhanced risk of coronary insufficiency in coronary artery disease.

EFFECTS ON DIAGNOSTIC TESTS
Blood lactic acid, serum glucose: elevated levels.
EKG: alterations, including decreased T-wave amplitude.

SPECIAL CONSIDERATIONS
• *Treatment of overdose:* Provide supportive care. Overdose may cause renal shutdown and circulatory collapse. Overdose or prolonged use can produce severe metabolic acidosis because of elevated lactic acid levels. Rapid-acting vasodilators, such as nitrites or sodium nitroprusside, may counteract marked pressor effects. Alpha- or beta-adrenergic blockers may treat symptoms.
• Monitor vital signs. Drug can widen pulse pressure.
• May contain sulfites.

---

epoetin alfa (erythropoietin)
Epogen, Eprex♦♦, Procrit

Pregnancy Risk Category: C

PHARMACOKINETICS
Distribution: throughout the plasma; animal studies reveal that the drug distributes to bone marrow, kidney, spleen, and liver.
Metabolism: not fully understood; animal studies are inconclusive regarding the importance of hepatic metabolism.
Excretion: elimination half-life ranges from 4 to 11 hours, depending upon dose. Higher doses are associated with a longer half-life. Less than 5% of the drug is eliminated by renal excretion, and half-life is not affected by end-stage renal disease.

Unmarked trade names available in the United States only.
♦Also available in Canada.   ♦♦Available in Canada only.

MECHANISM OF ACTION
An amino acid glycoprotein synthesized using recombinant DNA technology, epoetin alfa mimics naturally occurring erythropoietin, which is produced by the kidney. It stimulates the division and differentiation of cells within the bone marrow to produce RBCs.

INDICATIONS & DOSAGE
• Treatment of anemia associated with chronic renal failure. *Adults:* initiate therapy at 50 to 100 units/kg three times weekly. Patients receiving dialysis should receive the drug I.V.; patients with chronic renal failure who aren't on dialysis may receive the drug S.C.

Reduce dosage when target hematocrit is reached or if hematocrit rises more than 4 points within any 2 week period. Increase dosage if hematocrit doesn't rise by 5 to 6 points after 8 weeks of therapy and target range of 30% to 33% hasn't been reached. Individualize dosage for maintenance range. Usually, dosage is changed by 25 units/kg three times weekly.

• Treatment of anemia associated with zidovudine (AZT) therapy in patients infected with human immunodeficiency virus and low endogenous erythropoietin levels. *Adults:* Initiate therapy with 100 units/kg three times weekly for 8 weeks. If response is not adequate, increase dosage to 150 or 200 units/kg three times a week. Reevaluate response every 1 to 2 months and increase dosage by 50 to 100 units/kg three times a week as needed. Patients are unlikely to respond to dosages higher than 300 units/kg three times a week. Doses should be cautiously adjusted based upon intercurrent infections or alterations in zidovudine therapy.

CONTRAINDICATIONS & CAUTIONS
• Contraindicated in patients hypersensitive to mammalian cell-derived products or to human albumin, and in patients with uncontrolled hypertension.
• During initiation of therapy, instruct patient to avoid driving or operating heavy machinery because of possible increased risk of seizures.
• Dialysis patients may require increased anticoagulation with heparin.

PREPARATION & STORAGE
Available in vials of 2,000 units/ml, 3,000 units/ml, 4,000 units/ml, and 10,000 units/ml. Vials also contain 2.5 mg human albumin. Refrigerate at 36° to 46° F. (2° to 8° C.). Do not shake because this may denature glycoprotein. Do not dilute solution, and use only one dose per vial (do not reenter vial) because it does not contain preservatives.

ADMINISTRATION
Direct injection: Administer through the I.V. access site after dialysis session.
Intermittent infusion: not recommended.
Continuous infusion: not recommended.

INCOMPATIBILITY
Avoid mixing with other drugs.

ADVERSE REACTIONS
Life-threatening: none reported.
Other: arthralgias, clotted venous access device, diarrhea, headache, hypertension, nausea, seizures (if hematocrit rises too rapidly), vomiting.

INTERACTIONS
None reported.

EFFECTS ON DIAGNOSTIC TESTS

BUN, serum creatinine, phosphorus, potassium, and uric acid: increased levels.

SPECIAL CONSIDERATIONS

• Monitor hematocrit at least twice weekly during initiation of therapy and during any dosage adjustment. Closely monitor blood pressure. During the initial therapy (when hematocrit is increasing), about 25% of patients require antihypertensive therapy or dosage adjustment in current therapy.

• A rapid rise in hematocrit can cause loss of control of blood pressure. Reduce dosage so hematocrit doesn't increase by more than 4 points within any 2 week period. Drug may have to be withheld until blood pressure is controlled.

• An interval of 2 to 6 weeks may be necessary before a dosage change is reflected in the hematocrit.

• If a patient fails to respond to epoetin alfa therapy, consider any of the following causes: vitamin deficiency (especially of folate or vitamin B_{12}), iron deficiency, underlying inflammatory disease or infection, occult blood loss, underlying hematologic disease (including thalassemia, refractory anemia, or myelodysplastic disorders), hemolysis, aluminum intoxication, osteitis fibrosa cystica, malignancy.

• Most patients require supplemental iron therapy. Before and during therapy, monitor the patient's iron stores, including serum ferritin and transferrin saturation.

• Discontinue drug if hematocrit rises beyond target range of 30% to 33%.

• Hemodialysis patients being treated with epoetin alfa may require increased heparin dosage to reduce risk of clogging dialysis machine.

• Epoetin alfa therapy may result in increased hematocrit and decreased plasma volume, which may reduce effectiveness of dialysis treatments.

• Maximum safe dosage has not been established. But doses up to 1,500 units/kg have been administered three times weekly for 3 weeks without causing direct toxic effects.

• Drug can cause polycythemia; phlebotomy may be used to restore the hematocrit to appropriate levels.

• Routine monitoring of CBC, with differential and platelet counts, is recommended.

• Explain to the patient and his family the importance of regularly monitoring blood pressure in light of the potential effects of this drug.

• Many patients report an improved sense of well-being.

• Advise patients to follow dietary restrictions and to report as directed for dialysis sessions during therapy.

• Remind dialysis patients that epoetin alfa will not affect the course of their renal failure.

• Determine endogenous erythropoietin levels in patients receiving the drug for zidovudine-induced anemia before therapy. They are unlikely to respond to epoietin alfa therapy if endogenous levels are greater than 500 milliunits per ml.

---

ergonovine maleate
Ergotrate Maleate♦

Pregnancy Risk Category: Not applicable

PHARMACOKINETICS

Distribution: rapidly, into plasma, extracellular fluid, and tissues.
Metabolism: presumably in the liver.
Excretion: primarily in feces via bile. Elimination may be prolonged in neonates. Ergonovine appears in breast milk but not enough to affect breast-feeding infants.

Action: onset, less than 1 minute; duration, up to 45 minutes, although rhythmic contractions may persist for 3 hours.

MECHANISM OF ACTION
Ergonovine directly stimulates uterine and vascular smooth muscle, causing uterine contraction and vasoconstriction.

INDICATIONS & DOSAGE
• Emergency treatment of postpartum or postabortion hemorrhage caused by uterine atony or subinvolution. *Adults:* 0.2 mg in a single dose, repeated q 2 to 4 hours, if necessary, up to five doses.
• Adjunct to coronary arteriography in diagnosis of coronary artery spasm in patients with variant angina and no coronary obstruction. *Adults:* 0.05 to 0.2 mg in a single dose, repeated q 5 minutes until chest pain occurs or a total dose of 0.4 mg has been given.

CONTRAINDICATIONS & CAUTIONS
• Contraindicated before placental expulsion because captivation of the placenta may occur.
• Contraindicated for induction of labor because of possible uterine tetany or rupture, cervical and perineal lacerations, amniotic fluid embolism, and fetal trauma; in threatened spontaneous abortion; and in hypersensitive or idiosyncratic reaction to ergonovine or methylergonovine.
• Contraindicated in hypertension, heart disease, atrioventricular shunts, mitral valve stenosis, and obliterative vascular disease because of adverse cardiovascular effects.
• Use cautiously in sepsis or in hepatic or renal impairment (drug can accumulate); and in hypocalcemia (may alter patient response).

PREPARATION & STORAGE
Supplied in 1 ml ampules containing 0.2 mg/ml. Dilute with 5 ml of 0.9% sodium chloride before infusion. Store below 46° F. (8° C.) in light-resistant containers. Discard discolored ergonovine injections (normally clear and colorless) or those that contain a precipitate. Avoid freezing.

ADMINISTRATION
Direct injection: Inject diluted drug directly into vein over at least 60 seconds. Avoid rapid injection because of severe cardiovascular effects.
Intermittent infusion: not recommended.
Continuous infusion: not recommended.

INCOMPATIBILITY
No incompatibilities reported, but drug shouldn't be mixed with any I.V. infusions.

ADVERSE REACTIONS
Life-threatening: anaphylaxis or hypersensitivity reaction, severe dysrhythmias and cerebrovascular accident in eclampsia.
Other: arm, back, chest, or leg pain; confusion; diaphoresis; dizziness; dyspnea; ergotism; gangrene of fingers and toes; headache; hypertension; nausea; palpitations; seizures; tinnitus; vomiting.

INTERACTIONS
Other ergot alkaloids, vasoconstrictors, vasopressors: enhanced vasoconstriction, requiring dosage adjustment.
Regional anesthetics, vasoconstrictors: heightened risk of hypertension and headache.
Tobacco: increased vasoconstriction with heavy smoking.

EFFECTS ON DIAGNOSTIC TESTS
Serum prolactin: possible decreased levels, which may impair lactation.

SPECIAL CONSIDERATIONS
• *Treatment of overdose:* Principal signs include seizures and gangrene. As ordered, administer an anticonvulsant and a vasodilator.
• Closely monitor blood pressure and pulse. I.V. hydralazine or chlorpromazine can effectively treat ergonovine-induced hypertension.
• Closely monitor contractions and uterine tone after administration. If appropriate, give analgesics.
• Review the patient's history. In a hypocalcemic patient, for instance, the uterus may not respond until I.V. calcium is administered.
• Unlike other ergot alkaloids, ergonovine isn't recommended for migraine headaches.

Erwinia asparaginase

Pregnancy Risk Category: C

PHARMACOKINETICS
Distribution: minimal outside vascular compartment. Not known if drug crosses the placenta.
Metabolism: unknown.
Excretion: minimal, with trace amounts in urine. Plasma elimination is biphasic: Initial half-life is about 4 to 9 hours; terminal half-life, about 1 to 5 days. Not known if drug appears in breast milk.
Action: onset, immediate; duration, 23 to 33 days (active enzyme detected in plasma).

MECHANISM OF ACTION
Derived from a plant parasite, this enzyme depletes neoplastic cells of exogenous asparagine, thus inhibiting the DNA and protein synthesis necessary for their survival.

INDICATIONS & DOSAGE
• Induction phase of acute lymphocytic leukemia. *Adults and children:* 200 IU daily for 28 days, followed by 6,000 IU/m² daily for 5 days, followed by 20,000 IU/m² once weekly for 2 weeks; when used as part of combination therapy, 1,000 IU/kg daily for 10 days.

CONTRAINDICATIONS & CAUTIONS
• Contraindicated in asparaginase hypersensitivity and in a history of pancreatitis.

PREPARATION & STORAGE
Available in 10,000 IU vials. Reconstitute with 2 ml of 0.9% sodium chloride or sterile water for injection to yield a concentration of 5,000 IU/ml. For infusion, dilute reconstituted drug in dextrose 5% in water or 0.9% sodium chloride.
  Refrigerate intact vials. Store reconstituted vials at room temperature or in refrigerator for up to 20 days. Discard turbid solutions.

ADMINISTRATION
Direct injection: not recommended.
Intermittent infusion: Give through newly started peripheral I.V., using 23G or 25G winged-tip needle. Administer through side port of rapidly infusing dextrose 5% in water or 0.9% sodium chloride solution.
Continuous infusion: not recommended.

INCOMPATIBILITY
None reported.

ADVERSE REACTIONS
Life-threatening: anaphylaxis.
Other: anorexia, drowsiness, hepatotoxicity, hyperglycemia, immunosup-

pression, lethargy, malaise, nausea, pancreatitis, renal failure.

INTERACTIONS
Cyclophosphamide, cytarabine, mercaptopurine: altered activation or detoxification.
Mercaptopurine, methotrexate, prednisone: increased risk of hepatotoxicity and therapeutic antagonism or synergism, depending on schedule.
Prednisone: magnified risk of hyperglycemia.
Vincristine: increased risk of hyperglycemia, neuropathy, and altered erythropoiesis; altered activation or detoxification.

EFFECTS ON DIAGNOSTIC TESTS
Serum albumin, calcium, cholesterol; plasma fibrinogen: possible decreased levels.
Serum alkaline phosphatase, bilirubin, SGOT, SGPT: possible increased levels.
Serum ammonia, gamma globulin: possible elevated levels.
Thyroid function tests: possible reduced serum thyroxine and increased thyroxine-binding globulin levels.

SPECIAL CONSIDERATIONS
• To help prevent life-threatening hypersensitivity, perform skin tests and desensitization before first treatment or if 1 week or more has elapsed between treatments. Inject 2 IU of reconstituted drug intradermally, and observe patient for at least 1 hour for flare or wheal. If skin test is positive or if the patient with a heightened risk of hypersensitivity must be retreated, desensitize by gradually increasing the I.V. dose until reaching the ordered daily dosage. Be aware that a negative skin test doesn't rule out hypersensitivity. Keep emergency resuscitation equipment nearby.

• Incidence of hypersensitivity is lower with *Erwinia* asparaginase than with L-asparaginase. Also, a daily dosage schedule carries less risk than a weekly one.
• Monitor liver function tests. Teach patient to recognize signs of hepatic impairment, such as jaundice, dark orange urine, and clay-colored stools.
• Resistance to cytotoxic effects of *Erwinia* asparaginase develops rapidly.

erythromycin gluceptate
Ilotycin Gluceptate♦

erythromycin lactobionate
Erythrocin♦

Pregnancy Risk Category: B

PHARMACOKINETICS
Distribution: in most body tissues and fluids, with high concentrations in liver and bile and extremely low concentrations in cerebrospinal fluid. Erythromycin may appear in pleural and peritoneal spaces and in inflamed meninges. Drug is 73% to 81% protein-bound. It crosses the placenta, and fetal levels are about 5% to 20% as high as maternal levels.
Metabolism: partly changed in the liver to inactive metabolites.
Excretion: in bile, mainly as unchanged drug, and in urine with 10% to 15% excreted unchanged. Some drug is reabsorbed after biliary excretion. It appears in breast milk in concentrations that are about 50% as high as maternal levels. In normal renal function, plasma half-life is 1 to 3 hours; in anuria, it may extend to 6 hours.
Action: peak serum levels, immediately after administration.

MECHANISM OF ACTION

A bacteriostatic antibiotic, erythromycin inhibits protein synthesis of sensitive microorganisms by binding to the 50S ribosomal subunit.

The drug is active against gram-positive cocci and gram-positive bacilli, including *Bacillus anthracis, Corynebacterium, Clostridium, Erysipelothrix,* and *Listeria monocytogenes.* It acts against gram-negative cocci, such as *Neisseria,* and some gram-negative bacilli, including strains of *Haemophilus influenzae, Legionella pneumophilia, Pasteurella,* and *Brucella.* It also acts against strains of *Chlamydia, Actinomyces, Mycoplasma pneumoniae, Ureaplasma urealyticum, Rickettsia, Treponema,* and *Entamoeba histolytica.* Against *Mycobacterium kansasii* and *M. scrofulaceum,* the drug is somewhat effective.

INDICATIONS & DOSAGE

• Systemic infections caused by susceptible organisms. *Adults:* 15 to 20 mg/kg daily in divided doses q 6 hours; do not to exceed 6 g daily. *Children:* 300 to 600 mg/m² daily in divided doses q 6 hours.
• Acute pelvic inflammatory disease caused by *Neisseria gonorrhoeae. Adults:* 500 mg q 6 hours for 3 days, then given P.O.
• Legionnaires' disease. *Adults:* 1 to 4 g daily in divided doses, alone or with rifampin.

CONTRAINDICATIONS & CAUTIONS

• Contraindicated in erythromycin hypersensitivity.
• Use cautiously in hepatic impairment because of the enhanced risk of toxicity.

PREPARATION & STORAGE

Erythromycin gluceptate is available in 250 mg, 500 mg, and 1 g vials; erythromycin lactobionate, in 500 mg and 1 g vials. Reconstitute with sterile water for injection (without preservatives). Add at least 10 ml of sterile water for injection to the 250 and 500 mg vials and at least 20 ml to the 1 g vial. For intermittent infusion, dilute reconstituted erythromycin gluceptate with 100 ml of dextrose 5% in water or Normosol-R solution, or erythromycin lactobionate to a maximum concentration of 5 mg/ml with 0.9% sodium chloride or Ringer's lactate. For continuous infusion, dilute erythromycin lactobionate to a concentration of 1 g/1,000 ml of 0.9% sodium chloride or Ringer's lactate.

Store intact vials at room temperature. Reconstituted drug remains stable for 14 days if refrigerated. Diluted drug for infusion remains stable for 8 hours at room temperature, for 24 hours if refrigerated, and for 30 days if frozen.

ADMINISTRATION

Direct injection: not recommended.
Intermittent infusion: Infuse diluted solution through a patent I.V. line over 20 to 60 minutes.
Continuous infusion: Infuse diluted solution over 4 to 8 hours. Longer infusion risks loss of potency.

INCOMPATIBILITY

Erythromycin gluceptate is incompatible with amikacin, aminophylline, cephapirin, chloramphenicol sodium succinate, heparin sodium, oxytetracycline, pentobarbital sodium, phenytoin sodium, secobarbital sodium, streptomycin, and tetracycline hydrochloride.

Erythromycin lactobionate is incompatible with ampicillin sodium, ascorbic acid injection, colistimethate sodium, dextrose 2.5% in half-strength Ringer's lactate, dextrose 5% in Ringer's lactate, dextrose 5%

in 0.9% sodium chloride, dextrose 5% and 10% in water, heparin sodium, metaraminol bitartrate, Normosol-M in dextrose 5%, Ringer's injection, tetracycline hydrochloride, and vitamin B complex with C.

ADVERSE REACTIONS
Life-threatening: anaphylaxis.
Other: bacterial and fungal superinfection, dark amber urine, diarrhea, hepatic dysfunction (reversible), jaundice, nausea, ototoxicity (reversible), pale stools, rash, sore mouth or tongue, thrombophlebitis, urticaria, venous irritation, vomiting.

INTERACTIONS
Alfentanil: with perioperative use of erythromycin, reduced plasma clearance and prolonged action.
Carbamazepine: possible increased serum levels, leading to toxicity.
Chloramphenicol, lincomycin: diminished bactericidal action.
Cyclosporine: possible enhanced risk of nephrotoxicity.
Digoxin: increased serum levels.
Ergotamine: increased vasospasm associated with ergotamine.
Hepatotoxic drugs: increased risk of hepatotoxicity.
Ototoxic drugs: possible heightened risk of ototoxicity.
Penicillins: possible antagonized bactericidal action if used with low doses of erythromycin.
Warfarin: possible excessively prolonged prothrombin time.
Xanthine derivatives: increased serum levels and risk of toxicity.

EFFECTS ON DIAGNOSTIC TESTS
Serum alkaline phosphatase, bilirubin, SGOT, SGPT: increased levels.
Urine catecholamines, 17-hydroxycorticosteroids, 17-ketosteroids: possible falsely elevated levels.

SPECIAL CONSIDERATIONS
● Obtain specimens for culture and sensitivity tests before first dose. Therapy may begin before results are known.
● Monitor liver function studies.
● Reduce venous irritation by diluting drug, slowing infusion rate, or applying ice to infusion site.
● Only small amounts of drug may be removed by dialysis.
● Oral therapy should replace I.V. as soon as possible.
● May contain benzyl alcohol.
● Observe patient for signs of superinfection during prolonged use.
● Monitor patient for hearing loss.

esmolol hydrochloride
Brevibloc

Pregnancy Risk Category: C

PHARMACOKINETICS
Distribution: rapidly, into plasma, with 55% bound to plasma proteins. Probably crosses placenta.
Metabolism: rapid hydrolysis by RBC esterases.
Excretion: in urine in 24 hours. Half-life is about 9 minutes. Renal dysfunction prolongs elimination.
Action: onset, 2 minutes; duration, 10 to 20 minutes.

MECHANISM OF ACTION
An ultra-short-acting cardioselective beta blocker, esmolol possesses no sympathomimetic activity. The drug blocks the agonist effect of sympathetic neurotransmitters by competing for beta$_1$-receptor sites, chiefly in the cardiac muscle.

INDICATIONS & DOSAGE
● Rapid, short-term control of atrial fibrillation or flutter. *Adults:* loading dose of 500 mcg/kg/minute infused

over 1 minute, followed by a 4 minute maintenance infusion of 50 mcg/kg/minute. If response isn't adequate within 5 minutes, repeat loading dose and increase maintenance infusion to 100 mcg/kg/minute over 4 minutes. Repeat this regimen until desired heart rate or lowered blood pressure is achieved. Usually, maintenance dose shouldn't exceed 200 mcg/kg/minute. Can be given for up to 48 hours. Depending on response, titration intervals may be increased to 10 minutes.

CONTRAINDICATIONS & CAUTIONS
• Contraindicated in sinus bradycardia or second- or third-degree heart block because of the chronotropic effects of beta blockade, and in cardiogenic shock or overt heart failure because beta blockade further depresses myocardial contractility.
• Use cautiously in bronchospastic disease because of possible exacerbation; in diabetes mellitus and hypoglycemia because drug may mask tachycardia during hypoglycemia.
• Use cautiously in elderly patients and in patients with renal impairment because of increased risk of toxicity; base dosage on clinical response. Safe use in children hasn't been established.

PREPARATION & STORAGE
Available in 10 ml ampules containing 250 mg/ml. Before infusion, reconstitute 2 ampules with 20 ml of diluent to yield a concentration of 10 mg/ml. Concentrations of 20 mg/ml or higher are associated with venous irritation and thrombophlebitis.

Compatible solutions include dextrose 5% in water, dextrose 5% in Ringer's lactate, Ringer's lactate, dextrose 5% in 0.45% sodium chloride, and 0.45% or 0.9% sodium chloride. Diluted solution stable for 24 hours at room temperature. Freezing doesn't alter drug effect, but don't expose to high temperatures.

ADMINISTRATION
Direct injection: not recommended.
Intermittent infusion: not recommended.
Continuous infusion: Using an I.V. catheter and an infusion pump, give loading dose over 1 minute and maintenance dose over 4 minutes. If reaction occurs at infusion site, stop infusion and resume at another site. Avoid using winged infusion needle.

INCOMPATIBILITY
Incompatible with sodium bicarbonate and furosemide.

ADVERSE REACTIONS
Life-threatening: none reported.
Other: agitation, anxiety, bradycardia, bronchospasm, chest pain, cold hands and feet, confusion, depression, dizziness, drowsiness, dyspnea, fatigue, headache, hypotension, nausea, seizures, sweating, thrombophlebitis, venous irritation, vomiting.

INTERACTIONS
Antihypertensives: potentiated effects.
Cardiac glycosides: increased serum digoxin concentrations.
Catecholamine-depleting drugs, such as reserpine: possible enhanced effects of both drugs.
Insulin: possible masked symptoms of hypoglycemia (except sweating and dizziness).
MAO inhibitors: significant hypertension may occur if taken within 14 days of each other.
Morphine: esmolol levels increased by 50%.
Nondepolarizing neuromuscular blockers: possible prolonged action.
Phenytoin: possible additive cardiac depression.

Sympathomimetics: possible inhibited esmolol and sympathomimetic effects.
Xanthines (especially aminophylline and theophylline): impaired esmolol and xanthine effects.

EFFECTS ON DIAGNOSTIC TESTS
None reported.

SPECIAL CONSIDERATIONS
• *Treatment of overdose:* Discontinue drug and, if necessary, treat symptomatically. As ordered, give atropine or another anticholinergic for severe bradycardia, a theophylline derivative for bronchospasm, and a diuretic or a cardiac glycoside for cardiac failure. Closely monitor blood pressure and heart rate and rhythm, and frequently assess for signs of neurologic deficit.
• Once heart rate stabilizes, substitute a longer-acting antiarrhythmic, as ordered. After starting new drug, gradually reduce esmolol infusion over 1 hour.

---

estrogens, conjugated
Premarin Intravenous

Pregnancy Risk Category: X

PHARMACOKINETICS
Distribution: in cells of female genitalia, breasts, hypothalamus, and pituitary. Drug is moderately to highly protein-bound. It crosses the placenta.
Metabolism: primarily in the liver.
Excretion: primarily in urine. Drug appears in breast milk.
Action: peaks at end of injection.

MECHANISM OF ACTION
Conjugated estrogenic substances bind to cytoplasmic proteins, forming a complex that promotes synthesis of DNA, RNA, and other proteins in responsive tissues. They also reduce pituitary gonadotropin production, curtailing release of follicle-stimulating hormone and luteinizing hormone.

INDICATIONS & DOSAGE
• Abnormal uterine bleeding (hormonal imbalance) in the absence of disease. *Adults:* 25 mg repeated in 6 to 12 hours, if necessary.

CONTRAINDICATIONS & CAUTIONS
• Contraindicated in known or suspected estrogen-dependent neoplasia or breast cancer (except for selected patients being treated for metastatic disease) because drug may exacerbate these conditions.
• Also contraindicated in undiagnosed vaginal bleeding or active or past thrombophlebitis or thromboembolic disorders because estrogens can worsen these disorders.
• Avoid use during pregnancy because of increased risk of fetal malignancy and abnormalities.
• Use cautiously in renal insufficiency or in metastatic bone disease associated with hypercalcemia (affects calcium and phosphorus metabolism); and in hepatic impairment (drug may be poorly metabolized).
• Safety and efficacy in children haven't been established.

PREPARATION & STORAGE
Available in a package containing 25 mg vial of drug and 5 ml ampule of sterile water for injection and 2% benzyl alcohol. To reconstitute, withdraw air from vial and slowly inject provided diluent against inside wall of vial. Swirl gently; don't shake vigorously.

Intact vial remains stable for 5 years if refrigerated. Reconstituted drug stays stable for 60 days if refrigerated and protected from light, although the manufacturer recommends immediate use. Don't use if drug darkens or precipitates. Compatible with dextrose, saline, and invert sugar solutions.

ADMINISTRATION
Direct injection: Inject reconstituted drug directly into a vein over 1 to 5 minutes or into an established I.V. line containing a free-flowing compatible solution; inject just distal to the infusion needle.
Intermittent infusion: not recommended.
Continuous infusion: not recommended.

INCOMPATIBILITY
Incompatible with ascorbic acid, protein hydrolysate, or any solution with an acid pH.

ADVERSE REACTIONS
Most reactions occur with long-term therapy.
Life-threatening: none reported.
Other: flushing, perineal or vaginal burning with overly rapid injection.

INTERACTIONS
Adrenocorticosteroids: enhanced therapeutic and toxic effects.
Anticoagulants: reduced effects.
Carbamazepine, primidone, other anticonvulsants: reduced effectiveness because of altered metabolism.
Dantrolene, other hepatotoxic drugs: heightened risk of hepatotoxicity.
Insulin: increased requirements for diabetic patients.
Tricyclic antidepressants: increased toxicity.

EFFECTS ON DIAGNOSTIC TESTS
Factors VII, VIII, IX, and X, platelet aggregation: possible increased levels.
Metyrapone test: reduced response.
Phospholipids, triglycerides: possible elevated levels.
Prothrombin time: possibly prolonged.
Sulfobromophthalein test: possible increased sulfobromophthalein retention.
Thyroid-binding protein: possible elevated levels, leading to increased T_4 and decreased T_3 levels.
Urine and serum glucose: possible elevated levels.

SPECIAL CONSIDERATIONS
• Drug may inhibit lactation.
• Diluent contains benzyl alcohol.

---

ethacrynate sodium
Edecrin♦

Pregnancy Risk Category: B

PHARMACOKINETICS
Distribution: readily dispersed but probably accumulates only in the liver. Highly protein-bound; doesn't cross the blood-brain barrier. Not known if drug crosses placenta or is distributed into breast milk.
Metabolism: primarily in the liver.
Excretion: about 30% to 65% secreted by proximal renal tubules and excreted in urine. As urine pH rises, urine excretion increases. About 35% to 40% excreted in bile.
Action: onset, 5 minutes; duration, 2 hours.

MECHANISM OF ACTION
Ethacrynate sodium inhibits reabsorption of electrolytes, including sodium and chloride, in the proximal tubule and ascending loop of Henle

and increases potassium excretion in the distal tubule. Drug may also directly affect electrolyte transport at the proximal tubule.

INDICATIONS & DOSAGE
• Edema associated with congestive heart failure, cirrhosis, renal disease, ascites in malignancy, lymphedema, or nephrotic syndrome.
Adults: 50 mg or 0.5 to 1 mg/kg; may be repeated in 2 to 4 hours if necessary, then in 4 to 6 hours. In emergency use, may be repeated hourly. Maximum, 100 mg/dose.
Children: 1 mg/kg.

CONTRAINDICATIONS & CAUTIONS
• Contraindicated in hypersensitivity to ethacrynate and thimerosal (a preservative).
• Also contraindicated in electrolyte imbalance, hypotension, dehydration with low serum sodium concentrations, and metabolic alkalosis with hypokalemia because the drug worsens these conditions.
• Avoid use in anuria, azotemia, or oliguria because of the heightened risk of toxicity.
• Use with caution in diabetes mellitus because drug may impair glucose tolerance; in hyperuricemia or gout because drug may raise serum uric acid levels; in hepatic impairment because possible dehydration and electrolyte imbalance may precipitate hepatic coma; and in acute myocardial infarction because diuresis may precipitate shock.
• Because drug may exacerbate pancreatitis or lupus erythematosus, use cautiously in patients with a history of these disorders.

PREPARATION & STORAGE
Supplied in 50 mg vials. Reconstitute with 50 ml of 0.9% sodium chloride or dextrose 5% in water to a concentration of 1 mg/ml. Don't use cloudy solution (a sign of pH below 5.0). Compatible solutions include Dextran 75 6% in 0.9% sodium chloride, dextrose 5% in 0.9% sodium chloride, dextrose 5% in water, Normosol-R, Ringer's injection, Ringer's lactate, and 0.9% sodium chloride. Store at room temperature and discard any unused solution after 24 hours.

ADMINISTRATION
Direct injection: Inject drug directly into vein over several minutes, or infuse slowly over 20 to 30 minutes through I.V. tubing of free-flowing compatible solution. In repeated doses, change I.V. sites to reduce risk of thrombophlebitis.
Intermittent infusion: not recommended.
Continuous infusion: not recommended.

INCOMPATIBILITY
Incompatible with hydralazine, Normosol-M, procainamide, reserpine, tolazoline, triflupromazine, whole blood and its derivatives, and any solution or drug with a pH below 5.0.

ADVERSE REACTIONS
Life-threatening: acute necrotizing pancreatitis, hepatic coma, profound diuresis.
Other: carbohydrate intolerance, chills, diarrhea (severe, profuse, watery), fever, fluid and electrolyte depletion, GI bleeding, hematuria, local irritation, metabolic alkalosis, orthostatic hypotension, ototoxicity, pain, rash, thrombophlebitis, tinnitus, vertigo.

INTERACTIONS
Alcohol, antihypertensive drugs: enhanced hypotensive and diuretic effects.

Aminoglycosides, amphotericin B, other ototoxic and nephrotoxic drugs: increased risk of ototoxicity and nephrotoxicity and intensified electrolyte imbalance.

Amiodarone, cardiac glycosides: increased risk of dysrhythmias associated with hypokalemia.

Anticoagulants, thrombolytics: enhanced anticoagulant effects and risk of GI bleeding.

Antidiabetic agents, insulin: interference with hypoglycemic effects.

Antigout drugs: possible elevated serum uric acid levels.

Antihistamines, antivertigo agents, phenothiazines, thioxanthenes, trimethobenzamide: masked symptoms of ototoxicity.

Corticosteroids: possible decreased natriuretic and diuretic effects and intensified electrolyte imbalance.

Dopamine: increased diuresis.

Lithium: heightened risk of toxicity because of reduced clearance.

Neuromuscular blocking drugs: prolonged blockade resulting from hypokalemia.

NSAIDs, probenecid: antagonized natriuresis and diuresis and heightened risk of renal failure.

Sodium bicarbonate: enhanced risk of hypochloremic alkalosis.

Sympathomimetics: reduced antihypertensive effects of ethacrynate.

EFFECTS ON DIAGNOSTIC TESTS

BUN, serum uric acid, urine uric acid: elevated levels.

Serum calcium, chloride, magnesium, potassium, sodium: diminished levels.

Serum and urine glucose: increased levels.

SPECIAL CONSIDERATIONS

• *Treatment of overdose:* Signs include excessive diuresis with dehydration and electrolyte depletion.

Correct fluid and electrolyte imbalance and treat symptomatically.

• Monitor blood pressure, BUN and electrolyte levels, intake and output, and weight.

• Severe, watery diarrhea may necessitate discontinuing drug.

• In patients with renal edema and hypoproteinemia, administer salt-poor albumin, as ordered, to enhance response to ethacrynate sodium.

• In patients at high risk for metabolic alkalosis, administer ammonium chloride or arginine chloride, as ordered.

• Drug has been successfully used in hypertensive crisis, with mannitol in ethylene glycol poisoning, in nephrogenic diabetes insipidus unresponsive to vasopressin or chlorpropamide, in hypercalcemia to promote calcium excretion, and in bromide intoxication to promote bromide excretion.

etomidate
Amidate, Hypnomidate

Pregnancy Risk Category: C

PHARMACOKINETICS

Distribution: 76% bound to albumin. Drug appears in cerebrospinal fluid and probably crosses the placenta.

Metabolism: rapidly metabolized by hepatic microsomal enzymes and plasma esterases to its carboxylic acid ester.

Excretion: about 85% in urine, 15% in bile. Half-life is 2 to 5 hours. Not known if drug appears in breast milk.

Action: onset, 30 to 60 seconds; duration (dose-dependent), usually 3 to 5 minutes.

MECHANISM OF ACTION
This short-acting hypnotic depresses the reticular-activating system and, like the barbiturates, blocks acetylcholine-dependent synaptic transmission. It also mimics the action of gamma-aminobutyric acid.

INDICATIONS & DOSAGE
• Induction of anesthesia. *Adults:* usually, 300 mcg/kg (dosage ranges from 200 to 600 mcg/kg).

CONTRAINDICATIONS & CAUTIONS
• Contraindicated in hypersensitivity to etomidate.
• Use cautiously in seizures because the drug may stimulate irritable foci, leading to myotonic activity.
• Use cautiously in immunosuppression, sepsis, or organ transplant because of potential effects on adrenal function.

PREPARATION & STORAGE
Available in 2 mg/ml concentrations in 10 and 20 ml ampules and 20 ml prefilled syringes. Store at room temperature; avoid freezing. No need to dilute further for direct injection.

ADMINISTRATION
Only properly trained staff should administer this general anesthetic.
Direct injection: Inject drug into I.V. tubing containing a free-flowing compatible solution over 30 to 60 seconds.
Intermittent infusion: not recommended.
Continuous infusion: not recommended.

INCOMPATIBILITY
No incompatibilities reported.

ADVERSE REACTIONS
Life-threatening: none reported.

Other: bradycardia, bradypnea, extreme pain at injection site, hiccups, hypertension, hypotension, involuntary muscle movements, nausea, tachycardia, tachypnea, temporary adrenal failure, transient apnea, vomiting.

INTERACTIONS
CNS depressants: possible increased CNS effects.
Ketamine: especially with high doses or rapid administration, possible heightened risk of hypotension or respiratory depression.
Other antihypertensives: possible potentiated hypotensive effects.

EFFECTS ON DIAGNOSTIC TESTS
None reported.

SPECIAL CONSIDERATIONS
• Before use, administer a narcotic analgesic to reduce injection pain and diazepam to reduce involuntary muscle movements.
• Patients with low albumin levels may experience significantly higher levels of free form of drug.

---

etoposide
(VP-16, VP-16-213)
VePesid♦

Pregnancy Risk Category: D

PHARMACOKINETICS
Distribution: minimally distributed into pleural fluid, liver, spleen, kidneys, and CNS. Drug apparently crosses the placenta. Drug is 94% bound to plasma proteins.
Metabolism: unknown, but probably in the liver.
Excretion: primarily in urine as unchanged drug and metabolites, with 40% to 60% excreted unchanged in

48 to 72 hours; 2% to 16% is excreted in feces in 72 hours. Not known if drug appears in breast milk.

Action: peak plasma level, at end of infusion.

MECHANISM OF ACTION
Etoposide inhibits or alters DNA synthesis. It arrests the cell cycle at the G_2 phase, killing cells in that phase or in late S phase.

INDICATIONS & DOSAGE
• Induction of remission in refractory testicular cancer. *Adults:* 50 to 100 mg/m² daily on days 1 to 5 or 100 mg/m² daily on days 1, 3, and 5.
• Small-cell lung cancer. *Adults:* 35 mg/m² daily for 4 days or 50 mg/m² daily for 5 days, repeated q 3 to 4 weeks.
• Other malignant neoplasms and leukemias and in preparation for bone marrow transplant. *Adults:* in high-dose regimens, 300 to 800 mg/m² daily for 3 days.
• Kaposi's sarcoma in acquired immune deficiency syndrome (investigational). *Adults:* 150 mg/m² daily for 3 days q 4 weeks, repeated as necessary.

CONTRAINDICATIONS & CAUTIONS
• Contraindicated in etoposide hypersensitivity and in patients with known or recent chicken pox or herpes zoster because of the risk of generalized infection.
• Also contraindicated in patients with platelet counts less than 50,000/mm³ or with a neutrophil count less than 500/mm³, because drug increases myelosuppression.
• Use with caution in patients with hepatic or renal impairment because of the heightened risk of toxicity.

• Drug's safety and efficacy in children haven't been established.

PREPARATION & STORAGE
Exercise extreme caution when preparing or giving etoposide to avoid mutagenic, teratogenic, and carcinogenic risks. Use a biological containment cabinet and avoid contact with skin. Wear mask and gloves. If solution comes in contact with skin or mucosa, immediately wash thoroughly with soap and water. Use syringes with Luer-lok fittings to handle etoposide concentrate for injection. Dispose of needles, syringes, ampules, and any unused drug correctly. Avoid contaminating work surfaces.

Etoposide is supplied in 5 ml ampules containing 20 mg/ml. Unopened ampules remain stable at room temperature for 2 years; diluted solutions, up to 48 hours. Dilute with 5% dextrose in water or 0.9% sodium chloride to a concentration of 0.2 or 0.4 mg/ml. Discard discolored solutions or those that contain precipitates.

ADMINISTRATION
Direct injection: not used because of delayed and possibly fatal toxicity.
Intermittent infusion: Give diluted drug over at least 30 to 60 minutes. Administer through a 21G or 23G needle directly into vein, taking care to avoid extravasation. Monitor blood pressure during administration. If hypotension occurs, stop infusion, administer fluids and other supportive treatment, and restart the infusion at a slower rate.
Continuous infusion: not recommended.

INCOMPATIBILITY
No incompatibilities reported.

ADVERSE REACTIONS
Life-threatening: anaphylaxis, leukopenia (nadir of 7 to 14 days), thrombocytopenia (nadir of 9 to 16 days).
Other: abdominal pain, alopecia, anemia, anorexia, back pain, bronchospasm, chills, constipation, coryza, diarrhea, dysphagia, dyspnea, fever, flushing, generalized aching and hearing loss (in hypersensitivity), headache, hepatotoxicity, hypertension or hypotension, lacrimation, muscle cramps, nausea, parotitis, peripheral neuropathy, pigmentation, pruritus, rash, sneezing, stomatitis, substernal chest pain, sweating, swelling and erythema at injection site, tachycardia, throat pain, transient cortical blindness, vomiting.

INTERACTIONS
Drugs causing myelosuppression or blood dyscrasias: worsened bone marrow depression.
Live virus vaccines: potentiated virus replication.

EFFECTS ON DIAGNOSTIC TESTS
Serum alkaline phosphatase, bilirubin, SGOT: possible increased levels.

SPECIAL CONSIDERATIONS
• Etoposide is usually given with other chemotherapeutic agents.
• Therapeutic response to drug is usually associated with toxic effects.
• To control nausea and vomiting, give antiemetics. As ordered, treat anaphylaxis with pressor agents, adrenocorticosteroids, antihistamines, or volume expanders.
• Monitor CBC at least weekly.
• Used investigationally to treat refractory acute myelogenous and lymphocytic leukemia.
• May contain benzyl alcohol.

Factor VIII concentrate (antihemophilic factor)
Heat-Treated Profilate, Hemofil T, H.T. Factorate, Humate P, Koate-H.T.

Pregnancy Risk Category: C

COMPOSITION
This product is a sterile, dried concentrate derived from pooled human plasma. One IU equals the Factor VIII clotting activity of 1 ml of normal plasma.

INDICATIONS & DOSAGE
• Factor VIII deficiency (hemophilia A). The specific dosage needed to provide hemostasis depends on the patient's weight, the severity of bleeding and deficiency, the presence of inhibitors, and the desired Factor VIII level. Minor bleeding episodes require a circulating Factor VIII level equal to 20% to 30% of normal; major bleeding episodes, a level equal to 70% to 100% of normal. *Adults and children:* To calculate dose, multiply 0.4 by body weight (kg). Then multiply this figure by the percentage of normal Factor VIII desired. Dose may be repeated in 8 to 12 hours.

CONTRAINDICATIONS & CAUTIONS
• Avoid using drug in von Willebrand's disease because of its ineffectiveness.

PREPARATION & STORAGE
Available in vials of 250 to 1,500 IUs with sterile water for injection. Refrigerate or store at room temperature for up to 6 months. Avoid freezing; diluent bottle will break.
  If refrigerated, warm concentrate to room temperature before use. Re-

constitute with diluent, using sterile technique and following manufacturer's directions. Gently swirl vial (don't shake vigorously), allowing 5 to 10 minutes for contents to dissolve completely. Don't refrigerate reconstituted drug. Administer within 3 hours.

ADMINISTRATION
Direct injection: Using the filter needle provided, draw reconstituted drug into a plastic syringe (don't use glass; drug may adhere to ground glass surfaces). Inject about 5 ml per minute, using a 21G or 23G winged infusion set. To minimize adverse reactions, reduce rate if ordered.
Intermittent infusion: not recommended.
Continuous infusion: Using an infusion pump, complete administration within 3 hours of reconstituting drug.

INCOMPATIBILITY
Incompatible with all drugs and solutions except 0.9% sodium chloride.

ADVERSE REACTIONS
Life-threatening: acquired immune deficiency syndrome (AIDS), anaphylaxis, intravascular hemolysis, viral hepatitis.
Other: back pain, burning at infusion site, chest tightness, chills, clouding or loss of consciousness (rare), drowsiness, flushing, headache, hypotension, jaundice (rare), lethargy, mild nausea, paresthesias, tachycardia, urticaria, visual disturbances, vomiting.

INTERACTIONS
None reported.

EFFECTS ON DIAGNOSTIC TESTS
Coombs' test: possible positive results.
Factor VIII coagulant activity: increased levels.
Partial thromboplastin time (PTT): shortened, if prolonged PTT resulted from Factor VIII deficiency.

SPECIAL CONSIDERATIONS
• I.V. administration of 1 IU/kg increases plasma antihemophilic activity by about 2%.
• Carefully monitor therapy, especially if surgery is necessary. About 5% to 8% of patients develop inhibitors to Factor VIII, requiring larger doses or alternate therapy.
• If patient has received multiple infusions, regularly check liver function tests and screen for hepatitis.
• Monitor hematocrit in patients with type A, B, or AB blood who require large doses for a prolonged period. Hemolysis is possible. Factor VIII concentrate contains naturally occurring blood group–specific antibodies. Alternative therapy includes administration of a concentrate that's blood group specific, if circulating isohemagglutinins are positive. If RBC replacement is necessary, use compatible type O packed RBCs.
• Prepared from pooled plasma and treated to minimize viral transmission, Factor VIII concentrate still carries the risk of transmitting severe infection, especially non-A, non-B hepatitis. Before administration, its benefits and risks should be weighed against those of using single-donor cryoprecipitate.
• Educate patients about HIV, and encourage immunization against hepatitis B in HBsAg-negative patients. Explain that the risk of infection with human immunodeficiency virus is low in patients receiving

heat-treated Factor VIII concentrates from screened donors.
- Humate P has been found to contain von Willebrand's factor.
- New technologies continue to improve factor replacement products. For example, new Factor VIII concentrates use a monoclonal antibody purification method. Although still made from human blood products, these highly purified concentrates may further reduce the risk of viral transmission and protein exposure.

Factor VIII:C, heat-treated (antihemophilic factor)
Hemofil-M, Monoclate

Pregnancy Risk Category: C

COMPOSITION
Factor VIII:C is a sterile, lyophilized concentrate of Factor VIII:C (coagulant portion of Factor VIII complex) and small amounts of Factor VIII:R (the protein responsible for von Willebrand factor activity).

This highly purified concentrate of pooled human plasma is tested for hepatitis and human immunodeficiency virus. Also, a monoclonal antibody purification method washes away undesirable or therapeutically unnecessary blood components and other noncoagulant proteins and viruses. This process sharply lowers the risk of hepatitis or acquired immune deficiency syndrome (AIDS).

INDICATIONS & DOSAGE
Drug provides hemostasis in Factor VIII deficiency (hemophilia A). The specific dosage depends on the patient's weight, the severity of hemorrhage, and the presence of inhibitors. Mild bleeding episodes require a circulating Factor VIII:C level of 30% or more of normal;

moderate bleeding episodes and minor surgery, a level of 30% to 50% of normal; severe bleeding or major surgery, a level of 80% to 100% of normal. The following dosages provide guidelines.
- Mild bleeding. *Adults and children:* 15 to 25 IU/kg.
- Moderate bleeding and minor surgery. *Adults and children:* 15 to 25 IU/kg initially, then 10 to 15 IU/kg q 8 to 12 hours p.r.n.
- Severe bleeding and bleeding near vital organs. *Adults and children:* 40 to 50 IU/kg initially, then 20 to 25 IU/kg q 8 to 12 hours p.r.n.
- Major surgery. *Adults and children:* 40 to 50 IU/kg 1 hour before surgery, then 20 to 25 IU/kg 5 hours after first dose. Maintain circulating factor levels at 30% of normal for 10 to 14 days after surgery.

CONTRAINDICATIONS & CAUTIONS
- Contraindicated in hypersensitivity to mouse protein.
- Avoid use in von Willebrand's disease because drug doesn't provide effective treatment.

PREPARATION & STORAGE
Available in a kit, including single-dose vial with diluent, sterile needles for reconstitution and withdrawal, winged infusion set with microbore tubing, and alcohol swabs. Refrigerate unreconstituted drug; avoid freezing.

Reconstitute by using the double-ended needle to transfer diluent into vial (drawn in by vacuum). Gently swirl vial until contents dissolve. Use within 3 hours.

ADMINISTRATION
Direct injection: Using a plastic syringe (concentrate may adhere to

glass) and the winged infusion set, inject into vein at 2 ml/minute.
Intermittent infusion: not recommended.
Continuous infusion: not recommended.

INCOMPATIBILITY
No incompatibilities reported.

ADVERSE REACTIONS
Life-threatening: AIDS, anaphylaxis, viral hepatitis.
Other: chest tightness, hypotension, mild chills, nausea, stinging at infusion site, urticaria, wheezing.

INTERACTIONS
None reported.

SPECIAL CONSIDERATIONS
• I.V. administration of 1 IU/kg increases circulating antihemophilic activity by about 2%.

Factor IX complex
Konyne-HT, Profilnine Heat-Treated, Proplex SX-T, Proplex T

Pregnancy Risk Category: C

COMPOSITION
Derived from pooled plasma, this sterile, dried concentrate contains vitamin K–dependent coagulation Factors II, IX, and X and low levels of Factor VII (higher levels in Proplex T). One international unit (IU) of Factor IX concentrate equals the amount of Factor IX in 1 ml of normal plasma.

INDICATIONS & DOSAGE
• Hemostasis in Factor IX deficiency (hemophilia B). Specific dosage depends on the patient and the type of bleeding episode. About 15 minutes after giving 2 IU/kg of Fac-

tor IX, plasma levels rise by about 3% and Factor VII levels by about 4%. Minor bleeding episodes require a circulating Factor IX level of 20% to 30% of normal; major bleeding episodes, 70% to 100% of normal. Doses are usually given q 24 hours. International units required equal 0.6 to 1 multiplied by body weight (kg), multiplied by the desired percentage of increase.
• Hemostasis in patients with Factor VIII inhibitors. *Adults and children:* usually, 75 IU/kg repeated q 12 hours p.r.n.
• Hemostasis in severe Factor II or Factor X deficiency when fresh frozen plasma isn't warranted. *Adults and children:* initial dose of Factor II, 40 IU/kg; maintenance dosage, 15 to 20 IU/kg daily. Initial dose of Factor X, 10 to 50 IU/kg; maintenance dosage, 10 IU/kg daily.
• Hemostasis in Factor VII deficiency (Proplex T only). *Adults and children:* international units required equal 0.5 multiplied by body weight (kg), multiplied by the desired percentage of increase. Dose is repeated in 6 to 8 hours p.r.n.
• Reversal of coumarin anticoagulant effects. *Adults and children:* 15 IU/kg.

CONTRAINDICATIONS & CAUTIONS
• Contraindicated in patients with hepatic disease who show signs of intravascular coagulation or fibrinolysis.
• Also contraindicated in patients undergoing elective surgery, especially if predisposed to thrombosis, because of the risk of postoperative thrombosis. If drug must be used, give prophylactic anticoagulant, as ordered.
• Use cautiously in patients receiving multiple infusions of blood or plasma products for first time be-

---

Unmarked trade names available in the United States only.
♦ Also available in Canada.   ♦ ♦ Available in Canada only.

cause of the risk of transmitting a virus, especially non-A, non-B hepatitis.

PREPARATION & STORAGE

Available in kit that includes concentrate, diluent (from 10 to 30 ml, depending on manufacturer), and filter needle. Number of international units of Factor IX per vial appears on label. Refrigerate but avoid freezing; diluent bottle will break.

After warming concentrate and diluent to room temperature, reconstitute using aseptic technique. Add diluent, and swirl bottle to dissolve contents. Using the filter needle, draw concentrate into syringe. Administer within 3 hours. Don't refrigerate after reconstitution.

ADMINISTRATION

Direct injection: Using a 21G or 23G winged infusion set, inject slowly (don't exceed 3 ml/minute). Slow injection minimizes the risk of thrombosis. If facial flushing or tingling occurs during infusion, stop momentarily and resume at a slower rate.
Intermittent infusion: not recommended.
Continuous infusion: not recommended.

INCOMPATIBILITY

Incompatible with all drugs and solutions except 0.9% sodium chloride.

ADVERSE REACTIONS

Life-threatening: AIDS, anaphylaxis, thrombosis (especially in hepatic disease), viral hepatitis.
Other: chills, facial flushing, fever, headache, pulse and blood pressure changes, tingling, urticaria.

INTERACTIONS

Aminocaproic acid: increased risk of thrombotic complications if given within 12 hours of Factor IX infusion.

EFFECTS ON DIAGNOSTIC TESTS

Factors II, VII, IX, X: elevated levels.

SPECIAL CONSIDERATIONS

• Prepared from pooled plasma and treated to minimize viral transmission, Factor IX concentrate still carries the risk of transmitting severe infection, especially non-A, non-B hepatitis. Before the drug is administered, its benefits and risks should be weighed against those of single-donor fresh frozen plasma.
• Educate patients about AIDS, and encourage immunization against hepatitis B in HBsAg-negative patients. Explain that the risk of infection with human immunodeficiency is low in patients receiving heat-treated Factor IX concentrate from screened donors.
• Perform coagulation assays before and during treatment.
• To reduce the risk of thrombosis, the International Committee on Thrombosis and Hemostasis recommends adding 5 units of heparin per milliliter of diluent when treating Factor IX–deficient patients. This practice isn't recommended for patients with Factor VIII inhibitors.

famotidine
Pepcid I.V.

Pregnancy Risk Category: B

PHARMACOKINETICS
Distribution: about 15% to 20% bound to plasma proteins. Drug probably crosses the placenta.
Metabolism: in the liver.
Excretion: in urine, with 65% to 70% excreted as unchanged drug and 30% to 35% as metabolites. Elimination half-life is about 3 hours in normal renal function, 11 hours in moderate renal failure, and over 20 hours in severe renal failure. Drug may appear in breast milk.
Action: peak effect, 30 minutes.

MECHANISM OF ACTION
Famotidine competitively inhibits histamine (H_2) receptors, thereby suppressing acid concentration and gastric secretion volume in basal, nocturnal, and stimulated states.

INDICATIONS & DOSAGE
• Active duodenal ulcer in N.P.O. patients. *Adults:* 20 mg q 12 hours.
• Hypersecretory conditions, including Zollinger-Ellison syndrome and multiple endocrine adenomas.
Adults: 20 mg q 6 hours. May require up to 160 mg q 6 hours.

CONTRAINDICATIONS & CAUTIONS
• Contraindicated in famotidine hypersensitivity and during breast-feeding.
• Use cautiously in patients with severe renal or hepatic impairment because of decreased plasma clearance.

PREPARATION & STORAGE
Available in 2 ml single-dose vials and 4 ml multidose vials with a concentration of 10 mg/ml. Refrigerate vials but avoid freezing.

For injection, reconstitute with 5 or 10 ml of diluent; for infusion, use 100 ml of diluent. Compatible with sterile water for injection, 0.9% sodium chloride, 5% or 10% dextrose in water, Ringer's lactate, or 5% sodium bicarbonate. Diluted solution remains stable for 48 hours at room temperature.

ADMINISTRATION
Direct injection: Inject 5 or 10 ml of reconstituted drug over at least 2 minutes.
Intermittent infusion: Infuse drug diluted in 100 ml over 15 to 30 minutes.
Continuous infusion: not recommended.

INCOMPATIBILITY
No incompatibilities reported.

ADVERSE REACTIONS
Life-threatening: none reported.
Other: abdominal discomfort, acne, alopecia, altered taste, anorexia, arthralgias, asthenia, bronchospasm, chest tightness, conjunctival injection, constipation, diarrhea, drowsiness, dry mouth or skin, fatigue, fever, flushing, generalized tonic-clonic seizures, headache, insomnia, musculoskeletal pain, nausea, orbital edema, palpitations, paresthesias, pruritus, psychic disturbances (anxiety, depression, hallucinations), rash, thrombocytopenia, tinnitus, transient irritation at I.V. site, vomiting.

INTERACTIONS
None reported.

EFFECTS ON DIAGNOSTIC TESTS
Gastric acid stimulation test: possible antagonism of pentagastrin or histamine.

Unmarked trade names available in the United States only.
♦ Also available in Canada.   ♦♦ Available in Canada only.

Liver function tests: possible elevated levels.
Skin tests: false-positive results.

SPECIAL CONSIDERATIONS
• Check I.V. sites for irritation.
• Discontinue drug for 24 hours before diagnostic skin tests.
• Closely monitor patient with gastric ulcers. Gastric cancer must be ruled out before famotidine therapy.
• Warn patient that smoking may increase gastric acid secretion.
• Famotidine has been used to treat gastric ulcers and severe reflux esophagitis and to treat or prevent stress ulcers, hemorrhagic gastritis, and other upper GI hemorrhage.

fat emulsions
Intralipid 10%♦, Intralipid 20%, Liposyn 10%, Liposyn 20%, Soyacal 10%, Soyacal 20%, Travamulsion 10%, Travamulsion 20%

Pregnancy Risk Category: C
(B for Soyacal 10%)

COMPOSITION
Although the percentage of components varies, fat emulsions contain soybean oil (Intralipid, Soyacal, Travamulsion) or safflower oil (Liposyn) and provide neutral triglycerides and primarily unsaturated fatty acids (linoleic, oleic, palmitic, stearic, and linolenic). Fatty acids are an energy source, essential to the normal structure and function of cell membranes.

Preparations also contain glycerol to adjust tonicity and 1.2% egg yolk to emulsify fat particles. Ten percent solutions contain 1.1 calories/ml; 20% solutions, 2 calories/ml. All fat emulsions are isotonic.

INDICATIONS & DOSAGE
• Source of calories and fatty acids adjunctive to intravenous hyperalimentation (IVH). *Adults:* using 10% solution, up to 500 ml on day 1, gradually increased on following days to 60% of daily caloric intake; using 20% solution, up to 500 ml of Intralipid or Travamulsion on day 1 or up to 250 ml of Liposyn or Soyacal on day 1, gradually increased on following days. Maximum daily dosage for Liposyn is 3 g/kg; for Intralipid and Soyacal, 2.5 g/kg; and for Travamulsion, 4 g/kg. *Children:* using 10% solution, 1 g/kg of Intralipid, Soyacal, or Travamulsion given over 4 hours on day 1, gradually increased to 4 g/kg daily; or 100 ml/hour of Liposyn on day 1, gradually increased to 5 to 10 ml/kg daily. Using 20% solution, 1 g/kg of Intralipid or Soyacal given over 4 hours on day 1, gradually increased to 4 g/kg daily; or 100 ml/hour of Liposyn on day 1, gradually increased to 2.5 to 5 ml/kg daily. *Neonates:* maximum dosage, 1 g/kg given over 4 hours.
• Fatty acid deficiency. *Adults and children:* 8% to 10% of caloric intake.

CONTRAINDICATIONS & CAUTIONS
• Contraindicated in impaired fat metabolism (for example, hyperlipemia, lipoid nephrosis, and acute pancreatitis with hyperlipemia); in bone marrow dyscrasias because fat emulsions may induce blood dyscrasias; in infants with hyperbilirubinemia because fat emulsions may worsen jaundice; and in hypersensitivity to solution components.
• Use cautiously in severe hepatic or pulmonary disease, coagulation disorders, anemia, thrombocytopenia, diabetes mellitus, gastric ulcer, or a risk for fat embolism because the

solution may exacerbate these disorders; and in premature infants or infants who are small for their gestational age.

PREPARATION & STORAGE

Ready-to-use, sterile, nonpyrogenic emulsions are available in single-dose glass bottles. Intralipid 10% comes in 50, 100, and 500 ml bottles; Intralipid 20%, in 100, 250, and 500 ml bottles. Liposyn 10% is supplied in 25, 50, 100, 200, and 500 ml bottles; Liposyn 20%, in 200 and 500 ml bottles. Soyacal 10% and 20% come in 250 and 500 ml bottles. Travamulsion 10% is available in a 500 ml bottle.

Store fat emulsions at room temperature and discard if accidentally frozen. Inspect the bottle for cracks or separation at the seams; check expiration date and integrity of closure. Discard bottle for any problem.

ADMINISTRATION

Direct injection: not recommended.
Intermittent infusion: Give once daily as part of IVH. See guidelines for continuous infusion.
Continuous infusion: Administer the solution through the nonphthalate infusion set provided by the manufacturer. Fat emulsions may extract phthalates from phthalate-plasticized PVC tubing. Do not use an in-line filter when administering drug because fat particles (0.5-micron diameter) are larger than the 0.22-micron in-line filter.

Use a new I.V. line for each bottle of fat emulsion, infusing solution through peripheral or central venous line. Control flow rates with infusion pump, using a separate pump for solutions running simultaneously.

Infuse fat emulsions intermittently, alternating with a protein–calorie solution for IVH. Or infuse fat emulsions into same vein with carbohydrate–amino acid solution, using a Y connector near the infusion site. To facilitate flow, hang the fat emulsion container higher than the other one.

Begin infusing 10% fat emulsion at 0.1 ml/minute or 20% emulsion at 0.5 ml/minute. Closely monitor patient, and if no adverse reactions occur within 15 minutes, increase infusion rate. For adults, infuse 500 ml of 10% solution or 250 ml of 20% solution over 4 to 6 hours. If patient develops fever, chills, or other reactions, especially in first 15 minutes, or if infusion bottle shows evidence of contamination or instability, discontinue infusion and notify the doctor.

INCOMPATIBILITY

Incompatible with aminophylline, ampicillin sodium, ascorbic acid injection, calcium chloride, calcium gluconate, cephalothin, gentamicin, magnesium chloride, methicillin, penicillin G, phenytoin sodium, potassium chloride, sodium bicarbonate, sodium chloride, tetracycline hydrochloride, and vitamin B complex.

Only the Intralipid brand of fat emulsion can be mixed with amino acid solution, dextrose, electrolytes, or vitamins in the same I.V. container. Because of potential incompatibility, do not mix electrolytes, other nutrient solutions, drugs, vitamins, or any other additives with other brands of fat emulsions in the infusion bottle.

ADVERSE REACTIONS

Life-threatening: cardiac arrest, pulmonary edema.
Other: agitation, anemia, back and chest pain, bleeding, blood dyscrasias (leukopenia, thrombocytopenia),

---

cyanosis, diaphoresis, dilated non-reactive pupils, drowsiness, fever, flushing, focal seizures, headache, hepatosplenomegaly, hypercoagulability, hyperlipemia, hyperthermia, hyperventilation, intravenous fat pigment syndrome (brown pigment deposits in the reticuloendothelial system), irritation at infusion site, jaundice, leukocytosis, metabolic acidosis, nausea, overhydration, pressure over eyes, pruritus, sepsis, shock, urticaria, vomiting.

INTERACTIONS
None reported.

EFFECTS ON DIAGNOSTIC TESTS
Liver function tests: with long-term therapy, transient elevations.
Mean corpuscular hemoglobin, mean corpuscular hemoglobin concentration: possible increased levels during and shortly after infusion.
Serum bilirubin: possible increased levels in neonates.

SPECIAL CONSIDERATIONS
• Before administration, perform a complete nutritional assessment.
• Obtain baseline CBC, platelet count, coagulation studies, liver function tests, and serum lipid (especially triglycerides and cholesterol) levels.
• After 4 to 6 hours of infusion, collect serum samples for triglyceride and cholesterol determinations because transient lipemia must clear after each daily dose. In long-term therapy, monitor liver function tests and repeat other baseline studies once or twice weekly.
• Administer fat emulsions to adults during the day to avoid interrupting sleep.
• During administration, frequently check the infusion site for signs of inflammation or infection.

• Neonates and premature infants receive fat emulsions over 24 hours because they metabolize fats more slowly than adults. Monitor triglyceride and free fatty acid levels daily. Also obtain daily platelet counts during the first week of therapy because neonates are susceptible to thrombocytopenia. In succeeding weeks, obtain platelet counts on alternate days.

fentanyl citrate
Sublimaze♦

Controlled Substance Schedule II
Pregnancy Risk Category: C

PHARMACOKINETICS
Distribution: rapidly dispersed to inactive tissue sites, such as skeletal muscle, fat, and lungs. Drug is highly protein-bound, probably crosses the placenta, and readily crosses the blood-brain barrier.
Metabolism: extensively metabolized in the liver to inactive metabolites. Rate depends on hepatic blood flow and release from body tissues.
Excretion: primarily renal, with 10% to 25% excreted in urine as unchanged drug; 70% of dose is excreted within 4 days. Not known if drug appears in breast milk.
Action: onset, immediate; duration, 30 to 60 minutes, depending on dose.

MECHANISM OF ACTION
Fentanyl acts as an agonist at stereospecific opioid receptor sites in the CNS (probably the mu receptors). Drug alters perception of pain and emotional response to it. Administered in high doses, it will produce loss of consciousness.

INDICATIONS & DOSAGE

Dosage depends on concurrently given drugs (especially anesthetics), type and anticipated length of surgery, and the patient's age, weight, body size, physical status, underlying disorder, and response to the drug.

● Short-term perioperative analgesia. *Adults:* up to 2 mcg/kg in divided doses.

● General anesthesia (as sole agent with 100% oxygen). *Adults:* 50 to 100 mcg/kg; up to 150 mcg/kg may be required.

● Induction and maintenance of general anesthesia. *Children age 2 to 12:* 1.7 to 3.3 mcg/kg.

● Adjunct in general anesthesia. *Adults:* low dose, 2 mcg/kg in divided doses; moderate dose before major surgery, 2 to 20 mcg/kg initially, then 25 to 100 mcg p.r.n.; high dose before complicated surgery, 20 to 50 mcg/kg initially, then 25 mcg to half initial dose p.r.n.

● Adjunct in regional anesthesia. *Adults:* 50 to 100 mcg.

CONTRAINDICATIONS & CAUTIONS

● Contraindicated in hypersensitivity to fentanyl derivatives and in children under age 2.

● In patients with poor pulmonary reserve, give drug cautiously because it may further diminish respiratory drive and increase airway resistance.

● Use cautiously in patients with head injury and increased intracranial pressure because fentanyl may interfere with neurologic assessment. The drug may also raise intracranial pressure resulting from hypoventilation and hypercarbia.

● Administer carefully in bradydysrhythmias because drug may exacerbate the condition.

● Because of the increased risk of toxicity, use cautiously in patients with hepatic, renal, or respiratory dysfunction.

● Also use cautiously in patients with hypothyroidism because of the risk of prolonged respiratory and CNS depression.

● Administer carefully to elderly, young, or debilitated patients because of heightened sensitivity to drug effects.

PREPARATION & STORAGE

Available in 2, 5, 10, 20, and 50 ml containers in concentrations of 50 mcg/kg. Store at room temperature, avoid excessive heat or freezing, and protect from light. Drug is compatible with most common I.V. solutions.

ADMINISTRATION

Only staff trained in administering I.V. anesthetics and managing their potential adverse reactions should give this drug.

Direct injection: Inject drug over at least 1 minute to avoid muscle rigidity. If rapid injection is necessary, administer a neuromuscular blocker beforehand to prevent rigidity.

Intermittent infusion: not recommended.

Continuous infusion: sometimes used for induction of general anesthesia. Use high-dose concentrations to rapidly and smoothly achieve initial induction dose.

INCOMPATIBILITY

Incompatible with methohexital, pentobarbital sodium, and thiopental.

ADVERSE REACTIONS

Life-threatening: apnea, respiratory depression.

Other: blurred vision, bradycardia, diaphoresis, dizziness, dyspnea, hy-

pertension, hypotension, laryngospasm, muscle rigidity (especially
intercostal), nausea, postoperative
depression, restlessness, seizures,
vomiting.

INTERACTIONS
Antihypertensives: possible potentiated hypotension.
Benzodiazepines: substantially decreased induction time when administered for preoperative sedation.
Beta-adrenergic blocking agents:
decreased frequency and severity of
hypertensive response to surgery.
*Buprenorphine and other partial
mu-receptor agonists:* decreased
therapeutic effects of fentanyl.
Cimetidine: possible increased CNS
toxicity.
MAO inhibitors: possible unpredictable, severe hypertension and tachycardia if fentanyl citrate is given
within 14 days of receiving MAO inhibitors.
Nalbuphine, pentazocine: partially
antagonized effect of fentanyl.
Naloxone: antagonized analgesic,
hypotensive, CNS, and respiratory
effects of fentanyl.
Naltrexone: blocked therapeutic effects of fentanyl.
Neuromuscular blockers: deepened
respiratory depression and alleviated
muscle rigidity.
Nitrous oxide: cardiovascular depression when combined with high-
dose fentanyl.
Other CNS depressants: deepened
CNS and respiratory depression.

EFFECTS ON DIAGNOSTIC TESTS
Lumbar puncture: possible increased cerebrospinal fluid pressure
resulting from respiratory depression–induced carbon dioxide retention.
Serum amylase, lipase: possible increased levels.

SPECIAL CONSIDERATIONS
● *Treatment of overdose:* For hypoventilation or apnea, give oxygen
and positive pressure ventilation via
bag and mask or endotracheal tube
to maintain a patent airway and ventilation. To reverse respiratory depression, as ordered, administer
naloxone in divided doses. Continue
supportive therapy until the drug is
metabolized.
● Monitor patient's respiratory, cardiovascular, and neurologic status
before, during, and after surgery.
● May cause muscle rigidity in the
chest wall, leading to problems with
ventilation. Note that these problems
may occur during emergence from
anesthesia.
● Following recovery from anesthesia, the patient may experience delayed respiratory depression,
respiratory arrest, bradycardia, asystole, dysrhythmias, and hypotension.
● When used in high doses, respiratory depression may persist for several hours after the patient awakens,
making ventilatory support necessary.
● Patients who receive repeated
doses or are tolerant of other opiates
may become tolerant of fentanyl.

fentanyl citrate with droperidol
Innovar

Controlled Substance Schedule II
Pregnancy Risk Category: C

PHARMACOKINETICS
Distribution of fentanyl: rapidly dispersed to skeletal muscle, lungs, and
fat and slowly into blood. Drug is
highly bound to plasma proteins,
probably crosses the placenta, and
readily crosses the blood-brain barrier.

Distribution of droperidol: not fully understood but known to cross the blood-brain barrier and the placenta.
Metabolism: in the liver.
Excretion: in urine and feces. Not known if drug appears in breast milk.
Action of fentanyl: onset, immediate; duration, 30 to 60 minutes.
Action of droperidol: onset, 3 to 10 minutes; duration, 2 to 4 hours for sedation and up to 12 hours for altered consciousness.

MECHANISM OF ACTION
Fentanyl acts at stereospecific opioid receptor sites in the CNS to depress ventilation, decrease heart rate, and produce euphoria. *Droperidol* blocks postsynaptic alpha-adrenergic and dopaminergic receptor sites. Their combination produces neuroleptanalgesia, characterized by general quiescence, reduced motor activity, and profound analgesia.

INDICATIONS & DOSAGE
Dosage depends on concurrently given drugs (especially anesthetics), the surgical procedure, and the patient's age, weight, physical status, and underlying disorder.
• Adjunct in general anesthesia induction. *Adults:* 1 ml/20 to 25 lb (9 to 11 kg) body weight. *Children over age 2:* 0.5 ml/20 lb body weight.
• Adjunct in regional anesthesia. *Adults:* 1 to 2 ml.

CONTRAINDICATIONS & CAUTIONS
• Contraindicated in hypersensitivity to fentanyl or droperidol.
• In high-risk patients and in those with hepatic or renal impairment, administer drug carefully because of the increased potential for toxicity.
• Use cautiously in hypotensive and hypovolemic patients because fentanyl citrate with droperidol can exacerbate hypotension.
• Because of the heightened risk of respiratory depression, give cautiously in ventilatory impairment, such as chronic obstructive pulmonary disease, or poor respiratory reserve.
• Also give cautiously to patients with bradyarrhythmias because the drug can exacerbate this condition and to patients with head injury because it may cause unreliable neurologic assessment findings. Drug may also raise intracranial pressure resulting from hypoventilation and hypercarbia.
• In hypothyroidism, administer carefully because of the magnified risk of prolonged respiratory and CNS depression.

PREPARATION & STORAGE
Available in 2 and 5 ml ampules containing 50 mcg/ml of fentanyl and 2.5 mg/ml of droperidol. For infusion, dilute 10 ml in 250 ml of dextrose 5% in water. Store at room temperature and protect from light. Don't use discolored drug or drug that contains particulates. Fentanyl citrate with droperidol is compatible with all I.V. solutions.

ADMINISTRATION
Only staff specially trained in giving I.V. anesthetics and managing potential adverse reactions should administer this drug.
Direct injection: Inject undiluted drug directly into vein or into I.V. tubing containing a free-flowing compatible solution.
Intermittent infusion: not recommended.
Continuous infusion: Rapidly infuse diluted drug until onset of drowsiness. Then slow infusion or stop drip and administer general anesthetic, as ordered.

INCOMPATIBILITY
Incompatible with barbiturates and diazepam.

ADVERSE REACTIONS
Life-threatening: respiratory depression, which, if untreated, may lead to respiratory arrest, circulatory depression, and cardiac arrest.
Other: blurred vision, bradycardia, bronchospasm, chills, diaphoresis, dizziness, emergence delirium, extrapyramidal symptoms (akathisia, anxiety, dystonia, hyperactivity, oculogyric crisis, restlessness), hypertension, hypotension, laryngospasm, muscle rigidity, nausea, postoperative drowsiness, postoperative hallucinations, tachycardia, twitching, vomiting.

INTERACTIONS
Antihypertensives: possible potentiated hypotensive effects of fentanyl.
Benzodiazepines: substantially decreased induction time when administered for preoperative sedation.
Beta-adrenergic blocking agents: decreased frequency and severity of hypertensive response to surgery.
Buprenorphine and other partial mu-receptor agonists: decreased therapeutic effects of fentanyl.
Cimetidine: possible increased CNS toxicity.
CNS depressants: additive and potentiated effects.
Epinephrine: paradoxically reduced blood pressure because of droperidol's alpha-adrenergic blocking action.
MAO inhibitors: possible unpredictable, severe hypertension and tachycardia if fentanyl citrate with droperidol is given within 14 days of receiving MAO inhibitors.
Nalbuphine, pentazocine: partially antagonized effect of fentanyl.

Naloxone: antagonized analgesic, hypotensive, CNS, and respiratory effects of fentanyl.
Naltrexone: blocked therapeutic effects of fentanyl.
Neuromuscular blockers: possible enhanced effects. Reduce dosage, if necessary.
Nitrous oxide: cardiovascular depression when used with high-dose fentanyl.

EFFECTS ON DIAGNOSTIC TESTS
Lumbar puncture: possible increased cerebrospinal fluid pressure resulting from respiratory depression–induced carbon dioxide retention.
EEG: altered pattern for up to 12 hours after last dose.
Hemodynamic measurements: possible decreased pulmonary artery pressure.
Serum amylase, lipase: increased levels.

SPECIAL CONSIDERATIONS
• *Treatment of overdose:* Take supportive measures. Treat respiratory depression by maintaining a patent airway and giving oxygen and assisted ventilation if needed. To treat hypotension, provide volume expansion with I.V. fluids and pressor agents (except epinephrine). Have naloxone available to antagonize the narcotic component of fentanyl citrate with droperidol.
• Keep resuscitation equipment nearby, and monitor patient's neurologic, cardiovascular, and respiratory status.
• Move and position patient slowly during anesthesia because of the risk of orthostatic hypotension.
• Patients who receive repeated doses or are tolerant of other opioids may become tolerant of fentanyl citrate with droperidol.

- Following recovery from anesthesia, the patient may experience delayed respiratory depression, respiratory arrest, bradycardia, asystole, dysrhythmias, and hypotension.
- When used in high doses, respiratory depression may persist for several hours after the patient awakens, making ventilatory assistance necessary.

fluconazole
Diflucan

Pregnancy Risk Category: C

PHARMACOKINETICS
Distribution: at steady state, the drug penetrates all compartments well, including central nervous system. Apparent volume of distribution is similar to that of total body water; plasma protein binding is low (11% to 12%).
Metabolism: 11% of drug appears in urine as metabolites.
Excretion: primarily by kidneys. Dosage needs adjustment in patients with renal failure. Plasma elimination half-life is about 30 hours (range 20 to 50 hours).

MECHANISM OF ACTION
Selectively inhibits fungal cytochrome P-450 sterol C-14 alpha-demethylation, thus preventing the production of normal sterols. Drug is active in vitro against *Cryptococcus neoformans* and *Candida*; animal studies also confirm activity against *Aspergillus flavus* and *A. fumigatus, Blastomyces dermatitidis, Coccidiodes immitis,* and *Histoplasma capsulatum.*

INDICATIONS & DOSAGE
- Oropharyngeal candidiasis. *Adults:* 200 mg on the first day, followed by 100 mg once daily. Therapy should continue for 2 weeks.
- Esophageal candidiasis. *Adults:* 200 mg on the first day, followed by 100 mg once daily. Higher doses (up to 400 mg daily) have been used, depending upon patient's condition and tolerance of treatment. Patients should receive the drug for at least 3 weeks and for 2 weeks after symptoms resolve.
- Systemic candidiasis. *Adults:* 400 mg on the first day, followed by 200 mg once daily. Treatment should continue for at least 4 weeks or 2 weeks after symptoms resolve.
- Cryptococcal meningitis. *Adults:* 400 mg on the first day, followed by 200 mg once daily. Higher doses (up to 400 mg daily) may be used. Treatment should continue for 10 to 12 weeks after cerebrospinal fluid cultures are negative.
- Suppression of relapse of cryptococcal meningitis in patients with human immunodeficiency virus (HIV) infection. *Adults:* 200 mg daily.
Note: Adjust dosage in renal failure. For adults, give an initial loading dose of 50 to 400 mg. If the creatinine clearance is 21 to 50 ml/minute, dosage should be reduced 50%. If it ranges from 11 to 20 ml/minute, reduce dosage by 75%.

CONTRAINDICATIONS & CAUTIONS
- Contraindicated in patients hypersensitive to the drug.
- Use cautiously in patients hypersensitive to other antifungal azole compounds because no information exists regarding cross sensitivity.
- Also use cautiously in patients with abnormal liver function tests. Evaluate these patients for serious liver injury and discontinue the drug if liver function continues to deteriorate.

PREPARATION & STORAGE

Available in glass bottles or plastic I.V. bags with 200 mg/100 ml or 400 mg/200 ml. Store glass bottles at 41° to 86° F. (5° to 30° C.), and plastic bags at 41° to 77° F. (5° to 25° C.). Protect from freezing. Brief exposure of plastic containers to temperatures up to 104° F. (40° C.) will not adversely affect the drug.

I.V. bags of fluconazole are shipped with a protective overwrap that shouldn't be removed until just before use. This helps ensure product sterility. The plastic container may show some opacity from moisture absorbed during sterilization. This is normal, doesn't affect the drug, and diminishes over time.

ADMINISTRATION

Direct injection: not recommended.
Intermittent infusion: not recommended.
Continuous infusion: Administer ordered dose at a rate of approximately 200 mg/hour.

INCOMPATIBILITY

Do not mix with other drugs.

ADVERSE REACTIONS

Life-threatening: hepatotoxicity (rare), Stevens-Johnson syndrome (rare).
Other: abdominal pain, diarrhea, elevated liver enzymes, headache, nausea, rash, vomiting.

INTERACTIONS

Cyclosporine, oral antidiabetic agents (tolbutamide, glyburide, glipizide), phenytoin: possible increased plasma concentrations of these drugs.
Hydrochlorothiazide: possible decreased renal clearance of fluconazole.
Isoniazid, oral sulfonylureas, phenytoin, rifampin, valproic acid: increased incidence of abnormally elevated hepatic transaminase levels.
Rifampin: enhances fluconazole metabolism.
Warfarin: increased prothrombin time.

EFFECTS ON DIAGNOSTIC TESTS

SGOT: increased levels (rare).

SPECIAL CONSIDERATIONS

• Oral bioavailability of fluconazole is greater than 90% and is unaffected by gastric pH. Dosage is the same for oral or I.V. use.
• Since the drug is excreted unchanged by the kidneys, the dosage should be adjusted in patients with impaired renal function.
• Patients receiving regular hemodialysis treatment should receive the usual dose after each dialysis session. Additional dosage adjustments may be needed, depending on the patient's clinical condition.
• Patients who develop a rash in response to the drug should be monitored closely. Discontinue the drug if rash worsens.
• The incidence of adverse reactions appears to be greater in patients with severe underlying disease, including malignancies, and in patients with HIV infection, especially if such patients are taking other medications that are known to be hepatotoxic or associated with exfoliative skin disorders.
• Safety and effectiveness guidelines in children have not been established, but a small number of children ages 3 to 13 have received 3 to 6 mg/kg/day.
• Do not use I.V. bags in series connections, to prevent air embolism resulting from residual air being drawn from primary container before infusion of fluid from secondary container is complete.

• When preparing the I.V. bag, check for leaks by squeezing the inner bag firmly. If leaks appear, discard the solution, which may not be sterile.

fluorouracil
(5-FU)
Adrucil♦, Fluorouracil Injection

Pregnancy Risk Category: D

PHARMACOKINETICS
Distribution: by diffusion to all areas of body water (tumors, intestinal mucosa, bone marrow, liver, CNS, and other tissues). Fluorouracil also crosses the placenta.
Metabolism: in the liver. Up to 80% is rapidly detoxified to an active metabolite by metabolic degradation.
Excretion: about 60% to 80% eliminated through the lungs as carbon dioxide. About 15% is removed unchanged in urine within 6 hours (mostly within the first hour). Drug half-life is 10 to 20 minutes, extending to 20 hours for metabolites. Not known if drug appears in breast milk.
Action: peak serum levels, immediately after injection.

MECHANISM OF ACTION
This antimetabolite interferes with DNA synthesis by inhibiting thymidylate synthetase. Drug also incorporates in RNA, producing a fraudulent RNA. It inhibits utilization of preformed uracil in RNA synthesis by blocking uracil phosphatase.

INDICATIONS & DOSAGE
Dosage depends on protocol and patient's weight.
• Palliative treatment of colorectal, stomach, and advanced breast cancer. _Adults:_ initially, 12 mg/kg daily for 4 days. Maximum daily dosage, 800 mg. If no toxicity occurs, 6 mg/kg given on days 6, 8, 10, and 12. Maintenance dosage: initial dose repeated in 30 days, then 10 to 15 mg/kg weekly. _High-risk adults:_ initially, 6 mg/kg daily for 3 days. Maximum daily dosage, 400 mg. If no toxicity occurs, 3 mg/kg given on days 5, 7, and 9. Maintenance dosage is reduced.

CONTRAINDICATIONS & CAUTIONS
• Avoid use in patients with poor nutrition because of the increased risk of toxicity and in patients with myelosuppression because of the heightened risk of hematologic toxicity.
• Contraindicated in patients with serious infection, especially recent or existing chicken pox or herpes zoster, because of the magnified risk of severe generalized disease.
• Also contraindicated in patients who've had surgery within the past month.
• Use cautiously in hepatic or renal impairment because of the increased risk of toxicity.
• Also use cautiously in patients with previous metastasis to the bone marrow and after high-dose radiation therapy or use of alkylating agents because of the heightened risk of hematologic toxicity.

PREPARATION & STORAGE
Exercise extreme caution when preparing fluorouracil to avoid mutagenic, teratogenic, and carcinogenic risks. Use a biological containment cabinet and wear gloves and mask. Use syringes with Luer-lok tips to avoid drug leakage. Correctly dispose of needles, ampules, and unused drug, and avoid contaminating work surfaces.

Fluorouracil is available in 10 ml glass ampules containing 500 mg of drug in a clear pale yellow aqueous solution. Store at room temperature and protect from direct sunlight. Don't use dark yellow solutions; potency may be affected.

For injection, the drug requires no further dilution. For infusion, dilute with dextrose 5% in water or 0.9% sodium chloride in an appropriate volume based on the patient's condition. Use a filtered needle to prevent injection of any glass particles that may enter the solution when opening the ampule.

ADMINISTRATION
Direct injection: Administer by a 23G or 25G winged infusion set at any convenient rate. Consider using distal rather than major veins to allow for repeated venipunctures if needed. Use a new site for each injection.
Intermittent infusion: not recommended.
Continuous infusion: Infuse appropriately diluted drug via central line over 2 to 24 hours.

INCOMPATIBILITY
Incompatible with cytarabine, diazepam, doxorubicin, droperidol, and methotrexate.

ADVERSE REACTIONS
Life-threatening: GI hemorrhage, severe hematologic toxicity.
Other: acute cerebellar syndrome, alopecia, anemia, anorexia, ataxia, bone marrow depression, diarrhea, diffuse erythema, dry skin, epistaxis, esophagitis, euphoria, fever, hyperpigmentation of nail beds and skin, hypotension, leukopenia, loss of nails, maculopapular rash, nausea, neurotoxicity, paralytic ileus, photophobia, proctitis, skin scaling,

stomatitis, thrombocytopenia, vomiting.

INTERACTIONS
Cimetidine: altered fluorouracil pharmacokinetics.
Live virus vaccines: possible virus replication.
Myelosuppressants and drugs causing blood dyscrasias: possible worsened bone marrow depression.
Thiazide diuretics: possible increased hematologic toxicity.

EFFECTS ON DIAGNOSTIC TESTS
Serum albumin: possible decreased levels.
Serum alkaline phosphatase, bilirubin, LDH, SGOT, SGPT: possible elevated levels.
Urine 5-hydroxyindoleacetic acid: possible increased levels.

SPECIAL CONSIDERATIONS
• Expect toxic effects with therapeutic doses of fluorouracil.
• Monitor CBC and liver and kidney function tests. If platelet count falls below 100,000/mm^3, or if WBC count falls below 3,500/mm^3 or rapidly declines, discontinue drug as ordered.
• WBC nadir usually occurs from 9th to 14th day after treatment, possibly up to 25th day. Recovery occurs by 30th day.
• Inform patient of expected adverse effects. Treat anorexia and nausea with antiemetics. Discontinue drug if the patient experiences intractable vomiting or diarrhea or if you find any evidence of GI bleeding.
• Administer antibiotics, as ordered, if myelosuppressed patient develops an infection.
• Examine the patient's mouth for ulceration before each dose.
• Advise the patient to avoid exposure to people with infections and to

report any unusual bleeding or bruising.
• Fluorouracil may be used with other chemotherapeutic drugs.
• Advise women not to become pregnant while on fluorouracil therapy.
• Advise mothers of infants not to breast-feed during therapy.

folic acid
Folvite♦

Pregnancy Risk Category: A
(C if greater than RDA)

PHARMACOKINETICS
Distribution: distributed into all body tissues, especially the liver, CNS, and erythrocytes. Drug crosses placenta.
Metabolism: in the liver to metabolically active tetrahydrofolic acid by dihydrofolate reductase.
Excretion: in urine as metabolites and small amounts of unchanged drug. With higher doses, larger amounts of unchanged drug are removed in the urine. Drug is found in breast milk.
Action: onset, unknown; duration, unknown.

MECHANISM OF ACTION
Tetrahydrofolic acid is necessary for normal erythropoiesis and nucleoprotein synthesis.

INDICATIONS & DOSAGE
• Megaloblastic and macrocytic anemias resulting from folate deficiency or tropical sprue. *Adults and children:* 250 mcg to 1 mg per day.

CONTRAINDICATIONS & CAUTIONS
• Contraindicated in neonates and immature infants because benzyl alcohol contained in preparation may lead to potentially fatal toxicity.
• Administer with caution to patients who may also suffer from vitamin B_{12} deficiency. Folic acid can mask the diagnosis of pernicious anemia by improving hematologic measurements. Neurologic damage, however, will continue to progress. Therefore do not use as sole treatment of pernicious anemia.

PREPARATION & STORAGE
Available in 10 ml vial containing concentrations of 5 mg/ml or 10 mg/ml. Store below 104° F. (40° C.), preferably between 59° and 86° F. (15° and 30° C.). Protect from light and freezing.
    For direct injection, dilute 1 ml of 5 mg/ml concentration with 49 ml of sterile water for injection to get a concentration of 0.1 mg/ml.

ADMINISTRATION
Direct injection: Slowly inject dose directly into vein or into the tubing of a free-flowing compatible I.V. solution.
Intermittent infusion: not recommended.
Continuous infusion: not recommended.

INCOMPATIBILITY
Incompatible with calcium gluconate, 40% dextrose in water, 50% dextrose in water, oxidizing and reducing agents, and heavy metal ions.

ADVERSE REACTIONS
Life-threatening: allergic bronchospasms, anaphylaxis.
Other: erythema, fever, general malaise, pruritus, rash, yellow discoloration of urine.

INTERACTIONS
Chloramphenicol: antagonized hematopoietic response to folic acid.

Methotrexate, pyrimethamine, triamterene, trimethoprim: reduced dihydrofolate reductase, resulting in antagonized folic acid effect.
Phenytoin: increased phenytoin metabolism resulting in decreased serum concentrations and increased seizures.

EFFECTS ON DIAGNOSTIC TESTS
Serum and erythrocyte folate levels: falsely low levels with the microbiological assay method when patient concurrently takes antibiotics.
Serum vitamin B_{12}: reduced levels.

SPECIAL CONSIDERATIONS
• Use only when oral administration is not acceptable; for example, with GI surgery or malabsorption syndromes.
• Monitor complete blood count to measure effectiveness of drug treatment.

fructose (levulose)

Pregnancy Risk Category: C

COMPOSITION
This source of carbohydrates resembles dextrose but doesn't require insulin for phosphorylation and conversion to glucose. Fructose tends to deplete hepatic adenosine triphosphate levels, which may make it unsuitable for long-term use.

INDICATIONS & DOSAGE
• Fluid and calorie replacement.
Adults: 1 to 3 liters of 10% solution.

CONTRAINDICATIONS & CAUTIONS
• Contraindicated in hereditary fructose intolerance because fructose precipitates renal dysfunction associated with Fanconi's syndrome.
• Also contraindicated in gout because fructose raises serum uric acid levels.
• Because lactic acid is a major product of fructose metabolism, use cautiously in patients at risk for lactic acidosis, such as those with diabetes mellitus or acidosis.
• Safety and efficacy in children age 12 and under have not been established.

PREPARATION & STORAGE
Available in 1,000 ml containers of 10% solution. Protect from freezing and extreme heat. Don't use solution if it's cloudy.

ADMINISTRATION
Direct injection: not recommended.
Intermittent infusion: not recommended.
Continuous infusion: Rate varies, depending on patient's age, weight, and condition. Usual maximum hourly rate is 1 g/kg. Faster infusion increases risk of lactic acid production.

INCOMPATIBILITY
Incompatible with aminophylline, ampicillin sodium, furosemide, hydralazine, thiopental, warfarin, and whole blood.

ADVERSE REACTIONS
Life-threatening: none reported.
Other: extravasation, fever, fluid or solute overload, hypovolemia, phlebitis or venous thrombosis.

INTERACTIONS
None reported.

EFFECTS ON DIAGNOSTIC TESTS
Serum uric acid: possible increased levels.

SPECIAL CONSIDERATIONS
• Fructose shouldn't be used to treat hypoglycemia.
• Monitor fluid, electrolyte, and acid-base balance during therapy.

---

furosemide
Lasix♦, Lasix Special♦

Pregnancy Risk Category: C

PHARMACOKINETICS
Distribution: not well understood. About 95% bound to plasma proteins. Drug crosses the placenta.
Metabolism: small amount metabolized in the liver.
Excretion: in urine by glomerular filtration and secretion from the proximal tubule; 80% to 88% of drug and metabolite are excreted in urine in 24 hours (mostly in first 4 hours). Twelve percent is eliminated in bile, some as unchanged drug. Half-life varies; in normal renal function, it's 1 to 1½ hours. Drug appears in breast milk.
Action: onset, 5 minutes; duration, 2 hours.

MECHANISM OF ACTION
Exact mechanism unknown. But furosemide does inhibit reabsorption of electrolytes, including sodium and chloride, in the ascending loop of Henle; increase excretion of potassium in the distal tubule; and affect electrolyte transport at the proximal tubule. Drug also may cause renal vasodilation and a transient rise in glomerular filtration rate.

INDICATIONS & DOSAGE
• Edema. *Adults:* initially, 20 to 40 mg, increased in 20 mg increments q 2 hours until desired response is achieved. Effective dose given once or twice daily p.r.n.

• Pulmonary edema. *Adults:* initially, 40 mg, increased to 80 mg in 1 hour, if needed. *Infants and children:* initially, 1 mg/kg, increased by 1 mg/kg q 2 hours, if needed. Maximum daily dosage, 6 mg/kg.
• Hypertensive crisis with pulmonary edema or renal failure. *Adults:* 100 to 200 mg.
• Hypercalcemia. *Adults:* 80 to 100 mg q 1 to 2 hours, repeated until desired response is obtained.

CONTRAINDICATIONS & CAUTIONS
• Contraindicated in anuria, in hypersensitivity to furosemide or sulfonamides, and in worsening azotemia or oliguria.
• Use cautiously in diabetes mellitus (drug may impair glucose tolerance); in patients with hyperuricemia or a history of gout (may raise serum uric acid levels); in hepatic impairment (potential dehydration and electrolyte imbalance may precipitate hepatic coma); and in acute myocardial infarction (diuresis may precipitate shock).
• Because drug may exacerbate pancreatitis or lupus erythematosus, use cautiously in patients with a history of these disorders.

PREPARATION & STORAGE
Available in 2, 4, and 10 ml ampules and single-use vials and in syringes with a 10 mg/ml concentration. For infusion, dilute in dextrose 5% in water, Ringer's lactate, dextrose 5% in Ringer's lactate, dextrose 5% in Ringer's injection, or 0.9% sodium chloride. Filter solution to remove any glass particles from ampules.
Store at room temperature and protect from light. Discard discolored (yellow) solution or solution that contains a precipitate.

ADMINISTRATION

Give slowly; overly rapid injection or infusion can cause ototoxicity.

Direct injection: Inject directly into vein or through tubing of a free-flowing compatible solution over 1 to 2 minutes.

Intermittent infusion: Infuse diluted drug at appropriate rate, but not to exceed 4 mg/minute.

Continuous infusion: not recommended.

INCOMPATIBILITY

Incompatible with bleomycin, dobutamine, esmolol, fructose 10% and water, gentamicin, highly acidic solutions, invert sugar 10% and electrolyte #2, metoclopramide, and netilmicin.

ADVERSE REACTIONS

Life-threatening: cardiac arrest.

Other: abdominal pain (in children), allergic interstitial nephritis, anemia, bladder spasm, blurred vision, dizziness, electrolyte depletion, erythema multiforme, exfoliative dermatitis, headache, hypovolemia, increased perspiration, leukopenia, light-headedness, metabolic alkalosis, muscle spasm, necrotizing angiitis, neutropenia, orthostatic hypotension, ototoxicity, paresthesias, photosensitivity, pruritus, purpura, rash, restlessness, thrombocytopenia, urinary frequency, urticaria, vertigo, weakness, xanthopsia.

INTERACTIONS

Alcohol, antihypertensive drugs: possible enhanced hypotensive and diuretic effects.

Aminoglycosides, amphotericin B, other nephrotoxic or ototoxic drugs: increased risk of nephrotoxicity and ototoxicity and intensified electrolyte imbalance.

Amiodarone, cardiac glycosides: enhanced risk of dysrhythmias associated with hypokalemia.

Anticoagulants, thrombolytics: possible increased anticoagulant effects and risk of GI bleeding.

Antidiabetic agents, insulin: possible interference with hypoglycemic effects.

Antigout agents: possible elevated serum uric acid levels.

Antihistamines, antivertigo agents, phenothiazines, thioxanthenes, trimethobenzamide: possible masked signs of ototoxicity.

Chloral hydrate: possible diaphoresis, hot flashes, and variable blood pressure.

Clofibrate: possible enhanced effect of both drugs.

Corticosteroids: possible increased natriuretic and diuretic effects and intensified electrolyte imbalance.

Dopamine: possible enhanced diuresis.

Lithium: heightened risk of toxicity because of reduced clearance.

Neuromuscular blockers: possible enhanced blockade because of furosemide-induced hypokalemia.

NSAIDs, probenecid: antagonism of natriuresis and diuresis and increased risk of renal failure.

Sympathomimetics: possible reduced antihypertensive effects of furosemide.

EFFECTS ON DIAGNOSTIC TESTS

BUN, serum glucose, uric acid: elevated levels.

Serum calcium, chloride, magnesium, potassium, sodium: decreased levels.

Urine glucose, uric acid: increased levels.

SPECIAL CONSIDERATIONS

• *Treatment of overdose:* Manifestations include excessive diuresis with

dehydration and electrolyte depletion. Correct fluid and electrolyte imbalance and treat symptomatically.
• Monitor BUN, serum uric acid, glucose, and electrolyte levels, and liver and kidney function tests; also patient's weight, intake and output, and vital signs.
• Drug may cause hypochloremic metabolic alkalemia and a compensatory respiratory acidemia (increased PCO_2).

---

gallamine triethiodide
Flaxedil♦

Pregnancy Risk Category: C

PHARMACOKINETICS
Distribution: initially distributed to active sites in muscle tissue, then redistributed. Gallamine binds appreciably to serum albumin, especially at pH levels of less than 7.0. Drug crosses the placenta.
Metabolism: not metabolized.
Excretion: in urine as unchanged drug. Elimination half-life is 150 minutes. Not known if drug appears in breast milk.
Action: onset, 3 minutes; duration, 15 to 20 minutes (dose-related).

MECHANISM OF ACTION
Inhibits acetylcholine action at the neuromuscular junction, thereby blocking depolarization.

INDICATIONS & DOSAGE
• Skeletal muscle relaxation as an adjunct to anesthesia. *Adults and children:* initially, 1 mg/kg (not to exceed 100 mg), then 50 mcg/kg to 1 mg/kg after 30 to 40 minutes if needed. *Neonates:* 0.25 to 0.75 mg/kg initially, then 0.1 to 0.5 mg/kg if needed.

Reduce dosage by 20% when halothane is used; by 20% if cyclopropane is used; by 33% if methoxyflurane or fluroxene is used; or by 40% if ether is used.

CONTRAINDICATIONS & CAUTIONS
• Contraindicated in conscious patients and in those with myasthenia gravis because of possible prolonged neuromuscular blockade.
• Also contraindicated in renal impairment because of decreased drug elimination; in shock because of prolonged drug effect; and in cardiac disorders because of a heightened risk of tachycardia.
• Use cautiously in bronchogenic carcinoma because of the risk of enhanced neuromuscular blockade; in hypertension because of exacerbation; and in severe obesity or neuromuscular disease because of possible airway problems.
• Administer carefully in hyperthermia because intensity or duration of drug action may increase.
• Also administer carefully in pulmonary impairment or respiratory depression because of the risk of worsened respiratory depression.
• Also use cautiously in infants who weigh less than 11 lb (5 kg).

PREPARATION & STORAGE
Available in 10 ml vials with a concentration of 20 mg/ml. No dilution necessary before injection.
Protect gallamine injection from light and store at room temperature. Don't freeze drug.

ADMINISTRATION
Only staff specially trained in administering anesthetics and managing adverse reactions should give gallamine, since respiratory depression and apnea will occur.
Direct injection: Inject undiluted drug through the tubing of an I.V.

---

line containing a free-flowing compatible solution. Administer at ordered rate or according to hospital guidelines.
Intermittent infusion: not recommended.
Continuous infusion: not recommended.

INCOMPATIBILITY
Incompatible with anesthetics, barbiturates, and meperidine.

ADVERSE REACTIONS
Life-threatening: acute bronchospasm, anaphylaxis, laryngeal edema.
Other: apnea, cyanosis, dyspnea, flushing, hypotension, respiratory depression, shocklike symptoms, tachycardia, urticaria, wheezing.

INTERACTIONS
Aminoglycosides, anesthetics, capreomycin, citrate-containing blood, clindamycin, lidocaine, lincomycin, polymyxin B, procaine, trimethaphan: enhanced neuromuscular blockade.
Antimyasthenics, edrophonium: antagonized gallamine and antimyasthenic effects.
Calcium salts: diminished gallamine effects.
Depolarizing neuromuscular blocking drugs, parenteral magnesium salts, potassium-depleting drugs, procainamide, quinidine: enhanced neuromuscular blockade.
Opioid analgesics: deepened respiratory depression, increased risk of tachycardia and hypertension.

EFFECTS ON DIAGNOSTIC TESTS
None reported.

SPECIAL CONSIDERATIONS
• *Treatment of overdose:* Provide symptomatic care. Give oxygen and ventilatory support for apnea, anticholinesterase drugs for weakness, and fluids and vasopressors for hypotension or shock.
• To avoid overdose, use a peripheral nerve stimulator to monitor gallamine effects.
• Drug has been used to increase pulmonary compliance during assisted or controlled respiration.
• Hemodialysis and peritoneal dialysis can remove drug.

---

gallium nitrate
Ganite

Pregnancy Risk Category: C

PHARMACOKINETICS
Distribution: to most tissues and plasma. It is not known if the drug crosses the placenta or enters breast milk.
Metabolism: not metabolized in either the liver or the kidneys.
Excretion: appears to be significantly excreted in the kidneys.
Action: steady state levels, within 24 to 48 hours.

MECHANISM OF ACTION
Although gallium nitrate's mechanism of action is not known, the drug appears to reduce hypercalcemia by inhibiting the resorption of bone, possibly by reducing bone turnover. The drug has no cytotoxic effects on bone cells in animal studies.

INDICATIONS & DOSAGE
• Hypercalcemia (cancer-related).
Adults: 200 mg/m^2 daily for 5 consecutive days, administered as a constant infusion over 24 hours. Lower doses (100 mg/m^2) may be given to patients with mild, symptomatic hy-

percalcemia. *Children:* Safety and efficacy have not been established.

CONTRAINDICATIONS & CAUTIONS
• Contraindicated in patients with severe renal impairment (serum creatinine greater than 2.5 mg/dl).
• Use with caution in patients taking other potentially nephrotoxic drugs (aminoglycosides, amphotericin B) because of increased risk of developing renal insufficiency.
• Rapid infusion of doses greater than 200 mg/m² may increase risk of nephrotoxicity or cause nausea and vomiting and substantially increase risk of renal insufficiency.
• Concomitant use of highly nephrotoxic drugs with gallium nitrate may increase the risk of renal insufficiency. Following administration of such drugs, discontinue gallium nitrate therapy and continue hydration for several days.
• Because it is not known whether gallium nitrate can cause fetal harm or affect reproductive capability, administer the drug to a pregnant woman only if clearly needed.

PREPARATION & STORAGE
Available as a clear, colorless, odorless solution in 500 mg (25 mg/ml) single-dose vial. For continuous infusion, dilute in 1,000 ml of 0.9% sodium chloride injection or 5% dextrose injection.

After reconstitution, the drug is stable for at least 48 hours at 59° to 86° F. (15° to 30° C.) and for 7 days if it is stored under refrigeration at 36° to 46° F. (2° to 8° C.). Store the drug carefully. Because the vials contain no preservative, discard the unused portion.

ADMINISTRATION
Direct injection: not recommended.

Intermittent infusion: not recommended.
Continuous infusion: Infuse diluted daily dosage over 24 hours.

INCOMPATIBILITY
None reported.

ADVERSE REACTIONS
Life-threatening: acute renal failure.
Other: acute optic neuritis, anemia, confusion, constipation, decreased mean systolic and diastolic blood pressure, decreased serum bicarbonate, diarrhea, dyspnea, hearing impairment, hypocalcemia, hypophosphatemia, increased BUN, increased creatinine, lethargy, leukopenia, lower extremity edema, nausea and vomiting, pleural effusion, pulmonary infiltrates, rales and rhonchi, skin rash, tachycardia, visual impairment.

INTERACTIONS
Aminoglycosides, amphotericin B, other potentially nephrotoxic drugs: increased risk of renal insufficiency in patients with cancer-related hypercalcemia.

EFFECTS ON DIAGNOSTIC TESTS
Serum calcium and phosphorus: decreased levels.

SPECIAL CONSIDERATIONS
• *Treatment of overdose:* Discontinue drug and give patient vigorous I.V. hydration (with diuretics, if ordered) for 2 to 3 days. Carefully monitor patient's intake and output to make sure fluid intake and output are balanced. Carefully monitor renal function and serum calcium.
• Before starting therapy, make sure that the patient is adequately hydrated and that a satisfactory urine output (at least 2 liters per day) is established.

• Maintain adequate hydration throughout the treatment period. Pay careful attention to the patient's fluid status, including his intake and output, to avoid overhydration in patients with compromised cardiovascular function.

• Monitor renal function (serum creatinine and BUN) closely during gallium nitrate therapy. After baseline assessment, determine calcium levels daily and phosphorus levels twice weekly.

• Monitor serum calcium levels daily and phosphorus levels at least twice weekly during therapy. Frequent renal function studies (BUN and creatinine) are also recommended. Discontinue therapy if serum creatinine rises above 2.5 mg/dl.

• Assess patient for signs of hypocalcemia (including a positive Chvostek's sign). If hypocalcemia occurs, discontinue gallium nitrate therapy. Short-term calcium therapy may be necessary.

• Transient hypophosphatemia is common (may occur in up to 79% of patients). Patient may require oral phosphorus supplements.

• Warn nursing mothers of the potential for serious adverse reactions in nursing infants from gallium nitrate.

• Advise patient to report hearing or vision problems.

• A small number of patients have developed optic neuritis or changes in auditory acuity. The relationship to gallium nitrate therapy is unclear because these patients were taking other antineoplastic drugs.

• For any given level of hypercalcemia, a rapid rise in serum calcium may cause more symptoms.

• Cancer-related hypercalcemia may affect up to 20% of all patients hospitalized with malignancy. The incidence appears higher in patients with multiple myeloma, kidney cancer, cancer of the head and neck, breast cancer, and non-small-cell cancer of the lung.

• Signs and symptoms of hypercalcemia include anorexia, lethargy, fatigue, nausea, vomiting, constipation, dehydration, impaired mental status, renal insufficiency, coma, and cardiac arrest.

ganciclovir
Cytovene

Pregnancy Risk Category: C

PHARMACOKINETICS
Distribution: drug concentrates in cells infected with cytomegalovirus (CMV) because of the action of cellular kinases that convert it to ganciclovir triphosphate. It crosses the blood-brain barrier.
Metabolism: more than 90% of drug excreted unchanged.
Excretion: elimination half-life is about 3 hours. Primary route of excretion is by kidneys. Not known if drug appears in breast milk.

MECHANISM OF ACTION
Ganciclovir is a synthetic nucleoside analog of $2'$-deoxyguanosine. It competitively inhibits viral DNA polymerase and may be incorporated within viral DNA to cause early termination of DNA replication. It has shown activity against CMV, herpes simplex viruses 1 and 2 (HSV-1 and HSV-2), varicella-zoster virus, and Epstein-Barr virus.

INDICATIONS & DOSAGE
• Treatment of CMV retinitis.
Adults: 2.5 to 5 mg/kg I.V. q 8 hours for 10 to 14 days, followed by a maintenance dose of 5 to 7.5 mg/

kg once or twice daily for 5 to 7 days per week.

Note: Adjust dosage in renal failure. For adults, dosage should reflect creatinine clearance. If clearance exceeds 80 ml/minute, give 5 mg/kg q 12 hours; if it ranges from 50 to 79 ml/minute, give 2.5 mg/kg q 12 hours; if it ranges from 25 to 49 ml/minute, give 2.5 mg/kg q 24 hours; if clearance is less than 25 ml/minute, give 1.25 mg/kg q 24 hours.

CONTRAINDICATIONS & CAUTIONS

• Contraindicated in patients hypersensitive to ganciclovir or acyclovir.
• About 40% of the patients that receive the drug experience some form of hematologic toxicity, including granulocytopenia or thrombocytopenia. Granulocytopenia usually occurs during the first week but may occur anytime during therapy. Patients with drug-induced immunosuppression seem more likely to develop thrombocytopenia than those infected with human immunodeficiency virus (HIV). Cell counts usually recover 3 to 7 days after discontinuing the drug.
• Drug has shown carcinogenic and mutagenic activity in animal tests and has also caused aspermatogenesis in animal studies. Indicated only for treatment of immunocompromised patients with CMV retinitis.
• Rarely used in children under age 12. Use with extreme caution, keeping in mind the drug's potential for carcinogenic and reproductive toxicity.

PREPARATION & STORAGE

Available in vials of 500 mg. Store between 59° and 86° F. (15° and 30° C.) and do not exceed 104° F. (40° C.). Add 10 ml of sterile water without preservatives to one 500 mg vial to produce a solution of 50 mg/ml. Shake vial until solution is clear to ensure complete dissolution of particles. After reconstitution, solutions with a concentration of 50 mg/ml retain potency for 12 hours at room temperature. Do not refrigerate.

Dilute further to a final concentration of 10 mg/ml with 100 ml of 0.9% sodium chloride, dextrose 5% in water, Ringer's injection, or lactated Ringer's injection. Use diluted solutions within 24 hours. Keep them refrigerated until use. Do not freeze.

ADMINISTRATION

Direct injection: not recommended.
Intermittent infusion: Administer the drug over 1 hour.
Continuous infusion: not recommended.

INCOMPATIBILITY

Do not mix with other drugs.

ADVERSE REACTIONS

Life-threatening: granulocytopenia, hepatotoxicity, neutropenia, thrombocytopenia.
Other: anemia, confusion, diarrhea, disorientation, dizziness, fever, headaches, nausea, rash, seizures, vomiting.

INTERACTIONS

Imipenem and cilastatin: generalized seizures have been reported in patients taking imipenem/cilastatin ganciclovir combination.
Immunosuppressive agents: additional bone marrow suppression.
Probenecid: reduced renal clearance of ganciclovir.
Zidovudine: possible higher incidence of neutropenia.

EFFECTS ON DIAGNOSTIC TESTS

Serum alkaline phosphatase, serum bilirubin, SGOT, SGPT: possible increased levels.

SPECIAL CONSIDERATIONS

• Monitor complete blood count (CBC) to detect neutropenia, which may occur in up to 40% of patients. This complication usually appears after about 10 days of therapy and may be associated with higher doses (15 mg/kg/day). Neutropenia is reversible but may necessitate discontinuation of therapy. Patient may restart the drug when CBC returns to normal.

• Thrombocytopenia may develop in up to 20% of patients treated with the drug.

• Tell the patient that maintenance infusions are necessary to prevent recurrence of the disease.

• Advise the patient to immediately report any signs or symptoms of infection (fever, sore throat) or easy bruising or bleeding.

• Tell the patient to take extra care when brushing teeth and when using dental floss or toothpicks.

• Animal studies reveal some evidence of carcinogenicity and reproductive toxicity.

• Breast-feeding during treatment is not recommended. Instruct patients to refrain from breast-feeding until at least 72 hours after their last ganciclovir treatment.

• Because ganciclovir should be considered a potential carcinogen, consider handling it according to institutional guidelines developed for cytotoxic drugs.

• Because ganciclovir solutions are alkaline (about pH 11.0), use caution in handling and preparing the drug. Latex gloves and safety glasses are recommended. If solution contacts skin or mucous membranes, wash area thoroughly with soap and water; irrigate eyes with plain water.

• Patients on dialysis should receive their dose of ganciclovir after the dialysis session, since plasma levels will be substantially reduced by the treatment.

• Patients with HIV infection, as well as organ and bone marrow transplant recipients, appear to be at increased risk of CMV infections. Drug is under investigation for other forms of CMV infections, including pneumonitis and GI disease.

---

gentamicin sulfate
Garamycin♦, Jenamicin

Pregnancy Risk Category: C

PHARMACOKINETICS

Distribution: mostly distributed in extracellular fluid; also found in sputum and in abscess, pleural, synovial, peritoneal, and pericardial fluids. Small amounts appear in bile, inner ear, kidneys, and ocular tissue. Cerebrospinal fluid concentrations are low, reflecting dose, penetration rate, and extent of meningeal inflammation. Drug crosses the placenta.

Metabolism: not metabolized.

Excretion: in urine, principally unchanged by glomerular filtration; 70% removed within 24 hours in adults. About 10% excreted within 12 hours in neonates less than 3 days old. Serum half-life is 2 to 3 hours in adults (24 to 60 hours in renal impairment), 6 to 12 hours in children, about 3 hours in infants between age 1 week and 6 months, and nearly 6 hours in younger neonates.

Not known if drug appears in breast milk.

Action: peak serum level, 30 to 60 minutes.

MECHANISM OF ACTION

Inhibits protein synthesis by binding to the 30S ribosomal subunit. The drug's spectrum of action includes gram-negative aerobic bacteria, such as *Acinetobacter, Enterobacter, Escherichia coli, Klebsiella, Proteus, Providencia, Pseudomonas, Salmonella, Serratia,* and *Shigella.* Susceptible gram-positive bacteria include *Staphylococcus aureus* and *S. epidermidis.*

INDICATIONS & DOSAGE

• Life-threatening infections caused by susceptible organisms. *Adults:* 2.5 mg/kg q 6 to 8 hours. Reduce dosage to 3 mg/kg daily as soon as possible.
• Severe infections caused by susceptible organisms. *Adults:* 1 mg/kg q 8 hours. *Children age 1 and older:* 2 to 2.5 mg/kg q 8 hours. *Infants:* 2.5 mg/kg q 8 hours. *Neonates age 1 week and under:* 2.5 mg/kg q 12 hours.
• Endocarditis prophylaxis in GI or GU procedures. *Adults:* 1.5 mg/kg 30 to 60 minutes before procedure, then q 8 hours afterward for up to two doses. *Children:* 2 to 2.5 mg/kg 30 to 60 minutes before procedure, then q 8 hours afterward for up to two doses.
Note: Adjust dosage in renal failure. For adults, adjust dosage to keep peak levels between 4 and 10 mcg/ml and trough levels between 1 and 2 mcg/ml. If patient is undergoing hemodialysis, measure serum levels after each session; dialysis may remove half of the drug. If serum levels aren't measured, give 1 to 1.7 mg/kg for adults and 2 to 2.5 mg/kg for children, depending on infection's severity.

CONTRAINDICATIONS & CAUTIONS

• Contraindicated in aminoglycoside hypersensitivity or previous severe toxic reaction.
• Use cautiously in renal impairment because of the risk of nephrotoxicity. Also use cautiously in elderly patients, in infants and neonates, and in patients who've had previous aminoglycoside therapy because of the heightened risk of nephrotoxicity and ototoxicity.
• Administer cautiously in patients with hearing impairment or a history of noise exposure or ear infections because of an increased risk of further cranial nerve VIII damage.
• Because of the risk of further weakness, give cautiously to infants with botulism and to patients with neuromuscular disorders (especially myasthenia gravis).
• Use cautiously in hypomagnesemia, hypocalcemia, and hypokalemia to avoid exacerbation.

PREPARATION & STORAGE

Available as a clear, colorless to slightly yellow aqueous solution in 2 ml vials with a 10 or 40 mg/ml concentration, in 20 ml vials with a 40 mg/ml concentration, in 1.5 ml disposable syringes with a 40 mg/ml concentration, and in 2 ml disposable syringes with a 10 mg/ml concentration. Also available in 60, 80, and 100 ml containers (with a concentration of 1 mg/ml) diluted with dextrose 5% in water for intermittent infusion and in 50 and 100 ml bags (with a concentration of 0.4 to 2.4 mg/ml) diluted with 0.9% sodium chloride for intermittent infusion. The containers and bags have no preservatives and must be used promptly once the seal is broken. Discard unused portions.

Don't use a discolored or precipitated solution. Store solution between 36° and 86° F. (15° and 30° C.). Stability usually holds for 24 hours at room temperature.

ADMINISTRATION

Direct injection: not recommended, but used for adults if necessary. Slowly inject drug directly into vein or an established I.V. line. Don't use infusion units.

Intermittent infusion: Infuse solution (with a concentration not exceeding 1 mg/ml) over 30 minutes to 2 hours.

Continuous infusion: not used.

INCOMPATIBILITY

Do not mix with other drugs.

ADVERSE REACTIONS

Life-threatening: anaphylaxis, respiratory paralysis (rare).

Other: acute organic brain syndrome, agranulocytosis, alopecia, anemia (transient), anorexia, bacterial or fungal superinfection, blurred vision, burning sensation (generalized), confusion, depression, encephalopathy, eosinophilia, fever, flaccidity, granulocytopenia, headache, hepatomegaly, hypertension, hypocalcemia, hypokalemia, hypomagnesemia, hyponatremia, hypotension, increased salivation, injection site pain, joint pain, laryngeal edema, lethargy, leukopenia, metabolic acidosis, muscle twitching, myasthenia gravis–like syndrome, nausea, nephrotoxicity, optic neuritis, ototoxicity (possibly irreversible), paresthesias, peripheral neuritis, pruritus, pseudotumor cerebri, pulmonary fibrosis, rash, respiratory depression, scotoma, seizures, splenomegaly, stomatitis, stupor, thrombocytopenia, thrombocytopenic purpura, thrombophlebitis at injection site, tremors, urticaria, vomiting, weakness, weight loss.

INTERACTIONS

Antihistamines, phenothiazines, thioxanthenes: possible masked symptoms of ototoxicity.

Beta-lactam antibiotics, vancomycin: possible synergistic effect against certain organisms.

Chloramphenicol, clindamycin, tetracycline: antagonized bactericidal effects of gentamicin.

General anesthetics, neuromuscular blocking drugs, opioid analgesics, parenteral polymyxin B: possible potentiated neuromuscular blockade and respiratory paralysis.

Indomethacin I.V.: increased risk of gentamicin toxicity in neonates.

Nephrotoxic, neurotoxic, and ototoxic drugs: heightened risk of toxicity.

EFFECTS ON DIAGNOSTIC TESTS

Serum bilirubin, creatinine, LDH; BUN, nonprotein nitrogen: possible elevated levels.

CBC: reduced RBC and WBC counts.

Reticulocyte count: increased or decreased.

Serum calcium, magnesium, potassium, sodium: possible reduced levels.

SGOT, SGPT: possible increased levels.

Urinalysis: possible decreased specific gravity, elevated protein levels, hematuria, presence of cells or casts.

SPECIAL CONSIDERATIONS

• *Treatment of overdose:* Support respiratory and renal function. Hemodialysis or peritoneal dialysis may help to remove drug. In neonates, exchange transfusions may be used.

• Collect specimens for culture and sensitivity tests before first dose; therapy may begin before results are available.

- Weigh patient and test renal function before therapy.
- During therapy, monitor renal function and intake and output. Keep patient well hydrated to minimize risk of toxicity and chemical irritation of renal tubules.
- Obtain peak and trough serum levels and adjust dosage, as ordered, especially in patients with renal impairment. Coordinate specimen collection times with laboratory. Peak levels above 10 mcg/ml and trough levels above 2 mcg/ml increase risk of toxicity.
- Treatment usually lasts for 7 to 10 days. If improvement doesn't occur within 5 days, stop drug and collect new specimens for culture and sensitivity tests.
- Risk of neuromuscular blockade is greatest after rapid, direct injection.
- Ask patient about tinnitus or hearing loss. An audiogram may be ordered if ototoxicity occurs.
- May contain sulfites.

glucagon

Pregnancy Risk Category: B

PHARMACOKINETICS
Distribution: to most tissues and plasma. Not known if drug crosses the placenta.
Metabolism: primarily in the liver; also in kidneys, tissues, and plasma through enzymatic proteolysis.
Excretion: by the kidneys, mostly as metabolites. Not known if drug appears in breast milk. Half-life is about 3 to 10 minutes.
Action for diagnostic use: onset, within 1 minute; duration, 9 to 25 minutes, depending on dose.
Action for hypoglycemic use: onset, 5 to 30 minutes; duration, 1 to 2 hours.

MECHANISM OF ACTION
Drug promotes hepatic glycogenolysis and gluconeogenesis, raising serum glucose levels. It also relaxes GI smooth muscle and produces a positive inotropic and chronotropic myocardial effect.

INDICATIONS & DOSAGE
- Severe hypoglycemia. *Adults:* 0.5 to 1 unit (0.5 to 1 mg). Larger doses may be necessary. *Children:* 0.025 unit/kg to a maximum of 1 unit. If patient doesn't awaken within 20 minutes, repeat dose. Can be repeated again.
- Diagnostic aid for GI, urologic, and radiologic examinations. *Adults:* 0.25 to 2 units, depending on desired onset time and duration of effect.

CONTRAINDICATIONS & CAUTIONS
- Contraindicated for treating asphyxia at birth or hypoglycemia in premature infants or those with intrauterine growth retardation.
- Use cautiously in patients who are allergic to proteins; they also may be allergic to glucagon.
- Also use cautiously in patients with a history of insulinoma because severe hypoglycemia may occur, and in patients with pheochromocytoma because of the risk of a marked increase in blood pressure.

PREPARATION & STORAGE
Potency of glucagon is expressed in USP units. One USP unit equals 1 IU and about 1 mg.
  Drug is available as a powder in 1 and 10 unit vials; store at room temperature. Reconstitute with provided diluent, which is clear and sterile and contains 0.2% phenol as a preservative and 1.6% glycerin. Preparation contains lactose.

Although reconstituted solution should be used immediately, it remains stable for up to 3 months when stored at 36° to 46° F. (2° to 8° C.).

ADMINISTRATION
Direct injection: Give directly into vein or into I.V. tubing of a free-flowing compatible solution over 2 to 5 minutes. Interrupt primary infusion during glucagon injection if you're using the same I.V. line.
Intermittent infusion: not recommended.
Continuous infusion: not recommended.

INCOMPATIBILITY
Incompatible with saline solution and other solutions having a pH of 3 to 9.5 because drug may cause precipitation.

ADVERSE REACTIONS
Life-threatening: none reported.
Other: dizziness, dyspnea, light-headedness, nausea, rash, tachycardia, vomiting.

INTERACTIONS
Anticoagulants (such as coumarin or indanedione derivatives): possible potentiated anticoagulant effects.
Epinephrine: enhanced and prolonged hyperglycemic effect.

EFFECTS ON DIAGNOSTIC TESTS
None reported.

SPECIAL CONSIDERATIONS
• Monitor patient's blood pressure. Rapid glucagon administration can reduce blood pressure.
• Monitor serum glucose levels.
• If hypoglycemic patient doesn't respond to glucagon, give I.V. dextrose. Glucagon may fail to relieve coma because of markedly depleted hepatic stores of glycogen or irreversible brain damage caused by prolonged hypoglycemia.
• Teach the hypoglycemic patient's family how to give glucagon in an emergency. Instruct them to use a standard insulin syringe, employing a 90-degree approach (rather than the usual subcutaneous one) to deliver a deeper injection and achieve a faster response.
• Glucagon causes a smooth, gradual termination of insulin coma. When used to terminate insulin shock therapy in a psychiatric patient, give dose 1 hour after coma induction.
• Once hypoglycemia resolves, give carbohydrate- and protein-containing foods to prevent recurrence.
• Drug may cause both hyperglycemia and hypoglycemia.
• If drug is given to patient who is taking coumadin, monitor prothrombin time.
• Drug has been used as a cardiac stimulant in managing toxicity resulting from use of beta-adrenergic blockers, quinidine, and tricyclic antidepressants.

glycopyrrolate
Robinul♦

Pregnancy Risk Category: B

PHARMACOKINETICS
Distribution: rapid and widespread, with high levels found in stomach and intestines. Drug crosses the placenta and appears in cerebrospinal fluid in low concentrations.
Metabolism: metabolized in small amounts to several metabolites.
Excretion: removed primarily as unchanged drug in feces and urine. Half-life is less than 5 minutes. Not

known if drug appears in breast milk.

Action: onset, about 1 minute; duration, 2 to 3 hours for vagal effect, up to 7 hours for salivary inhibition, and 8 to 12 hours for anticholinergic effect.

MECHANISM OF ACTION

Glycopyrrolate competitively inhibits the muscarinic effects of acetylcholine on autonomic effectors innervated by postganglionic cholinergic nerves. Drug curtails GI motility and gastric, nasal, bronchial, and oropharyngeal secretions. It reduces the tone and amplitude of ureteral and bladder contractions and decreases motility. Cardiac responses include vagal stimulation.

INDICATIONS & DOSAGE

• Adjunctive treatment of peptic ulcers. *Adults and children age 12 and over:* 0.1 to 0.2 mg q 6 to 8 hours (daily maximum, 4 doses).

• Intraoperative medication. *Adults:* 0.1 mg, repeated q 2 to 3 minutes, as needed. *Children:* 0.0044 mg/kg (0.1 mg maximum), repeated q 2 to 3 minutes, as needed.

• Blockage of adverse muscarinic effects of neostigmine or pyridostigmine. *Adults and children:* 0.2 mg for each 1 mg of neostigmine or 5 mg of pyridostigmine. Give in same syringe.

CONTRAINDICATIONS & CAUTIONS

• Contraindicated in glycopyrrolate hypersensitivity.

• Also contraindicated in severe ulcerative colitis, toxic megacolon, obstructive GI disease, cardiospasm, paralytic ileus, and intestinal atony because the drug diminishes intestinal motility and heightens the risk of obstruction; in angle-closure glaucoma because the drug may raise intraocular pressure; and in obstructive uropathy or prostatic hypertrophy because urinary retention may worsen.

• Avoid use in tachycardia stemming from cardiac insufficiency, thyrotoxicosis, or acute hemorrhage with unstable cardiovascular status because the drug will block vagal inhibition of the sinoatrial node, and in myasthenia gravis because of possible exacerbated weakness.

• Use glycopyrrolate cautiously in febrile patients and in those exposed to high temperatures because of the risk of hyperthermia.

• Administer the drug carefully to children, especially those under age 2, because of the increased risk of adverse reactions. Give carefully to children with brain damage because CNS effects may be exacerbated, and to children with spastic paralysis because of a possible increased response to drug.

• In Down's syndrome, give carefully because of the risk of tachycardia. In elderly patients, give cautiously because drug may cause paradoxical excitement, agitation, increased drowsiness, or acute glaucoma.

• Administer glycopyrrolate cautiously in hyperthyroidism because tachycardia may worsen; in hypertension because of possible aggravation; in tachydysrhythmias, congestive heart failure, or coronary artery disease because the drug will block vagal inhibition of the sinoatrial node; in hepatic or renal impairment because of the heightened risk of adverse reactions; and in chronic pulmonary disease because the drug may promote mucous plug formation.

• Also administer the drug cautiously in esophageal reflux or hiatal hernia because it promotes gastric retention and aggravates reflux; in gastric ulcer because delayed gastric emptying may cause antral stasis; in known or suspected GI infection because diminished GI motility prolongs retention of causative organisms or toxins; in diarrhea because this sign may be an early indicator of intestinal obstruction; and in mild or moderate ulcerative colitis because decreased GI motility may produce paralytic ileus or toxic megacolon.

• In autonomic or partial obstructive uropathy, give glycopyrrolate carefully because it may aggravate or precipitate urine retention.

• In xerostomia, also give the drug carefully because salivary flow may be further curtailed.

PREPARATION & STORAGE
Available as a clear, colorless sterile solution in 1, 2, 5, and 20 ml vials with a concentration of 0.2 mg/ml. Drug can be given diluted or undiluted. Having a pH of 2 to 3, glycopyrrolate is stablest in acidic solutions and unstable in solutions with a pH exceeding 6. Store at room temperature.

For infusion, solutions containing glycopyrrolate concentrations of 0.8 mg/liter remain stable at room temperature for 48 hours when mixed with dextrose 5% in water, dextrose 5% in 0.45% sodium chloride, 0.9% sodium chloride, or Ringer's lactate.

ADMINISTRATION
Direct injection: Inject drug at ordered rate into vein or into an I.V. line containing a free-flowing compatible solution.
Intermittent infusion: Infuse at ordered rate or according to hospital guidelines.
Continuous infusion: not recommended.

INCOMPATIBILITY
Incompatible with drugs having an alkaline pH and with chloramphenicol sodium succinate, dexamethasone sodium phosphate, diazepam, dimenhydrinate, methohexital sodium, methylprednisolone sodium succinate, pentazocine lactate, pentobarbital sodium, secobarbital sodium, sodium bicarbonate, and thiopental sodium.

ADVERSE REACTIONS
Incidence and severity are dose-dependent.
Life-threatening: anaphylaxis, respiratory paralysis.
Other: anhidrosis, bloated sensation, blurred vision, breathing difficulty, confusion, constipation, cycloplegia, decreased lactation, dizziness, drowsiness, dysphagia, dysuria, excitement, fever, flushing, headache, hypertension, hypotension, increased ocular tension, insomnia, loss of taste, memory loss (especially in elderly), mydriasis, nausea, palpitations, marked photophobia, rash, tachycardia, thirst, urinary hesitancy or retention, urticaria, vomiting, weakness, xerostomia.

INTERACTIONS
Alphaprodine, amantadine, antidyskinetics, antihistamines, phenothiazines, quinidine, tricyclic antidepressants, other antimuscarinics: additive anticholinergic effects.
Antimyasthenics: reduced intestinal motility.
Antipsychotics, benzodiazepines, disopyramide, glutethimide, MAO inhibitors: increased anticholinergic effects.
Cyclopropane anesthetics: ventricular dysrhythmias.
Guanadrel, guanethidine, reserpine: antagonized inhibitory action of glycopyrrolate on gastric acid.

Ketoconazole: impaired absorption because of increased gastric pH.
Metoclopramide: antagonized effect on GI motility.
Opioid analgesics: heightened risk of severe constipation and additive anticholinergic effects.
Potassium chloride (wax-matrix preparations, Slow-K): increased severity of GI mucosal lesions.
Urinary alkalizers (such as antacids, carbonic anhydrase inhibitors): delayed excretion.

EFFECTS ON DIAGNOSTIC TESTS
Gastric acid secretion test: antagonized effects of pentagastrin.
Serum uric acid: decreased levels in patients with hyperuricemia or gout.

SPECIAL CONSIDERATIONS
• *Treatment of overdose:* Provide symptomatic and supportive care. Physostigmine may act as an antidote, but this is controversial.
• Monitor intake, output, vital signs, and bowel habits.
• Encourage good oral hygiene. Provide gum or sugarless candy to help relieve dry mouth.
• Elderly or debilitated patients usually require lower doses.
• High doses over a prolonged period may cause CNS stimulation, resulting in a curare-like action.
• Avoid giving drug for 24 hours before gastric acid secretion tests.
• May contain benzyl alcohol.

---

gonadorelin hydrochloride
Factrel♦

Pregnancy Risk Category: B

PHARMACOKINETICS
Distribution: unknown.
Metabolism: unknown.

Excretion: by kidneys as metabolites. Half-life is a few minutes.
Action: peak effects, 13 to 41 minutes in men and 12 to 60 minutes in premenopausal women; duration, 3 to 5 hours.

MECHANISM OF ACTION
A synthetic hormone structurally identical to luteinizing hormone releasing hormone, drug stimulates release of luteinizing hormone (LH) and follicle-stimulating hormone (FSH) from anterior pituitary.

INDICATIONS & DOSAGE
• Evaluation of functional capacity and response of anterior pituitary gonadotropin to aid diagnosis of hypogonadism. *Adults and children over age 12:* 0.1 mg in a single dose. Prolonged or repeated doses help to evaluate pituitary gonadotropin reserve.

CONTRAINDICATIONS & CAUTIONS
• Administer cautiously to patients with gonadorelin hypersensitivity, other drug allergies, or chronic renal failure.

PREPARATION & STORAGE
Available in 100 and 500 mg vials. Just before use, add 1 ml of diluent provided by manufacturer to 100 mg vial or 2 ml to 500 mg vial. Reconstituted mixture remains stable for 24 hours at room temperature. Discard unused portions.

ADMINISTRATION
Direct injection: Inject directly into vein over 3 to 5 minutes. Alternatively, inject into an I.V. line containing a free-flowing compatible solution.
Intermittent infusion: not recommended.

Unmarked trade names available in the United States only.
♦Also available in Canada.   ♦♦Available in Canada only.

Continuous infusion: not recommended.

INCOMPATIBILITY
No incompatibilities reported.

ADVERSE REACTIONS
Life-threatening: none reported.
Other: abdominal discomfort, dizziness, flushing, headache, light-headedness, nausea.

INTERACTIONS
Digoxin, oral contraceptives: possible depressed gonadotropin levels.
Levodopa, spironolactone: possible elevated gonadotropin levels.
Phenothiazines, dopamine agonists: possible blunted response to gonadorelin.

EFFECTS ON DIAGNOSTIC TESTS
Serum estradiol (females): fluctuating levels for 18 hours after injection.
Serum testosterone: transiently elevated levels.

SPECIAL CONSIDERATIONS
• To test women, give drug early in the follicular phase of the menstrual cycle (day 1 to day 7).
• Collect serum samples for LH determinations 15 minutes before gonadorelin injection, immediately before injection, and at regular intervals after injection (usually at 15, 30, 45, 60, and 120 minutes).
• Gonadorelin test can be performed with other studies of pituitary function, such as serum tests of LH and FSH levels.
• A subnormal response may indicate impaired function of the pituitary, hypothalamus, or both.

granulocytes
Granulocyte Concentrate

Pregnancy Risk Category: C

COMPOSITION
Derived from 7 liters of whole blood by granulocytapheresis, this product contains at least 1×10^{10} granulocytes, varying amounts of lymphocytes (about 30%), 6 to 10 units of platelets, 30 to 50 ml of RBCs, and about 200 to 400 ml of plasma.

INDICATIONS & DOSAGE
• Treatment of bacterial infections that fail to respond to conventional therapy in patients with chronic granulomatous disease or profound neutropenia (less than 500 neutrophils/microliter). *Adults:* 1 unit daily for 1 week or longer. *Children:* same dosage as adults, but daily infusion volume mustn't exceed 10 ml/kg.

CONTRAINDICATIONS & CAUTIONS
• Contraindicated in patients in whom recovery of bone marrow function appears unlikely.

PREPARATION & STORAGE
Granulocyte concentrate is prepared by granulocytapheresis. In this process, donor blood flows into a centrifuge located within an automated cell separator, WBCs are removed, and the remaining blood is returned to the donor.
    Granulocytes can be stored at room temperature for up to 24 hours. However, because of their short survival time, they should be transfused as soon as possible after collection. To prevent graft-versus-host disease (GVHD), a rare complication, granulocytes can be exposed to 1,500 rad.

ADMINISTRATION
Direct injection: not recommended.
Intermittent infusion: not recommended.
Continuous infusion: Using a standard transfusion set with a 170-micron filter and a 19G needle, infuse 200 ml over 1 to 2 hours. Don't use a microaggregate or depth-type filter because this may trap granulocytes. Begin the infusion slowly, according to institutional recommendations. Record the patient's vital signs. If there's no evidence of a reaction, adjust flow to the prescribed rate. Observe the patient closely throughout transfusion.

INCOMPATIBILITY
Incompatible with all drugs and solutions except for 0.9% sodium chloride.

ADVERSE REACTIONS
Life-threatening: AIDS, GVHD, viral hepatitis.
Other: cytomegalovirus infection; febrile, nonhemolytic reaction; severe pulmonary reaction (cough, dyspnea, fever, increased respiratory rate).

INTERACTIONS
Amphotericin B: possible pulmonary insufficiency.

EFFECTS ON DIAGNOSTIC TESTS
Platelet count: elevated.
Human lymphocyte antigen (HLA) antibody: possibly present after repeated exposure to foreign HLA antigens.

SPECIAL CONSIDERATIONS
• Confirm ABO compatibility before transfusion. Granulocyte concentrates contain a significant number of RBCs, making crossmatching necessary.

• Describe the procedure, product, duration of transfusion, and expected outcome to the patient. Instruct him to report any unusual symptoms immediately.
• Check vital signs and establish patent venous catheter before requesting granulocytes from blood bank.
• If a severe pulmonary reaction occurs, discontinue the transfusion immediately, keep vein open with 0.9% sodium chloride, and notify the doctor. Treatment may include diuretics, oxygen, and corticosteroids.
• If a febrile, nonhemolytic reaction occurs, discontinue the transfusion, keep vein open with 0.9% sodium chloride, and contact the doctor. Treatment and prophylaxis include acetaminophen, meperidine, or diphenhydramine.
• Instruct the patient to report fever, rash, or symptoms of hepatitis—indicators of GVDH that appear 2 to 3 weeks after transfusion.

heparin calcium
Calcilean♦, Calciparine♦

heparin sodium
Hepalean♦, Hep-Flush, Hep-Lock, Hep-Pak, Liquaemin, Minihep♦♦

Pregnancy Risk Category: C

PHARMACOKINETICS
Distribution: in plasma with extensive protein binding. Drug doesn't cross the placenta.
Metabolism: apparently partly metabolized in the liver but mainly removed from circulation by the reticuloendothelial system.
Excretion: in urine as unchanged drug (up to 50%), especially after large doses, and as metabolites. Serum half-life averages 1 to 6

hours. Drug doesn't appear in breast milk.

Action: peak plasma level, steady with continuous infusion.

MECHANISM OF ACTION

An anticoagulant, heparin potentiates the effects of antithrombin, which inhibits conversion of fibrinogen to fibrin. Drug also inhibits the action of Factors IX, X, XI, and XII. It inactivates fibrin-stabilizing factor and prevents formation of a stable fibrin clot. Heparin doesn't have fibrinolytic action and so won't dissolve existing clots.

INDICATIONS & DOSAGE

Dosage depends on the patient's weight, disease, hepatorenal function, and activated partial thromboplastin time (APTT). Dosages given are guidelines.

• Venous thrombosis or pulmonary embolism. *Adults:* 5,000 units initially, then continuous infusion of 20,000 to 40,000 units in 1,000 ml of 0.9% sodium chloride over 24 hours; or 10,000 units initially, then 5,000 to 10,000 units q 4 to 6 hours. *Children:* 50 units/kg initially, then continuous infusion of 100 units/kg q 4 hours or 20,000 units/m² over 24 hours; or 100 units/kg initially, then 50 to 100 units/kg q 4 hours.

• Disseminated intravascular coagulation (DIC). *Adults:* 50 to 100 units/kg q 4 hours. Discontinue after 4 to 8 hours if no improvement occurs. *Children:* 25 to 50 units/kg q 4 hours. Discontinue after 4 to 8 hours if no improvement occurs.

• I.V. flush to maintain indwelling catheter patency. *Adults and children:* 10 to 100 units after use or at designated intervals.

CONTRAINDICATIONS & CAUTIONS

• Contraindicated in heparin hypersensitivity, except in life-threatening situations.

• Also contraindicated in severe thrombocytopenia because of possible exacerbation; in uncontrollable bleeding (except when caused by DIC) because of the risk of severe hemorrhage; and in severe, uncontrolled hypertension because of the increased risk of cerebral hemorrhage.

• Avoid using heparin if coagulation tests can't be performed regularly.

• In neonates, avoid using commercially available heparin sodium injections and heparin lock flush solutions that contain benzyl alcohol. This preservative has caused death in premature infants.

• Use with extreme caution in patients with hemorrhage or at risk for hemorrhage (surgery, GI conditions such as ulcerative colitis); in patients with a history of allergies because of a possible hypersensitivity reaction; during pregnancy (especially the last trimester) and immediately postpartum because of the risk of maternal hemorrhage; in women over age 60 because of heightened susceptibility to hemorrhage; and in patients with mild hepatic disease because of the heightened risk of toxicity.

• Because of possible hyperkalemia, give heparin cautiously in hypoaldosteronism.

• In renal insufficiency, use heparin carefully because of decreased renal clearance.

• Because of the risk of bleeding, use heparin cautiously in diabetic patients undergoing medical or dental procedures.

PREPARATION & STORAGE

Available in 0.5 to 1 ml ampules, vials, or prefilled syringes and in 1,

2, 5, 10, and 30 ml multidose vials, with concentrations ranging from 1,000 to 40,000 units/ml. Heparin flush concentrations range from 10 to 100 units/ml.

For infusion, dilute with 0.9% sodium chloride or another compatible solution, such as dextrose and Ringer's combination, dextrose 2.5% in water, dextrose 5% in water, fructose 10%, Ringer's injection, or Ringer's lactate, to achieve the prescribed concentration and volume. When diluting heparin solutions for continuous infusion, invert the container at least six times to ensure adequate mixing and to prevent pooling of heparin in the solution.

Store commercially available heparin preparations at room temperature. Avoid exposure to excessive heat. Don't freeze heparin solutions.

Before administration, inspect heparin for particles or discoloration. Discard solution if you find particulate matter or marked discoloration. Slight discoloration doesn't affect potency.

ADMINISTRATION

Direct injection: Give diluted or undiluted drug through intermittent infusion device or into I.V. tubing containing a free-flowing compatible solution.
Intermittent infusion: Give drug undiluted or diluted in 50 to 100 ml of 0.9% sodium chloride. Using an infusion pump, administer through a peripheral or central venous line over prescribed duration.
Continuous infusion: Using an infusion pump, give diluted solution over 24 hours.

INCOMPATIBILITY

Incompatible with amikacin, ampicillin sodium, codeine phosphate, dobutamine, erythromycin glucceptate, erythromycin lactobionate, gentamicin, hyaluronidase, hydrocortisone sodium succinate, hydroxyzine hydrochloride, kanamycin, levorphanol tartrate, meperidine, methadone, morphine, oxytetracycline, penicillin G sodium, polymyxin B, prochlorperazine edisylate, promethazine hydrochloride, ⅙ M sodium lactate, streptomycin sulfate, tetracycline hydrochloride, and vancomycin.

May also be incompatible with solutions containing a phosphate buffer, sodium carbonate, or sodium oxalate.

ADVERSE REACTIONS

Life-threatening: acute thrombocytopenia, anaphylaxis, gasping syndrome in neonates, new thrombus formation (white clot syndrome), severe hemorrhage.
Other: allergic vasospastic reaction, alopecia (delayed, transient), arthralgia, asthma (rare), chest pain, chills, cutaneous necrosis, fever, headache, hypertension, lacrimation, nausea, priapism, rebound hyperlipidemia, rhinitis, suppressed aldosterone synthesis and renal function, urticaria, vomiting.

INTERACTIONS

ACTH, corticosteroids, insulin: possible antagonized action.
Antihistamines, cardiac glycosides, nicotine, tetracyclines: diminished anticoagulant effect.
Aspirin, chloroquine, dextran, dipyridamole, hydrochloroquine, ibuprofen and other NSAIDs, indomethacin, penicillins (high doses), phenylbutazone: impaired platelet aggregation and possible heightened risk of bleeding.
Cefamandole, cefoperazone, moxalactam, plicamycin: possible platelet inhibition or damage and enhanced risk of bleeding.

Coumarin or indanedione anticoagulants: possible prolonged prothrombin time (PT).

Diazepam: possible increased levels.

Dihydroergotamine mesylate: potentiated heparin effects.

Nitroglycerin I.V.: possible diminished heparin effects.

Probenecid: possible increased and prolonged anticoagulant effect.

Streptokinase, urokinase: heightened risk of hemorrhage.

EFFECTS ON DIAGNOSTIC TESTS

Activated coagulation time (ACT), APTT, plasma recalcification time, PT, thrombin time, whole blood clotting time: prolonged.

Arterial blood gas analysis: inaccurate measurement of carbon dioxide pressure, bicarbonate concentration, and base excess if heparin makes up 10% or more of sample.

Free fatty acids: possible elevated levels.

I^{125} fibrinogen uptake test: false-negative results.

Serum alkaline phosphatase, bilirubin, LDH, SGOT, SGPT: possible elevated levels.

Serum cholesterol, triglycerides: possible reduced levels.

Serum thyroxine: possible elevated levels when competitive protein-binding methods are used.

Sulfobromophthalein test: false-positive findings.

SPECIAL CONSIDERATIONS

• *Treatment of overdose:* Give 1% solution of protamine sulfate by slow infusion. Don't infuse more than 50 mg in any 10-minute period.

• Monitor the patient for bleeding, which may occur at any site and is often difficult to detect. Frequently monitor hematocrit and check stools for occult blood to detect asymptomatic bleeding.

• Frequently monitor platelet count and coagulation tests, such as PT, APTT, and ACT. The therapeutic range for APTT is 1½ to 2½ times the control value; for ACT, 2 to 3 times the control value.

• If signs of acute adrenal hemorrhage and insufficiency appear, discontinue heparin, give I.V. corticosteroids, and draw samples for plasma cortisol determinations.

• If white clot syndrome or severe thrombocytopenia occurs, promptly discontinue heparin and substitute a coumarin anticoagulant.

• Observe bleeding precautions. Test all exudates for blood, regularly inspect I.V. and wound sites and the skin, and promote safety. Teach the patient the signs and symptoms of bleeding.

• Exercise caution when transfusing blood collected in heparin sodium and later converted to acid-citrate-dextrose blood because this may alter coagulation.

• Major bleeding episodes occur more frequently with intermittent infusion than with continuous infusion.

• Not removed by hemodialysis.

• Hep-Lock, Hep-Pak, and Liquaemin contain benzyl alcohol.

---

hetastarch
Hes, Hespan, Volex

Pregnancy Risk Category: C

COMPOSITION
A synthetic hydroxyethyl starch similar to human glycogen, hetastarch consists almost entirely of amylopectin. A hypertonic solution, hetastarch has a pH of 5.5 (adjusted with sodium hydroxide), an osmolarity of 310 mOsm, and an average

molecular weight of 450,000 daltons. Each commercially prepared bottle contains 77 mEq of sodium and 77 mEq of chloride.

INDICATIONS & DOSAGE
Dosage reflects amount of fluid loss and hemoconcentration.
• Plasma volume expansion and fluid replacement. *Adults:* 500 to 1,000 ml. Maximum daily infusion is 20 ml/kg, or 1,500 ml. In hemorrhagic shock, the maximum hourly infusion is 20 ml/kg. Lower dosages are used in burns and septic shock.

In mild to moderate renal impairment (creatinine clearance of less than 10 ml/minute), administer usual adult dosage initially. Expect to reduce subsequent dosages by 25% to 50%, depending on response. In severe renal impairment, infuse 0.3 to 0.6 g/kg/hour (5 to 10 ml/hour).
• Continuous flow centrifugation leukapheresis. *Adults:* 250 to 700 ml infused at a fixed ratio of 1 part hetastarch to 8 parts whole blood.

CONTRAINDICATIONS & CAUTIONS
• Manufacturer warns against use during pregnancy, especially the first trimester, unless the potential benefits outweigh the risk.
• Contraindicated in thrombocytopenia because the drug interferes with platelet function.
• Also contraindicated in elderly patients and in those with pulmonary edema, congestive heart failure, or renal impairment because of increased susceptibility to circulatory overload.
• Use cautiously in liver disease because hetastarch can raise indirect serum bilirubin levels.
• Safety and effectiveness in children haven't been established.

PREPARATION & STORAGE
Available in 500 ml ready-to-use, sterile, and nonpyrogenic bottles. Each bottle contains 6% hetastarch in 0.9% sodium chloride injection, but no preservative. Store at room temperature; avoid excessive heat or freezing.

Normally clear pale yellow to amber, the solution shouldn't be used if it turns a turbid deep brown or contains a crystalline precipitate. Discard any unused solution.

ADMINISTRATION
Direct injection: not recommended.
Intermittent infusion: not recommended.
Continuous infusion: Infuse at rate determined by patient's condition and therapeutic response.

INCOMPATIBILITY
Incompatible with ampicillin sodium.

ADVERSE REACTIONS
Life-threatening: anaphylaxis.
Other: chills, fever, headache, myalgia, parotid and submaxillary gland swelling, pruritus, vomiting.

INTERACTIONS
None reported.

EFFECTS ON DIAGNOSTIC TESTS
Bleeding time, clotting time, partial thromboplastin time, prothrombin time: possibly prolonged.
Erythrocyte sedimentation rate: possibly increased.
Fibrinogen: possible reduced levels.
Indirect serum bilirubin: possible elevated levels.
Serum albumin, calcium, total protein: possible reduced levels.
Serum amylase: possible increased levels.

Unmarked trade names available in the United States only.
♦ Also available in Canada.   ♦♦Available in Canada only.

SPECIAL CONSIDERATIONS

• Measure intake and output and report significant changes in their ratio. Also report oliguria.

• Monitor blood pressure and vital signs frequently, and check for signs of circulatory overload.

• Report dyspnea, wheezing, coughing, crackles, chest pressure, increased pulse and respirations, and elevated central venous pressure.

• Monitor hematocrit and notify the doctor if it drops appreciably.

• Observe patient for bruising or bleeding.

• If the patient's sodium intake is restricted, keep in mind that each bottle of hetastarch contains 77 mEq of sodium.

• Continuous flow centrifugation procedures, such as leukapheresis, using hetastarch up to twice weekly for 5 weeks have been reported safe and effective.

---

hydralazine hydrochloride
Apresoline Hydrochloride♦

Pregnancy Risk Category: C

PHARMACOKINETICS

Distribution: throughout tissues, with high concentrations in plasma, liver, kidneys, and arterial walls and low concentrations in heart, lungs, brain, muscle, and fat; 85% of drug binds to plasma proteins. Hydralazine crosses the placenta.

Metabolism: in the liver and GI mucosa, through acetylation, hydroxylation, and conjugation. Metabolites have no therapeutic effects.

Excretion: rapidly removed in urine, primarily as metabolites. Small amounts of drug appear in breast milk.

Action: onset, 10 to 20 minutes; duration, 3 to 8 hours.

MECHANISM OF ACTION

A phthalazine-derivative antihypertensive, hydralazine directly relaxes arterial smooth muscle (but has little effect on the veins), thereby reducing peripheral vascular resistance. Drug also increases heart rate and cardiac output, possibly as a compensatory response to decreased peripheral resistance.

INDICATIONS & DOSAGE

• Emergency treatment of hypertension. *Adults:* 10 to 40 mg, as needed. *Children:* 1.7 to 3.5 mg/kg q 4 to 6 hours. Maximum initial dose is 20 mg.

• Pregnancy-induced hypertension. *Adults:* 5 mg initially, then 5 to 10 mg q 20 to 30 minutes, as required.

CONTRAINDICATIONS & CAUTIONS

• Contraindicated in hydralazine hypersensitivity.

• Also contraindicated in dissecting aortic aneurysm and rheumatic disease affecting the mitral valve because the drug may exacerbate these conditions.

• Give hydralazine cautiously in patients with coronary artery disease because of possible myocardial ischemia.

• In patients with cerebrovascular accident or increased intracranial pressure (ICP), administer cautiously because cerebral ischemia may occur or worsen.

• Also administer cautiously and in reduced amounts in renal impairment.

PREPARATION & STORAGE

Available in 1 ml ampules with a concentration of 20 mg/ml. Store ampules at room temperature; don't freeze.

Avoid contact with metal syringe parts because discoloration and change in stability may result. Prepare just before use. Discard unused portion.

ADMINISTRATION
Direct injection: Inject undiluted drug directly into vein or as close to I.V. insertion site as possible. Give at rate of 10 mg/minute.
Intermittent infusion: not recommended.
Continuous infusion: not recommended.

INCOMPATIBILITY
Avoid mixing with any other drug in same container. Incompatible with aminophylline, ampicillin sodium, chlorothiazide, dextrose 10% in Ringer's lactate, dextrose 10% in 0.9% sodium chloride, edetate calcium disodium, ethacrynate sodium, fructose 10% in water, hydrocortisone sodium succinate, mephentermine sulfate, methohexital, nitroglycerin, phenobarbital sodium, and verapamil.

ADVERSE REACTIONS
Typically, adverse reactions are reversible when dose is reduced or drug discontinued.
Life-threatening: anaphylaxis, cerebral ischemia (in patients with elevated ICP), myocardial ischemia.
Other: angina pectoris, anorexia, anxiety, arthralgia, asthenia, blood dyscrasias (agranulocytosis, leukopenia, thrombocytopenia with or without purpura), chills, conjunctivitis, constipation, depression, diarrhea, disorientation, dizziness, dyspnea, dysrhythmias, edema, eosinophilia, fever, flushing, headache, hypotension, impotence, lacrimation, lymphadenopathy, malaise, muscle cramps, myalgia, nasal congestion, nausea, orthostatic hypotension, palpitations, paralytic ileus, peripheral neuritis, pleuritic chest pain, pruritus, rash, sodium retention, splenomegaly, systemic lupus erythematosus (SLE)–like syndrome, tachycardia, tremors, urticaria, vomiting, weakness, weight gain.

INTERACTIONS
Diazoxide, diuretics, MAO inhibitors: potentiated hypotensive effects.
Epinephrine: orthostatic hypotension resulting from reduced pressor response.
Estrogens, NSAIDs (especially indomethacin), sympathomimetics: possible antagonized hydralazine effects.

EFFECTS ON DIAGNOSTIC TESTS
Antinuclear antibody test, Coombs' test: possible positive response without signs of rheumatic disorder.
Hemoglobin level, RBC and WBC counts: reduced.

SPECIAL CONSIDERATIONS
• *Treatment of overdose:* Signs of overdose include dysrhythmias, headache, hypotension, shock, and tachycardia. Give volume expanders to support blood pressure; if a vasopressor is needed, select one that doesn't aggravate dysrhythmias. Digitalize the patient and monitor his renal function as needed.
• Check the patient's vital signs every 5 to 10 minutes for 1 hour, every hour for the next 2 hours, and then every 4 hours after injection. Continuously monitor EKG.
• Instruct the patient to report headache or chest pain. Headache and tachycardia are common; they can be minimized by starting with a small dose and gradually increasing dosage.
• Monitor the patient's CBC, LE cell preparation, and antinuclear an-

tibody titer before therapy and at regular intervals during prolonged use, to detect SLE-like syndrome. Discontinue drug if this syndrome develops.
• Discontinue drug if blood dyscrasias occur.
• Withdraw drug gradually in patients with marked reduction in blood pressure to avoid rebound hypertension.
• Control sodium retention and weight gain with a thiazide diuretic.
• Slow acetylation increases the risk of adverse reactions.
• Use of a beta blocker and diuretic may prevent myocardial ischemia in patients with coronary artery disease who must receive hydralazine.

hydrochloric acid, dilute

Pregnancy Risk Category: C

PHARMACOKINETICS
Distribution: unknown.
Metabolism: unknown.
Excretion: unknown.
Action: variable.

MECHANISM OF ACTION
Hydrochloric acid (HCl) replaces gastric acid by stimulating H + -sensitive peripheral or central chemoreceptors.

INDICATIONS & DOSAGE
• Severe systemic metabolic alkalosis. *Adults:* 150 ml/liter of isotonic fluid; may be repeated once. Or dosage may reflect chloride deficit. To calculate the HCl dose, multiply 0.2 liters/kg by the patient's body weight (in kg). Then multiply the product by the difference obtained by subtracting the patient's serum chloride level from 103.

CONTRAINDICATIONS & CAUTIONS
• Contraindicated in metabolic acidosis.

PREPARATION & STORAGE
A clear, colorless solution, HCl has a pungent odor. Store below 86° F. (30° C.) in a sealed, sterile glass container.
    Exercise extreme caution when handling because the drug is corrosive and irritating and can cause burns.

ADMINISTRATION
Direct injection: not recommended.
Intermittent infusion: not recommended.
Continuous infusion: Give total concentration over 12 to 24 hours, preferably through a central venous line.

INCOMPATIBILITY
No incompatibilities reported.

ADVERSE REACTIONS
Life-threatening: acidosis.
Other: hyperventilation.

INTERACTIONS
None reported.

EFFECTS ON DIAGNOSTIC TESTS
None reported.

SPECIAL CONSIDERATIONS
• Monitor arterial blood gas, BUN, and serum electrolyte levels every 4 hours during infusion.
• HCl is used when sodium or potassium chlorides are contraindicated; when hepatic failure precludes safe use of ammonium chloride or arginine chloride; or in severe renal failure.

hydrocortisone sodium phosphate
Hydrocortone Phosphate

hydrocortisone sodium succinate
A-HydroCort, Lifocort-100, Solu-Cortef

Pregnancy Risk Category: C

PHARMACOKINETICS
Distribution: rapidly dispersed to muscles, liver, skin, intestines, and kidneys. Extensively bound to plasma proteins.
Metabolism: metabolized in the liver to inactive compounds; also in the kidneys and in most tissues.
Excretion: inactive metabolites removed by kidneys as glucuronides and sulfates. Small amounts of unmetabolized drug are excreted in urine and negligible amounts in bile. Drug appears in breast milk.
Action: onset, rapid; duration, varies with dosage and duration of therapy.

MECHANISM OF ACTION
A naturally occurring corticosteroid, hydrocortisone affects virtually all body systems. Given systemically, it decreases inflammation by stabilizing leukocyte lysosomal membranes. It also suppresses pituitary release of corticotropin; so the adrenal cortex stops secreting corticosteroids.

INDICATIONS & DOSAGE
• Severe inflammation, adrenal insufficiency. *Adults:* depending on disease, 15 to 240 mg of hydrocortisone sodium phosphate daily; or 100 to 500 mg of hydrocortisone sodium succinate initially, repeated q 2 to 10 hours, as needed. *Children:* 0.16 to 1 mg/kg or 6 to 30 mg/m² of hydrocortisone sodium succinate.

• Shock. *Adults:* 50 mg/kg of hydrocortisone sodium succinate initially, repeated in 4 hours or q 24 hours. Alternatively, 0.5 to 2 g initially, repeated q 2 to 6 hours, as required.

CONTRAINDICATIONS & CAUTIONS
• Use cautiously in hypothyroidism or cirrhosis because an exaggerated drug response may occur.
• Also use cautiously in seizure disorders because of an increased risk of seizures; in renal insufficiency because of a magnified risk of edema; in osteoporosis because of possible exacerbation; and in patients with a history of tuberculosis because of possible disease reactivation.
• Because drug may mask infection, give it cautiously in recent intestinal anastomosis or in diverticulitis or nonspecific ulcerative colitis if patient is at risk for perforation, abscess, or other pyogenic infection.
• In patients with uncontrolled viral or bacterial infections, give drug carefully; it may mask infection and increase susceptibility to it.
• In children, give carefully because of possible bone growth retardation, pancreatitis and pancreatic destruction, and increased intracranial pressure, resulting in papilledema, oculomotor or abducens nerve paralysis, vision loss, and headache.

PREPARATION & STORAGE
Hydrocortisone sodium phosphate is available in 2 and 10 ml multidose vials and 2 ml disposable syringes, with concentrations of 50 mg/ml.
   Available in 100 mg vials that require reconstitution with no more than 2 ml of bacteriostatic water for injection or bacteriostatic 0.9% sodium chloride for injection. Drug is also supplied in 100 mg, 250 mg, 500 mg, and 1 g containers that require dilution with dextrose 5% in

water, 0.9% sodium chloride, or dextrose 5% in 0.9% sodium chloride to a concentration of 0.1 to 1 mg/ml.

Store solutions at 77° F. (25° C.) or below for up to 3 days. Discard thereafter or if solutions aren't clear.

ADMINISTRATION
Direct injection: Inject directly into vein or into an I.V. line containing a free-flowing compatible solution over 30 seconds to several minutes.
Intermittent infusion: Give diluted solution over prescribed duration.
Continuous infusion: Infuse diluted solution over 24 hours.

INCOMPATIBILITY
Incompatible with ampicillin sodium; amobarbital sodium; bleomycin; cephalothin sodium with aminophylline; colistimethate sodium; diazepam; dimenhydrinate; diphenhydramine; doxorubicin; ephedrine; ergotamine; fructose 10% in 0.9% sodium chloride; heparin sodium; hydralazine; Ionosol B, D, or G in invert sugar 10%; kanamycin; metaraminol; methicillin; nafcillin; oxytetracycline; pentobarbital sodium; phenobarbital sodium; prochlorperazine edisylate; promethazine hydrochloride; secobarbital sodium; tetracycline hydrochloride; vancomycin; and vitamin B complex with C.

ADVERSE REACTIONS
Life-threatening: anaphylaxis.
Other: acne, adrenal insufficiency, anorexia, cataracts, delayed wound healing, edema, euphoria, fever, fluid and electrolyte disturbances, glaucoma, headache, hyperglycemia, hypertension, hypokalemia, hypotension, infection, joint pain, lethargy, nausea, peptic ulcer, psychotic behavior, vomiting, weakness, weight loss.

INTERACTIONS
Alcohol, NSAIDs, ulcerogenic drugs: heightened risk of GI ulcers.
Amphotericin B, carbonic anhydrase inhibitors, potassium-depleting diuretics, other potassium-depleting drugs: possible enhanced potassium loss.
Anabolic steroids, androgens: increased risk of edema.
Anticholinesterase drugs: severe weakness in myasthenia gravis patients.
Anticoagulants, thrombolytics: altered effects and increased risk of GI ulcers or hemorrhage.
Antithyroid drugs, thyroid hormones: altered hydrocortisone removal. Adjust thyroid or antithyroid dosage.
Cardiac glycosides: heightened risk of toxicity or dysrhythmias.
Drugs that induce hepatic microsomal enzymes: possible enhanced hydrocortisone metabolism.
Ephedrine: increased hydrocortisone metabolism.
Estrogens, oral contraceptives: enhanced therapeutic and toxic effects of hydrocortisone.
Immunosuppressants: magnified risk of infection, lymphomas, or lymphoproliferative disorders.
Mexiletine: reduced serum levels.
Mitotane: suppressed adrenocortical function. Give higher hydrocortisone dosages if necessary.
Nondepolarizing neuromuscular blocking drugs: enhanced neuromuscular blockade.
Potassium-sparing diuretics, potassium supplements: diminished hypokalemic effects of hydrocortisone.
Sodium-containing foods, drugs: possible hypernatremia.
Streptozocin: heightened risk of hyperglycemia.
Toxoids, vaccines: diminished response.

EFFECTS ON DIAGNOSTIC TESTS

ACTH stimulation test, plasma cortisol: possible decreased levels.

Basophil, eosinophil, lymphocyte, monocyte counts: possible decline.

Gonadorelin test: altered results.

Nitroblue tetrazolium test: possible false-negative results.

Platelet count: increased or decreased.

Polymorphonuclear leukocyte count: possible rise.

Protein-bound iodine and serum calcium, potassium, thyroxine: possible reduced levels.

Radioactive iodine test: reduced uptake of ^{123}I or ^{131}I.

Radionuclide brain and bone scans: diminished uptake of sodium pertechnetate Tc 99m or technetium Tc 99m gluceptate, pentetate, medronate, oxidronate, or pyrophosphate.

Serum cholesterol, fatty acids: possible increased levels.

Serum glucose, urine glucose: possible elevated levels.

Serum sodium, uric acid: possible heightened levels.

Skin tests: possible suppressed reaction.

Urine 17-hydroxycorticosteroids, urine 17-ketosteroids: possible diminished levels.

SPECIAL CONSIDERATIONS

• Before long-term therapy, evaluate baseline EKGs, blood pressure, chest and spinal X-rays, glucose tolerance tests, serum potassium levels, and hypothalamic and pituitary function.

• Instruct the patient to report any signs of infection during therapy and for 12 months after it.

• Diabetic patients may need an adjustment in antidiabetic drug dosage because of hydrocortisone's hyperglycemic effects.

• Increased protein intake may be needed to keep pace with drug-induced protein catabolism.

• Give a phenothiazine or lithium for depression or psychotic behavior.

• Avoid abrupt withdrawal after high-dose therapy.

• Adrenal recovery may occur within 1 week after short-term therapy.

• Hydrocortone Phosphate contains sulfites. A-HydroCort and Solu-Cortef contain benzyl alcohol.

---

hydromorphone hydrochloride
Dilaudid♦, Dilaudid HP♦

Controlled Substance Schedule II
Pregnancy Risk Category: C

PHARMACOKINETICS

Distribution: throughout body tissues, with highest concentrations in skeletal muscle, kidneys, liver, intestines, lungs, spleen, and brain. Drug readily crosses the placenta.

Metabolism: chiefly metabolized in the liver but also altered in the CNS, kidneys, lungs, and placenta. At all sites, drug undergoes conjugation with glucuronic acid, hydrolysis, oxidation, or N-dealkylation to form metabolites.

Excretion: in urine, primarily as unchanged drug. Small amounts of drug and its metabolites are also eliminated in feces.

Action: onset, 10 to 15 minutes; duration, 2 to 3 hours.

MECHANISM OF ACTION

Hydromorphone binds with opiate receptors throughout the CNS, altering the perception of pain and the emotional response to it.

INDICATIONS & DOSAGE

• Moderate to severe pain. *Adults:* 0.5 to 1 mg as needed for moderate pain; 3 to 4 mg q 4 to 6 hours for severe pain.

CONTRAINDICATIONS & CAUTIONS

• Contraindicated in known hypersensitivity to hydromorphone.
• Also contraindicated in diarrhea caused by poisons or toxins because drug may slow GI motility, decreasing elimination of toxins.
• Avoid use in acute respiratory depression because of possible exacerbation.
• In patients with head injury and increased intracranial pressure (ICP), use hydromorphone carefully because it can mask changes in level of consciousness and further raise ICP.
• Give the drug cautiously in acute abdominal conditions because of possibly unreliable assessment findings; in respiratory impairment because of reduced respiratory drive and increased airway resistance; in hepatic or renal impairment because of slowed drug clearance; in gallbladder disease because of drug-induced biliary contraction; and in severe inflammatory bowel disease because of the heightened risk of toxic megacolon.
• In patients with a history of drug dependence or emotional instability, administer carefully because of the risk of dependence.
• Because hydromorphone can cause urinary retention, use it cautiously in prostatic hypertrophy or urethral stricture and after recent urinary tract surgery.
• Also use cautiously after recent GI surgery because of slowed GI motility.
• In patients with dysrhythmias or a history of seizures, give hydromor-
phone carefully because of possible exacerbation.
• Because of the risk of respiratory depression and prolonged CNS depression, administer drug carefully to elderly patients and to patients with hypothyroidism or Addison's disease.
• Because of possible potentiated hypotension, give drug carefully in hypovolemia.
• Safety and efficacy haven't been established for children.

PREPARATION & STORAGE

Available in preservative-containing multidose vials and syringes in concentrations of 1, 2, 3, 4, and 10 mg/ml. Also available in preservative-free ampules in a concentration of 2 mg/ml.

Dilution isn't necessary, but most common I.V. solutions may be used as diluents. Store between 59° and 86° F. (15° and 30° C.). Protect from freezing and light. Slight yellowish tint may develop but doesn't indicate loss of potency.

ADMINISTRATION

Keep in mind that rapid administration has been associated with anaphylaxis, respiratory failure, and cardiac arrest.
Direct injection: Inject directly into a vein or into an I.V. line containing a free-flowing compatible solution over 2 to 3 minutes, especially if the 10 mg/ml preparation is used.
Intermittent infusion: Give diluted drug over prescribed duration.
Continuous infusion: Using an infusion pump, give at the ordered dilution and rate.

INCOMPATIBILITY

Incompatible with alkalies, bromides, iodides, prochlorperazine edisylate, sodium bicarbonate, and thiopental.

Unmarked trade names available in the United States only.
♦ Also available in Canada.   ♦ ♦ Available in Canada only.

ADVERSE REACTIONS

Life-threatening: apnea, bradycardia, hypotension, tachycardia.

Other: anorexia; anxiety; blurred or double vision; cold, clammy skin; confusion; constipation; diaphoresis; dizziness; drowsiness; dry mouth; euphoria; facial flushing; faintness; unusual fatigue or weakness; headache; malaise; nausea; pinpoint pupils; seizures; urinary retention; vomiting.

INTERACTIONS

Antidiarrheals, antiperistaltics: heightened risk of severe constipation and CNS depression.

Antihypertensives: increased risk of orthostatic hypotension.

Antimuscarinics: magnified risk of severe constipation, paralytic ileus, or urinary retention.

Buprenorphine: reduced therapeutic effects of hydromorphone if given before it; also, depending on dose, possible reversal or potentiation of respiratory depression and precipitation or suppression of narcotic withdrawal symptoms.

Diuretics: heightened risk of orthostatic hypotension; antagonized effects in congestive heart failure.

Metoclopramide: slowed GI motility.

Naloxone, naltrexone: antagonized analgesic, CNS, and respiratory depressant effects of hydromorphone.

Neuromuscular blocking agents: possible deepened respiratory depression.

Other CNS depressants, hydroxyzine, MAO inhibitors, opioid agonists: possible potentiated CNS, respiratory, and hypotensive effects.

Scorpion venoms: potentiated effects of *Centruroides sculpturatus Ewing* and *C. gertschi stahnke.*

EFFECTS ON DIAGNOSTIC TESTS

Gastric emptying studies: possible delayed gastric emptying.

Hepatobiliary imaging: delayed or misleading visualization because hydromorphone may constrict the sphincter of Oddi and raise biliary tract pressure, as in common bile duct obstruction.

Lumbar puncture: increased cerebrospinal fluid pressure secondary to carbon dioxide retention.

Serum amylase, lipase: unreliable results for up to 24 hours after hydromorphone administration.

SPECIAL CONSIDERATIONS

• *Treatment of overdose:* Maintain airway patency and provide respiratory support. Give 0.4 mg of naloxone by I.V. push, as needed, to reverse respiratory depression. Administer I.V. fluids and vasopressors to maintain blood pressure.

• Monitor respiratory status frequently for at least 1 hour after dose. Keep resuscitation equipment and naloxone readily available. If respiratory rate drops below 8 breaths/minute, arouse patient to stimulate breathing. Notify the doctor; naloxone or respiratory support may be ordered.

• Check access site before giving drug by I.V. push. Local tissue irritation can occur with infiltration.

• Give drug with patient lying down, to minimize hypotensive effects. After administration, tell him to get up slowly to reduce dizziness and avoid fainting.

• Because hydromorphone can cause drowsiness, advise patient to avoid activities that require alertness.

• Give smallest effective dose to reduce tolerance and physical dependence. However, high doses may be required for severe chronic or cancer

pain. Adjust dosage based on patient response and severity of pain.
• Give concentrate (10 mg/ml) only to patients tolerant of opiate agonists who are receiving high doses.
• Duration of effects lengthens with repeated doses because of drug accumulation.
• Habituation and psychic dependence can develop with long-term use.
• If necessary, reduce dosage in elderly patients, in patients with renal or hepatic impairment, and in those receiving other opioid analgesics.
• Monitor shock patient (overdose may occur when circulation is restored).
• Atropine may control bradycardia or other cholinergic effects.
• Assess bowel function. A stool softener may be indicated.

---

hyoscyamine sulfate
Levsin

Pregnancy Risk Category: C

PHARMACOKINETICS
Distribution: throughout the body, with 50% bound to plasma proteins. Drug crosses the blood-brain barrier and, in small amounts, the placenta.
Metabolism: by the liver to the metabolites tropic acid, tropine, and hyoscyamine glucuronide.
Excretion: in urine, with about 30% to 50% removed unchanged. Phases of biphasic half-life last for about 3½ and 12½ hours in normal renal function, longer in renal impairment. Small amounts of drug appear in breast milk.
Action: onset, 2 to 3 minutes; duration, up to 4 hours.

MECHANISM OF ACTION
Hyoscyamine competitively inhibits the muscarinic effects of acetylcholine and other cholinergic stimuli on autonomic effectors innervated by postganglionic cholinergic nerves. Drug curtails GI secretions and motility, diminishes tone and amplitude of ureter and bladder contraction, and reduces nasal, oropharyngeal, and bronchial secretions.

INDICATIONS & DOSAGE
• Adjunctive treatment of peptic ulcer disease. *Adults:* 0.25 to 0.5 mg q 4 hours, three to four times a day.
• Acute GI symptoms. *Adults:* 0.25 to 0.5 mg as a single dose.
• Preoperative reduction of salivation and respiratory secretions.
Adults and children age 2 and over: 5 mcg/kg, 30 to 60 minutes before induction of anesthesia.
• Prevention of cholinergic effects during surgery. *Adults:* 0.125 mg, repeated as needed.
• Treatment of muscarinic toxicity. *Adults:* 1 to 2 mg initially, then 1 mg q 3 to 10 minutes until symptoms subside.
• Blockage of adverse muscarinic effects. *Adults:* 0.2 mg for each 1 mg of neostigmine or equivalent dose of physostigmine or pyridostigmine.
• Reduction of duodenal motility in GI radiographic procedures. *Adults:* 0.25 to 0.5 mg 5 to 10 minutes before procedure.

CONTRAINDICATIONS & CAUTIONS
• Contraindicated in hyoscyamine or other anticholinergic drug hypersensitivity.
• Also contraindicated in severe ulcerative colitis, toxic megacolon, obstructive GI disease, cardiospasm, paralytic ileus, and intestinal atony because drug diminishes intestinal motility and heightens the risk of obstruction; in angle-closure glaucoma because drug may raise intra-

---

ocular pressure; in obstructive uropathy or prostatic hypertrophy because urinary retention may worsen; in myasthenia gravis because drug may exacerbate the condition; and in tachycardia stemming from cardiac insufficiency, thyrotoxicosis, or acute hemorrhage with unstable cardiovascular status because drug may block vagal inhibition of sinoatrial node.

• Use hyoscyamine cautiously in febrile patients and those exposed to high temperatures because of the risk of hyperthermia.

• In children, especially those under age 2, administer the drug carefully because of the heightened risk of adverse reactions. In children with brain damage, give carefully because CNS effects may be exacerbated. In those with spastic paralysis, also give carefully because of a possible increased response to drug.

• In Down's syndrome, administer hyoscyamine carefully because of the risk of tachycardia.

• Give the drug cautiously to elderly patients because it may cause paradoxical excitement, agitation, increased drowsiness, or acute glaucoma.

• Use hyoscyamine cautiously in hyperthyroidism because tachycardia may worsen; in hypertension because of possible aggravation; in tachydysrhythmias, congestive heart failure, or coronary artery disease because the drug will block vagal effects at the sinoatrial node; in hepatic or renal impairment because of the heightened risk of adverse reactions; and in chronic pulmonary disease because the drug may promote bronchial mucous plug formation.

• Use with caution in esophageal reflux or hiatal hernia because the drug promotes gastric retention and aggravates reflux; in gastric ulcer because delayed gastric emptying may cause antral stasis; in known or suspected GI infection because diminished GI motility prolongs retention of causative organisms or toxins; in diarrhea because this sign may be an early indicator of intestinal obstruction; and in mild or moderate ulcerative colitis because decreased GI motility may produce paralytic ileus or toxic megacolon.

• Administer hyoscyamine carefully in autonomic or partial obstructive uropathy because drug may aggravate or precipitate urinary retention.

• Use cautiously in xerostomia because salivary flow may be further curtailed.

PREPARATION & STORAGE
Available in 1 and 10 ml vials, with a concentration of 0.5 mg/ml. Store in tight, light-resistant containers at room temperature. Drug is compatible with dextrose 5% in water, dextrose 5% in Ringer's lactate, and 0.9% sodium chloride.

ADMINISTRATION
Direct injection: Inject directly into vein or into an I.V. line containing a free-flowing compatible solution at prescribed rate.
Intermittent infusion: not recommended.
Continuous infusion: not recommended.

INCOMPATIBILITY
Incompatible with metaraminol bitartrate, methohexital sodium, norepinephrine bitartrate, and sodium bicarbonate.

ADVERSE REACTIONS
Most adverse reactions are dose-related.
Life-threatening: anaphylaxis, respiratory paralysis.
Other: anhidrosis, bloated sensation, blurred vision, breathing difficulty,

confusion, constipation, cycloplegia, decreased lactation, dizziness, drowsiness, dysphagia, dysuria, excitement, fever, flushing, headache, hypertension, hypotension, increased ocular tension, insomnia, loss of taste, memory loss (especially in elderly patients), mydriasis, nausea, palpitations, marked photophobia, rash, tachycardia, thirst, urinary hesitancy or retention, urticaria, vomiting, weakness, xerostomia.

INTERACTIONS

Alphaprodine, amantadine, antidyskinetics, antihistamines, disopyramide, quinidine: additive anticholinergic effects.
Antimyasthenics: reduced intestinal motility.
Antipsychotics, benzodiazepines, glutethimide, MAO inhibitors, phenothiazines, tricyclic antidepressants: additive anticholinergic effects.
Cyclopropane anesthetics: ventricular dysrhythmias.
Guanadrel, guanethidine, reserpine: antagonized inhibitory action of hyoscyamine on gastric acid.
Ketoconazole: impaired absorption because of increased gastric pH.
Metoclopramide: antagonized effect on GI motility.
Opioid analgesics: heightened risk of severe constipation and additive anticholinergic effects.
Potassium chloride (wax-matrix preparations, Slow-K): increased severity of GI mucosal lesions.
Urinary alkalizers (such as antacids, carbonic anhydrase inhibitors): delayed excretion.

EFFECTS ON DIAGNOSTIC TESTS

Gastric acid secretion test: antagonized effects of pentagastrin.

SPECIAL CONSIDERATIONS

• ***Treatment of overdose:*** Provide symptomatic and supportive care. Physostigmine can be used as an antidote but this practice is controversial.
• For peptic ulcer therapy, follow I.V. dose with I.M. or S.C. administration.
• Monitor intake, output, vital signs, and bowel habits.
• Encourage good oral hygiene. Provide gum or sugarless candy to help relieve dry mouth.
• Elderly patients usually require lower dosages.
• Avoid giving drug for 24 hours before gastric acid secretion tests.

---

ifosfamide
Haloxan, Isophosphamide

Investigational Drug
Pregnancy Risk Category: D

PHARMACOKINETICS
Distribution: throughout the body and across the placenta.
Metabolism: in the liver by microsomal enzymes. Drug must be metabolized to be active.
Excretion: in urine, with 50% to 60% removed unchanged and the remainder excreted as metabolites. Half-life is about 15 hours for high doses and 6 to 7 hours for low ones. Not known if drug appears in breast milk.
Action: peak serum level, immediately upon administration.

MECHANISM OF ACTION
An alkylating agent, ifosfamide interferes with cell division primarily by cross-linking strands of DNA.

INDICATIONS & DOSAGE

● Germ cell testicular cancers, soft tissue sarcomas, pancreatic and lung carcinoma. *Adults:* 1,200 mg/m^2 for 5 consecutive days. Repeat q 3 weeks or after recovery from hematologic toxicity (platelets ≥ 100,000/mcl, WBC > 4,000/mcl). Administer with mesna, a protective agent used to prevent hemorrhagic cystitis.

CONTRAINDICATIONS & CAUTIONS

● Use cautiously in patients with renal impairment, with previous or current radiation therapy, with severely depressed bone marrow, or with hypersensitivity to drug.

PREPARATION & STORAGE

Use caution when preparing and giving drug because of mutagenic, teratogenic, and carcinogenic risks. Use a biological containment cabinet, and wear gloves and mask. If drug comes in contact with skin or mucosa, immediately wash the area with soap and water. Use syringes with tight fittings (Luer-lok) to prevent leakage of solution, and correctly dispose of needles, syringes, vials, and unused drug. Avoid contaminating work surfaces.

Drug is available as an off-white powder in 1 and 3 g vials. Vials remain stable for 5 years if refrigerated. Reconstitute the 1 g vial with 20 ml of sterile water, yielding a concentration of 50 mg/ml. Reconstitute the 3 g vial with 30 ml of sterile water for a concentration of 100 mg/ml.

For intermittent infusion, dilute with at least 75 ml of sterile 0.9% sodium chloride. For continuous infusion, dilute with ordered amount of sterile 0.9% sodium chloride. Use within 8 hours because vials don't contain preservatives.

ADMINISTRATION

Direct injection: not recommended.
Intermittent infusion: Using a 23G or 25G winged-tip needle, infuse solution over at least 30 minutes. Use a new I.V. site for each infusion, if possible.
Continuous infusion: Give solution over 24 hours.

INCOMPATIBILITY

No incompatibilities reported.

ADVERSE REACTIONS

Life-threatening: none reported.
Other: alopecia, confusion, lethargy, myelosuppression, nausea, urologic toxicity, vomiting.

INTERACTIONS

Allopurinol: possible worsened myelosuppression.
Chloral hydrate, phenobarbital, phenytoin: enhanced ifosfamide conversion to active and toxic metabolites.
Cisplatin: synergistic effect.
Corticosteroids: possible impaired metabolism and diminished effectiveness of ifosfamide.
Succinylcholine: possible increased effects.

EFFECTS ON DIAGNOSTIC TESTS

Serum alkaline phosphatase, SGOT, SGPT: elevated levels.

SPECIAL CONSIDERATIONS

● Maintain daily fluid intake of at least 2 liters during and after therapy to reduce risk of urologic toxicity. Along with increased fluids, use of oral ascorbic acid, 250 mg t.i.d. and 500 mg h.s., further reduces toxicity risk.
● Warn the patient to report immediately signs of urologic toxicity, such as hematuria, dysuria, and burning on urination.

---

imipenem/cilastatin sodium
Primaxin

Pregnancy Risk Category: C

PHARMACOKINETICS
Distribution: widely and rapidly distributed throughout the body. Low concentrations appear in CSF. Both imipenem and cilastatin cross the placenta.
Metabolism: when given alone, imipenem is hydrolyzed in the proximal renal tubule. Cilastatin is partly metabolized by the kidneys but prevents imipenem metabolism.
Excretion: 5% to 40% of imipenem is excreted by kidneys when given alone; 70% to 78% of cilastatin is removed by kidneys when given alone. When given together, 70% to 76% is excreted by kidneys, 20% to 25% by an unknown nonrenal mechanism, and up to 2% in bile. Elimination half-life is about 1 hour. Not known if drugs appear in breast milk.
Action: peak serum level, about 20 minutes.

MECHANISM OF ACTION
Imipenem joins with penicillin-binding proteins to inhibit bacterial cell wall synthesis. The broadest-spectrum antibiotic available, it's effective against most gram-positive cocci, including staphylococci and *Streptococcus pneumoniae*. It's also used against such gram-positive and gram-negative organisms as *Acinetobacter, Bacteroides, Bifidobacterium, Citrobacter, Clostridium, Enterobacter, Escherichia coli, Eubacterium, Fusobacterium, Gardnerella vaginalis,* Group B and D streptococci, *Haemophilus influenzae, Klebsiella, Morganella morganii, Peptococcus, Peptostreptococcus, Pseudomonas aeruginosa,* and *Serratia*.

Cilastatin inhibits renal hydrolysis of imipenem, thus raising urine concentrations of active imipenem. Cilastatin has no antibacterial activity and doesn't affect imipenem's mechanism of action.

INDICATIONS & DOSAGE
• Infections of the lower respiratory tract, urinary tract, intra-abdominal infections, gynecologic infections, bone and joint infections, skin and skin structure infections, bacterial septicemia, endocarditis, and polymicrobic infections involving susceptible organisms. *Adults and children over age 12 with normal renal function:* 250 to 500 mg q 6 hours for mild infections; 500 mg or 1 g q 6 to 8 hours for severe infections. Maximum daily dosage is 4 g or 50 mg/kg, whichever is lower.
Adults and children over age 12 with impaired renal function: Dosage based on creatinine clearance. If creatinine clearance is 30 to 70 ml/minute, give 500 mg q 6 to 8 hours; if 20 to 29 ml/minute, 500 mg q 8 to 12 hours; and if less than 20 ml/minute, 250 to 500 mg q 12 hours.

CONTRAINDICATIONS & CAUTIONS
• Contraindicated in hypersensitivity to either imipenem or cilastatin. Use cautiously in patients with hypersensitivity to cephalosporins or penicillins or who have a history of seizure disorders or multiple allergies.
• Give cautiously to elderly patients and to patients with renal impairment or CNS disorders because of an increased risk of toxicity.
• Also give cautiously to patients with GI disorders (particularly colitis) because of increased risk of pseudomembranous colitis.

PREPARATION & STORAGE

Available as a white or yellow powder in 13 ml vials and 120 ml infusion bottles. These contain 250 mg imipenem and 250 mg cilastatin or 500 mg imipenem and 500 mg cilastatin. Reconstitute 13 ml vial with 10 ml of a compatible solution, such as 0.9% sodium chloride, dextrose 5% or 10% in water, dextrose 5% in 0.9% sodium chloride, or dextrose 5% in 0.02% sodium bicarbonate. Shake until dissolved. Using a new needle, transfer reconstituted solution into container of remaining 90 ml of solution. Reconstitute 120 ml vial with 100 ml of compatible diluent.

Solutions containing 0.9% sodium chloride as sole diluent and having a concentration no greater than 5 mg/ml remain stable for 4 hours at room temperature or for 24 hours when refrigerated. Other solutions remain stable half as long. Solutions may turn deep yellow. Discard if brown.

ADMINISTRATION

Direct injection: not recommended.
Intermittent infusion: Give diluted solution into an I.V. line containing a free-flowing compatible solution. Infuse 250 or 500 mg doses over 20 to 30 minutes and 1 g doses over 40 to 60 minutes. Reduce rate if nausea, vomiting, hypotension, dizziness, or sweating occurs.
Continuous infusion: not recommended.

INCOMPATIBILITY

Do not mix drug with any other antibiotics.

ADVERSE REACTIONS

Life-threatening: anaphylaxis.
Other: abdominal pain, acute renal failure, agranulocytosis, bacterial and fungal superinfection, confusion, diarrhea, dizziness, dyspnea, encephalopathy, eosinophilia, erythema multiforme, facial edema and flushing, glossitis, headache, heartburn, hyperventilation, hypotension, increased salivation, leukocytosis, leukopenia, myoclonus, nausea, neutropenia, oliguria, palpitations, paresthesias, pharyngeal pain, phlebitis, pseudomembranous colitis, psychic disturbances, rash, seizures, somnolence, tachycardia, thrombocytopenia, thrombocytosis, thrombophlebitis, tinnitus, tremor, urticaria, vertigo, vomiting.

INTERACTIONS

Aminoglycosides: possible synergistic effect when given concomitantly.
Other beta-lactam antibiotics: antagonized effects.
Probenecid: decreased excretion of imipenem/cilastatin sodium.

EFFECTS ON DIAGNOSTIC TESTS

BUN, serum creatinine: increased levels.
Coombs' test: positive findings.
Electrolytes: decreased sodium levels; increased potassium and chloride levels.
Hematocrit, hemoglobin level: reduced.
Prothrombin time: prolonged.
Serum alkaline phosphatase, bilirubin, LDH, SGOT, SGPT: elevated levels.
Urinalysis: proteinuria, urine casts, RBCs or WBCs in urine.
Urine glucose: false-positive results when tested with cupric sulfate (Benedict's solution, Clinitest).

SPECIAL CONSIDERATIONS

• Treat overdose symptomatically. Hemodialysis can reduce drug blood levels.
• Check for previous penicillin or cephalosporin hypersensitivity before first dose. Negative history doesn't rule out future allergic reaction.

• Obtain specimens for culture and sensitivity testing before first dose. Therapy may start before results are available.

• If diarrhea persists during therapy, discontinue drug and collect stool specimens for culture to rule out pseudomembranous colitis.

• If patient has a history of seizures, monitor anticonvulsant drug levels carefully. Keep in mind that the risk of seizures rises when imipenem doses exceed 2 g daily.

• Monitor BUN and serum creatinine levels to assess renal function.

• Reduce dosage in renal impairment if needed.

• When used with other anti-infectives, monitor for signs of bacterial or fungal superinfection.

• When administering with aminoglycosides, use separate solution containers. However, drug can be infused through same I.V. line.

• Use Clinistix or Tes-Tape for urine glucose determinations to avoid spurious results.

• If the patient is undergoing hemodialysis, give a supplemental dose after the treatment unless the next dose is scheduled within 4 hours.

• If the patient has sodium restrictions, keep in mind that each gram of imipenem and cilastatin contains 3.2 mEq (75.2 mg) of sodium.

---

immune globulin
Gamimune N, Gammagard, Sandoglobulin

Pregnancy Risk Category: C

PHARMACOKINETICS
Distribution: remains in intravascular space. Probably crosses the placenta.
Metabolism: not metabolized.

Excretion: not excreted; cleared by the spleen. Drug appears in breast milk. Half-life is 21 to 24 days.
Action: highly variable—onset, 1 to 5 days; duration, 2 to 4 weeks.

MECHANISM OF ACTION
Provides passive immunity by increasing antibody titer and antigen-antibody reaction potential.

INDICATIONS & DOSAGE
• Immunodeficiency diseases, such as congenital agammaglobulinemia, common variable hypogammaglobulinemia, X-linked immunodeficiency with hyper-IgM, and combined immunodeficiency. *Adults:* 200 to 400 mg/kg of Gammagard monthly, with dosage adjusted to ensure adequate serum IgG levels; 100 to 200 mg/kg or 2 to 4 ml/kg of Gamimune N monthly, or up to 400 mg/kg or 8 ml/kg monthly or more frequently to ensure adequate serum IgG levels; 200 mg/kg of Sandoglobulin monthly, or up to 300 mg/kg monthly or more frequently to ensure adequate serum IgG levels.

• Idiopathic thrombocytopenic purpura. *Adults and children:* 400 mg/kg of Gamimune N or Sandoglobulin daily for 5 days. Maintenance dosage, 400 mg/kg of Gamimune N once every several weeks, or 1 g/kg daily for 3 days.

CONTRAINDICATIONS & CAUTIONS
• Contraindicated in hypersensitivity to immune globulin.

• Also contraindicated in certain IgA deficiencies because of the heightened risk of anaphylaxis.

• Use Gamimune N cautiously in patients with compromised acid-base compensatory mechanisms because it has a pH of 4 to 4.5.

PREPARATION & STORAGE

Produced by different isolation and purification methods, each immune globulin has a different constitution. Gammagard contains about 50 mg of protein/ml and no less than 90% IgG. Gamimune N contains 50 mg of protein/ml and no less than 96% IgG; Sandoglobulin contains no less than 96% IgG.

Before use, refrigerate Gamimune N at 36° to 46° F. (2° to 8° C.). May be diluted in 5% dextrose, but don't use solution that has been frozen.

Before reconstitution, refrigerate Gammagard at 36° to 46° F. Reconstitute with sterile water for injection (make sure the powder and sterile water have been warmed to room temperature). Use the transfer device provided to prepare a solution containing 50 mg of protein/ml. Administer as soon as possible after reconstitution.

Before reconstitution, store Sandoglobulin at room temperature, below 77° F. (25° C.). Reconstitute with the 0.9% sodium chloride provided to prepare a solution containing 30 or 60 mg of protein/ml. Use promptly.

Don't administer turbid solutions. Discard unused drug.

ADMINISTRATION

Direct injection: not recommended.
Intermittent infusion: not recommended.
Continuous infusion: Infuse Gamimune N at a rate of 0.01 to 0.02 ml/kg/minute for 30 minutes. If no adverse reactions occur, increase up to 0.08 ml/kg/minute.

Give Gammagard using the manufacturer's administration set, which contains a 15-micron filter. Start at a rate of 0.5 ml/kg/hour and, if no adverse reactions occur, increase up to 4 ml/kg/hour.

Infuse initial dose of Sandoglobulin at a rate of 0.5 to 1 ml/minute for 15 to 30 minutes, increasing to 1.5 to 2.5 ml/minute. Give subsequent doses at a rate of 2 to 2.5 ml/minute. If additional high doses are necessary, infuse a 60 mg/ml solution at a rate of 1 to 1.5 ml/minute for 15 to 30 minutes, increasing up to 2.5 ml/minute.

INCOMPATIBILITY

Don't mix with other drugs or fluids.

ADVERSE REACTIONS

Life-threatening: none reported.
Other: chest tightness; chills; dyspnea; faintness; fatigue; fever; headache; hypotension; light-headedness; malaise; mild back, chest, or hip pain; nausea; vomiting. Gamimune N may also cause a burning sensation in the head, local reactions (such as erythema, pain, phlebitis, and eczema), mild diuresis, and tachycardia.

INTERACTIONS

Live-virus vaccine for measles, mumps, rubella (MMR): possible impaired response.

EFFECTS ON DIAGNOSTIC TESTS

IgG antibody screening tests: false-positive results.

SPECIAL CONSIDERATIONS

• Currently available preparations of immune globulin don't have a discernible risk of transmitting human immunodeficiency virus.
• Monitor vital signs continuously during infusion.
• Most adverse reactions are related to infusion rate. If patient becomes symptomatic, reduce rate. Use of corticosteroids before infusion may prevent adverse reactions.

• Signs of an allergic reaction may occur 30 to 60 minutes after the start of infusion.
• Don't give live-virus MMR vaccines for 2 weeks before or 6 weeks after giving immune globulin.
• Drug has been used to treat Kawasaki's disease, pediatric human immunodeficiency virus (HIV), cytomegalovirus infection, and neonatal sepsis.

indomethacin sodium trihydrate
Indocid PDA♦♦, Indocin I.V.

Pregnancy Risk Category: B (D in last trimester)

PHARMACOKINETICS
Distribution: throughout body tissues, with 99% bound to plasma proteins. Drug readily crosses the blood-brain barrier and placenta.
Metabolism: undergoes hepatic metabolism to glucuronide conjugates as well as to desmethyl and desbenzoyl derivatives and their metabolites. Some drug is N-deacylated by nonmicrosomal enzymes.
Excretion: about 60% is removed in urine by renal tubular secretion within 48 hours, primarily as metabolites. About one third is excreted in feces, primarily as metabolites. In premature infants, plasma half-life ranges from 15 to 21 hours, declining with increasing age and weight. Drug appears in breast milk.
Action: peak serum level varies by infant's age and weight. Duration may be especially long for a single dose given shortly after birth.

MECHANISM OF ACTION
Inhibits the enzyme cyclooxygenase, thereby permitting prostaglandin synthesis.

INDICATIONS & DOSAGE
• Patent ductus arteriosus. *Infants less than 2 days old:* 0.2 mg/kg initially, then 0.1 mg/kg 12 to 14 hours later. Give 0.1 mg/kg again after another 12 to 14 hours. *Infants 2 to 7 days old:* 0.2 mg/kg q 12 to 14 hours for three doses. *Infants over 7 days old:* 0.2 mg/kg initially, then 0.25 mg/kg 12 to 14 hours later. Give 0.25 mg/kg again after another 12 to 14 hours.

CONTRAINDICATIONS & CAUTIONS
• Contraindicated in intracranial hemorrhage, GI bleeding, thrombocytopenia, and coagulation defects because of possible worsened bleeding.
• Also contraindicated in infection or necrotizing enterocolitis because signs and symptoms may be masked, leading to unrecognized, overwhelming sepsis; in severe renal impairment because of the risk of hypercalcemia; and in infants who need a patent ductus arteriosus to maintain pulmonary or systemic blood flow.
• Use cautiously in premature infants because of the risk of intraventricular hemorrhage. Also use cautiously in cardiac dysfunction and hypertension because of possible fluid retention and peripheral edema; in congestive heart failure because of possible exacerbation; and in volume depletion or hepatic dysfunction because of the heightened risk of acute renal failure.
• Administer carefully to patients with controlled infection because the drug may mask symptoms.

PREPARATION & STORAGE
Available as a white or yellow powder in single-dose vials containing indomethacin sodium trihydrate equivalent to 1 mg of indomethacin. Protect from sunlight and store be-

low 86° F. (30° C.). Reconstitute with 1 ml of preservative-free sterile 0.9% sodium chloride or preservative-free sterile water for injection to yield a concentration of 1 mg/ml. Or reconstitute with 2 ml to yield a concentration of 0.5 mg/ml. Although drug concentrations of 1 mg/ml remain stable for 16 days, prepare them just before use because diluent is preservative-free and risks contamination.

Don't dilute drug. Discard unused portion.

ADMINISTRATION
Direct injection: Give drug over 5 to 10 seconds through the tubing of a compatible I.V. solution. Avoid extravasation because drug irritates tissues.
Intermittent infusion: not recommended.
Continuous infusion: not recommended.

INCOMPATIBILITY
Incompatible with solutions having a pH of less than 6.

ADVERSE REACTIONS
Life-threatening: disseminated intravascular coagulation, intracranial bleeding, necrotizing enterocolitis, pulmonary hemorrhage.
Other: abdominal distention, acid-base imbalance, apnea, bradycardia, decreased urine volume, epistaxis, exacerbated pulmonary infection, fever, fluid retention, gastric perforation, minor GI bleeding, headache, hematuria, hyperkalemia, hypoglycemia, hyponatremia, ileus, kernicterus, pulmonary hypertension, reduced platelet aggregation, retrolental fibroplasia, skin changes (redness, peeling, thickening, scales), thrombocytopenia.

INTERACTIONS
ACE inhibitors, potassium-sparing diuretics, potassium supplements: heightened risk of hyperkalemia.
Acetaminophen: worsened renal effects.
Adrenocorticosteroids, alcohol, anticoagulants, sulfinpyrazone: heightened risk of GI bleeding or hemorrhage.
Aminoglycosides, cardiac glycosides: increased levels because of reduced renal clearance. Reduce indomethacin dose.
Antihypertensives, especially beta-adrenergic blockers: possible reduced effects.
Aspirin, other salicylates: heightened risk of severe GI bleeding and other adverse reactions.
Azlocillin, carbenicillin (parenteral), dextran, dipyridamole, mezlocillin, piperacillin, ticarcillin, valproic acid: possible increased risk of bleeding.
Cefamandole, cefoperazone, moxalactam, plicamycin: possible hypoprothrombinemia and enhanced platelet aggregation.
Diflunisal, probenecid: diminished excretion, leading to increased risk of toxicity.
Diuretics, especially triamterene: reduced effects.
Furosemide: diminished effect on plasma renin activity and increased urine output, sodium and chloride excretion, and GFR.
Hydantoins, oral anticoagulants, sulfonamides, sulfonylureas: heightened risk of adverse reactions because of displacement from binding sites.
Lithium: may reduce renal clearance.
Methotrexate: possible increased renal and systemic toxicity from reduced renal clearance.
Nephrotoxic drugs: magnified risk of nephrotoxicity.

Oral antidiabetics: possible enhanced hypoglycemic effect.
Phenylbutazone: increased risk of renal failure.
Phenylpropanolamine: possible severe hypertension.
Verapamil: possible displacement of indomethacin or verapamil from binding sites, increasing therapeutic or adverse effects.

EFFECTS ON DIAGNOSTIC TESTS
Bleeding time: possibly prolonged because of suppressed platelet aggregation.
BUN; serum creatinine, potassium; urine glucose, protein: possible elevated levels.
Creatinine clearance, glomerular filtration rate: possible reduction.
Liver function tests, especially SGOT, SGPT: possible increased levels.
Plasma renin activity: possibly diminished.
Platelet, WBC counts: reduced.
Serum glucose: possible increased or decreased levels.
Serum sodium: possible diminished levels.
Urine chloride, osmolality, potassium, sodium, volume: possible decline.
Urine 5-hydroxyindoleacetic acid: unreliable results (Goldenberg-Underfriend method).

SPECIAL CONSIDERATIONS
• Carefully monitor hemodynamic indicators, such as vital signs, central venous pressure, cardiac output, pulmonary artery wedge pressure, and pulmonary artery pressure.
• Check for changes in coagulation studies, such as prothrombin time, partial thromboplastin time, and fibrinogen level.
• Closely monitor urine output and BUN and serum creatinine levels.

Restrict fluids and compare output with fluid intake.
• If renal function declines significantly after dose, hold next dose until urine volume or renal studies indicate a return to normal function.
• Discontinue drug if severe hepatic reactions occur.
• Be alert for signs of infection.
• Give lowest dose that provides symptomatic relief.
• Surgery may be indicated if infant doesn't respond to two courses of therapy (three doses per course).
• Ductus may reopen, possibly requiring additional indomethacin, or surgery. However, spontaneous reclosure often occurs.
• Drug isn't removed by hemodialysis.

---

insulin (regular)
Humulin R, Novolin R, Regular, Regular Iletin I, Regular Iletin II, Velosulin, Velosulin Human

Pregnancy Risk Category: B

PHARMACOKINETICS
Distribution: rapid, throughout extracellular fluids.
Metabolism: rapid, primarily in the liver and, to a lesser extent, in the kidneys and muscles.
Excretion: only small amounts excreted in the urine unchanged.
Action: onset, immediately after injection; duration, 30 to 60 minutes.

MECHANISM OF ACTION
Stimulates carbohydrate metabolism in skeletal and cardiac muscle and adipose tissue, aiding glucose transport to these cells. Drug stimulates protein synthesis and lipogenesis and inhibits lipolysis and release of free fatty acids from adipose tissue; also promotes intracellular shifts of potassium and magnesium, temporarily

reducing elevated serum levels of electrolytes.

INDICATIONS & DOSAGE

• **Severe ketoacidosis and diabetic coma.** *Adults:* 50 to 100 units I.V. along with similar dose S.C.; additional doses based on response and serum glucose level. Alternatively, 2.4 to 7.2 units initially, then 2.4 to 7.2 units/hour by continuous infusion, based on response and serum glucose level. *Children:* 0.5 to 1 unit/kg initially along with same dose S.C.; additional doses based on response and serum glucose level. Alternatively, 0.1 unit/kg initially, then 0.1 unit/kg/hour by continuous infusion.
• **Growth hormone secretion test.** *Adults:* 0.05 to 0.15 units/kg.

CONTRAINDICATIONS & CAUTIONS

None reported.

PREPARATION & STORAGE

Available in 10 ml vials in concentrations of 40 and 100 units/ml. Can be added to most I.V. and hyperalimentation solutions.

Store insulin at 36° to 46° F. (2° to 8° C.); avoid freezing. Don't use cloudy, discolored, or unusually viscous preparations. Use only syringes calibrated for the specific insulin concentration being given.

ADMINISTRATION

Direct injection: Inject directly into vein, through an intermittent infusion device, or into a port close to I.V. access site at ordered rate.
Intermittent infusion: not recommended.
Continuous infusion: Infuse drug diluted in 0.9% sodium chloride at a rate sufficient to reverse ketoacidosis.

INCOMPATIBILITY

Incompatible with aminophylline, amobarbital sodium, chlorothiazide sodium, cytarabine, dobutamine, methylprednisolone sodium succinate, pentobarbital sodium, phenobarbital sodium, phenytoin sodium, secobarbital sodium, sodium bicarbonate, and thiopental sodium.

ADVERSE REACTIONS

Life-threatening: hypoglycemia.
Other: anxiety, aphasia, blurred vision, chills, cold sweats, concentration difficulty, confusion, cool and pale skin, drowsiness, excessive hunger, fatigue, headache, irritability, maniacal behavior, nausea, pallor, paresthesias, personality changes, shallow breathing, tachycardia, tremors, unconsciousness, unusual tiredness or weakness, yawning.

INTERACTIONS

Adrenocorticosteroids, amphetamines, baclofen, corticotropin, danazol, dextrothyroxine, epinephrine, estrogen-containing oral contraceptives, estrogens, ethacrynic acid, furosemide, glucagon, glucocorticoids: heightened hyperglycemic effects, requiring dosage adjustment of one or both interacting drugs.
Alcohol, anabolic steroids, androgens, disopyramide, guanethidine, MAO inhibitors: enhanced hypoglycemic effects of insulin.
Appetite suppressants: possible alteration in serum glucose levels.
Beta-adrenergic blockers, propranolol: heightened risk of hypoglycemia or hyperglycemia.
Carbonic anhydrase inhibitors: reduced hypoglycemic response.
Edetate calcium disodium, edetate disodium: possible chelation of zinc in zinc-insulin preparations, requiring higher insulin dosage.
Molindone, phenytoin, thiazides, thiazide-like diuretics, thyroid hor-

mones, triamterene: enhanced hyperglycemic effects, requiring dosage adjustment of one or both interacting drugs.
Nicotine resin complex, smoking cessation, smoking deterrents (lobeline sulfate, silver acetate): enhanced therapeutic effect of insulin.
NSAIDs, oral antidiabetics, salicylates (large doses): heightened hypoglycemic effects of insulin.
Parenteral diazoxide: reversed hypoglycemic effect.

EFFECTS ON DIAGNOSTIC TESTS
Serum magnesium, phosphate, potassium: possible reduced levels.

SPECIAL CONSIDERATIONS
• *Treatment of overdose (hypoglycemia):* Give orange juice, sugar, or candy to conscious patient. In severe hypoglycemia or coma, give 10 to 30 ml of dextrose 50%. Alternatively, give 1 unit of glucagon if hepatic glycogen stores are adequate. Severe, untreated hypoglycemia can cause irreversible brain damage.
• Monitor serum and urine glucose and ketone levels before administration.
• During therapy, monitor serum glucose levels by reflectance meter every hour and serum acetone or ketone levels every 1 to 2 hours.
• Assess the patient for signs of hypoglycemia and dehydration.
• Increased dosages may be required in high fever, hyperthyroidism, severe infections, trauma, or surgery. Reduced dosages may be required in diarrhea, hepatic or renal impairment, hypothyroidism, nausea, and vomiting.
• Large single doses of insulin aren't recommended because of short half-life.
• Insulin (regular) has been added to dextrose infusions to promote intracellular potassium shift in hyperkalemia.

---

intravascular perfluorochemical emulsion
Fluosol

Pregnancy Risk Category: B

PHARMACOKINETICS
Distribution: perfluorotri-n-propylamine and perfluorodecalin are taken up by the reticuloendothelial system (liver, spleen, bone marrow), but do not penetrate the central nervous system. The circulating half-life is about 8 hours at a dose of 10 ml/kg, but traces of emulsion components may be found in the liver and spleen for up to 80 days after the injection.
Metabolism: not metabolized.
Excretion: via the lungs.

MECHANISM OF ACTION
An emulsion of synthetic perfluorochemicals that acts as a carrier of oxygen.

INDICATIONS & DOSAGE
• To prevent or decrease myocardial ischemia during percutaneous transluminal coronary angioplasty (PTCA) in patients at high risk for ischemic complications of angioplasty (including patients with a low baseline ejection fraction; patients with large areas of the myocardium at risk; patients with recent MI; and patients who have unstable angina or refractory angina requiring hospitalization). *Adults:* Initially, give test dose of 0.5 ml of prepared solution I.V. in a peripheral vein. If no adverse effects occur within 10 minutes, give warmed, oxygenated emulsion by intracoronary injection at a rate of 60 to 90 ml/min. Admin-

ister through the central lumen of an angioplasty balloon catheter without removing the guide wire. Use an angiographic power injector with a warming jacket.

CONTRAINDICATIONS & CAUTIONS
• Contraindicated in patients with hypersensitivity to any components of the compound.
• Also contraindicated in patients with functionally critical secondary stenosis in areas distal to the lesion.
• If the patient reacts to the test dose (1.2% of the patients in clinical trials reacted), do not give the drug. Severe reactions can be managed with corticosteroids, such as methylprednisolone, or antihistamines, such as diphenhydramine hydrochloride.

PREPARATION & STORAGE
Available as 20% emulsion for injection. Supplied in kit form with materials to provide continuous oxygenation. Store the 400 ml container of perfluorochemical emulsion in the freezer between 23° and −22° F. (−5° and −30° C.). Store solutions 1 and 2 at room temperature, not exceeding 86° F. (30° C.). Allow 30 minutes to thaw the emulsion. Do not refreeze the thawed emulsion. The emulsion must be oxygenated and warmed to approximately 98.6° F. (37° C.) before administration.
The emulsion should be prepared by personnel familiar with the procedures specified by the manufacturer.

ADMINISTRATION
Direct injection: After a test dose, warmed, oxygenated solution is administered by intracoronary injection.
Intermittent infusion: not used.
Continuous infusion: not used.

INCOMPATIBILITY
No incompatibilities reported. Because the solution is an emulsion, don't add any other substances to it after preparation.

ADVERSE REACTIONS
Life-threatening: ventricular tachycardia or fibrillation.
Other: bradycardia, chest discomfort, coughing, dyspnea, hypotension, increased respiratory rate, mild pruritus.

INTERACTIONS
Anesthetics: emulsion may prolong the action of lipid-soluble anesthetics.
Carbon tetrachloride: animal studies have shown that perfluorochemicals enhance the hepatotoxic effects of carbon tetrachloride. The clinical significance of this finding is unknown.

EFFECTS ON DIAGNOSTIC TESTS
High concentrations (which will not be achieved during angioplasty) may alter the standard curve of some radioimmunoassays. Additionally, perfluorochemicals may interfere with some spectrophotometric assays because the plasma samples will be turbid.

SPECIAL CONSIDERATIONS
• Drug may accumulate in the body following repeated doses. As a result, intravascular perfluorochemical emulsion should not be given more than once every 6 months.
• Drug should be administered only by doctors familiar with PTCA. Be prepared to follow institutional standby protocols for emergency coronary artery bypass surgery.

Unmarked trade names available in the United States only.
♦Also available in Canada.   ♦♦Available in Canada only.

• When the drug is administered with an angiographic power injector reservoir of 260 ml and a flow rate of 60 ml/minute, more than 4 minutes of perfusion time is allowed. Perfusion time is limited by patient's tolerance and doctor's judgment.

• Discard emulsions that appear to have thawed partially before use.

• Use a warming cabinet or water bath set at 98.6° F. to thaw the emulsion. Avoid using a microwave oven because the device may heat the emulsion unevenly.

• Keep in mind that infusion of solutions at room temperature has been associated with ventricular fibrillation.

• Do not add anything other than solutions 1 and 2 or carbogen gas (95% oxygen, 5% carbon dioxide) to perfluorochemical emulsion. Do not oxygenate with 100% oxygen, because this will adversely affect the solution's final pH.

• When administering perfluorochemical emulsion, do not use a filter. Never administer any solution that shows emulsion separation.

• Studies have shown that perfluorochemicals are excreted in breast milk. Therefore, breast-feeding after administration of intravascular perfluorochemical emulsion isn't recommended.

• When blood samples from patients given perfluorochemicals are centrifuged, a layer of perfluorochemicals may be found at the bottom of the tube. The volume percent of the perfluorochemicals in this layer is the fluorocrit.

invert sugar
Travert 5%, Travert 10%

Pregnancy Risk Category: C

COMPOSITION
A proportionally equimolar mixture of dextrose and fructose, invert sugar comes in hypertonic 10% solutions having a pH of 3.7 to 4. Each liter of 10% solution contains 375 calories and 555 mOsm.

Invert sugar is also available with electrolytes: Ionosol B, D, or G with Invert Sugar 10% Injection, Multiple Electrolyte No. 2 with Invert Sugar 5% Injection, Multiple Electrolyte No. 1 or 2 with Invert Sugar 10% Injection, and Travert 5% or 10% with Electrolyte No. 2 Injection.

INDICATIONS & DOSAGE
• Nonelectrolyte fluid replacement and calorie supplement. *Adults and children:* 1 to 3 liters daily. Specific dosage based on patient's weight and age.

CONTRAINDICATIONS & CAUTIONS
• Contraindicated in hereditary fructose intolerance because renal abnormalities of Fanconi's syndrome may occur.

• Use cautiously in patients susceptible to congestive heart failure, hypertension, or renal disease because fluid overload may occur.

PREPARATION & STORAGE
Available in 1 liter ready-to-use, sterile, nonpyrogenic bottles or bags. Store at room temperature.

ADMINISTRATION
Direct injection: not recommended. *Intermittent infusion:* not recommended.

Continuous infusion: Using an infusion pump, administer into a large peripheral vein or through a central venous line at an hourly rate not exceeding 1 g/kg. Carefully monitor flow rate. Overly rapid administration can cause lactic acidosis and hyperuricemia.

INCOMPATIBILITY
Incompatible with aminophylline, amobarbital sodium, ampicillin sodium, blood products, penicillin G sodium, thiopental sodium, and warfarin sodium.

ADVERSE REACTIONS
Life-threatening: none reported.
Other: extravasation; fever; hyperuricemia; hypervolemic, osmotic diuresis; infection at injection site; lactic acidosis; rebound hyperinsulinemia; reduced insulin production (prolonged use).

INTERACTIONS
None reported.

EFFECTS ON DIAGNOSTIC TESTS
Laboratory values may vary depending on patient's hydration status.

SPECIAL CONSIDERATIONS
• Measure intake and output. Report significant changes to doctor.
• Take vital signs frequently and report symptoms of fluid overload.
• Monitor serum glucose levels.
• Keep dextrose 10% available if rebound hyperinsulinemia develops.
• Because of fructose component, invert sugar possesses advantages over dextrose: It minimizes glycogenesis and promotes anabolism in fasting patients.

iron dextran injection
Feostat, Feronim, Hematran, Hydextran, Imfergen, Imferon♦, Irodex, K-Feron, Nor-Feron, Proferdex

Pregnancy Risk Category: C

PHARMACOKINETICS
Distribution: in reticuloendothelial system, with high levels in the liver, spleen, and bone marrow. Small amounts of iron cross the placenta.
Metabolism: by reticuloendothelial cells, which separate iron from dextran, allowing iron to become part of body stores. Ferric iron, slowly released into plasma, combines with transferrin for transport to bone marrow, where it's incorporated into hemoglobin.
Excretion: not easily eliminated. Small amounts are lost in the shedding of skin, hair, and nails and in perspiration. Trace amounts of unmetabolized drug appear in urine and feces. Drug has a half-life of 5 to 20 hours. Small amounts appear in breast milk.
Action: peak levels, immediately upon administration.

MECHANISM OF ACTION
Iron is essential for hemoglobin formation, effective erythropoiesis, and, ultimately, the blood's oxygen transport capacity. It may promote synthesis of myoglobin or nonhemoglobin heme units.

INDICATIONS & DOSAGE
• Iron-deficiency anemias. *Adults and children weighing over 14 kg:* Dosage depends on iron requirements and hemoglobin deficit. To calculate total iron dosage in milliliters, multiply 0.0476 by the patient's weight (in kilograms). Now multiply

this product by the difference between normal (14.8) and the patient's actual hemoglobin level. Next, add this volume to the amount required to replace iron stores (1 ml/ 5 kg, maximum of 14 ml) to obtain total volume.

To calculate total iron dosage in milligrams, multiply 0.3 by the patient's weight (in pounds). Now multiply the patient's hemoglobin level (in grams per deciliter) by 100, then divide by 14.8 and subtract from 100. Next, multiply the hemoglobin figure by the weight figure. Divide by 50 to calculate the dose in milliliters. *Children weighing 14 kg or under:* 80% of dosage obtained by the formula above, or by the first formula, using a normal hemoglobin level of 12.

• Iron replacement resulting from blood loss. *Adults and children:* To calculate total iron dosage in milliliters, multiply 0.02 by the blood loss (in milliliters). Then multiply the product by the hematocrit percentage (a hematocrit of 21, for instance, would be expressed as 0.21). To calculate total iron dosage in milligrams, multiply blood loss (in milliliters) by the hematocrit percentage. Divide by 50 to get the volume in milliliters.

CONTRAINDICATIONS & CAUTIONS
• Contraindicated in iron hypersensitivity and in infants age 4 months or younger.
• Also contraindicated in hemochromatosis and hemosiderosis because existing iron load may increase; in acute renal infection because of impaired metabolism; and in multiple blood transfusions because erythrocytes contain considerable iron.
• Avoid concurrent use with oral iron preparations because of possible overdose.

• Also avoid use in anemias not caused by iron deficiency because of lack of therapeutic value.
• Use cautiously—and only after test dose—in patients with a history of significant allergies or asthma because of possible hypersensitivity.
• Use with extreme caution in hepatic impairment because of delayed metabolism and in rheumatoid arthritis because drug may cause fever and trigger or exacerbate joint pain and swelling.

PREPARATION & STORAGE
Available as a dark brown slightly viscous liquid in 2 ml ampules containing a 50 mg/ml concentration. Store at room temperature, preferably below 77° F. (25° C.). Administer undiluted. Be sure not to use iron dextran with phenol or other preservatives for I.V. injection.

Although manufacturers don't recommend dilution, iron dextran can be infused after dilution with 250 to 1,000 ml of 0.9% sodium chloride injection, depending on dose.

ADMINISTRATION
Direct injection: After initial test dose, give undiluted dose of 2 ml (or less) over at least 2 minutes.
Intermittent infusion: After initial test dose, infuse solution over 1 to 6 hours, using an appropriate dilution. On completion, infuse 0.9% sodium chloride to flush vein.
Continuous infusion: not recommended.

INCOMPATIBILITY
Incompatible with oxytetracycline and sulfadiazine sodium. Manufacturers recommend that iron dextran not be mixed with other drugs or parenteral nutrition solutions.

ADVERSE REACTIONS
Life-threatening: anaphylaxis.

Other: arthralgia, backache, bronchospasm, brown serum (with high doses), brown skin, chest pain, chills, diarrhea, dizziness, dyspnea, faintness, fever, headache, hypotension, iron toxicity, leukocytosis, malaise, muscle pain, myalgia, nausea, transient paresthesias, peripheral vascular flushing, phlebitis, purpura, rheumatoid arthritis reactivation, urticaria, vomiting, weakness.

INTERACTIONS
Chloramphenicol: delayed reticulocyte response to iron dextran injection.
Oral iron: additive effects.
Penicillamine: diminished effects. Give 2 hours apart from iron dextran.
Vitamin E: impaired hematologic response in iron-deficiency anemia. Increased vitamin dosage may be necessary.

EFFECTS ON DIAGNOSTIC TESTS
Bone marrow iron: unreliable findings because residual iron dextran may remain in reticuloendothelial cells.
Orthotoluidine test: possible false-positive results.
Partial thromboplastin time: prolonged if blood sample is mixed with anticoagulant citrate dextrose solution.
Radionuclide bone scan: reduced uptake of technetium Tc 99m in bone after iron dextran administration or when serum ferritin levels are high.
Serum bilirubin: falsely elevated levels.
Serum calcium: possible falsely depressed levels.
Serum ferritin: elevated levels starting 7 to 9 days after administration and slowly declining to normal after 3 weeks.

Serum iron, total iron binding capacity: altered for 3 weeks after iron dextran administration.

SPECIAL CONSIDERATIONS
• Because of the risk of anaphylaxis, inject a test dose of 0.5 ml (25 mg) over 5 minutes. Observe patient for 1 hour and, if no adverse reactions occur, proceed with full dose.
• Keep epinephrine and resuscitation equipment readily available to treat possible anaphylaxis.
• I.V. route is used only when oral route is unsatisfactory or impossible or when rapid replenishment of iron stores is necessary.
• Be sure diagnosis of iron-deficiency anemia is definitive before giving drug. Otherwise, excess iron storage, hemosiderosis, or iron toxicity may occur.
• Because toxicity may not cause acute signs, monitor serum ferritin and hemoglobin levels, hematocrit, and reticulocyte count. Late signs of toxicity include bluish lips, fingernails, and palms; drowsiness; pale, clammy skin; tachycardia; and unusual tiredness or weakness.
• Warn patient not to take over-the-counter vitamin preparations containing iron.
• Delayed reactions (1 to 2 days) are more common with parenteral administration. Such reactions include arthralgia, backache, chills, dizziness, headache, malaise, moderate to high fever, myalgia, nausea, and vomiting.
• Hemodialysis removes only negligible amounts of drug.

isoproterenol hydrochloride
Isuprel♦

Pregnancy Risk Category: C

PHARMACOKINETICS
Distribution: throughout the body.
Metabolism: primarily in the liver and lungs, and in other tissues by the enzyme catechol-O-methyl transferase. Drug is metabolized more rapidly and extensively in children.
Excretion: in urine, with about 40% to 50% removed unchanged and the remainder excreted as the metabolite 3-O-methylisoproterenol. In children, small amounts of unidentified metabolites appear in feces. About 75% of drug is excreted within 15 hours. Not known if drug appears in breast milk.
Action: onset, immediately upon administration; duration, less than 1 hour.

MECHANISM OF ACTION
This sympathomimetic amine acts predominantly on $beta_1$-receptors in smooth muscle and on $beta_2$-receptors in blood vessels. Its direct action on the heart causes tachycardia, elevated systolic pressure related to increased contractility and cardiac output, and diminished diastolic pressure related to arteriolar dilation and reduced peripheral vascular resistance.

Acting on $beta_2$-receptors in the bronchi, the drug relaxes bronchial smooth muscle, thereby relieving bronchospasm, increasing vital capacity, and reducing residual volume.

INDICATIONS & DOSAGE
• Acute asthma unresponsive to inhalation therapy. *Adults:* 0.01 to 0.02 mg (0.5 to 1 ml of a 1:50,000 dilution). Repeat as necessary. *Children:* 0.08 to 1.7 mcg/kg/minute.
• Bronchospasm during anesthesia. *Adults:* 0.01 to 0.02 mg (0.5 to 1 ml of a 1:50,000 dilution). *Children:* individualized.
• Dysrhythmias. *Adults:* bolus of 0.02 to 0.06 mg (1 to 3 ml of a 1:50,000 dilution) initially, then 0.01 to 0.2 mg (0.5 to 10 ml of a 1:50,000 dilution). Alternatively, infuse 20 mg diluted in 500 ml of dextrose 5% in water at a rate of 0.5 to 5 mcg/minute. Adjust subsequent doses based on patient response. *Children:* 2.5 mcg/minute. Adjust subsequent doses based on patient response.
• Shock. *Adult:* 0.5 to 5 mcg/minute. In advanced shock, give 5 to 30 mcg/minute.

CONTRAINDICATIONS & CAUTIONS
• Contraindicated in hypersensitivity to sympathomimetics or isoproterenol.
• Also contraindicated in tachydysrhythmias (especially ventricular tachycardia and dysrhythmias that require increased inotropic activity).
• Avoid use in shock patients who haven't received fluid replacement.
• Also avoid use in uncorrected hypoxia, acidosis, hypokalemia, hyperkalemia, or hypercapnia because the drug may have reduced effects or may increase the risk of adverse reactions.
• Use cautiously in elderly patients and in patients with cardiovascular disease, hyperthyroidism, or cardiac glycoside–induced tachycardia because of the heightened risk of adverse cardiovascular effects.
• Also use cautiously in sulfite hypersensitivity if the isoproterenol preparation contains this element; in Parkinson's disease because the drug

may temporarily exacerbate symptoms; and in diabetes mellitus. Dosage adjustment of insulin or hypoglycemic agents may be necessary.

PREPARATION & STORAGE
Available in a dilution of 1:5,000 in 1 ml (0.2 mg) and 5 ml (1 mg) ampules and in 5 ml (1 mg) and 10 ml (2 mg) vials. For direct injection, add 1 ml of isoproterenol to 10 ml of 0.9% sodium chloride or dextrose 5% in water to yield a 1:50,000 dilution (20 mcg/ml). For infusion, dilute 10 ml of isoproterenol with 500 ml of dextrose 5% in water to yield a dilution of 1:250,000 (4 mcg/ml). Drug is also compatible with Ringer's lactate and dextrose 5% in Ringer's lactate.

Store in a cool place, protect from light, and keep in an opaque container until used. Don't use if pink or brown or if a precipitate forms.

ADMINISTRATION
Direct injection: Inject diluted solution (1:50,000) directly into vein or into an I.V. line containing a free-flowing compatible solution. Usual initial dose: 1 to 3 ml (20 to 60 mcg).
Intermittent infusion: not recommended.
Continuous infusion: Using an infusion pump, give appropriate dose and dilution (1:250,000) at ordered rate. Usual initial dose is 5 mcg/minute (1.25 ml/minute).

INCOMPATIBILITY
Incompatible with alkalies, aminophylline, metals, and sodium bicarbonate.

ADVERSE REACTIONS
Life-threatening: anaphylaxis, dysrhythmias.

Other: angina, anxiety, asthenia, diaphoresis, dizziness, excitement, fear, flushed face, headache, hypotension, insomnia, light-headedness, nausea, palpitations, restlessness, tachycardia, tinnitus, trembling, vomiting, weakness.

INTERACTIONS
Antihypertensives: reduced effects.
Beta-blockers: inhibited effects of isoproterenol and beta-blockers.
Cardiac glycosides: heightened risk of dysrhythmias.
CNS stimulants: excessive stimulation.
Epinephrine, other sympathomimetics: severe dysrhythmias; administer at least 4 hours apart.
Inhalation hydrocarbon anesthetics: severe dysrhythmias.
Levodopa: dysrhythmias.
MAO inhibitors, tricyclic antidepressants: dysrhythmias, tachycardia, severe hypertension.
Nitrates: reduced effects.
Oxytocic drugs: severe persistent hypertension and possible cerebral hemorrhage.
Thyroid hormones: heightened effects of isoproterenol and these hormones; increased risk of coronary insufficiency in patients with coronary artery disease.
Xanthines: possible enhanced CNS effects.

EFFECTS ON DIAGNOSTIC TESTS
Serum bilirubin; urine catecholamines, vanillylmandelic acid: increased levels.

SPECIAL CONSIDERATIONS
• *Treatment of overdose:* Symptoms include severe, persistent chest pain and irregular heartbeat, elevated blood pressure, headache, and dizziness. If these symptoms occur, dis-

---

continue drug immediately. Cumulative effects haven't been reported.

• In cardiac arrest, dysrhythmias, shock, and heart block, closely observe EKG to help adjust dosage.

• Monitor blood PCO_2, bicarbonate, and pH. For shock patients, also monitor central venous pressure, heart rate, blood pressure, and urine output.

• Adjust infusion rate according to heart rate and blood pressure.

• Drug may aggravate ventilation-perfusion abnormalities.

• Give sedatives, if ordered, to reduce CNS stimulation.

• With high doses, systolic pressure falls because of a marked reduction in peripheral vascular resistance.

• Drug isn't useful if peripheral vascular bed is already dilated.

• Lower dosages are recommended for elderly patients.

• Isoproterenol has been used successfully to treat status asthmaticus in children.

---

kanamycin sulfate
Kantrex◆, Klebcil

Pregnancy Risk Category: D

PHARMACOKINETICS
Distribution: primarily distributed to extracellular fluids (ascitic, pericardial, peritoneal, pleural, synovial, and abscess fluids) and tissues. Kanamycin doesn't bind to plasma proteins or reach ocular tissue. It achieves 50% of serum concentrations in cerebrospinal fluid when meninges are inflamed. Drug crosses the placenta.
Metabolism: not metabolized.
Excretion: in urine by glomerular filtration. In adults, half-life is 2 to 4 hours with normal renal function and 27 to 80 hours with severe impairment. In premature infants, half-life is about 9 hours. Complete elimination takes 10 to 20 days with normal renal function. Small amounts of drug appear in breast milk.
Action: peak serum level, about 1 hour.

MECHANISM OF ACTION
This bactericidal antibiotic inhibits protein synthesis by binding directly to the 30S ribosomal subunit in susceptible microorganisms. It's effective against such gram-negative aerobic bacteria as *Escherichia coli, Proteus, Enterobacter, Citrobacter aerogenes, Klebsiella, Acinetobacter, Providencia, Salmonella, Serratia,* and *Shigella.* Susceptible gram-positive aerobic bacteria include *Staphylococcus aureus* and *S. epidermidis.*

INDICATIONS & DOSAGE
• Severe infections caused by susceptible organisms. *Adults and children:* 5 to 7.5 mg/kg q 8 to 12 hours for 7 to 10 days; maximum dosage, 1.5 g/day. In renal impairment, give 7.5 mg/kg initially and base subsequent doses on serum levels and creatinine clearance. Typically, the dosage interval (hours) is equivalent to the serum creatinine level (in mg/dl) multiplied by 9. *Infants 7 days old or younger weighing 2 kg or less:* 7.5 mg/kg q 12 hours. *Infants 7 days old or younger weighing more than 2 kg:* 10 mg/kg q 12 hours.

CONTRAINDICATIONS & CAUTIONS
• Contraindicated in hypersensitivity to kanamycin or other aminoglycosides.
• Give cautiously in patients with myasthenia gravis, infant botulism, or parkinsonism because drug may cause neuromuscular blockage, worsening weakness.

• Because of an increased risk of hearing loss, administer kanamycin cautiously to elderly patients, especially those with preexisting tinnitus, vertigo, or subclinical deafness; to patients who previously received ototoxic drugs; and to patients receiving a total dose of 15 g or more.
• Use cautiously in patients with cranial nerve VIII dysfunction because of a heightened risk of ototoxicity and in patients with renal impairment because of the risk of nephrotoxicity. Reduce daily dosage and lengthen interval between doses.
• In infants younger than 6 weeks old, use cautiously because of immature renal function.

PREPARATION & STORAGE

Available in 3 ml vials containing 1 g (333 mg/ml), 2 ml vials and disposable syringes containing 500 mg (250 mg/ml), and 2 ml vials containing 75 mg (37.5 mg/ml). For infusion, mix 100 to 200 ml of dextrose 5% in water or 0.9% sodium chloride with contents of 500 mg vial, or mix 200 to 400 ml with contents of 1 g vial. Children require a proportionately smaller diluent volume.

Store between 59° and 86° F. (15° and 30° C.). Solution remains stable for 24 hours at room temperature. Protect from freezing. Darkened vial doesn't indicate loss of potency.

ADMINISTRATION

Direct injection: not recommended.
Intermittent infusion: Using an appropriate dilution, infuse drug over 30 to 60 minutes.
Continuous infusion: not recommended.

INCOMPATIBILITY

Incompatible with ampicillin sodium, carbenicillin sodium, cephalothin sodium, chlorpheniramine maleate, colistimethate sodium, heparin sodium, hydrocortisone sodium succinate, methicillin sodium, and methohexital sodium.

ADVERSE REACTIONS

Life-threatening: anaphylaxis.
Other: anorexia, bacterial and fungal superinfection, dizziness, drowsiness, encephalopathy, fever, headache, hearing loss, hematuria, nephrotoxicity (albuminuria; RBCs, WBCs, and granular casts in urine; azotemia; oliguria), paresthesias, rash, scotomas, seizures, thrombophlebitis, tinnitus, tremors, unusual thirst, vertigo, visual disturbances, weakness.

INTERACTIONS

Antihistamines, loxapine, phenothiazines, thioxanthenes: possible masked signs of ototoxicity.
Antimyasthenics: antagonized effects. Adjust dosage.
Beta-lactam antibiotics, vancomycin: additive or synergistic effects against certain organisms.
Chloramphenicol, clindamycin, tetracycline: possible antagonized bactericidal activity.
Citrated blood, general anesthetics, neuromuscular blockers, opioid analgesics: potentiated neuromuscular blockade, causing respiratory depression and paralysis.
Ethacrynic acid, furosemide, mannitol (parenteral): possible rapid loss of hearing in renal impairment.
Indomethacin (parenteral): increased risk of toxicity.
Methoxyflurane, polymyxins: possible heightened risk of nephrotoxicity and neuromuscular blockade.
Nephrotoxic, neurotoxic, and ototoxic drugs: possible enhanced risk of toxicity.
Penicillins (broad-spectrum): synergistic effects against some Enterobacteriaceae.

EFFECTS ON DIAGNOSTIC TESTS

BUN, serum bilirubin, creatinine, LDH, SGOT, SGPT: possible elevated levels.
Serum calcium, magnesium, potassium, sodium: possible reduced levels.

SPECIAL CONSIDERATIONS

• *Treatment of overdose:* Hemodialysis or peritoneal dialysis aids drug removal. An exchange transfusion may be used in neonates.
• Check for previous aminoglycoside hypersensitivity before giving first dose.
• Collect specimens for culture and sensitivity testing before giving first dose. Therapy may begin before results are available.
• Obtain a baseline audiogram before therapy and ensure that audiometric tests are performed during it. Discontinue drug if patient reports tinnitus or hearing difficulty or if follow-up audiograms show high-frequency hearing loss.
• Provide adequate hydration because drug irritates renal tubules.
• Monitor BUN and serum creatinine levels and urinalysis during therapy. Adjust dosage accordingly. If azotemia occurs or urine output declines, discontinue drug.
• Obtain peak and trough serum levels to adjust dosages. Coordinate specimen collection with the laboratory. For systemic infection, desirable peak levels are 15 to 30 mcg/ml and desirable trough levels are 5 to 10 mcg/ml.
• If beta-lactam antibiotics must be given concurrently, administer at a separate site. Don't mix with kanamycin or use same I.V. line.
• May contain sulfites.
• Observe patient for superinfections during prolonged use.

ketamine hydrochloride
Ketalar♦

Pregnancy Risk Category: C

PHARMACOKINETICS

Distribution: rapidly dispersed into tissues, including brain. Drug achieves high concentrations in adipose tissue, liver, and lungs. Not known if it crosses the placenta.
Metabolism: in the liver.
Excretion: about 90% removed in urine as metabolites and about 5% eliminated in feces. Half-life is 2 to 3 hours.
Action: onset, 15 to 30 seconds; duration, about 20 minutes.

MECHANISM OF ACTION

Ketamine selectively interrupts cerebral pathways, causing dissociative anesthesia.

INDICATIONS & DOSAGE

• Induction of anesthesia. Can be used as sole anesthetic for diagnostic and surgical procedures (especially short ones) that don't require skeletal muscle relaxation, as a preanesthetic, or as an adjunct to low-potency anesthetics, such as nitrous oxide. *Adults and children:* initially, 1 to 2 mg/kg, then 0.01 to 0.03 mg/kg by continuous infusion. Adjust dosage based on patient's response.

CONTRAINDICATIONS & CAUTIONS

• Contraindicated in ketamine hypersensitivity.
• Also contraindicated as the sole anesthetic for laryngeal, pharyngeal, or bronchial surgery or for diagnostic procedures because of active laryngeal and pharyngeal reflexes.
• Because ketamine raises intracranial pressure, don't give drug for in-

---

Unmarked trade names available in the United States only.
♦ Also available in Canada.   ♦♦ Available in Canada only.

tracranial procedures or to patients with an intracerebral mass or hemorrhage, increased cerebrospinal fluid (CSF) pressure, or cerebral trauma.
• Avoid use in hypertension and in conditions in which an appreciable rise in blood pressure would be harmful.
• Also avoid use in eye surgery because drug often causes nystagmus and raises intraocular pressure.
• Use cautiously in alcoholism because of possible exacerbated withdrawal symptoms; in psychiatric disorders because of the high incidence of postoperative hallucinations; and in thyrotoxicosis because of the heightened risk of tachycardia and hypertension.

PREPARATION & STORAGE
Available in multidose vials with concentrations of 10 mg/ml, 50 mg/ml, and 100 mg/ml. For direct injection, dilute 100 mg/ml concentration with an equal volume of sterile water for injection, 0.9% sodium chloride, or dextrose 5% in water. For continuous infusion, prepare a 1 mg/ml solution by adding 10 ml from the 50 mg/ml vial or 5 ml from the 100 mg/ml vial to 500 ml of dextrose 5% in water or 0.9% sodium chloride. If the patient must restrict fluids, prepare a 2 mg/ml solution by adding 10 ml of 50 mg/ml or 5 ml of 100 mg/ml of drug to 250 ml of diluent.
Store at room temperature, and protect from light and heat.

ADMINISTRATION
Only staff specially trained in administering anesthetics and managing their adverse reactions should give ketamine.
Direct injection: Over 1 minute, inject initial dose directly into vein or into I.V. tubing containing a free-flowing compatible solution.

Intermittent infusion: not recommended.
Continuous infusion: Infuse diluted drug at a rate of 1 to 2 mg/minute.

INCOMPATIBILITY
Incompatible with barbiturates and diazepam.

ADVERSE REACTIONS
Life-threatening: apnea, respiratory depression.
Other: altered body image or mood, bradycardia, bradypnea, breathing difficulty, delirium, dissociation, hypertension, hypotension, severe emergence reaction (vivid dreams or hallucinations usually limited to duration of drug effects, but flashbacks may occur for several weeks postoperatively), tachycardia, uncontrolled muscle movements, visual illusions, vomiting.

INTERACTIONS
Antihypertensives, CNS depressants: possible heightened risk of hypotension or respiratory depression.
Halogenated inhalation anesthetics: possible prolonged elimination half-life of ketamine.
Thyroid hormones: increased risk of hypertension and tachycardia.

EFFECTS ON DIAGNOSTIC TESTS
Lumbar puncture: possible increased CSF pressure.
Ophthalmic examination: possible altered results because of drug-induced rise in intraocular pressure.

SPECIAL CONSIDERATIONS
• *Treatment of overdose:* Maintain a patent airway and provide ventilatory support until drug effects subside.

• Before giving drug, make sure patient hasn't eaten because of the risk of aspirating vomitus.
• Monitor EKG during administration, especially in patients with hypertension or cardiac decompensation.
• Emergence reactions occur in about 12% of patients, but least often in the young and elderly. If severe, give a small dose of a short-acting sedative.
• Reduce incidence of emergence reactions by lowering ketamine dose and giving with I.V. diazepam and by reducing postoperative sensory stimulation.
• When using ketamine for an outpatient, don't release him until effects wear off and then only if he's accompanied by a responsible adult.
• Warn patient not to drive or perform other tasks that require alertness for 24 hours because of the risk of psychomotor impairment.
• Can use as anesthetic if accident victim's limb must be amputated at the scene.

labetalol hydrochloride
Normodyne, Trandate Injection

Pregnancy Risk Category: C

PHARMACOKINETICS
Distribution: rapid and widespread into extravascular space, with highest concentrations in the lungs, liver, and kidneys. Distribution declines in hepatic impairment. Drug is about 50% bound to plasma proteins. Small amounts cross the placenta and blood-brain barrier.
Metabolism: primarily changed in the liver through conjugation to glucuronide metabolites, such as O-alkylglucuronide.

Excretion: 55% to 60% eliminated in urine within 24 hours and 30% excreted in feces within 4 days. Less than 5% excreted as unchanged drug. Small amounts of drug appear in breast milk.
Action: onset, 2 to 5 minutes; duration, 2 to 4 hours.

MECHANISM OF ACTION
Competitively blocks stimulation of myocardial beta$_1$-receptors, bronchial beta$_2$-receptors, and alpha- and beta$_2$-receptors of the vascular smooth muscle. The drug reduces blood pressure in 5 to 10 minutes, and also depresses renin secretion.

INDICATIONS & DOSAGE
• Severe hypertension and hypertensive crisis. *Adults:* 20 mg initially, then 20 to 80 mg q 10 minutes, up to 300 mg.
• Hypotension control during halothane anesthesia. *Adults:* 10 to 25 mg after induction of anesthesia. Hypotension will then be controlled by inspired halothane.
• Hypotension control with use of other anesthetics. *Adults:* 30 mg initially, then 5 to 10 mg if needed.

CONTRAINDICATIONS & CAUTIONS
• Contraindicated in patients with second- or third-degree heart block, overt congestive heart failure, cardiac ischemia, cardiogenic shock, or severe bradycardia because of the risk of further myocardial depression.
• Also contraindicated in asthma or bronchospastic disease because drug may inhibit bronchodilation.
• Avoid use in children.
• Use cautiously in diabetes mellitus controlled by hypoglycemic agents because drug may mask signs of hypoglycemia.

Unmarked trade names available in the United States only.
♦Also available in Canada.   ♦♦Available in Canada only.

- Also use cautiously in myasthenia gravis, depression, or psoriasis because of possible exacerbation.
- In pheochromocytoma, give carefully because paradoxical hypertension may occur.
- In hepatic impairment, also give carefully because of the heightened risk of toxicity.

PREPARATION & STORAGE

Available as a clear, colorless to light yellow solution in 20 ml ampules with a concentration of 5 mg/ml. Store at room temperature.

For infusion, add two 20 ml ampules to 160 ml of dextrose 5% in water, 0.9% sodium chloride, dextrose 2.5% in 0.45% sodium chloride, dextrose 5% in Ringer's lactate, or Ringer's lactate to yield a concentration of 1 mg/ml. To obtain a concentration of 2 mg/3 ml, add two 20 ml ampules to 250 ml of diluent. Solutions remain stable for at least 24 hours at room temperature or when refrigerated.

ADMINISTRATION

Direct injection: Over 2 minutes, inject directly into vein or into an I.V. line containing a free-flowing compatible solution.
Intermittent infusion: not recommended.
Continuous infusion: Give 2 mg/minute until satisfactory response is obtained, then stop infusion. May repeat in 6 to 8 hours.

INCOMPATIBILITY

Incompatible with sodium bicarbonate.

ADVERSE REACTIONS

Life-threatening: intensified atrioventricular block, severe hypotension.
Other: agranulocytosis, increased airway resistance, alopecia (reversible), atrioventricular conduction delay, bradycardia, bronchospasm, chest pain, decreased libido, diaphoresis, diarrhea, dizziness, dyspepsia, dyspnea, facial erythema, fatigue, fever, headache, hyperglycemia (mild), impotence, infusion site pain, laryngospasm, lethargy, leukopenia, memory loss, muscle cramps, nasal congestion, nausea, orthostatic hypotension, Peyronie's disease, pruritus, rash, skin or scalp tingling, systemic lupus erythematosus–like illness, urinary difficulty or retention, ventricular dysrhythmias, vivid dreams, vomiting, wheezing.

INTERACTIONS

Antihypertensives: potentiated effects.
Anti-inflammatory drugs: reduced labetalol effects.
Cardiac glycosides: extreme bradycardia.
Diazoxide: potentiated hypotension.
Estrogens: reduced antihypertensive effect.
Halothane anesthetics: synergistic hypotensive effects.
Insulin, oral hypoglycemics: possible altered dosage requirements.
Lidocaine: possible prolonged metabolism and heightened risk of toxicity.
MAO inhibitors: severe hypertension for up to 2 weeks after discontinuation.
Nitroglycerin: reduced reflex tachycardia and potentiated hypotension.
Nondepolarizing neuromuscular blockers: possible prolonged action.
Phenothiazines: increased serum levels of labetalol and phenothiazines.
Phenoxybenzamine, phentolamine: enhanced alpha-adrenergic blocking action.

Sympathomimetics, xanthine derivatives: inactivation of labetalol and these drugs.

EFFECTS ON DIAGNOSTIC TESTS

Antinuclear antibody test: positive titer.
BUN, serum creatinine: transient rise in levels.
Intraocular pressure: possible altered pressure.
Radionuclide ventriculography: possible bradycardia.
Urine catecholamines: falsely increased levels when measured by a nonspecific trihydroxyindole reaction.

SPECIAL CONSIDERATIONS

• Avoid reducing blood pressure rapidly. Adjust dosage according to supine blood pressure.
• Higher initial doses commonly cause nausea and severe hypotension.
• Keep patient supine for 3 hours after administration to prevent severe orthostatic hypotension. Frequently monitor blood pressure.
• Advise patient that transient scalp tingling may occur during initial therapy.
• Labetalol is less likely than other beta blockers to decrease heart rate or cardiac output.
• Steady-state plasma levels aren't attained during infusion. Follow with oral therapy when supine blood pressure begins to rise.
• Drug masks common signs of shock and hypoglycemia.
• In severe renal impairment, adjust dosage as necessary.
• Dialysis removes less than 1% of drug.

leucovorin calcium (citrovorum factor, folinic acid)
Wellcovorin

Pregnancy Risk Category: C

PHARMACOKINETICS
Distribution: throughout body tisues, with highest concentrations in the liver. Drug crosses the placenta; moderate amounts cross the blood-brain barrier.
Metabolism: more than half metabolized by the liver, primarily to the active metabolite 5-methyltetrahydrofolate, the major transport and storage form of folate.
Excretion: in urine primarily as two metabolites, with 5% to 8% removed in feces. Not known if drug appears in breast milk.
Action: onset, less than 5 minutes; duration, 3 to 6 hours.

MECHANISM OF ACTION
The active form of folic acid, leucovorin calcium acts as a cofactor for 1-carbon transfer reactions in purine and pyrimidine biosynthesis. The drug is thought to limit the action of methotrexate and other folic acid antagonists by competing for transport into cells. It rescues bone marrow and GI cells from methotrexate but has no effect on existing methotrexate nephrotoxicity.

INDICATIONS & DOSAGE
• Treatment of methotrexate overdose. *Adults:* Up to 75 mg within 12 hours or a dosage sufficient to produce serum levels at least equal to serum methotrexate levels.
• Treatment of hematologic toxicity caused by other folic acid antagonists, such as trimethoprim. *Adults and children:* 5 to 15 mg/day.

• Neutralization of methotrexate's toxic effects (leucovorin rescue). Used investigationally in various regimens. Specific dosage depends on extent of systemic toxicity. *Adults and children:* 10 mg/m². About 10 to 50 mg can be given q 6 hours for six doses or 96 hours after methotrexate.

CONTRAINDICATIONS & CAUTIONS

• Contraindicated in leucovorin hypersensitivity.
• Also contraindicated in undiagnosed anemia because drug may mask signs of pernicious anemia, leading to severe CNS damage.
• Use cautiously in pernicious anemia. Hemolytic remission may accompany progressive neurologic effects.
• For leucovorin rescue, use cautiously in patients with a urine pH less than 7, ascites, dehydration, pleural or peritoneal effusions, or renal dysfunction because of the heightened risk of toxicity.

PREPARATION & STORAGE

Available as a yellow-white solution in 1, 3, and 5 mg/ml ampules and as a powder in 50 mg vials. Store at room temperature. Reconstitute powder for injection by adding 5 ml of sterile or bacteriostatic water to 50 mg vial, yielding a solution of 10 mg/ml. For intermittent infusion, add 15 to 50 mg of reconstituted drug to 50 ml of a compatible solution, such as Ringer's lactate or dextrose 5% or 10% in water. For continuous infusion, add up to 200 mg of reconstituted drug to 1 liter of a compatible solution.

Use solutions containing sterile water immediately. Use those containing bacteriostatic water within 1 week if refrigerated.

ADMINISTRATION

Direct injection: Using a 21G or 23G needle, inject into vein or into I.V. tubing containing a free-flowing compatible solution over 5 minutes.
Intermittent infusion: Using a 21G or 23G needle, infuse solution over 15 minutes.
Continuous infusion: Infuse over 24 hours at a rate of about 40 ml/hour.

INCOMPATIBILITY

Incompatible with droperidol.

ADVERSE REACTIONS

Life-threatening: anaphylaxis.
Other: erythema, flushing, pruritus, rash, warm sensation, wheezing.

INTERACTIONS

Barbiturate and hydantoin anticonvulsants, primidone: reduced effects with large leucovorin doses.
CNS depressants: possible deepened CNS depression because of alcohol in leucovorin preparation.

EFFECTS ON DIAGNOSTIC TESTS

None reported.

SPECIAL CONSIDERATIONS

• Monitor serum methotrexate and serum creatinine levels, creatinine clearance, and urine pH every 6 to 24 hours during leucovorin rescue.
• Begin leucovorin rescue within 24 hours of high-dose methotrexate regimen. If the patient's serum creatinine level is at least 50% of his baseline level after 24 hours of leucovorin therapy, increase dosage to 100 mg/m² q 3 hours until serum methotrexate falls below specified levels.
• If needed, increase leucovorin dosage or lengthen duration of therapy in patients with aciduria, ascites, dehydration, GI obstruction, renal impairment, or pleural or peri-

---

Unmarked trade names available in the United States only.
♦ Also available in Canada.   ♦ ♦ Available in Canada only.

toneal effusion. Duration of therapy depends on serum methotrexate levels.
• Treat overdoses of folic acid antagonists within 1 hour if possible. Drug is usually ineffective after 4-hour delay.
• Drug may increase seizures in susceptible children. Adjust anticonvulsant drug dose if necessary.
• Parenteral administration is recommended when oral doses are poorly absorbed because of nausea and vomiting.
• Don't give leucovorin simultaneously with methotrexate. Encourage fluids during rescue.
• Drug has been used to treat pediatric osteosarcoma and to improve tumor response in combination with methotrexate and fluorouracil. Rarely, it has been used with methotrexate for trophoblastic disease and persistent ectopic pregnancy.
• Do not use as the sole antianemic agent in treating vitamin B_{12} deficiencies.
• Generic forms of drug may contain benzyl alcohol.

levothyroxine sodium (T_4, L-thyroxine sodium)
Levothroid, Synthroid

Pregnancy Risk Category: A

PHARMACOKINETICS
Distribution: not fully understood but thought to be distributed to most body tissues and fluids, with highest levels in the liver and kidneys. Drug is more than 99% bound to plasma proteins. It doesn't readily cross the placenta.
Metabolism: about 85% deiodinated in peripheral tissues. Smaller amounts are conjugated with glucuronic and sulfate acids in the liver.

Excretion: in feces and urine. Half-life is 6 to 7 days, shorter in hyperthyroidism and longer in hypothyroidism. Minimal amounts of drug appear in breast milk.
Action: onset, 6 to 8 hours; duration, 1 to 3 weeks.

MECHANISM OF ACTION
Although levothyroxine's mechanism of action isn't clearly established, the drug's catabolic and anabolic effects are mediated at the cellular level by triiodothyronine (T_3). Thyroxine (T_4) is crucial to normal metabolism, growth, and development.

INDICATIONS & DOSAGE
• Hypothyroidism. *Adults:* 50 to 100 mcg daily as a single dose. *Children age 6 to 12:* 75 to 115.5 mcg or 3 to 3.75 mcg/kg daily. *Children age 1 to 5:* 56.25 to 75 mcg or 3.75 to 4.5 mcg/kg daily. *Infants age 6 to 12 months:* 37.5 to 56.25 mcg or 4.5 to 6 mcg/kg daily. *Healthy infants up to age 6 months:* 6 to 7.5 mcg/kg daily. *Premature infants weighing less than 2 kg and infants at risk for cardiac failure:* initially, 18.66 mcg daily, increased to 37.5 mcg daily after 4 to 6 weeks.
• Myxedema coma. *Adults:* initially, 200 to 500 mcg. Give 100 to 300 mcg on next day to obtain necessary improvement. *Children:* See schedule for hypothyroidism.

CONTRAINDICATIONS & CAUTIONS
• Use cautiously in angina, coronary artery disease, or hypertension because of possible exacerbation from increased metabolic demands.
• Also use cautiously in patients undergoing surgery or emergency treatment because of heightened metabolic demands.

• In adrenocortical insufficiency, administer carefully to avoid exacerbation and possible adrenal crisis.
• Also administer carefully in diabetes mellitus because of possible reduced glucose tolerance.
• In elderly patients, give levothyroxine cautiously because of possible undiagnosed cardiac disease.

PREPARATION & STORAGE
Available as a buff-colored, odorless powder in 6 ml vials (concentrations of 200 or 500 mcg) that remain stable at room temperature. Store in light-resistant containers; otherwise, powder may turn light pink.

Reconstitute Levothroid powder by adding 2 to 5 ml of 0.9% sodium chloride injection (without preservative) to the 200 or 500 mg vial. Shake until clear. This solution contains 40 or 100 mcg/ml.

To reconstitute Synthroid powder, add 5 ml of 0.9% sodium chloride injection or bacteriostatic sodium chloride injection with benzyl alcohol to the 200 or 500 mg vial. Shake to dissolve. The solution contains 40 or 100 mcg/ml.

Reconstitute drug immediately before use and discard any unused portions.

ADMINISTRATION
Direct injection: Inject into vein over 1 to 2 minutes.
Intermittent infusion: not recommended.
Continuous infusion: not recommended.

INCOMPATIBILITY
Don't mix with any solution for I.V. infusion.

ADVERSE REACTIONS
Life-threatening: congestive heart failure, craniosynostosis (in infants given high doses).

Other: accelerated bone growth (in infants given high doses), alopecia (in children), angina, anxiety, clumsiness, cold sensation, constipation, diarrhea, dyspnea, fever, headache (severe), heat intolerance, hypertension, insomnia, ischemia, leg cramps, lethargy, nausea, rash, skin dryness and puffiness, tachydysrhythmias, tremors, urticaria, weakness, weight loss or gain.

INTERACTIONS
Anticoagulants, sympathomimetics, tricyclic antidepressants: possible enhanced effects of levothyroxine and these drugs, worsened coronary insufficiency, dysrhythmias.
Antidiabetics: altered levothyroxine and antidiabetic drug effects. Monitor serum glucose levels.
Beta blockers: possible diminished peripheral conversion of T_4 to T_3.
Corticosteroids: altered metabolic clearance, possibly requiring a dosage adjustment.
Estrogens: reduced levothyroxine effectiveness because of increased serum thyroxine-binding globulin.
Hepatic enzyme inducers: enhanced hepatic degradation of levothyroxine.
Ketamine: possible hypertension and tachycardia.
Maprotiline: possible increased dysrhythmias.
Somatrem, somatropin: possible accelerated epiphyseal maturation.

EFFECTS ON DIAGNOSTIC TESTS
Radionuclide thyroid scan: possible diminished uptake of ^{123}I, ^{131}I, and sodium pertechnate Tc 99m.

SPECIAL CONSIDERATIONS
• *Treatment of overdose:* Withdraw drug for 2 to 6 days. Resume administration at a lower dose.
• In myxedema coma, give levothyroxine with hydrocortisone to pre-

vent adrenal crisis, and monitor the EKG for ventricular dysrhythmias. Hydrocortisone dosage starts at 300 mg/day in divided doses and should be tapered over the next 4 or 5 days.
• If adrenal insufficiency occurs during therapy, correct it promptly to prevent adrenal crisis.
• Reduce adult levothyroxine dosage by about 25% in patients over age 60. Also give smaller doses in cardiovascular disease and hyperthyroidism.
• Monitor vital signs to detect adverse effects early.
• Be alert for tachydysrhythmias and signs of ischemia.
• Monitor thyroid function tests: serum free T_4 index, total serum T_4, T_3 resin uptake, serum free T_4, and serum thyroid-stimulating hormone.
• Regularly assess bone growth and psychomotor development in pediatric congenital hypothyroidism.

lidocaine hydrochloride
LidoPen, Xylocaine, Xylocard♦♦

Pregnancy Risk Category: B

PHARMACOKINETICS
Distribution: throughout body tissues, with rapid dispersal to the kidneys, lungs, liver, and heart and slower dispersal to skeletal muscle and fat. Sixty to eighty percent binds to plasma proteins. Drug crosses the blood-brain barrier and placenta.
Metabolism: 90% in the liver.
Excretion: in urine, primarily as metabolites. Initial phase half-life is 7 to 30 minutes; terminal phase half-life, 1.5 to 2 hours. Drug appears in breast milk.
Action: onset, 45 to 90 seconds; duration, 10 to 20 minutes.

MECHANISM OF ACTION
A Class IB antiarrhythmic (fast sodium channel blocker), lidocaine reduces automaticity in the His-Purkinje system and suppresses ventricular depolarization. The drug also acts as a CNS anesthetic, producing sedative, analgesic, and anticonvulsant effects.

INDICATIONS & DOSAGE
• Acute ventricular dysrhythmias (premature ventricular contractions, ventricular tachycardia) associated with acute MI, cardiac glycoside toxicity, cardioversion, cardiac manipulation from trauma or surgery, or drug side effects. *Adults:* 50 to 100 mg initial bolus, repeated after 5 minutes if dysrhythmias continue. For maintenance, infuse 20 to 50 mcg/kg/minute (1 to 4 mg/minute in 70-kg adult). Don't exceed 300 mg within 1 hour. Keep rate below 30 mcg/kg/minute in patients with congestive heart failure or liver disease. *Children:* 0.5 to 1 mg/kg initial bolus, repeated as necessary. For maintenance, infuse 10 to 50 mcg/kg/minute. Maximum dosage, 5 mg/kg.
• Status epilepticus unresponsive to all other measures. *Adults and children:* initial bolus of 1 mg/kg. If seizure doesn't stop after 2 minutes, give 0.5 mg/kg bolus. For maintenance, infuse 30 mcg/kg/minute.

CONTRAINDICATIONS & CAUTIONS
• Contraindicated in hypersensitivity to lidocaine or amidelike anesthetics, in Adams-Stokes disease and Wolff-Parkinson-White syndrome, and in second- or third-degree heart block.
• Use cautiously in children, the elderly, and patients with severe kidney or liver disease, congestive heart

failure, or shock because drug may accumulate.

• Also use cautiously in patients with sinus bradycardia or incomplete heart block who haven't received isoproterenol or a pacemaker because lidocaine may increase premature ventricular contractions and ventricular escape beats, leading to ventricular tachycardia.

• In children, dosage ranges and drug efficacy haven't been determined through controlled studies.

PREPARATION & STORAGE

Available for injection in 5 ml ampules and prefilled syringes with concentrations of 10 and 20 mg/ml.

Available for continuous infusion in 40 mg, 1 g, and 2 g single-use 25 or 50 ml vials and in 5 and 10 ml syringes that require mixing with dextrose 5% in water. Dilute 1 g of drug in 250 ml of dextrose 5% in water to obtain a 0.4% solution (4 mg/ml). Drug also comes in premixed 250 ml bottles of 0.4% or 0.8% solution or 500 ml bottles of 0.2%, 0.4%, or 0.8% solution.

Store at room temperature. Be sure to use only solutions marked for treating dysrhythmias.

ADMINISTRATION

Direct injection: Inject undiluted drug into large vein or cannula at a rate of 25 to 50 mg/minute.
Intermittent infusion: not recommended.
Continuous infusion: Using an infusion pump and microdrop tubing, titrate dose according to suppression of ventricular ectopy.

INCOMPATIBILITY

Incompatible with amphotericin B, ampicillin sodium, cefazolin sodium, methohexital, and phenytoin.

ADVERSE REACTIONS

Life-threatening: anaphylaxis, bradycardia, cardiac arrest, coma, hypotension, respiratory arrest, seizures.
Other: agitation, anxiety, apprehension, blurred or double vision, confusion, dizziness, drowsiness, dysphagia, dyspnea, euphoria, lethargy, light-headedness, nausea, paresthesias, psychosis, restlessness, seizures, slurred speech, thrombophlebitis, tinnitus, tremors, twitching, unconsciousness, vomiting.

INTERACTIONS

Aminoglycosides, polymyxin B: enhanced neuromuscular blockade.
Beta blockers, cimetidine: reduced metabolism and heightened risk of lidocaine toxicity.
Hydantoin anticonvulsants: excessive respiratory depression.
Phenytoin, procainamide, propranolol, quinidine: potentiated or antagonized antiarrhythmic effects.

EFFECTS ON DIAGNOSTIC TESTS

None reported.

SPECIAL CONSIDERATIONS

• *Treatment of overdose:* Stop infusion immediately and notify doctor. Ensure an adequate airway and oxygenation. Give oxygen by nasal cannula if appropriate. Be prepared to initiate cardiopulmonary resuscitation. Continue to monitor EKG for underlying ventricular dysrhythmias, and prepare to give an alternate antiarrhythmic, such as procainamide. Monitor respirations and blood pressure every 5 minutes for 20 minutes. If the patient develops bradycardia, give atropine and be alert for tachycardia. If he experiences seizures, give diazepam and monitor carefully for respiratory depression.

- Monitor EKG continuously during administration to titrate continuous infusion and detect prolonged PR interval (more than 0.2 second), widened QRS complex (more than 0.12 second), or worsened ventricular dysrhythmias. Keep resuscitation equipment, including a defibrillator, nearby.
- If patient is alert, instruct him to report symptoms of toxicity during infusion. Also, assess frequently for signs of toxicity.
- Use smallest lidocaine dose possible to control dysrhythmias. Therapeutic levels range from 1.5 to 5 mcg/ml; toxic level is greater than 5 mcg/ml.
- Monitor SGOT, SGPT, BUN, and serum creatinine and electrolyte levels. Report abnormalities to doctor.
- Treat underlying causes of ventricular dysrhythmias.

lincomycin hydrochloride
Lincocin

Pregnancy Risk Category: B

PHARMACOKINETICS
Distribution: rapid and widespread to most body fluids and tissues, with moderate to high protein binding; poor distribution in normal cerebrospinal fluid and only up to 18% of serum levels when meninges are inflamed. Drug readily crosses the placenta, producing cord levels that are 25% of maternal serum levels.
Metabolism: partly in the liver. Rate rises in children.
Excretion: 2% to 30% in urine and 4% to 14% in feces. Half-life ranges from about 4 to 6 hours in normal renal and hepatic function to 9 to 13 hours in impaired function. Drug appears in breast milk.

Action: peak plasma levels, 2 to 4 hours.

MECHANISM OF ACTION
Bacteriostatic or bactericidal depending on the organism's susceptibility and the drug's concentration, lincomycin inhibits protein synthesis by binding to bacterial ribosomes. Drug is effective against most aerobic gram-positive cocci, including staphylococci and *Streptococcus pneumoniae*. It's also used against such anaerobic and microaerophilic gram-negative and gram-positive organisms as *Actinomyces, Bacteroides, Eubacterium, Fusobacterium, Propionibacterium,* microaerophilic streptococci, *Peptococcus, Peptostreptococcus, Veillonella, Clostridium perfringens, Clostridium tetani, Corynebacterium diphtheriae,* and *Mycoplasma.*

INDICATIONS & DOSAGE
- Severe infections caused by susceptible organisms. *Adults:* 600 mg to 1 g q 12 to 24 hours. Maximum dosage, 8 g/day. *Children older than age 1 month:* 3.3 to 6.7 mg/kg q 8 hours or 5 to 10 mg/kg q 12 hours. *Note:* Adjust dosage in renal failure. In adult patients, if creatinine clearance is 10 to 50 ml/min, give 50% of the usual dose. If creatinine clearance is less than 10 ml/min, give 25% of the usual dose.

CONTRAINDICATIONS & CAUTIONS
- Contraindicated in neonates and in patients with lincomycin or clindamycin hypersensitivity; and in hepatic or severe renal disease.
- Use cautiously in elderly or debilitated patients or those with GI disorders (especially colitis); and in patients with a history of asthma or allergies.

PREPARATION & STORAGE
Available as a clear, colorless to slightly yellow solution in 2 and 10 ml vials with a concentration of 300 mg/ml. Store vials at room temperature; don't freeze.

For infusion, dilute drug with 100 to 400 ml of dextrose 5% or 10% in water, 0.9% sodium chloride, or Ringer's lactate. Solution remains stable for 24 hours at room temperature.

ADMINISTRATION
Direct injection: not recommended.
Intermittent infusion: Infuse solution over at least 1 hour, preferably over 2 to 4 hours for 200 to 400 ml volumes. Rapid infusion may cause cardiac arrest or severe hypotension.
Continuous infusion: not recommended.

INCOMPATIBILITY
Incompatible with ampicillin, carbenicillin, kanamycin, novobiocin, penicillin G potassium or sodium, and phenytoin.

ADVERSE REACTIONS
Life-threatening: anaphylaxis, angioneurotic edema, cardiac arrest, hypotension, Stevens-Johnson syndrome.
Other: abdominal cramps; agranulocytosis; anal pruritus; aplastic anemia; azotemia; diarrhea; enterocolitis; exfoliative, vesiculobullous dermatitis (rare); glossitis; headache; leukopenia; myalgia; nausea; neutropenia; oliguria; pain at infusion site; pancytopenia; proteinuria; pseudomembranous colitis; rash; stomatitis; superinfection; syncope; thrombocytopenic purpura; thrombophlebitis at injection site; tinnitus; unusual thirst; urticaria; vaginitis; vertigo; vomiting; weight loss.

INTERACTIONS
Antimyasthenics: possible antagonized effects.
Chloramphenicol, erythromycins: antagonized lincomycin effects.
Hydrocarbon inhalation anesthetics, neuromuscular blockers: enhanced neuromuscular blockade.
Neurotoxic drugs: enhanced risk of toxicity.
Opioid analgesics: possible deepened respiratory depression.

EFFECTS ON DIAGNOSTIC TESTS
SGOT, SGPT: possible elevated levels.

SPECIAL CONSIDERATIONS
• Use lincomycin only when penicillin is contraindicated or in patients with infections unresponsive to other antibiotics.
• Obtain specimens for culture and sensitivity testing before first dose. Therapy may start before results are available.
• If diarrhea persists during therapy, discontinue drug and collect stool specimens for culture to rule out pseudomembranous colitis.
• Frequently monitor blood pressure.
• Check infusion site for signs of phlebitis. Rotate sites regularly.
• Monitor hepatic function (SGOT, SGPT, bilirubin).
• Monitor CBC and platelet count. Stop drug if blood dyscrasias develop.
• If patient has a monilial infection, give an antifungal drug along with lincomycin.
• Drug isn't appreciably removed by hemodialysis or peritoneal dialysis.
• May contain benzyl alcohol.
• Observe patient for signs of bacterial or fungal superinfection during prolonged use.

Unmarked trade names available in the United States only.
♦Also available in Canada.   ♦♦Available in Canada only.

lorazepam
Ativan

Controlled Substance Schedule IV
Pregnancy Risk Category: D

PHARMACOKINETICS
Distribution: widespread, with 85% of drug bound to plasma proteins. Drug crosses the blood-brain barrier and placenta.
Metabolism: in the liver.
Excretion: in urine as conjugated drug. Half-life is 10 to 20 hours. Drug appears in breast milk.
Action: onset, 1 to 5 minutes; duration, usually 6 to 8 hours but sedation may last for up to 24 hours.

MECHANISM OF ACTION
Lorazepam's sites and mechanism of action aren't completely understood. But it is thought to enhance or facilitate the action of the neurotransmitter gamma-aminobutyric acid, which depresses the CNS at the limbic and subcortical levels, producing an antianxiety effect. It also possesses skeletal muscle–relaxant, anticonvulsant, and amnesic properties.

INDICATIONS & DOSAGE
• Short-term symptomatic relief of anxiety in N.P.O. patient. *Adults:* 0.044 mg/kg. Maximum total dose is 2 mg.
• Preoperative sedation. *Adults:* 0.044 to 0.5 mg/kg 15 to 20 minutes before surgery. Maximum total dose is 4 mg.
• Prevention of nausea and vomiting associated with chemotherapy. *Adults:* 2 mg 30 minutes before chemotherapy, followed by 2 mg q 4 hours as needed.

CONTRAINDICATIONS & CAUTIONS
• Contraindicated in hypersensitivity to benzodiazepines, polyethylene glycol, propylene glycol, or benzyl alcohol; in acute narrow-angle glaucoma because of possible anticholinergic effect; in shock or coma because drug's hypotensive or hypnotic effects may be prolonged or worsened; in acute alcohol intoxication because drug deepens CNS depression; and in hepatic or renal failure.
• Avoid use in respiratory depression because of the heightened risk of airway obstruction.
• Give cautiously to psychotic patients because of possible paradoxical reaction; to depressed patients because of possible worsened depression; and to patients with myasthenia gravis or porphyria because of possible exacerbation.
• Also administer cautiously to patients with renal or hepatic impairment because of delayed drug elimination; to patients with hypoalbuminemia because of a higher incidence of adverse effects; to elderly or debilitated patients because of increased CNS effects; to seizure patients because withdrawal may precipitate seizures; and to addiction-prone patients.
• Pediatric safety hasn't been established.

PREPARATION & STORAGE
Available in 1 and 10 ml vials and single-dose prefilled syringes with concentrations of 2 and 4 mg/ml. Refrigerate drug (but don't freeze) and protect from light. Discard if drug becomes discolored or contains precipitate. Immediately before administration, dilute drug with an equal volume of sterile water for injection, 0.9% sodium chloride, or dextrose 5% in water. Rotate syringe gently to ensure complete mixing.

ADMINISTRATION
Direct injection: Inject into vein or into an I.V. line containing a free-flowing compatible solution at a maximum rate of 2 mg/minute.
Intermittent infusion: not recommended.
Continuous infusion: not recommended.

INCOMPATIBILITY
No incompatibilities reported.

ADVERSE REACTIONS
Life-threatening: airway obstruction, apnea, cardiac arrest, hypotension.
Other: anorexia, anxiety, ataxia, blurred or double vision, carpal tunnel syndrome, confusion, constipation, depression, dizziness, double or blurred vision, drowsiness, dry mouth, dysarthria, dyspnea, edema, esophageal dilation, euphoria, excitation, fatigue, hallucinations, headache, hearing loss, hiccups, hypertension, hypotension, increased salivation and bronchial secretions, metallic taste, muscle spasticity, nausea, nightmares, pain or redness at injection site, palpitations, paresthesias, photosensitivity, pruritus, purpura, rage, rash, sleep disturbances, syncope, tachycardia, talkativeness, thrombophlebitis, tongue swelling, tremulousness, urinary incontinence or retention, urticaria, vertigo, vomiting, weakness.

INTERACTIONS
Alcohol, other CNS depressants: increased effects.
Antihypertensives: heightened risk of severe hypotension.
Digoxin: possible enhanced effects.
Fentanyl derivatives: reduced amounts required for induction of anesthesia.
Ketamine: increased risk of hypotention or respiratory depression.

Levodopa: decreased therapeutic effects of levodopa.

EFFECTS ON DIAGNOSTIC TESTS
Serum alkaline phosphatase, SGOT, SGPT: elevated levels.
WBC count and differential: reduced levels.

SPECIAL CONSIDERATIONS
● *Treatment of overdose:* Maintain a patent airway and adequate ventilation, and give I.V. fluids to enhance drug excretion. If hypotension occurs, administer norepinephrine or metaraminol.
● Always keep emergency resuscitation equipment nearby when giving I.V. lorazepam. Obtain baseline respiratory rate before administration, and notify doctor if rate falls below 12 breaths/minute. Also obtain baseline blood pressure, and carefully monitor blood pressure during and after administration.
● Monitor respiratory rate for 1 hour after administration. If rate falls below 8 breaths/minute, arouse patient and encourage him to breathe at a rate of 10 to 12 breaths/minute. If you can't arouse patient, maintain airway patency and manually ventilate the patient to maintain rate of 10 to 12 breaths/minute. Notify doctor; he may decide to intubate patient.
● Observe infusion site for signs of phlebitis.
● Overly rapid infusion can cause apnea, hypotension, bradycardia, or cardiac arrest.
● Maintain bed rest. Adjust the bed to lowest position and raise the bed's side rails to prevent falls.
● Discontinue drug if paradoxical reaction occurs, typified by anxiety, acute excitation, hallucinations, increased muscle spasticity, insomnia, or rage.

• Warn patient that drug diminishes alertness and coordination.
• Lorazepam has been used successfully to terminate status epilepticus.

---

magnesium sulfate

Pregnancy Risk Category: A

PHARMACOKINETICS
Distribution: widely distributed; readily crosses the placenta.
Metabolism: not metabolized.
Excretion: in urine by glomerular filtration. Drug appears in breast milk.
Action: onset, immediately after administration; duration, 30 minutes.

MECHANISM OF ACTION
Produces anticonvulsant effects by depressing the CNS; also blocks peripheral neuromuscular transmission.

INDICATIONS & DOSAGE
• Preeclampsia or eclampsia. *Adults:* 4 g, followed by either 1 to 2 g/hour given by continuous infusion or 4 to 11 g given I.M. Dosage over next 24 hours depends on serum magnesium levels and urine output. Maximum dosage is 30 to 40 g q 24 hours; in renal disease, it's 20 g q 48 hours.
• Prevention and control of seizures in severe preeclampsia or eclampsia, epilepsy, glomerulonephritis, or hypothyroidism. *Adults:* 1 to 4 g (8 to 32 mEq of magnesium) of 10% to 20% solution.
• Severe hypertension, encephalopathy, and seizures caused by nephritis. *Children:* 100 to 200 mg/kg of 1% to 3% solution. Give total dose within 1 hour, half within the first 15 to 20 minutes.
• Severe magnesium deficiency. *Adults:* 5 g.

• Magnesium supplement in total parenteral nutrition. *Adults:* 0.5 to 3 g daily (4 to 24 mEq of magnesium). *Infants:* 0.25 to 1.25 g daily (2 to 10 mEq of magnesium).
• Barium poisoning. *Adults:* 1 to 2 g.
• Paroxysmal atrial tachycardia. *Adults:* 3 to 4 g.

CONTRAINDICATIONS & CAUTIONS
• Contraindicated in myocardial damage and heart block because drug depresses cardiac muscle.
• Also contraindicated within 2 hours of expected delivery because neonate may show signs of magnesium toxicity.
• Use cautiously in renal impairment.

PREPARATION & STORAGE
Available as a 10% concentration in 10 and 20 ml ampules (100 mg/ml), and in 20 and 50 ml vials; 12.5% concentration in 20 ml vials (125 mg/ml); and 50% concentration in 2 ml ampules (500 mg/ml), 2, 5, 10, 30, and 50 ml vials, and 10 ml syringes. Store at room temperature and avoid freezing.
   In seizures, dilute dose in 250 ml dextrose 5% in water. In magnesium deficiency, dilute dose in 1 liter of dextrose 5% in water or dextrose 5% in 0.9% sodium chloride. For all indications, don't use concentrations over 20% (200 mg/ml).

ADMINISTRATION
Direct injection: Inject directly into vein, not exceeding 150 mg/minute.
Intermittent infusion: Administer diluted drug over 1 to 3 hours.
Continuous infusion: Give by infusion pump, not exceeding 150 mg/minute (1.2 mEq/minute).

INCOMPATIBILITY
Incompatible with alcohol, alkali carbonates and bicarbonates, calcium gluceptate, calcium gluconate, clindamycin phosphate, dobutamine, hydrocortisone sodium succinate, 10% intravenous fat emulsion, polymyxin B, procaine, and soluble phosphates.

ADVERSE REACTIONS
Life-threatening: cardiac arrest, hypermagnesemia (serum level greater than 4 mEq/liter), respiratory paralysis, severe bradycardia, severe hypotension.
Other: depressed reflexes, diaphoresis, flushing, hypothermia, hypotonia, prolonged PR interval, widened QRS complex.

INTERACTIONS
Calcium salts: possible neutralization of magnesium sulfate.
CNS depressants: additive CNS depression.
Neuromuscular blocking agents: possible excessive neuromuscular blockade.

EFFECTS ON DIAGNOSTIC TESTS
Reticuloendothelial cell imaging: unreliable results when using technetium Tc 99m sulfur colloid.

SPECIAL CONSIDERATIONS
• *Treatment of overdose:* Disappearance of patellar reflexes signals onset of toxicity. Treat with 5 to 10 mEq of calcium (10 to 20 ml of 10% calcium gluconate), as ordered. In severe overdose, peritoneal dialysis or hemodialysis may be necessary.
• Keep I.V. calcium gluconate available; however, use cautiously in patients undergoing digitalization because dysrhythmias may develop.
• Monitor vital signs every 15 minutes. Be alert for respiratory depression and signs of heart block. Also monitor intake and output. Before each dose, respirations should be about 16 per minute, and urine output should be 100 ml or more for 4 hours.
• Monitor serum magnesium levels.
• Rapid administration causes uncomfortable sensation of heat.
• In pediatric hypertension and encephalopathy, I.M. administration precedes I.V.
• Observe neonate for signs of magnesium toxicity, such as neuromuscular or respiratory depression, especially when drug has been given to toxemic mothers within 24 hours before delivery.

mannitol
Osmitrol♦♦

Pregnancy Risk Category: C

PHARMACOKINETICS
Distribution: confined to extracellular space. Drug doesn't cross the blood-brain barrier, except in high concentrations or in acidosis, or reach the eye. Not known if it crosses the placenta.
Metabolism: metabolized slightly (if at all) to glycogen in the liver.
Excretion: in urine, with about 80% eliminated unchanged in 3 hours. Half-life is about 100 minutes. Clearance decreases in renal disease.
Action: onset, 15 minutes for reduction of cerebrospinal fluid (CSF), 30 to 60 minutes for intraocular pressure, and 1 to 3 hours for diuresis; duration, 3 to 8 hours for reduction of CSF or intraocular pressure.

MECHANISM OF ACTION
Mannitol increases osmotic pressure of glomerular filtrate, which inhibits renal tubular reabsorption of water

and solutes, thus promoting diuresis. This aids excretion of sodium, potassium, chloride, calcium, phosphates, lithium, magnesium, and some toxins. Drug also elevates plasma osmolality, aiding water flow from tissues (including brain, CSF, and eye) into interstitial fluid and plasma, thereby reducing CSF, intracranial, and intraocular pressure.

INDICATIONS & DOSAGE

• Prevention of oliguric phase in acute renal failure. *Adults:* 50 to 100 g, followed by infusion of a 5% or 10% solution.

• Test dose for marked oliguria or suspected inadequate renal function. *Adults and children over age 12:* 200 mg/kg, or 12.5 g as a 15% or 20% solution given over 3 to 5 minutes. *Children age 12 and under:* 0.2 g/kg given over 3 to 5 minutes, then 2 g/kg.

• Treatment of oliguria. *Adults:* 100 g of a 15% to 20% solution given over 90 minutes to several hours.

• Reduction of intracranial and intraocular pressure. *Adults:* 1.5 to 2 g/kg of a 15%, 20%, or 25% solution given over 30 to 60 minutes. *Children age 12 and under:* 1 to 2 g/kg of a 15% or 20% solution given over 30 to 60 minutes.

• Reduction of nephrotoxic effects of amphotericin B. *Adults:* 12.5 g given immediately before and after each dose of amphotericin B.

• Promotion of diuresis in drug intoxication (adjunct). *Adults:* 50 to 200 g of a 5% to 25% solution, followed by infusion to maintain urine output at 100 to 500 ml/hour.

• Adjunctive treatment of edema and ascites. *Adults:* 100 g of a 10% to 20% solution given over 2 to 6 hours. *Children age 12 and under:* 2 g/kg of a 15% or 20% solution given over 2 to 6 hours.

CONTRAINDICATIONS & CAUTIONS

• Contraindicated in anuria because circulatory overload may occur.

• Also contraindicated in intracranial bleeding (except during craniotomy) because of possible exacerbation.

• Avoid use in severe dehydration because mannitol worsens the condition, and in severe pulmonary congestion and congestive heart failure because increased circulating volume aggravates these conditions.

• Use cautiously in cardiopulmonary impairment because of the risk of congestive heart failure.

• Also use cautiously in hyperkalemia or hyponatremia because drug may worsen electrolyte imbalance; in hypovolemia because drug may mask the condition and enhance hemoconcentration; and in severe renal impairment because of possible circulatory overload.

PREPARATION & STORAGE

Available in strengths of 5%, 10%, 15%, 20%, and 25% in 150, 250, 500, and 1,000 ml glass and plastic I.V. containers. Store at room temperature; avoid freezing. Mannitol may crystallize, especially if chilled. If crystals form, dissolve according to manufacturer's directions. Avoid using any solution that contains undissolved crystals.

ADMINISTRATION

When giving mannitol solutions with concentrations of 15% or above, make sure the administration set includes a filter. Rapid administration of large doses may lead to drug accumulation and circulatory overload.

Avoid extravasation to prevent edema and necrosis.

Direct injection: not recommended.

Intermittent infusion: Infuse appropriate dose and concentration at ordered rate.

Continuous infusion: Infuse appropriate dose and concentration at ordered rate.

INCOMPATIBILITY
Incompatible with imipenem/cilastatin and blood products. If blood must be given with mannitol, add 20 mEq of sodium chloride to each liter of mannitol.

ADVERSE REACTIONS
Life-threatening: acute renal failure, dysrhythmias, vacuolar nephrosis.
Other: acidosis, arm pain, backache, blurred vision, chest pain, chills, confusion, dizziness, dry mouth, extravasation (localized edema, necrosis), fever, headache, hypertension, hypotension, muscle rigidity, nausea, paresthesias, pulmonary congestion (dyspnea, wheezing), rhinitis, seizures, tachycardia, thirst, thrombophlebitis, uricosuria, urine retention, urticaria, vomiting, weakness in extremities.

INTERACTIONS
Cardiac glycosides: enhanced risk of hypokalemia-induced toxicity.
Diuretics, including carbonic anhydrase inhibitors: possible potentiation of diuretic and intraocular effects.
Lithium: decreased effects.

EFFECTS ON DIAGNOSTIC TESTS
Blood ethylene glycol: altered results.
Inorganic phosphorus: increased or decreased blood levels.
Serum electrolytes: altered levels.

SPECIAL CONSIDERATIONS
• Give test dose of mannitol to determine if adequate response is possible. Infuse 200 mg/kg of 15% to 25% solution over 3 to 5 minutes. Urine flow should increase to at least 30 ml/hour for 2 to 3 hours after giving drug.
• Before giving mannitol, obtain baseline blood pressure, heart and lung sounds, and EKG.
• Monitor vital signs frequently during first hour of infusion and hourly thereafter or as needed. Also monitor intake and output, BUN, and serum electrolytes, especially sodium and potassium.
• Large doses may cross the blood-brain barrier and cause CNS damage or death.
• Small or debilitated patients may require lower doses.
• Advise patients to change position slowly to avoid dizziness from orthostatic hypotension.
• Maintain hemostasis with adequate hydration and electrolytes.
• Lower mannitol concentrations and solutions containing sodium chloride reduce the risk of dehydration and electrolyte depletion.
• Rebound increase in intracranial and intraocular pressure may occur about 12 hours after mannitol administration.
• Alkalinization of urine with sodium bicarbonate may be necessary to help treat salicylate or barbiturate poisoning.

mechlorethamine hydrochloride (nitrogen mustard)
Mustargen♦

Pregnancy Risk Category: D

PHARMACOKINETICS
Distribution: widely distributed to body fluids and tissues. Not known if drug crosses the placenta.

Metabolism: rapidly metabolized in body fluids and tissues.

Excretion: by the kidneys apparently, but not well characterized. More than 50% of inactive metabolites are excreted in urine.

Action: peak serum level, within a few minutes.

MECHANISM OF ACTION

An alkylating agent, mechlorethamine inhibits rapid cell division by interfering with DNA replication and RNA transcription.

INDICATIONS & DOSAGE

Dosage is based on patient response and degree of toxicity.

• Hodgkin's disease. *Adults and children:* 6 mg/m^2 daily on days 1 and 8 of 28-day cycle in combination with other antineoplastics (MOPP regimen). Dosage repeated for six cycles. Subsequent doses reduced by 50% in MOPP regimen when WBC count is between 3,000 and 3,999/mm^3 and by 75% when WBC count is between 1,000 and 2,999/mm^3 or platelet count is between 50,000 and 100,000/mm^3.

• Other neoplastic disorders. *Adults and children:* 0.4 mg/kg as single dose or 0.1 to 0.2 mg/kg divided in two or four successive daily doses during each course of therapy.

CONTRAINDICATIONS & CAUTIONS

• Contraindicated in chicken pox, herpes, or other infections because of the risk of generalized disease.

• Also contraindicated in acute or chronic suppurative inflammation because drug may contribute to development of amyloidosis.

• Use cautiously in concurrent anticoagulant therapy, radiation therapy, or other chemotherapy, and in prexisting myelosuppression or tumor cell infiltration of bone marrow be-

cause further myelosuppression may occur.

• Also use cautiously in patients with gout or a history of urate renal stones because of the increased risk of hyperuricemia.

PREPARATION & STORAGE

Exercise extreme caution when preparing or administering mechlorethamine to avoid mutagenic, teratogenic, and carcinogenic risks. Use a biological containment cabinet, wear gloves and mask, and use syringes with Luer-Lok fittings to prevent leakage of drug solution. Also correctly dispose of needles, vials, and unused drug, and avoid contaminating work surfaces.

Avoid inhalation of mechlorethamine dust or vapors or contact with skin or mucous membranes. If eye contact occurs, irrigate with liberal amounts of water or saline solution and consult an ophthalmologist immediately. If skin contact occurs, irrigate for at least 15 minutes with water and then with 2% sodium thiosulfate solution.

Mechlorethamine is available in 10 mg vials. Store at room temperature. Reconstitute with 10 ml sterile water for injection or 0.9% sodium chloride for a concentration of 1 mg/ml. Shake vial several times to dissolve. Administer within 15 minutes. Highly unstable, the solution decomposes while standing. Don't use if it's discolored or if water droplets appear in vial. Discard any unused drug.

ADMINISTRATION

Direct injection: Use one sterile needle to aspirate reconstituted drug from the vial and another for direct injection. Inject reconstituted solution directly into vein or, preferably, into a free-flowing I.V. solution over a few minutes or according to proto-

col. After administration, flush vein with I.V. solution for 2 to 5 minutes.
Intermittent infusion: not recommended.
Continuous infusion: not recommended.

INCOMPATIBILITY
Incompatible with methohexital sodium.

ADVERSE REACTIONS
Life-threatening: cerebral degeneration, hemorrhagic diathesis, myelosuppression.
Other: alopecia, amenorrhea (temporary or permanent), anemia, anorexia, black tarry stools, chills, confusion, dehydration (secondary to vomiting), delayed menses, dependent edema, diarrhea, drowsiness, dyspnea, extravasation (induration, local inflammation, possible sloughing of tissues, thrombophlebitis, thrombosis, tissue necrosis), fever, flank pain, headache, hyperuricemia, impaired spermatogenesis or azospermia, jaundice, lymphocytopenia, maculopapular rash, metallic taste, nausea, oligomenorrhea, pain or redness at injection site, paresthesias, progressive muscle paralysis, seizures, stomach pain, stomatitis, thrombocytopenia, tinnitus, vertigo, vomiting, weakness, wheezing.

INTERACTIONS
Antigout drugs: diminished effectiveness. Increased doses may be necessary.
Myelosuppressive drugs: additional myelosuppression.

EFFECTS ON DIAGNOSTIC TESTS
Serum cholinesterase: possible decreased levels.
Serum isocitric acid dehydrogenase, uric acid: possible increased levels.

SPECIAL CONSIDERATIONS
• Mechlorethamine is used almost exclusively in combination chemotherapy. Lower dosages are required when it's used with other myelosuppressive drugs.
• If infiltration occurs, inject area with sterile isotonic sodium thiosulfate (⅙ M), and apply ice compresses for 6 to 12 hours. Use 4.14 g of sodium thiosulfate per 100 ml of sterile water for injection, or dilute 4 ml of sodium thiosulfate (10%) with 6 ml of sterile water for injection.
• Administer with hydrocortisone, as ordered, to reduce risk of phlebitis or painful administration.
• Expect some evidence of toxicity with a therapeutic response. Mechlorethamine is highly toxic and has a low therapeutic index.
• Give antiemetics to reduce severity of nausea and vomiting, which usually begin 1 to 3 hours after administration.
• Monitor WBC and platelet counts, and BUN, hematocrit, SGPT, SGOT, bilirubin, creatinine, LDH, and uric acid levels.
• Also closely monitor patient for potentially fatal infections or hemorrhagic complications noted by fever, sore throat, or unusual bruising or bleeding. Advise the patient to avoid exposure to people with infections.
• Give antibiotics, as ordered, to patients with leukopenia who develop an infection.
• Adequate hydration, alkalization of urine, and administration of allopurinol may prevent uric acid nephropathy.
• In lymphocytopenia, nadirs occur 1 to 3 weeks after drug administration.
• Interval between courses of therapy is usually 3 to 6 weeks.

---

menadiol sodium diphosphate (menadione, vitamin K₃)
Synkayvite

Pregnancy Risk Category: C

PHARMACOKINETICS
Distribution: unknown. Drug crosses the placenta
Metabolism: in the liver.
Excretion: in urine and feces. Drug doesn't appear in breast milk.
Action: onset, 8 to 24 hours; duration, unknown.

MECHANISM OF ACTION
Similar to that of naturally occurring vitamin K. A fat-soluble vitamin, menadiol promotes hepatic synthesis of prothrombin and other clotting factors.

INDICATIONS & DOSAGE
• Hypoprothrombinemia. *Adults:* 5 to 15 mg once or twice daily. *Children:* 5 to 10 mg once or twice daily.
• Liver function testing. *Adults:* 75 mg.

CONTRAINDICATIONS & CAUTIONS
• Contraindicated in hypersensitivity to menadiol or sulfites.
• Use cautiously in glucose-6-phosphate dehydrogenase deficiency to avoid hemolysis and in hepatic impairment to prevent exacerbation.
• Menadiol isn't recommended for neonates.

PREPARATION & STORAGE
Available in 1 and 2 ml ampules containing 5, 10, or 37.5 mg/ml. Store at room temperature and protect from light. For direct injection, dilute with 10 ml of 0.9% sodium chloride; for intermittent infusion, dilute with a larger volume of 0.9% sodium chloride or dextrose 5% in water; for continuous infusion, add to total parenteral nutrition (TPN) solution. For liver function testing, dilute 75 mg in a compatible solution.

ADMINISTRATION
Direct injection: Using a 21G or 23G needle, inject drug into vein or into I.V. tubing at maximum rate of 1 mg/minute. Never inject more than 10 mg at once.
Intermittent infusion: Using a 21G or 23G needle, infuse solution at a maximum rate of 1 mg/minute. In liver function testing, infuse diluted solution over at least 2 hours. Control rate with infusion pump.
Continuous infusion: Add drug to TPN solution and infuse over 12 to 24 hours.

INCOMPATIBILITY
Incompatible with protein hydrolysate.

ADVERSE REACTIONS
Life-threatening: anaphylaxis, brain damage, hemolytic anemia, kernicterus in premature infants.
Other: facial flushing, pain at infusion site, rash, unusual taste, urticaria.

INTERACTIONS
Anticoagulants: decreased effects.
Primaquine: heightened risk of adverse reactions.

EFFECTS ON DIAGNOSTIC TESTS
Urine 17-hydroxycorticosteroids: falsely elevated levels when using modified Reddy-Jenkins-Thorn procedure.

SPECIAL CONSIDERATIONS
• Determine cause of hypoprothrombinemia. Aspirin, antibiotics,
or anticoagulants may induce it.
• Large doses may cause temporary
resistance to prothrombin-depressing
anticoagulants. When reinstituting
therapy, higher doses may be necessary. Perform coagulation studies 12
hours after initial dose and repeat as
needed.
• Menadiol isn't effective in treating
oral anticoagulant–induced hypoprothrombinemia and hereditary hypoprothrombinemia.
• Be careful not to confuse menadiol (K_3) with phytonadione (K_1).
• Vitamin K_1 preparations are safer
than menadiol for prophylaxis and
treatment of hemorrhagic disease.

---

meperidine hydrochloride (pethidine hydrochloride)
Demerol Hydrochloride♦

Controlled Substance Schedule: II
Pregnancy Risk Category: B
(D for prolonged use or high doses
at term)

PHARMACOKINETICS
Distribution: widespread. Drug is
highly bound to plasma proteins,
with highest concentrations in limbic
system, thalamus, striatum, hypothalamus, midbrain, and spinal cord.
Meperidine readily crosses the placenta.
Metabolism: occurs primarily in mi-
crosomes of the hepatic endoplasmic
reticulum. Also occurs in the CNS,
kidneys, lungs, and placenta. Nor-
meperidine, the primary metabolite,
is both active and toxic.
Excretion: primarily eliminated in
urine as metabolites. Small amounts
are removed in feces. Drug appears
in breast milk.

Action: onset, 1 minute; duration, 2
to 4 hours.

MECHANISM OF ACTION
A morphinelike agonist, meperidine
binds with opiate receptors in the
CNS to alter the perception of pain
and the emotional response to it.
Meperidine also exerts mild antitus-
sive action.

INDICATIONS & DOSAGE
• Moderate to severe pain. *Adults:*
10 to 50 mg q 2 to 4 hours or 15 to
35 mg hourly by infusion. Dosage
reflects patient response and severity
of pain.
• Adjunct in anesthesia. *Adults:*
fractional doses of a 10 mg/ml solution, repeated p.r.n., or 1 mg/ml by
infusion.

CONTRAINDICATIONS & CAUTIONS
• Contraindicated in sensitivity to
meperidine.
• Also contraindicated in diarrhea
resulting from poisons, toxins, or
use of cephalosporins or topical clindamycin until toxic substances clear
because meperidine may slow GI
motility.
• Avoid use in acute respiratory depression because drug may worsen
the condition.
• Give with extreme caution to patients with seizure disorders because
of possibility of exacerbating their
condition.
• Administer carefully in altered respiratory function because of the
risk of respiratory depression.
• Use cautiously in patients with
head injury and increased intracranial pressure (from intracranial lesions) because meperidine can mask
changes in level of consciousness
and elevate cerebrospinal fluid
(CSF) pressure.

• In prostatic hypertrophy, urethral stricture, or recent urinary tract surgery, use cautiously because meperidine can cause urinary retention. In renal or hepatic impairment, or renal failure, adjust dosage because of slowed drug clearance.

• Use cautiously in patients with atrial flutter or other supraventricular tachyarrhythmias; drug can increase ventricular response through a vagolytic action.

• Because of possible abuse, administer cautiously in patients with a history of drug abuse or emotional instability, or who show evidence of suicide potential.

• Give meperidine carefully in gallbladder disease because drug may increase biliary contractions; in abdominal disorders because drug may obscure diagnosis; and in inflammatory bowel disease because of the risk of toxic megacolon.

• Because meperdine may alter GI motility, use cautiously after recent GI surgery.

• In patients with hypothyroidism, give cautiously because of the risk of prolonged CNS and respiratory depression.

PREPARATION & STORAGE

Available in preservative-free ampules and vials and in preservative-containing syringes with strengths of 10, 25, 50, 75, and 100 mg/ml. Store vials and ampules at room temperature. Single doses in syringes remain stable at room temperature for 24 hours.

For direct injection, dilute dose with a compatible solution to a concentration of 10 mg/ml. For infusion, dilute with a compatible solution to a concentration of 1 mg/ml.

ADMINISTRATION

Direct injection: Inject diluted dose over 3 to 5 minutes. Rapid injection increases the risk of severe adverse reactions.

Intermittent infusion: not recommended.

Continuous infusion: Give at a rate of 15 to 35 mg/hour, using an infusion control device. Avoid rapid infusion.

INCOMPATIBILITY

Incompatible with aminophylline, amobarbital sodium, ephedrine, heparin, methicillin, morphine, oxytetracycline, phenobarbital sodium, phenytoin, sodium bicarbonate, sodium iodide, sulfadiazine, tetracycline, thiamylal, and thiopental.

ADVERSE REACTIONS

Life-threatening: anaphylaxis, bradycardia, circulatory depression, severe respiratory depression, tachycardia.

Other: abdominal pain, agitation, anorexia, coma, confusion, constipation, delirium, diaphoresis, dizziness, drowsiness, dry mouth, euphoria, facial flushing or redness, hallucinations, headache, insomnia, malaise, mental dullness, nausea, nervousness, nightmares, oliguria, pain, palpitations, phlebitis at injection site, pruritus, restlessness, sedation, seizures (with prolonged use), syncope, tachycardia, tremors, unusual dreams, urine retention, urticaria, visual disturbances, vomiting, weakness.

INTERACTIONS

Anticoagulants: increased effects.
Antidiarrheals: heightened risk of severe constipation.
Antihypertensives, diuretics: potentiated hypotension.

Unmarked trade names available in the United States only.
♦ Also available in Canada.   ♦♦ Available in Canada only.

Antimuscarinics: increased risk of constipation or urine retention.

Estrogens, oral contraceptives: inhibited meperidine metabolism.

Hydroxyzine: enhanced analgesia and CNS depression.

Isoniazid: aggravated adverse reactions to isoniazid.

Magnesium sulfate: potentiated CNS effects.

MAO inhibitors: severe respiratory depression, cyanosis, hypotension, coma, hyperexcitability, hypertension, hyperpyrexia, seizures, and tachycardia. Don't administer meperidine within 2 weeks of MAO inhibitor use.

Metoclopramide: decreased GI motility.

Naloxone: decreased CNS and respiratory depression and possible blocked analgesic effect.

Naltrexone: blocked analgesic effects.

Neuromuscular blocking agents: additive respiratory depression and severe constipation.

Other opioid analgesics and CNS depressants: additive CNS effects, respiratory depression, and hypotension. Reduce dose, as ordered.

EFFECTS ON DIAGNOSTIC TESTS

Gastric emptying studies: possible delayed or prolonged times.

Hepatobiliary imaging with technetium Tc 99m disofenin: delayed visualization, and spurious resemblance to biliary obstruction.

Lumbar puncture: elevated cerebrospinal fluid pressure secondary to respiratory depression–induced carbon dioxide retention.

Serum amylase, lipase: possible increased levels.

SPECIAL CONSIDERATIONS

• *Treatment of overdose:* Maintain airway patency and provide respiratory support. To reverse respiratory depression, give 0.4 mg of naloxone by I.V. push; repeat as necessary. Maintain blood pressure with I.V. fluids and vasopressors, as ordered.

• Check access site before administration. Keep in mind that inadvertent injection around a nerve trunk may cause transient sensorimotor paralysis.

• Give meperidine with the patient lying down to minimize hypotension. Tell him to rise slowly to reduce dizziness.

• Monitor respirations frequently during infusion and every 15 minutes for 1 hour after infusion. Remember to keep resuscitation equipment and naloxone nearby. If respirations drop below 8 breaths/minute, arouse patient to stimulate breathing. Notify doctor. He may order naloxone or respiratory support.

• For improved analgesia, give before patient has intense pain. Initially, a smaller daily dose given on a fixed schedule may help to reduce patient anxiety. Once pain control is adequate, you may individualize scheduling.

• Advise the patient to avoid alcoholic beverages, other CNS depressants, and activities that require alertness.

• Acidifying urine may enhance excretion of unchanged drug.

• Long-term use can lead to dependence. Withdrawal symptoms may begin 3 to 4 hours after last dose and usually peak within 8 to 12 hours.

• Assess the patient's bowel function and give a stool softener if necessary.

• Regular use of meperidine during pregnancy can lead to narcotic dependence in neonate. Monitor neonate closely.

• Meperidine isn't recommended for chronic pain because of potential for toxicity.

mesna
Mesnex

Pregnancy Risk Category: B

PHARMACOKINETICS
Distribution: remains intravascular.
Metabolism: rapidly oxidized to mesna disulfide in the blood and reduced to the free thiol compound, mesna, in the kidneys.
Excretion: in the kidneys, with 33% of the dose eliminated in the urine in 24 hours. The half-life of mesna is 0.36 hour; that of mesna disulfide, 1.17 hours. Not known if drug appears in breast milk.

MECHANISM OF ACTION
The free thiol compound, mesna, reacts with and detoxifies the urotoxic metabolites of ifosfamide.

INDICATIONS & DOSAGE
• Prevention of ifosfamide-induced hemorrhagic cystitis. *Adults:* 60% of ifosfamide dose. Administer in three bolus doses (each 20% of the ifosfamide dose) before and 4 and 8 hours after the ifosfamide dose is administered.

CONTRAINDICATIONS & CAUTIONS
• Contraindicated in patients with known hypersensitivity to mesna or other thiol compounds.

PREPARATION & STORAGE
Available in 2, 4, and 10 ml ampules at a concentration of 100 mg/ml. Store ampules at room temperature.

Dilute the appropriate dose in dextrose 5% in water, 0.9% sodium chloride injection, or Ringer's lactate to a concentration of 20 mg/ml.

Diluted solutions are stable for 24 hours at 77° F. (25° C.), but use within 6 hours is recommended. Because mesna becomes oxidized in the presence of oxygen, discard any unused drug from open ampules and prepare a new ampule for each administration.

ADMINISTRATION
Direct injection: Using a 21G or 23G needle, inject into vein or into I.V. tubing containing a free-flowing compatible solution.
Intermittent infusion: not recommended.
Continuous infusion: Dosage varies with protocol. Some doctors give loading dose of mesna, equal to 10% of total ifosfamide dose, infused over 15 minutes, followed by continuous infusion of mesna equal (100% w/w) to ifosfamide dose over 8 to 12 hours after end of ifosfamide infusion.

INCOMPATIBILITY
Incompatible with cisplatin.

ADVERSE REACTIONS
Life-threatening: allergic reaction.
Other: diarrhea, dysgeusia, fatigue, headache, hypotension, limb pain, nausea, soft stools, vomiting.

INTERACTIONS
None reported.

EFFECTS ON DIAGNOSTIC TESTS
Urine ketones: false-positive results.

SPECIAL CONSIDERATIONS
• Mesna will not prevent or alleviate other adverse reactions to ifosfamide.

---

metaraminol bitartrate
Aramine

Pregnancy Risk Category: C

PHARMACOKINETICS
Distribution: probably distributed widely to body tissues, with highest concentrations in the kidneys, lungs, heart, and peripheral vasculature. Drug doesn't cross the blood-brain barrier. Not known if it crosses the placenta.
Metabolism: not well characterized. Uptake into tissues and urine excretion (rather than metabolism) put an end to drug's effects.
Excretion: in urine and in feces, mostly as metabolites. Not known if drug appears in breast milk.
Action: onset, 1 to 2 minutes; duration, about 20 minutes.

MECHANISM OF ACTION
Although acting primarily on alpha-adrenergic receptors, metaraminol also has potent, indirect sympathomimetic effects, which causes release of norepinephrine from storage sites to react with adrenergic receptors. The result of this action is increased blood pressure and reflex bradycardia.

INDICATIONS & DOSAGE
• Severe shock (except hypovolemic shock). *Adults:* 0.5 to 5 mg, followed by infusion. *Children:* 0.01 mg/kg.
• Acute hypotension. *Adults:* 15 to 100 mg. *Children:* 0.4 mg/kg.

CONTRAINDICATIONS & CAUTIONS
• Contraindicated in hypersensitivity to sulfites.
• Also contraindicated in patients with peripheral or mesenteric vascular thrombosis because drug may worsen ischemia.
• Administer metaraminol carefully in acidosis, hypercapnia, or hypoxia because of decreased effectiveness and possible increased adverse effects.
• Because the drug's vasoconstrictive effects may aggravate symptoms or predispose the patient to adverse reactions, use cautiously in diabetes mellitus, Buerger's disease, peripheral vascular disease, hypertension, heart disease, hyperthyroidism, or hypercoagulability.
• Also use cautiously in cirrhosis because the drug can cause severe diuresis, and in patients with a history of malaria because relapse may occur.

PREPARATION & STORAGE
Available in a 10 ml vial with a concentration of 10 mg/ml. Store at room temperature and protect from freezing and light.
For infusion, add 15 to 100 mg of drug to 500 ml of dextrose 5% in water, 0.9% sodium chloride, Ringer's lactate, or Ringer's injection. (As much as 500 mg in 500 ml of solution has been used.) For pediatric solutions, dilute to a concentration of 1 mg/25 ml. Use solutions within 24 hours.

ADMINISTRATION
Direct injection: In severe shock, inject drug slowly into vein.
Intermittent infusion: Using an infusion pump, administer solution at a rate sufficient to maintain blood pressure.
Continuous infusion: Using an infusion pump, give drug at a rate sufficient to maintain blood pressure. Titrate to patient response.

INCOMPATIBILITY

Incompatible with amphotericin B, barbiturates, dexamethasone sodium phosphate, erythromycin lactobionate, fibrinogen, hydrocortisone sodium succinate, methicillin, methylprednisolone sodium succinate, penicillin G potassium, phenytoin sodium, prednisolone sodium phosphate, thiopental sodium, warfarin.

ADVERSE REACTIONS

Life-threatening: acute pulmonary edema, cardiac arrest, cerebral hemorrhage, dysrhythmias, hypertension. *Other:* anxiety, apprehension, chest pain, decreased cardiac output (with prolonged use), faintness, flushing, hypotension, nausea, pallor, pruritus, rash, respiratory distress, restlessness, seizures, severe dizziness, severe headache, severe peripheral and visceral vasoconstriction, sweating, tissue sloughing at injection site, trembling, urticaria, weakness, wheezing.

INTERACTIONS

Alpha-adrenergic blockers: decreased metaramimol pressor effects.
Antihypertensives, diuretics: possible reduced antihypertensive effects.
Atropine sulfate: blocked bradycardia and enhanced pressor effects of metaraminol.
Beta-adrenergic blockers: possible diminished effects of metaraminol and these drugs.
Cardiac glycosides, levodopa: increased risk of dysrhythmias.
Diatrizoates, iothalamate: during aortography, possible heightened neurologic effects. Concurrent use can force more of these contrast materials into spine, causing paralysis.
Doxapram: possible enhanced pressor effects of both drugs.
Ergonovine: possible potentiated pressor effects, including severe hy-

pertension and rupture of cerebral vessels.
Ergotamine: risk of peripheral vascular ischemia and gangrene.
Guanadrel, guanethidine: decreased antihypertensive effects of these drugs and possible potentiated pressor effects of metaraminol.
Hydrocarbon anesthetics (such as halothane and methoxyflurane): possible severe ventricular dysrhythmias.
MAO inhibitors (especially furazolidone): possible prolonged cardiac stimulation and vasopressor effects. Don't give metaraminol within 2 weeks of an MAO inhibitor.
Maprotiline, tricyclic antidepressants: potentiated cardiovascular effects of metaraminol—dysrhythmias, severe hypertension, tachycardia.
Mazindol: possible potentiated metaraminol pressor effects.
Mecamylamine, methyldopa, trimethaphan: possible decreased hypotensive effects of these drugs and increased pressor effects of metaraminol.
Methylergonovine, methysergide, oxytocin: possible enhanced vasoconstriction.
Nitrates: possible diminished pressor effects of metaraminol and reduced antianginal effects.
Rauwolfia alkaloids: possible decreased hypotensive effect.
Sympathomimetics: possible enhanced cardiovascular effects.
Thyroid hormones: possible enhanced coronary insufficiency.

EFFECTS ON DIAGNOSTIC TESTS

Urine catecholamines: possible elevated levels.

SPECIAL CONSIDERATIONS

• *Treatment of overdose:* Symptoms include severe chest pain, dizziness, dysrhythmias, nausea, and vomiting.

If these symptoms occur, discontinue infusion. If severe hypertension occurs, give an alpha-adrenergic blocker.
● Monitor central venous pressure to assess circulating volume. Correct fluid deficit before giving metaraminol.
● Infuse drug into a large vein. Don't use veins in the ankle or in the dorsum of the hand, especially in peripheral vascular disease, diabetes mellitus, or hypercoagulability. Avoid extravasation because of the danger of tissue necrosis and sloughing.
● If extravasation occurs, discontinue drug immediately. Infiltrate area with 10 to 15 ml of 0.9% sodium chloride containing 10 to 15 mg of phentolamine. If given within 12 hours, phentolamine should produce immediate local hyperemic changes.
● During infusion, monitor blood pressure every 5 minutes until stable, then every 15 minutes. Check pulse rate, urine output, and extremity color and temperature.
● Report persistent decline in urine output. Output may decrease initially, then should rise as blood pressure reaches normal level.
● Avoid inducing a sharp rise in blood pressure. Otherwise, acute pulmonary edema, dysrhythmias, or cardiac arrest may occur.
● Allow at least 10 minutes before increasing dose.
● Discontinue metaraminol slowly; abrupt withdrawal risks recurrent hypotension. Continue to monitor the patient's blood pressure after stopping drug.
● Prolonged use of metaraminol may cause cumulative effects, such as continued rise in blood pressure after drug discontinuation. It may also prevent expansion of circulating volume and perpetuate shock.

● Monitor patients with diabetes mellitus closely. Antidiabetic medications may require dosage adjustment.
● Acidifying urine may accelerate drug excretion.
● May contain sulfites.

methicillin sodium
Staphcillin

Pregnancy Risk Category: B

PHARMACOKINETICS
Distribution: into bone, bile, and most body fluids, including synovial, pleural, pericardial, and ascitic fluids. Concentration in cerebrospinal fluid, usually low, increases in meningeal inflammation. Drug is about 30% to 50% bound to serum proteins. Methicillin crosses the placenta.
Metabolism: in the liver, but only slightly.
Excretion: in urine, primarily by renal tubular secretion and glomerular filtration; 32% to 80% is eliminated unchanged within 12 hours. Half-life stands at approximately 30 minutes. Drug appears in breast milk.
Action: peak plasma level, immediately after infusion.

MECHANISM OF ACTION
A semisynthetic penicillinase-resistant penicillin, methicillin inhibits bacterial cell wall synthesis.
Its spectrum of activity includes gram-positive aerobic bacteria, including *Staphylococcus aureus, S. epidermis, S. saprophyticus,* groups A, B, C, and G streptococci, *Streptococcus pneumoniae,* and some strains of *Streptococcus viridans.* The drug is also effective against gram-negative aerobic bacteria, in-

cluding some strains of *Neisseria meningitidis, N. gonorrhoeae, Haemophilus influenzae, Bordetella pertussis,* and *Pasteurella multocida.* Susceptible gram-positive anaerobic bacteria include some strains of *Actinomyces, Clostridium, Peptococcus, Peptostreptococcus,* and *Bacteroides.*

INDICATIONS & DOSAGE
• Infections caused by susceptible organisms. *Adults:* 1 g q 6 hours. *Children over age 1 month:* 200 to 400 mg/kg in divided doses q 6 hours.
• Endocarditis or acute or chronic osteomyelitis caused by susceptible organisms. *Adults:* 1.5 to 2 g q 4 hours. *Children over 1 month of age:* 200 to 300 mg/kg in divided doses q 4 hours.
Note: Adjust dosage in renal impairment. For adults, dosage reflects creatinine clearance. If clearance is 10 ml/minute or less, give 1 g q 8 to 12 hours.

CONTRAINDICATIONS & CAUTIONS
• Contraindicated in hypersensitivity to penicillins or cephalosporins.
• Use cautiously in patients with GI disorders because of increased risk of pseudomembranous colitis.
• Also use carefully in patients with impaired renal function because of the heightened risk of toxicity.
• Use with caution in breast-feeding women because of the potential for adverse reactions in infants.

PREPARATION & STORAGE
Available in 1, 4, and 6 g vials and in 1 and 4 g piggyback units. Before reconstitution, store methicillin at room temperature. Reconstitute by adding 1.5 ml of sterile water for injection or 0.9% sodium chloride to 1 g vial, 5.7 ml to 4 g vial, or 8.6 ml to 6 g vial.

For direct injection, dilute each gram of drug in 50 ml of 0.9% sodium chloride.

For infusion, further dilute in 50 to 100 ml of dextrose 5% in 0.9% sodium chloride, dextrose 5% in water, fructose 10% in water, fructose 10% in 0.9% sodium chloride, invert sugar 10% in 0.9% sodium chloride, or Travert 10% and electrolyte #1, #2, or #3 for a concentration of 2, 10, or 20 mg/ml. Reconstitute glass piggyback unit with volume of diluent specified on the label for I.V. infusion.

Reconstituted solutions remain stable for 24 hours at room temperature and for 4 days if refrigerated.

ADMINISTRATION
Direct injection: Inject diluted drug at a rate of 10 ml/minute.
Intermittent infusion: Infuse diluted drug into an I.V. line containing a free-flowing compatible solution over 20 to 30 minutes.
Continuous infusion: not recommended.

INCOMPATIBILITY
Incompatible with amikacin, aminoglycosides, chlorpromazine, codeine phosphate, Dextran 40 10% in dextrose 5%, Dextran 40 10% in 0.9% sodium chloride, 10% fat emulsion, gentamicin, heparin sodium, hydrocortisone sodium succinate, kanamycin, levallorphan tartrate, levorphanol tartrate, lincomycin, metaraminol, methadone hydrochloride, methohexital, morphine, oxytetracycline, promethazine hydrochloride, sodium bicarbonate, tetracycline hydrochloride, and vancomycin.

ADVERSE REACTIONS
Life-threatening: acute interstitial nephritis, anaphylaxis, bone marrow depression.

Other: bacterial and fungal superinfection, black or hairy tongue, chills, eosinophilia, fever, glossitis, hemorrhagic cystitis (without renal damage), myalgia, neurotoxicity (with large doses in renal impairment), phlebitis, pruritus, pseudomembranous colitis, rash, stomatitis, thrombophlebitis.

INTERACTIONS
Aminoglycosides: possible synergistic action against some strains of methicillin-resistant *S. aureus.*
Chloramphenicol, erythromycin, sulfonamides, tetracyclines: possible decreased bactericidal effect of methicillin.
Heparin, oral anticoagulants: enhanced risk of bleeding.
Probenecid: higher and prolonged serum concentrations of methicillin.

EFFECTS ON DIAGNOSTIC TESTS
Coombs' test: possible false-positive results.
Serum alkaline phosphatase, SGOT, SGPT: transiently increased levels.
Serum uric acid: possible falsely elevated levels with copper-chelate method.
Urine 17-hydroxycorticosteroids: falsely elevated levels with Porter-Silber reagent.

SPECIAL CONSIDERATIONS
• Check for previous penicillin or cephalosporin hypersensitivity before administering first dose. Keep in mind that negative history doesn't rule out future allergic reaction.
• Obtain specimens for culture and sensitivity testing before first dose. Therapy may start before obtaining results.
• Monitor CBC, urinalysis, and BUN, SGOT, and SGPT levels during therapy to detect adverse effects.

• If diarrhea persists during therapy, collect stool specimens for culture to rule out pseudomembranous colitis.
• Duration of therapy depends on the type and severity of infection. In severe staphylococcal infection, therapy should last for at least 1 week. In osteomyelitis, endocarditis, and other severe infections, therapy may last longer (usually 4 to 8 weeks). Following therapy, the patient may receive oral penicillinase-resistant penicillin.
• Hemorrhagic cystitis occurs more commonly when drug is given in large doses to patients with low urine output.
• Elderly patients face a greater risk of thrombophlebitis from methicillin infusion.
• If patient has sodium restrictions, keep in mind that each gram of methicillin contains 2.9 to 3.1 mEq (67 to 71 mg) of sodium.
• Dialysis removes slight amounts of drug.

methocarbamol
Carbacot, Robaxin♦

Pregnancy Risk Category: C

PHARMACOKINETICS
Distribution: highest concentrations probably occur in the liver and kidneys; lowest concentrations in the lungs, heart, and skeletal muscle. Methocarbamol probably crosses the placenta.
Metabolism: extensively metabolized, presumably in the liver.
Excretion: rapidly eliminated in urine as unchanged drug and metabolites. Half-life is about 1 to 2 hours. Small amounts appear in breast milk.

Action: onset, immediately after administration; duration, variable.

MECHANISM OF ACTION
Unknown but probably related to CNS depressant effects. Drug has sedative and skeletal muscle relaxant effects.

INDICATIONS & DOSAGE
• Adjunct in severe musculoskeletal pain. *Adults:* 1 g q 8 hours. Maximum dosage, 3 g daily for 3 days.
• Tetanus. *Adults:* 1 to 2 g by direct injection, followed by 1 to 2 g by infusion q 6 hours. Doses should be repeated until nasogastric tube can be inserted. *Children:* 15 mg/kg q 6 hours if necessary.

CONTRAINDICATIONS & CAUTIONS
• Contraindicated in hypersensitivity to methocarbamol and in renal impairment because nephrotoxic component used in preparation may cause increased urea retention and acidosis.
• Use with caution in patients with CNS depression because of the risk of exacerbating the condition and in patients with epilepsy because of an increased risk of seizures.
• Give carefully to patients with hepatic impairment because of decreased drug metabolism.
• Drug isn't recommended for children under age 12.

PREPARATION & STORAGE
Available in 10 ml vials containing 100 mg/ml. Dilute single-dose vial in up to 250 ml of 0.9% sodium chloride or dextrose 5% in water for infusion. Store drug and diluted solution at room temperature.

ADMINISTRATION
Direct injection: Inject drug into vein or through the tubing of free-flowing I.V. solution at a maximum rate of 300 mg/minute. Keep in mind that slow injection will help to minimize adverse effects.
Intermittent infusion: Infuse diluted solution through tubing of free-flowing I.V. line at ordered rate.
Continuous infusion: not recommended.

INCOMPATIBILITY
No incompatibilities reported.

ADVERSE REACTIONS
Life-threatening: anaphylaxis.
Other: blurred vision, bradycardia, conjunctivitis with nasal congestion, diplopia, dizziness, drowsiness, fever, flushing, GI upset, headache, hypotension, leukopenia, light-headedness, metallic taste, mild muscular incoordination, nystagmus, pruritus, rash, seizures, sloughing at injection site, syncope, thrombophlebitis, urticaria, vertigo.

INTERACTIONS
Other CNS depressants: deepened CNS depression.
Pyridostigmine: severe weakness in myasythenia gravis patients. Give methocarbamol cautiously.

EFFECTS ON DIAGNOSTIC TESTS
Urinalysis: if color changes (brown, black, blue, or green), increased RBC count and hemoglobin level.
Urine 5-hydroxyindoleacetic acid: possible falsely elevated levels with nitrosonaphthol reagent.
Urine vanillylmandelic acid: with possible falsely increased levels with Gitlow screening method.

SPECIAL CONSIDERATIONS
• Avoid extravasation; solution is hypertonic and may cause thrombophlebitis. Administer methocarbamol

for no longer than 3 consecutive days.
• Keep patient lying down during administration and for 10 to 15 minutes afterward.
• Switch to oral administration of methocarbamol, if ordered, as soon as possible.
• Though known to precipitate seizures, methocarbamol has been used to terminate epileptic seizures.

---

methohexital sodium
Brevital, Brietal♦♦

Controlled Substance Schedule IV
Pregnancy Risk Category: D

PHARMACOKINETICS
Distribution: rapidly distributed to the CNS, then redistributed, first to lean tissue, and eventually to fatty tissue because drug is highly lipid. Methohexital crosses the placenta.
Metabolism: probably in the liver; exact metabolism unknown.
Excretion: in urine, although elimination is minimal because of extensive renal tubular reabsorption of drug. About 1% is excreted unchanged in urine, the rest as a byproduct of oxidative or conjugative metabolism. Half-life of methohexital is about 4 hours. With large doses, small amounts appear in breast milk.
Action: onset, 10 to 20 seconds; duration, 5 to 7 minutes.

MECHANISM OF ACTION
Not completely understood. Methohexital is thought to act selectively throughout the CNS. It inhibits polysynaptic responses of the reticular-activating system, suppressing its arousal mechanism. It also affects gamma-aminobutyric acid and gluta-

mate activity to reduce neuronal excitability.

INDICATIONS & DOSAGE
• Induction of anesthesia. Dosage must be individualized. Young patients may require larger doses than middle-aged or elderly patients.
Adults and children: 1 to 2 mg/kg or 20 to 40 mg of 1% solution. Subsequent injections may be given q 4 to 6 minutes.
• Maintenance of general anesthesia. *Adults:* 0.25 to 1 mg/kg (intermittent injection) or 1 drop/second of 0.2% solution.

CONTRAINDICATIONS & CAUTIONS
• Contraindicated in hypersensitivity to methohexital or barbiturates and in patients in whom general anesthesia is considered hazardous.
• Also contraindicated in acute intermittent porphyria and porphyria variegata because drug may aggravate symptoms.
• Administer with extreme caution in patients with status asthmaticus because methohexital's respiratory depressant effects aggravate symptoms.
• In debilitated or elderly patients and in patients with CNS depression, use cautiously because respiratory depression or hypotension may occur.
• Also use cautiously in myasthenia gravis because of the increased risk of respiratory depression.
• Because the drug can cause prolonged depressant and hypnotic effects, administer cautiously to patients with respiratory, circulatory, renal, hepatic, and endocrine disorders.

PREPARATION & STORAGE

Available in 500 mg, 2.5 g, and 5 g vials. Store at room temperature. Reconstitute with sterile water for injection, dextrose 5% in water, or 0.9% sodium chloride injection. Don't use Ringer's lactate.

For a 1% solution for direct injection, add 50 ml of diluent to the 500 mg vial, 250 ml to the 2.5 g vial, or 500 ml to the 5 g vial. For a 0.2% solution for continuous infusion, add 500 mg of drug to 250 ml of dextrose 5% in water or 0.9% sodium chloride.

Solutions containing sterile water for injection remain stable at room temperature for 6 weeks; those containing dextrose 5% in water or 0.9% sodium chloride remain stable for 24 hours. Solutions should remain clear and colorless; otherwise, discard.

ADMINISTRATION

Only staff who are specially trained in administering anesthetics and managing their adverse effects should give methohexital. Always keep resuscitation equipment readily available. Overdosage may occur from overly rapid or repeated injection.

Direct injection: Inject diluted drug directly into vein (or into a free-flowing I.V. solution) over 30 seconds. Repeat as needed to maintain anesthesia.

Intermittent infusion: not recommended.

Continuous infusion: Give 0.2% solution at prescribed rate (such as 1 drop/second).

INCOMPATIBILITY

Incompatible with atropine, bacteriostatic diluents, chlorpromazine, droperidol, fentanyl, glycopyrrolate, hydralazine, lidocaine hydrochloride, mechlorethamine, methicillin, meth-yldopate hydrochloride, metocurine iodide, pentazocine lactate, prochlorperazine mesylate, promazine, promethazine, propiomazine hydrochloride, Ringer's lactate, scopolamine, streptomycin, succinylcholine, tetracycline hydrochloride, or tubocurarine. Drug is also incompatible with silicone; avoid its contact with rubber stoppers or syringe parts treated with silicone.

ADVERSE REACTIONS

Life-threatening: anaphylaxis, bronchospasm, respiratory depression.
Other: abdominal pain, bradycardia, circulatory depression, dyspnea, emergence delirium, hallucinations, headache, hypotension, injection site reaction (including nerve injury near site, necrosis, pain, swelling, thrombophlebitis, ulceration), nausea, rash, restlessness, salivation, shivering, skeletal muscle hyperactivity (cough, hiccups), tachycardia, vomiting.

INTERACTIONS

Antihypertensives, diuretics: possible additive hypotensive effects.
CNS depressants, parenteral magnesium sulfate: possible deepened CNS depression.
131I: possible reduced thyroid uptake of methohexital.
Ketamine: possible heightened risk of hypotension or respiratory depression.
Phenothiazines: possible potentiated hypotensive and CNS excitatory effects.

EFFECTS ON DIAGNOSTIC TESTS

Radioactive iodine tests: possible decreased uptake of ^{123}I and ^{131}I.

SPECIAL CONSIDERATIONS

• Have patient fast before drug administration to reduce postoperative nausea and avoid aspiration.
• Monitor vital signs before, during, and after anesthesia.
• After administration, warn patient to avoid tasks that require alertness. Psychomotor skills may be impaired for 24 hours.
• Effects may be cumulative in continuous infusion.
• Methohexital has potential for abuse.
• Avoid extravasation. It may result in local irritation leading to ulceration and necrosis.
• Also avoid intraarterial injection, which can cause platelet aggregation and thrombosis distal to injection site. Intraarterial injection may lead to necrosis and gangrene, making amputation necessary.

---

methotrexate sodium
Folex, Folex PFS, Methotrexate LPF, Mexate, Mexate AQ

Pregnancy Risk Category: D

PHARMACOKINETICS
Distribution: widely distributed, with highest concentrations in the kidneys, gallbladder, spleen, liver, and skin. Methotrexate crosses the placenta and blood-brain barrier in minimal amounts.
Metabolism: not significantly metabolized.
Excretion: in urine via glomerular filtration and active transport, with 55% to 88% excreted within 24 hours. Small amounts are excreted in feces. Drug appears in breast milk.
Action: peak serum levels, 30 minutes to 2 hours after administration.

MECHANISM OF ACTION
An antineoplastic antimetabolite, methotrexate blocks folinic acid's role in DNA synthesis and cellular replication. Rapidly proliferating cells, such as bone marrow and malignant cells, are more sensitive to this effect. Drug acts in S phase of cell cycle.

INDICATIONS & DOSAGE
• Induction of remission in lymphoblastic leukemia. *Adults:* 25 mg/kg q 14 days. Dosage varies widely.
• Psoriasis. *Adults:* 10 to 25 mg once weekly. Up to 100 mg may be required; however, manufacturer recommends maximum weekly dose of only 50 mg.
• Adjuvant therapy for osteosarcoma. *Adults:* 12 g/m². May be increased to 15 g/m² if lower dose proves insufficient to meet a 10^{-3} mol/liter blood level at end of infusion.

CONTRAINDICATIONS & CAUTIONS
• Contraindicated in preexisting or recent exposure to chicken pox or herpes virus because of the increased risk of generalized disease.
• Avoid use in psoriasis patients with poor nutrition, renal or hepatic impairment, or blood dyscrasias because of the heightened risk of toxicity.
• Use cautiously in GI obstruction, ascites, or peritoneal or pleural effusions because impaired elimination magnifies the risk of toxicity.
• In myelosuppression, also use cautiously because the condition may worsen.
• Administer carefully to patients with gout or a history of urate stones because of an increased risk of hyperuricemia, and to patients with GI infection, peptic ulcer, ulcerative colitis, or oral mucositis be-

---

Unmarked trade names available in the United States only.
♦ Also available in Canada.   ♦♦ Available in Canada only.

cause the drug may exacerbate these disorders.
• Because secondary dehydration increases risk of toxicity, use cautiously in nausea and vomiting.

PREPARATION & STORAGE

Exercise extreme caution when preparing and administering methotrexate to avoid mutagenic, teratogenic, and carcinogenic risks. Use a biological containment cabinet, wear gloves and mask, and use syringes with Luer-Lok fittings. Also, correctly dispose of needles, vials, and unused drug, and avoid contaminating work surfaces.

Methotrexate is available in 20, 50, 100, and 250 mg single-dose vials of lyophilized sterile powder and in 2, 4, 8, and 10 ml vials containing 25 mg/ml solution. Reconstitute with 2 to 10 ml of sterile water for injection, 0.9% sodium chloride, or dextrose 5% in water. Reconstituted concentrations range from 2 to 50 mg/ml. Further dilute for injection with 0.9% sodium chloride or dextrose 5% in water.

Store methotrexate preparations at room temperature and protect from light.

ADMINISTRATION

Direct injection: Inject directly into vein or into side port of free-flowing I.V. line over prescribed duration.
Intermittent infusion: not recommended.
Continuous infusion: not recommended.

INCOMPATIBILITY

Incompatible with bleomycin, fluorouracil, metoclopramide, prednisolone, and sodium phosphate.

ADVERSE REACTIONS

Life-threatening: GI hemorrhage, hepatotoxicity, myelosuppression

(nadir in 6 to 10 days with rapid recovery).
Other: abdominal distress, alopecia, blurred vision, chills, cystitis, diabetes mellitus, dizziness, drowsiness, fatigue, fever, gingivitis, glossitis, headache, hyperuricemia, hypogammaglobulinemia, malaise, nausea, osteoporosis, pulmonary reactions, septicemia, severe nephropathy, ulcerative stomatitis, urticaria, vomiting.

INTERACTIONS

Alcohol, hepatotoxic drugs: increased risk of hepatotoxicity.
Anticoagulants: possible potentiated effects.
Antigout drugs: possible rise in serum uric acid levels, requiring dosage adjustment.
Asparaginase: possible blocked methotrexate effect.
Aspirin, para-aminobenzoic acid, phenytoin, sulfonamides, tetracycline, other protein-bound drugs: possible increased toxicity resulting from displacement of methotrexate and increased free drug.
Cytarabine: synergistic cytotoxic effect if given from 48 hours before to 10 minutes after methotrexate.
Folic acid–containing vitamins: possible decreased response to methotrexate.
Live virus vaccines: increased risk of generalized disease.
Myelosuppresive drugs, radiation therapy: possible increased myelosuppression.
NSAIDS: reduced renal tubular secretion and possible intensified methotrexate toxicity.
Probenecid: increased risk of methotrexate toxicity, resulting from inhibited renal excretion.
Pyrimethamine, triamterene, trimethoprim: heightened risk of toxicity.

EFFECTS ON DIAGNOSTIC TESTS

Serum folic acid: possible inhibition of organism used to detect folic acid deficiency.

Serum isocitric acid dehydrogenase, uric acid: possible elevated levels.

SGOT: in high-dose therapy, possible increased levels.

SPECIAL CONSIDERATIONS

• *Treatment of overdose:* Administer leucovorin calcium as soon as possible, preferably in the first hour of overdose. In massive overdose, urine alkalinization and hydration help to prevent precipitation of methotrexate or its metabolites in the renal tubules.

• Expect toxic reactions with therapeutic doses. Methotrexate is highly toxic and has a low therapeutic index.

• Do not repeat methotrexate therapy unless WBC count rises above 1,500/μl; neutrophil count rises above 200/μl; platelet count rises above 75,000/μl; serum bilirubin level is greater than 1.2 mg/dl; SGPT level is greater than 450 U/liter; serum creatinine level is normal; creatinine clearance is at least 60 mg/minute; and the patient shows evidence of healing (if he has mucositis). Also do not repeat therapy if the patient experiences pleural effusion.

• Leucovorin calcium is used in high-dose methotrexate therapy to minimize adverse hematologic and GI effects.

• When treating osteosarcoma, measure serum creatinine level before each course of therapy. If serum creatinine level increases by 50% or more over previous levels, measure creatinine clearance to be sure it equals 60 mg/minute. If creatinine clearance is below 60 mg/minute, reduce dosage or withhold therapy until renal function improves.

• Advise patients receiving methotrexate, especially those with psoriasis, to avoid alcohol, salicylates, people with infections, and prolonged exposure to sunlight.

• Advise male patients on methotrexate to use contraceptive measures during therapy and for at least 3 months after therapy ends.

• Women receiving methotrexate should avoid becoming pregnant during therapy and for at least one ovulatory cycle after methotrexate therapy ends.

• Monitor serum creatinine and BUN levels daily during high-dose methotrexate therapy.

• Monitor serum methotrexate levels daily during therapy. Continue monitoring until serum level falls below 5×10^{-8} mol/liter.

• Reduce dosage by 25% if serum bilirubin level falls between 3 and 5 mg/dl or SGOT level is greater than 180 U/liter, and omit therapy if serum bilirubin level rises above 5 mg/dl.

• Advise women not to breast-feed while on methotrexate therapy because of the potential for serious adverse effects in the infant.

• Advise patient to notify doctor if he notices changes in his breathing patterns or if he notices signs of liver dysfunction (jaundice, malaise, nausea).

• Methotrexate is commonly used with other antineoplastics.

• Administration of large volumes of fluids, alkalinization of urine, or use of allopurinol may prevent uric acid neuropathy.

• If blood cell counts fall, discontinue drug, as ordered. Antibiotic therapy may be needed if infection occurs during period of myelosuppression.

• Generic preparations may contain benzyl alcohol.

methoxamine hydrochloride
Vasoxyl♦

Pregnancy Risk Category: C

PHARMACOKINETICS
Distribution: unknown.
Metabolism: unknown.
Excretion: unknown.
Action: onset, immediate; peak, 0.5 to 2 minutes; duration, 5 to 15 minutes.

MECHANISM OF ACTION
Methoxamine acts directly on alpha-adrenergic receptors of peripheral vasculature to cause vasoconstriction, thereby increasing systolic and diastolic blood pressure. Increased blood pressure stimulates the carotid sinus reflex over the vagus nerve, terminating some paroxysmal supraventricular tachycardias.

INDICATIONS & DOSAGE
• Hypotension. *Adults:* 3 to 5 mg. *Children:* 0.08 mg/kg or 2.5 mg/m².
• Paroxysmal supraventricular tachycardia. *Adults:* 5 to 15 mg. Systolic blood pressure should not rise over 160 mm Hg.

CONTRAINDICATIONS & CAUTIONS
• Contraindicated in severe hypertension and hypersensitivity to drug or sulfites.
• Use cautiously in patients with bradycardia, partial heart block, and myocardial disease because of the potential to exacerbate these conditions and in patients with hyperthyroidism and pheochromocytoma because drug may exacerbate episodes of severe hypertension.
• Administer cautiously in vascular, peripheral, or mesenteric thrombosis because of the risk of extending area of ischemia and infarction and in severe arteriosclerosis because decreased cardiac output may prove dangerous to patients with poor perfusion.

PREPARATION & STORAGE
Available in 1 ml ampules containing 20 mg/ml concentration. Store below 104° F. (40° C.), preferably between 59° and 86° F. (15° and 30° C.). Protect from light and freezing.
    For infusion, dilute 30 to 40 mg in 250 ml of dextrose 5% in water.

ADMINISTRATION
Direct injection: Slowly inject ordered amount directly into vein or through the tubing containing a free-flowing compatible solution. When treating paroxysmal supraventricular tachycardia, inject ordered dose over 3 to 5 minutes.
Intermittent infusion: not recommended.
Continuous infusion: Infuse diluted drug at rate required to maintain blood pressure.

INCOMPATIBILITY
Incompatible with alkaline compounds.

ADVERSE REACTIONS
Life-threatening: cerebral hemorrhage, respiratory distress.
Other: anxiety; bradycardia; decreased cardiac output; decreased perfusion to vital organs; desire to void; dizziness; nausea and vomiting; nervousness; pallor; pilomotor response; precordial pain; seizures; severe headaches; severe, prolonged hypertension; tremors; ventricular ectopic beats; weakness.

INTERACTIONS

Alpha-adrenergic blocking agents: blocked pressor response to methoxamine, possibly causing severe hypotension.

Antidepressants, maprotiline: potentiated cardiovascular effects of methoxamine.

Antihypertensives and diuretics: reduced antihypertensive effects.

Atropine: blocked reflex bradycardia and enhanced pressor effect of methoxamine.

Beta-adrenergic blocking agents: may potentiate vasoconstrictive effects of methoxamine.

Diatrizoates, iothalamate, ioxaglate: increased neurologic effects of these drugs.

Digitalis glycosides, levodopa: increased risk of cardiac dysrhythmias.

Doxapram, guanadrel, guanethidine, mazindol, mecamylamine, methyldopa, methylphenidate, trimethaphan: increased pressor effects.

Ergot alkaloids, oxytocin: enhanced vasoconstriction.

Nitrates: reduced antianginal effects.

Rauwolfia alkaloids: decreased hypotensive effects.

Sympathomimetics: increased cardiovascular effects.

Thyroid hormones: increased effects of either drugs.

EFFECTS ON DIAGNOSTIC TESTS

Plasma cortisol and corticotropin: increased serum concentrations.

SPECIAL CONSIDERATIONS

• *Treatment of overdose:* As ordered, use atropine to treat excessive bradycardia. Use an alpha-adrenergic blocking agent to reverse excessive increases in blood pressure.

• For a prolonged effect, administer supplemental I.M. doses of methoxamine after administering emergency I.V. therapy.

• As needed, replace blood, plasma, fluids, and electrolytes before administering methoxamine when seeking to achieve vasopressor effects.

• Especially useful for maintaining blood pressure during spinal anesthesia, methoxamine has also been used successfully during general anesthesia.

• Extravasation may cause necrosis and sloughing of surrounding tissue. To avoid extravasation, use the large veins of the antecubital fossa.

• To prevent sloughing of infiltrated tissue, infiltrate area with a solution of 10 to 15 ml of 0.9% sodium chloride and 5 to 10 mg of phentolamine as soon as possible. Use a fine needle.

• May contain sulfites.

methyldopate hydrochloride
Aldomet♦

Pregnancy Risk Category: C

PHARMACOKINETICS

Distribution: chiefly to the heart, kidneys, and peripheral vessels. Methyldopate and its metabolites are weakly bound to plasma proteins. Drug crosses blood-brain barrier and the placenta.

Metabolism: hydrolyzed to methyldopa, which is extensively metabolized in the liver.

Excretion: in urine, largely by glomerular filtration, with 20% to 55% removed unchanged. Drug appears in breast milk in concentrations of 20% to 35% of maternal serum levels. Biphasic elimination has an initial half-life of about 2 hours and a much slower second phase. In im-

paired renal function, initial half-life is about 3½ hours.
Action: onset, 4 to 6 hours; duration, 10 to 16 hours.

MECHANISM OF ACTION
Not known, but the drug is thought to act as an alpha-adrenergic agonist that reduces sympathetic outflow from the CNS, thereby diminishing plasma renin levels and peripheral resistance.

INDICATIONS & DOSAGE
• Sustained mild to severe hypertension and, in combination therapy, acute hypertensive emergencies.
Adults: 250 to 500 mg q 6 hours, as necessary. Maximum dosage, 1 g q 6 hours. *Children:* 20 to 40 mg/kg q 24 hours or 0.015 to 0.3 g/m² q 6 hours. Maximum daily dosage, 65 mg/kg, 2 g/m², or 3 g, whichever is least.
Note: Adjust dosage in renal impairment.

CONTRAINDICATIONS & CAUTIONS
• Contraindicated in active hepatitis or cirrhosis and in hypersensitivity to methyldopa hydrochloride and polyoxyl 35 castor oil.
• Contraindicated in previous methyldopa therapy associated with liver abnormalities or hemolytic anemia (positive direct Coombs' test) because of an increased risk of adverse reactions.
• Administer carefully to dialysis patients because drug can be removed, leading to hypertension, and to sulfite-sensitive patients because preparation contains sulfites.
• Use with caution in pheochromocytoma because drug interferes with urine catecholamine testing and may cause pressor response; in coronary insufficiency or Parkinson's disease because drug may aggravate symp-

toms; in elderly or debilitated patients who may be more sensitive to drug's hypotensive and sedative effects; and in renal impairment because of the risk of drug accumulation.

PREPARATION & STORAGE
Available in concentrations of 50 mg/ml. For infusion, add the required dose to 100 ml of dextrose 5% in water for a concentration of 100 mg/10 ml. Drug remains stable for 24 hours in most I.V. solutions; however, exposure to air may accelerate decomposition. Protect from light and store at room temperature; avoid freezing.

ADMINISTRATION
Direct injection: not recommended.
Intermittent infusion: Infuse diluted dose through a patent I.V. line over 30 to 60 minutes.
Continuous infusion: not recommended.

INCOMPATIBILITY
Incompatible with amphotericin B, methohexital, tetracycline hydrochloride, and some total parenteral nutrition solutions. Mix cautiously with drugs that have poor solubility in acidic media, such as barbiturates and sulfonamides.

ADVERSE REACTIONS
Life-threatening: anaphylaxis, hepatic changes.
Other: abdominal pain, aggravated angina, amber urine, black tongue, bradycardia, chills, constipation, Coombs'-positive hemolytic anemia, depression, diarrhea, drowsiness, dry mouth, fever, immune thrombocytopenia, leukopenia (reversible), nasal stuffiness, nausea, nightmares, orthostatic hypotension, paradoxical pressor response, paresthesias, prolonged carotid sinus hypersensitivity,

sodium retention, sore tongue, vomiting, weight gain.

INTERACTIONS

Alcohol, CNS depressants: deepened CNS depression.
Anti-inflammatory agents, appetite suppressants, estrogens: reduced antihypertensive effect of methyldopa.
Bromocriptine: decreased effects.
Chlorpromazine, haloperidol: adverse CNS reactions.
Diuretics, fenfluramine, general anesthetics, hypotensive agents, methotrimeprazine: enhanced hypotensive effect.
Levodopa: enhanced hypotensive and toxic CNS effects.
Lithium carbonate: heightened risk of toxicity.
MAO inhibitors: hyperexcitability, severe hypertension, other CNS disturbances.
Phenothiazines, tricyclic antidepressants: diminished hypotensive effect.
Sympathomimetics: potentiated pressor effect of these drugs and decreased hypotensive effect of methyldopa.

EFFECTS ON DIAGNOSTIC TESTS

BUN, serum bilirubin, potassium, prolactin, sodium, uric acid: possible increased concentrations.
Coombs' test: possible false-positive results.
Serum alkaline phosphatase, SGOT, SGPT: may alter levels.
Serum creatinine: possible unreliable results with alkaline picrate method.
Urine catecholamines: possible falsely elevated levels resulting from fluorescence in urine specimens at the same wavelengths as catecholamines.

SPECIAL CONSIDERATIONS

• *Treatment of overdose:* Keep the patient supine and provide symptomatic care. Monitor heart rate, cardiac output, blood volume, electrolyte balance, GI motility, renal function, and cerebral activity. To reverse hypotension, administer I.V. fluids. Dialysis may be helpful.
• Perform Coombs' test before therapy.
• Monitor hemoglobin level, hematocrit, or CBC before and during therapy. If hemolytic anemia develops, discontinue drug.
• Also monitor liver function tests. Discontinue drug, as ordered, if patient develops fever, abnormal liver function, or jaundice.
• Regularly check blood pressure. Once blood pressure is stable, change to oral form of drug as ordered.
• Monitor for signs of drug-induced depression.

methylene blue

Pregnancy Risk Category: C

PHARMACOKINETICS

Distribution: not fully characterized. Not known if drug crosses the placenta.
Metabolism: in tissues by reduction to leukomethylene blue.
Excretion: in urine (some unchanged) and bile. Not known if drug appears in breast milk.
Action: peak concentration, at end of infusion.

MECHANISM OF ACTION

High concentrations oxidize the ferrous iron of reduced hemoglobin to ferric iron, forming methemoglobin. Low concentrations increase the conversion rate of methemoglobin to hemoglobin.

Unmarked trade names available in the United States only.
♦ Also available in Canada.   ♦♦ Available in Canada only.

INDICATIONS & DOSAGE
• Methemoglobin and cyanide poisoning. *Adults and children:* 1 to 2 mg/kg of 1% solution; may be repeated in 1 hour.

CONTRAINDICATIONS & CAUTIONS
• Contraindicated in severe renal impairment or methylene blue hypersensitivity.
• Use with caution in glucose-6-phosphate dehydrogenase deficiency because drug may cause hemolysis.

PREPARATION & STORAGE
Available in 1 and 10 ml ampules containing 10 mg/ml. No need to dilute before injection.

ADMINISTRATION
Direct injection: Administer over several minutes directly into vein or through an I.V. line containing a free-flowing compatible solution. Overly rapid injection causes additional methemoglobin production. Don't exceed recommended dosage.
Intermittent infusion: not recommended.
Continuous infusion: not recommended.

INCOMPATIBILITY
Incompatible with dichromates, iodides, and oxidizing and reducing substances.

ADVERSE REACTIONS
Life-threatening: none reported.
Other: abdominal pain, confusion, cyanosis, diaphoresis, dizziness, headache, hypertension, methemoglobin formation, nausea, precordial pain, vomiting.

INTERACTIONS
None reported.

EFFECTS ON DIAGNOSTIC TESTS
None reported.

SPECIAL CONSIDERATIONS
• Avoid extravasation. Subcutaneous injection may cause necrotic abscesses.
• Drug discolors urine and stools and stains skin. Remove stains with hypochlorite solution.
• In prolonged therapy, monitor for signs of anemia.

---

methylergonovine maleate
Methergine, Methylergabasine-Sandoz♦♦

Pregnancy Risk Category: Not applicable

PHARMACOKINETICS
Distribution: rapid, into plasma, extracellular fluid, and tissues.
Metabolism: presumably in the liver.
Excretion: mostly in feces, some in urine. Negligible amounts appear in breast milk. Elimination may be prolonged in neonates. Half-life is biphasic: initial phase, 1 to 5 minutes; terminal phase, 30 minutes to 2 hours.
Action: onset, upon administration; duration, up to 45 minutes.

MECHANISM OF ACTION
Drug produces vasoconstriction and directly stimulates uterine and vascular smooth muscle. It also increases cervical contraction.

INDICATIONS & DOSAGE
• Emergency treatment of severe postpartum and postabortion hemorrhage caused by uterine atony or subinvolution. *Adults:* 0.2 mg in single dose, repeated q 2 to 4 hours (up to five doses, if necessary).

CONTRAINDICATIONS & CAUTIONS

• Contraindicated before placental expulsion because drug may cause captivation of placenta.
• Also contraindicated for induction of labor because uterine tetany or rupture, amniotic fluid embolism, or fetal trauma can occur.
• Avoid use in hypersensitivity to ergot preparations.
• Use cautiously in hypertension or occlusive peripheral vascular disease because drug can aggravate symptoms.
• Because drug can cause ergotism, use cautiously in sepsis or hepatic or renal impairment.
• Also use cautiously in patients with coronary artery disease because of possible angina or myocardial infarction.

PREPARATION & STORAGE

Available in 1 ml ampules containing 0.2 mg/ml. Store drug below 46° F. (8° C.) in light-resistant containers. Avoid freezing. Ready-to-use injections are normally clear and colorless. Discard if solution is discolored or contains a precipitate.

Dilute with 5 ml of 0.9% sodium chloride, if appropriate. The drug may be administered with dextrose 5% in water, dextrose 5% in Ringer's lactate, Ringer's lactate, or 0.9% sodium chloride.

ADMINISTRATION

Direct injection: Administer directly into vein or into free-flowing compatible I.V. solution over at least 60 seconds. If desired, use diluted dosage to facilitate slow injection. Overly rapid administration can cause severe cardiovascular effects.
Intermittent infusion: not recommended.
Continuous infusion: not recommended.

INCOMPATIBILITY

None reported.

ADVERSE REACTIONS

Life-threatening: anaphylaxis, cerebrovascular accident, severe dysrhythmias, shock.
Other: blurred vision, chest pain, cool extremities, diaphoresis, dizziness, dyspnea, ergotism (agitation, confusion, dry mouth, hallucinations, muscle twitching, palpitations), fever, headache, hypertension, joint pain, nausea, rash, seizures, sore throat, tachycardia, tinnitus, unusual bruising, vomiting, weakness.

INTERACTIONS

Dopamine, I.V. oxytocin, regional anesthetics: possible increased vasoconstriction.
Other ergot alkaloids, vasoconstrictors, vasopressors: possible enhanced vasoconstriction.
Tobacco: with heavy smoking, possible enhanced vasoconstriction.

EFFECTS ON DIAGNOSTIC TESTS

Serum prolactin: possible decreased levels, which may hinder lactation.

SPECIAL CONSIDERATIONS

• Closely monitor blood pressure and pulse. Give I.V. hydralazine or chlorpromazine, as ordered, for hypertension.
• After administration, closely monitor uterine activity. (Contractions are sustained and uterine tone is high.) If appropriate, give analgesics for discomfort.
• Reduce dosage, as ordered, if severe uterine cramping occurs.

methylprednisolone sodium succinate
A-methaPred, Solu-Medrol♦

Pregnancy Risk Category: C

PHARMACOKINETICS
Distribution: rapidly distributed to muscle, liver, skin, intestines, and kidneys. Drug binds especially with the protein transcortin. It crosses the placenta.
Metabolism: in most tissues, but primarily in the liver, to inactive compounds.
Excretion: inactive metabolites excreted by the kidneys, primarily as glucuronides and sulfates but also as unconjugated products. Small amounts of unmetabolized drug are eliminated in urine, and negligible amounts are removed in bile. Drug probably appears in breast milk. Serum half-life is about 2 to 3½ hours; tissue half-life, up to 36 hours. Excretion may be prolonged in hypothyroidism.
Action: onset, rapid; duration, 3 days to 3 weeks, depending on dose.

MECHANISM OF ACTION
A synthetic glucocorticoid, methylprednisolone suppresses pituitary release of ACTH, preventing adrenocorticol secretion of corticosteroids. As a result, the drug suppresses immune responses, stimulates bone marrow, and alters protein, fat, and carbohydrate metabolism. It also decreases inflammation by stabilizing leukocyte lysosomal membranes.

INDICATIONS & DOSAGE
• Severe inflammation or immunosuppression. *Adults:* 10 mg to 1.5 g daily. Usual dosage, 10 to 250 mg up to q 4 hours.

• Severe shock. *Adults:* 30 mg/kg initially, repeated q 4 to 6 hours p.r.n.; or 100 to 250 mg initially, repeated q 2 to 6 hours p.r.n. Initial dose may be followed by 30 mg/kg infusion q 12 hours for 24 to 48 hours.
• Severe lupus nephritis. *Adults:* 1 g (intermittent infusion) for 3 days, followed by oral prednisolone or prednisone. *Children:* 30 mg/kg on alternate days for six doses, followed by oral prednisolone or prednisone.

CONTRAINDICATIONS & CAUTIONS
• Contraindicated in systemic fungal infection, sepsis syndrome, or septic shock because drug may mask symptoms and exacerbate these conditions.
• Also contraindicated in viral or bacterial infections uncontrolled by antibiotics (except in life-threatening situations) because drug may mask symptoms, and in peptic ulcer (except in life-threatening situations) because drug may exacerbate the disorder.
• Avoid use in neonates and in patients with hypersensitivity to any component of the drug.
• Use cautiously in hyperthyroidism, hypothyroidism, or cirrhosis because of possible exaggerated drug response.
• Also use cautiously in psychosis because drug may precipitate mental disturbances, and in diverticulitis, nonspecific ulcerative colitis, or recent intestinal anastomosis because of possible perforation, abscess, or other pyogenic infection.
• Administer drug carefully in seizure disorders, renal insufficiency, diabetes mellitus, osteoporosis, or ocular herpes simplex infections to prevent exacerbation of symptoms.

- In patients with a history of tuberculosis, give cautiously because drug may reactivate the disease.
- Use cautiously in children because drug may retard bone growth. It may also increase intracranial pressure, resulting in papilledema, oculomotor or abducens nerve paralysis, vision loss, and headache.
- Also use cautiously in renal dysfunction because of possible severe fluid retention; in hepatic dysfunction because of an enhanced risk of toxicity; and in open-angle glaucoma because of the risk of elevated intraocular pressure.
- In hypoalbuminemia, give carefully to prevent drug toxicity.

PREPARATION & STORAGE
Available in container of drug and diluent in the following strengths: 40 mg (1 ml), 125 mg (2 ml), 500 mg (8.8 ml), 1 g (17.6 ml), and 2 g (30.6 ml). Reconstitute with diluent provided and store at room temperature. Avoid freezing. Don't use solution if cloudy, and discard any unused portion after 48 hours. Dilute for infusion with dextrose 5% in water, 0.9% sodium chloride, or dextrose 5% in 0.9% sodium chloride.

ADMINISTRATION
Direct injection: Inject diluted drug into vein or free-flowing compatible I.V. solution over at least 1 minute. In life-threatening situations, administer initial massive dose over 3 to 15 minutes.
Intermittent infusion: Using appropriately diluted dose, adjust flow rate, depending on the disorder and the patient's response.
Continuous infusion: Using appropriately diluted dose, adjust flow rate, depending on the disorder and the patient's response.

INCOMPATIBILITY
Incompatible with calcium gluconate, cephalothin, cytarabine, glycopyrrolate, metaraminol, nafcillin, and penicillin G sodium.

ADVERSE REACTIONS
Life-threatening: anaphylaxis.
Other: bleeding, blurred vision, depression, dyspnea, facial flushing, fever, fluid and electrolyte imbalance, hypertension, increased susceptibility to infection, insomnia, pain at injection site, palpitations, rash, rectal irritation, seizures, steroid withdrawal syndrome (anorexia, headache, hypotension, joint pain, lethargy, nausea, vomiting, weight loss), tachycardia.

INTERACTIONS
Anticholinesterase drugs: severe weakness in patients with myasthenia gravis. Use cautiously.
Asparaginase: possible heightened risk of neuropathy and disturbances in erythropoiesis.
Barbiturates, phenytoin, rifampin: possible increased methylprednisolone metabolism.
Cardiac glycosides: enhanced risk of dysrhythmias or glycoside toxicity.
Estrogen: possible potentiated methylprednisolone effects.
^{131}I: reduced thyroid uptake.
Indomethacin, NSAIDs, other ulcerogenic drugs: heightened risk of GI ulcers.
Isoniazid: possible increased metabolism and excretion.
Mexiletine: accelerated metabolism.
Oral anticoagulants: possible increased blood coagulability.
Potassium-depleting diuretics, other potassium-depleting drugs: enhanced potassium loss.
Salicylates: decreased effects.
Sodium-containing drugs and foods: possible hypernatremia.

Streptozocin: enhanced risk of hyperglycemia.
Toxoids, live or inactivated vaccines: diminished response.

EFFECTS ON DIAGNOSTIC TESTS
Basophil, eosinophil, lymphocyte, and monocyte counts: reduced.
[123]I, serum protein-bound iodine, thyroxine: reduced levels.
Nitroblue tetrazolium test for systemic bacterial infections: possible false-negative results.
Platelet, polymorphonuclear counts: increased.
Radionuclide brain imaging: decreased uptake of contrast medium.
Serum calcium: diminished levels.
Serum lipids, urine glucose: possible increased levels.
Skin tests: unreliable response because drug suppresses inflammation.

SPECIAL CONSIDERATIONS
• Before therapy, obtain baseline EKG, blood pressure, chest and spinal X-rays, glucose tolerance test, evaluation of hypothalamic-pituitary-adrenal axis function, and results of upper GI series (in patients with predisposition to GI disorders).
• Because of the risk of anaphylaxis, keep resuscitation equipment nearby.
• Adjust dosage as needed for the patient taking insulin, antithyroid drugs, or thyroid hormones.
• Protein intake may need to be increased because the drug promotes protein catabolism.
• During long-term therapy, monitor height, weight, blood pressure, chest and spinal X-rays, hematopoietic and electrolyte tests, and tests for glucose tolerance and intraocular pressure.
• Adrenal function may recover within 1 week after high-dose therapy lasting for 1 to 5 days.

• Instruct patient to notify the doctor of any sign of infection or any injury received during therapy and for 12 months afterward.
• In all preparations, diluent contains benzyl alcohol.

metoclopramide hydrochloride
Maxeran♦♦, Reglan♦

Pregnancy Risk Category: B

PHARMACOKINETICS
Distribution: throughout tissues, with 13% to 22% bound to plasma proteins. Drug crosses the blood-brain barrier and placenta.
Metabolism: minimal, in the liver.
Excretion: in urine and feces, mostly as unchanged drug and metabolites. Half-life averages 3 to 6 hours in normal renal function. Drug appears in breast milk.
Action: onset, 1 to 3 minutes; duration, 1 to 2 hours.

MECHANISM OF ACTION
Although metoclopramide's exact mechanism of action is unknown, this dopamine antagonist may act at the chemoreceptor trigger zone in the CNS to inhibit vomiting. Drug also enhances gastric emptying and increases GI muscle tone and phasic contractile activity.

INDICATIONS & DOSAGE
• Nausea and vomiting during chemotherapy. *Adults:* 2 mg/kg q 2 hours for three doses, beginning 30 minutes before chemotherapy; then 1 mg/kg q 3 hours.
• Severe delayed gastric emptying in diabetic gastroparesis (in patients unable to take oral dose). *Adults:* 10

mg q.i.d. 30 minutes before meals and at bedtime.

• Passage of intestinal tubes for diagnostic tests. *Adults:* 10 mg. *Children age 6 to 14:* 2.5 to 5 mg. *Children under age 6:* 0.1 mg/kg.

• Radiologic examination of GI tract (in delayed gastric emptying that interferes with examination of stomach or intestine). *Adults:* 10 mg. *Children age 6 to 14:* 2.5 to 5 mg. *Children under age 6:* 0.1 mg/kg.

Note: Adjust dosage in renal impairment. For adults, dosage reflects creatinine clearance. If clearance is less than 10 ml/min, decrease dosage by 50%; if 10 to 50 ml/min, decrease dosage by 25%.

CONTRAINDICATIONS & CAUTIONS

• Contraindicated in hypersensitivity or intolerance to drug or sulfites.

• Also contraindicated when acceleration of GI motility may be hazardous.

• Avoid use in pheochromocytoma because the drug may cause hypertensive crisis and in patients with a history of seizures because the drug may increase their frequency and severity.

• Use cautiously in renal impairment because delayed excretion may prolong and intensify drug effects, and in hepatic impairment because of decreased drug conjugation.

• Also use cautiously in hypersensitivity to procainamide because of possible cross-sensitivity, and in Parkinson's disease because drug may exacerbate symptoms.

PREPARATION & STORAGE

Available with a concentration of 5 mg/ml in 2, 10, 30, 50, and 100 ml vials and in 2 and 10 ml ampules. For infusion, dilute with 50 ml of dextrose 5% in water, 0.9% sodium chloride, dextrose 5% in 0.45% sodium chloride, Ringer's injection, or Ringer's lactate.

Solutions remain stable for 48 hours when stored at 39° to 86° F. (4° to 30° C.) and protected from light. If diluted with 0.9% sodium chloride, solution may be frozen in PVC bags for up to 4 weeks. (Don't use dextrose 5% diluent with PVC bags if solution will be frozen.)

ADMINISTRATION

Direct injection: Inject over 1 to 2 minutes directly into vein or into I.V. tubing containing a free-flowing compatible solution.

Intermittent infusion: Cover solution with a brown paper bag to prevent exposure to light. Infuse over at least 15 minutes. Slow infusion prevents anxiety and restlessness.

Continuous infusion: not recommended.

INCOMPATIBILITY

Incompatible with calcium gluconate, cephalothin, chloramphenicol sodium succinate, cisplatin, erythromycin lactobionate, methotrexate sodium, penicillin G potassium, sodium bicarbonate, and tetracycline hydrochloride.

ADVERSE REACTIONS

Life-threatening: anaphylaxis (in sulfite-sensitive patients), hypertensive crisis (in pheochromocytoma).

Other: agitation, amenorrhea (reversible), anxiety, bradycardia, constipation, depression, diarrhea, disorientation, dizziness, drowsiness, dry mouth, dystonia, extrapyramidal symptoms, fatigue, transient fluid retention with glossal or periorbital edema, galactorrhea, headache, hirsutism, insomnia, lethargy, maculopapular rash, methemoglobinemia, nausea, nipple tenderness, parkinsonian symptoms, restlessness, tardive dyskinesia, urticaria.

INTERACTIONS

Anticholinergic drugs, opioid analgesics: antagonized metoclopramide effects on GI motility.
Apomorphine: decreased emetic response.
Bromocriptine: altered effects.
CNS depressants: possible potentiated sedative effects.
Drugs that cause extrapyramidal reactions: possible increased frequency and severity of extrapyramidal effects.
Oral drugs: altered absorption with impaired tablet disintegration or dissolution in stomach because of increased GI motility. Gastric absorption may decline and drug absorption by small intestine may increase.

EFFECTS ON DIAGNOSTIC TESTS

Gonadorelin test: decreased response because of increased serum prolactin levels.
Serum aldosterone, prolactin: possible elevated levels.

SPECIAL CONSIDERATIONS

• *Treatment of overdose:* To control extrapyramidal symptoms, give antimuscarinic-antiparkinson drugs or antihistamines with antimuscarinic properties.
• Adjust insulin dosage, as ordered, in patients with diabetic gastroparesis. Metoclopramide affects intestinal food absorption.

metocurine iodide
Metubine Iodide♦

Pregnancy Risk Category: C

PHARMACOKINETICS

Distribution: to plasma. Drug is 35% bound to plasma proteins and crosses the placenta.
Metabolism: in the liver.
Excretion: mainly in urine, with 50% removed unchanged. Another 2% is excreted unchanged in bile. Elimination half-life is about 3½ hours.
Action: onset, 1 to 4 minutes; duration, 15 to 90 minutes.

MECHANISM OF ACTION

Metocurine produces skeletal muscle relaxation by a nondepolarizing (competitive) blockade at the neuromuscular junction. It inhibits neuromuscular transmission by competing with acetylcholine for cholinergic receptors on the motor end plate.

INDICATIONS & DOSAGE

Dosages must be individualized. The following are guidelines.
• Adjunct in general anesthesia.
Adults: 0.1 to 0.4 mg/kg initially. Maintenance dosage, 0.5 to 1 mg every 30 to 90 minutes. If used with general anesthetics that have muscle relaxant properties, reduce dosage by one-third to one-half.
• Adjunct during electroconvulsive therapy. *Adults:* 2 to 3 mg (ranges from 1.75 to 5.5 mg) given slowly until head drop response occurs.

CONTRAINDICATIONS & CAUTIONS

• Contraindicated in hypersensitivity to metocurine or to its iodide component.

• In patients with myasthenia gravis or other neuromuscular disease, administer metocurine carefully because the drug exacerbates the condition.

• Use cautiously in renal disease or poor renal perfusion because decreased drug excretion prolongs neuromuscular blockade; in hepatic impairment because of reduced drug effect; and in impaired pulmonary function or respiratory depression because of the risk of additive respiratory depression.

• Also use cautiously in hyperthermia because of increased drug effect; in hypothermia because of possible decreased drug effects and duration of action; in hypotension because rapid I.V. administration or large doses may cause exacerbation; and in shock because of prolonged drug action.

• In patients with bronchogenic carcinoma, give carefully because of possible enhanced drug action.

• Similarly, give carefully to patients in whom histamine release is hazardous because the drug may cause histamine release.

• Use cautiously in elderly patients and in neonates because of heightened sensitivity to drug effects, and in hypokalemia, hypermagnesemia, and hypocalcemia because of potentiated drug effect.

• Also use cautiously in patients with severe obesity or neuromuscular disease because of possible airway or ventilation problems.

PREPARATION & STORAGE
Available in 20 ml multidose vials containing 2 mg/ml. Dilution isn't necessary. Store at room temperature; avoid freezing.

ADMINISTRATION
Only staff with special training in administering anesthetics and managing their adverse reactions should give metocurine.
Direct injection: Inject into vein over 30 to 60 seconds. Monitor neuromuscular blockade with a peripheral nerve stimulator.
Intermittent infusion: not recommended.
Continuous infusion: not recommended.

INCOMPATIBILITY
Incompatible with alkaline solutions, barbiturates, meperidine, methohexital, morphine, and thiopental.

ADVERSE REACTIONS
Life-threatening: anaphylaxis, apnea, bronchospasm, cardiac irregularities, circulatory collapse, hypotension.
Other: edema, erythema, flushing, tachycardia.

INTERACTIONS
Aminoglycosides, capreomycin, clindamycin, lincomycin, massive transfusions of citrated blood, polymyxins, I.V. procaine, or trimethaphan: enhanced neuromuscular blockade.
Antimyasthenics, edrophonium: antagonized metocurine effects.
Beta blockers: possible enhanced or prolonged neuromuscular blockade.
Calcium salts: reversal of metocurine effect.
Doxapram: possible masked residual neuromuscular blockade when given postoperatively.
Hydrocarbon inhalation anesthetics: possible potentiated neuromuscular blockade.
Opioid analgesics: additive respiratory depression and increased risk of bradycardia or hypotension.
Other muscle relaxants: possible synergistic or antagonistic effects.
Parenteral antibiotics: possible intensified neuromuscular blockade.

Parenteral magnesium sulfate, procainamide, quinidine: possible enhanced neuromuscular blockade.
Potassium-depleting drugs: heightened neuromuscular blockade.

EFFECTS ON DIAGNOSTIC TESTS
None reported.

SPECIAL CONSIDERATIONS
• *Treatment of overdose:* Prolonged apnea, cardiovascular collapse, and sudden histamine release can result from overly rapid I.V. administration or excessive or multiple doses. Reverse neuromuscular blockade by giving an anticholinesterase inhibitor, such as neostigmine or pyridostigmine, as ordered. To prevent bradycardia, administer atropine or glycopyrrolate.
• For severe obesity or residual neuromuscular blockade, maintain a patent airway and provide manual or mechanical ventilation.
• Administer fluids to correct severe hypotension or shock.
• Adequate anesthesia is necessary when using metocurine; drug has no effect on consciousness, pain threshold, or cerebration.
• Half-life is longer than duration of action, so repeated doses may be cumulative.

metoprolol tartrate
Lopresor♦♦, Lopressor

Pregnancy Risk Category: C

PHARMACOKINETICS
Distribution: widely distributed, with highest concentrations in the heart, liver, lungs, and saliva. Drug is 12% bound to serum albumin. It crosses the placenta, producing about equal fetal and maternal levels. It also crosses the blood-brain barrier, producing cerebrospinal fluid levels about 80% of those in plasma.
Metabolism: mainly hepatic, with three major, relatively inactive metabolites.
Excretion: in urine by glomerular filtration and, to a lesser extent, by renal tubular secretion and reabsorption. About 10% of drug is excreted unchanged, 85% as metabolites. Half-life in healthy or hypertensive patients is 3 to 7 hours. In poor hydroxylators, half-life extends to $7\frac{1}{2}$ hours. Drug appears in breast milk.
Action: peak serum level, 20 minutes after 10-minute infusion.

MECHANISM OF ACTION
A beta$_1$-adrenergic blocker, metoprolol binds to postganglionic receptors in the myocardium and blocks the sympathetic neurotransmitter norepinephrine. Drug binds to beta$_2$-adrenergic receptors in bronchial and vascular smooth muscle only when given in high doses.

INDICATIONS & DOSAGE
• Early treatment in suspected or definitive acute MI. *Adults:* three injections of 5 mg each q 2 minutes, followed by oral maintenance doses if I.V. doses are tolerated.
Note: Dosage may need to be reduced in patients with hepatic dysfunction.

CONTRAINDICATIONS & CAUTIONS
• Because of an increased risk of myocardial depression, metoprolol is contraindicated in first-degree heart block with PR interval greater than 0.2 second, in second- and third-degree heart block, in bradycardia (less than 45 beats/minute), in systolic pressure of less than 100 mm Hg, in moderate to severe con-

gestive heart failure (CHF), or in cardiogenic shock.
• In CHF controlled with digitalis and diuretics, give metoprolol carefully because it may exacerbate the condition.
• Use with caution in elderly patients or those with hepatic or renal disease because of an increased risk of toxicity and adverse effects.
• Also use with caution in bronchospastic disease because drug may aggravate symptoms, and in myasthenia gravis because drug may cause muscle weakness.
• In diabetes mellitus and hyperthyroidism, metoprolol may mask symptoms. Use cautiously in these disorders.
• Administer cautiously in depression and psoriasis because drug may worsen these conditions.

PREPARATION & STORAGE
Available in 5 ml ampules or prefilled syringes (1 mg/ml). Store at room temperature and protect from light. Discard solution if discolored or if particulates form.

ADMINISTRATION
Direct injection: Rapidly inject bolus into free-flowing I.V. line.
Intermittent infusion: not recommended.
Continuous infusion: not recommended.

INCOMPATIBILITY
None reported.

ADVERSE REACTIONS
Life-threatening: respiratory distress with laryngospasm, severe bradycardia or hypotension.
Other: abdominal pain, alopecia, CHF, cold extremities, confusion, depression, dizziness, dyspnea, fatigue, fever, first-degree heart block (PR interval greater than 0.2 sec-

ond), hallucinations, headache, insomnia, intensified dysrhythmias, lethargy, nausea, palpitations, rash, Raynaud's syndrome, sleep disturbances, sore throat.

INTERACTIONS
Barbiturates, rifampin: increased metabolism of metoprolol, decreasing its effectiveness.
Calcium channel blockers: potentiated hypotensive effect.
Cardiac glycosides, catecholamine-depleting drugs (such as reserpine): possible potentiation of hypotension or bradycardia.
Chlorpromazine, cimetidine: increased beta blockade resulting from inhibited metoprolol metabolism.
Diazoxide: prevention of tachycardia and enhanced hypotensive effect.
Estrogens, NSAIDs: possible decreased antihypertensive effect.
Hydrocarbon inhalation anesthetics: heightened risk of myocardial depression and hypotension.
Insulin, oral antidiabetics: amplified risk of hypoglycemia or hyperglycemia.
Lidocaine: increased effect and risk of toxicity, resulting from reduced clearance.
MAO inhibitors: severe hypertension if metoprolol is given within 14 days of last dose.
Molindone: enhanced metoprolol effects.
Nondepolarizing neuromuscular blockers: possible potentiated and prolonged action.
Other antihypertensive drugs: potentiated hypotensive effect.
Phenothiazines: possible increased plasma levels of both drugs.
Phenytoin I.V.: possible additive myocardial depression.
Ritodrine: decreased effects.
Sympathomimetics, xanthines: possible antagonized beta blockade.

EFFECTS ON DIAGNOSTIC TESTS
BUN, serum lipoproteins, potassium, triglycerides, uric acid: increased levels.

SPECIAL CONSIDERATIONS
• *Treatment of overdose:* Administer atropine or prepare for temporary pacemaker insertion for bradycardia. Further treatment is symptomatic and supportive.
• Give metoprolol as soon as MI patient is stable.
• Continuously monitor hemodynamic status, blood pressure, heart rate, and EKG during infusion.
• If patient develops bradycardia or hypotension before dosage is complete, notify doctor; he may stop injections or change to oral form.
• Observe patient for signs of drug-induced depression.

---

metronidazole, metronidazole hydrochloride
Flagyl I.V., Flagyl I.V. R.T.U., Metro I.V., Metronidazole Redi-Infusion

Pregnancy Risk Category: B

PHARMACOKINETICS
Distribution: distributed widely throughout all body tissues, including saliva; bile; cerebrospinal, pleural, peritoneal, seminal, and empyema fluids; bone; liver; liver and cerebral abscesses; lungs; and vaginal secretions. Drug crosses the blood-brain barrier and placenta. Less than 20% is bound to plasma proteins.
Metabolism: 30% to 60% in the liver.
Excretion: 60% to 80% removed in urine (20% unchanged) and 6% to 15% in feces. Drug appears in breast milk. Plasma clearance declines in hepatic impairment. Half-life is 6 to 12 hours, averaging 8 hours.
Action: peak serum level, immediately after administration.

MECHANISM OF ACTION
A systemic, synthetic antibacterial and protozoal agent that's bactericidal against most obligate anaerobic bacteria, metronidazole interacts with DNA to inhibition of nucleic acid synthesis, causing cell death. It's equally effective against dividing and nondividing cells.

The drug acts against gram-negative anaerobic bacteria, including *Bacteroides fragilis, B. melaninogenicus,* other *Bacteroides* species, *Fusobacterium,* and *Veillonella.* Susceptible gram-positive anaerobic bacteria include *Clostridium, Peptococcus,* and *Peptostreptococcus.* The drug is also effective against *Entamoeba histolytica, Trichomonas vaginalis, Giardia lamblia,* and *Balantidium coli.*

INDICATIONS & DOSAGE
• Severe infections caused by susceptible bacteria. *Adults:* 15 mg/kg initially, then 7.5 mg/kg q 6 hours, beginning 6 hours after loading dose. Maximum dosage, 4 g daily.
• Surgical prophylaxis. *Adults:* 15 mg/kg, completed 1 hour before surgery, then 7.5 mg/kg q 6 hours for two doses at 6 and 12 hours after initial dose.
Note: Adjust dosage in renal failure. For adults, dosage reflects creatinine clearance. If clearance is less than 10 ml/min, decrease dosage by 50%.

Dosage may need to be reduced in patients with severe hepatic dysfunction.

CONTRAINDICATIONS & CAUTIONS

• Contraindicated in hypersensitivity to metronidazole or other nitroimidazole derivatives.
• Use cautiously in CNS disorders because of the risk of CNS toxicity; in blood dyscrasias because of possible leukopenia; in impaired cardiac function or predisposition to edema because of the drug's sodium content; and in severe hepatic impairment because of the heightened risk of toxicity.
• Pediatric safety and effectiveness haven't been established.

PREPARATION & STORAGE

Flagyl I.V. is supplied as sterile, off-white, lyophilized powder in single-dose vials containing 500 mg of metronidazole and 415 mg of mannitol. Drug requires reconstitution, dilution, and neutralization.

Order of mixing is important. Reconstitute drug with 4.4 ml of sterile water for injection, bacteriostatic water for injection, 0.9% sodium chloride injection, or bacteriostatic 0.9% sodium chloride injection. Mix thoroughly. Resulting solution provides 5 ml (100 mg/ml).

Using a glass or plastic container, dilute Flagyl I.V. further with 0.9% sodium chloride injection, dextrose 5% injection, or Ringer's lactate injection. Concentration shouldn't exceed 8 mg/ml.

Neutralize final dilution with 5 mEq of sodium bicarbonate injection for each 500 mg of drug. Because this produces carbon dioxide, the container may require venting.

Before reconstitution, store Flagyl I.V. below 86° F. (30° C.) and protect from light. Reconstituted vials are stable for 96 hours in room light if stored below 86° F. Don't refrigerate when neutralized because a precipitate may form. Use diluted and neutralized solutions within 24 hours.

Flagyl I.V. R.T.U. is supplied in 100 ml single-dose plastic containers or glass vials, each containing 500 mg of drug. Don't dilute, change pH, or mix any additive with this solution. Also avoid using aluminum equipment (such as needles or cannulae) that would come in contact with drug. Although drug may cause opacity of plastic containers, needle hubs, or cannulae, this reaction will subside and doesn't affect solution.

Flagyl I.V. R.T.U. needs no dilution or neutralization. Store at controlled room temperature protected from light. Don't refrigerate or freeze.

ADMINISTRATION

Direct injection: not recommended.
Intermittent infusion: Give by slow infusion only, over 1 hour (30 to 60 minutes when used for surgical prophylaxis). Discontinue the primary solution during drug administration.
Continuous infusion: rarely used. Infuse diluted drug over ordered amount of time.

INCOMPATIBILITY

Incompatible with aluminum, 10% amino acid, and dopamine. Manufacturer recommends mixing no other drugs with metronidazole.

ADVERSE REACTIONS

Life-threatening: none reported.
Other: abdominal discomfort, ataxia, bacterial or fungal superinfection, confusion, darkened urine, diarrhea, dizziness, fever, headache, hypersensitivity (pruritus, rash, urticaria), leukopenia (reversible), metallic taste, nausea, neutropenia, peripheral neuropathy (numbness, paresthesia, or weakness of an extremity, usually with high doses or prolonged use), pseudomembranous

colitis, seizures, sore throat, syncope, thrombophlebitis at injection site, vomiting.

INTERACTIONS
Alcohol, alcohol-containing drugs: disulfiram-like reaction.
Barbiturates: enhanced metronidazole metabolism.
Disulfiram: acute psychosis and confusion.
Drugs that decrease hepatic microsomal enzyme activity: may increase adverse effects of metronidazole.
Drugs that induce hepatic microsomal enzyme activity: decreased metronidazole levels resulting from accelerated drug excretion.
Fluorouracil I.V.: transient neutropenia.
Neurotoxic drugs: heightened risk of neurotoxicity.
Oral anticoagulants: potentiated action, resulting in prolonged prothrombin time.

EFFECTS ON DIAGNOSTIC TESTS
CBC: leukopenia.
Serum cholesterol: possible decreased levels.
Serum glucose, LDH, SGOT, SGPT, triglycerides: unreliable results.

SPECIAL CONSIDERATIONS
• Obtain specimens for culture and sensitivity tests before first dose. Therapy may begin before results are available.
• Obtain CBC before and after therapy.
• Closely monitor metronidazole levels and observe for toxicity in patients with severe hepatic disease.
• Symptoms of known or previously undiagnosed candidiasis may become more prominent during therapy, requiring treatment with an antifungal agent.

• If diarrhea persists during therapy, collect stool specimens for culture to rule out pseudomembranous colitis.
• Inform patient that urine may darken.
• To minimize risk of thrombophlebitis, avoid prolonged use of I.V. catheters.
• Therapy usually lasts for 7 to 10 days; however, infections of bones and joints, lower respiratory tract, and endocardium may require longer treatment.
• Parenteral therapy may change to oral therapy, depending on severity of disease and patient response.
• Patients with Crohn's disease who are undergoing high-dose, prolonged treatment with metronidazole have a higher incidence of breast and colon cancer. However, a cause-and-effect relationship hasn't been established.
• R.T.U. form of metronidazole contains 14 mEq (322 mg) of sodium. Neutralized I.V. solution contains 5 mEq (115 mg) of sodium.
• Observe patient for fungal and bacterial superinfection with prolonged use.
• Advise patient to avoid alcohol for 48 hours after last dose.

mezlocillin sodium
Mezlin

Pregnancy Risk Category: B

PHARMACOKINETICS
Distribution: into peritoneal and pleural fluid, bronchial and wound secretions, bile, urine, bone, muscle, adipose tissue, heart, and prostatic and gallbladder tissue. Mezlocillin is 16% to 42% bound to plasma proteins, albumin, and gamma globulin. Drug crosses the blood-brain barrier in small amounts, increasing with

inflamed meninges. It readily crosses the placenta.

Metabolism: partially metabolized in the liver.

Excretion: primarily removed in urine by renal tubular secretion and glomerular filtration. Small amounts are excreted in feces. About 40% to 70% is excreted unchanged in urine in 24 hours (most within 2 to 6 hours). About 15% is excreted as metabolites. Small amounts appear in breast milk. Half-life ranges from 40 to 80 minutes. In higher doses, nonrenal clearance declines more than renal clearance. Excretion is delayed in neonates and in patients with hepatic or renal impairment.

Action: peak serum level, immediately after administration.

MECHANISM OF ACTION

By adhering to penicillin-binding proteins, this semisynthetic, bactericidal, extended-spectrum penicillin inhibits bacterial cell wall synthesis.

Its spectrum of activity includes gram-positive aerobic bacteria, including many strains of nonpenicillinase-producing bacteria, such as *Staphylococcus aureus* and *S. epidermidis;* groups A, B, C, and G streptococci; *Streptococcus pneumoniae; S. viridans;* and some strains of enterococci. Susceptible gram-negative aerobic bacteria include many strains of *Neisseria meningitidis* and *N. gonorrhoeae;* some strains of *Haemophilus influenzae, Escherichia coli, Morganella morganii, Proteus mirabilis, P. vulgaris, Providencia rettgeri, Salmonella, Shigella;* and some strains of *Citrobacter, Enterobacter, Klebsiella, Serratia, Pseudomonas, Acinetobacter, Moraxella, Flavobacterium,* and *Eikenella corrodens.* The drug is also active against the anaerobic bacteria *Actinomyces, Bifidobacterium, Clostridium, Eubacterium, Lactobacillus, Peptococcus,* *Peptostreptococcus, Propionibacterium,* and some strains of *Bacteroides, Fusobacterium,* and *Veillonella.*

INDICATIONS & DOSAGE

• Severe infections caused by susceptible organisms. *Adults:* 200 to 300 mg/kg daily in four to six divided doses; 3 g q 4 hours; or 4 g q 6 hours. *Children age 1 month to 12 years:* 50 mg/kg q 4 hours. *Neonates 8 days old or older weighing over 2 kg:* 75 mg/kg q 6 hours. *Neonates 8 days old or older weighing 2 kg or less:* 75 mg/kg q 8 hours. *Neonates 7 days old or younger:* 75 mg/kg q 12 hours.

• Life-threatening infections caused by susceptible organisms. *Adults:* 350 mg/kg daily or 4 g q 4 hours. Maximum dosage, 24 g daily. *Children and neonates:* Same as for severe infections, above.

• Uncomplicated urinary tract infection. *Adults:* 100 to 125 mg/kg daily in divided doses q 6 hours or 1.5 to 2 g q 6 hours. *Children and neonates:* Same as for severe infections, above.

• Complicated urinary tract infection. *Adults:* 150 to 200 mg/kg daily in six divided doses or 3 g q 6 hours. *Children and neonates:* Same as for severe infections, above.

• Acute, uncomplicated gonococcal urethritis caused by susceptible strains of *Neisseria gonorrhoeae.* *Adults:* 1 to 2 g. *Children and neonates:* Same as for severe infections, above.

Note: Adjust dosage in renal failure. For adults, dosage reflects creatinine clearance. If clearance is less than 10 ml/min, dosage is 2 g q 8 hours. If 10 to 30 ml/min, dosage is 3 g q 8 hours. Patients on hemodialysis should be given 3 to 4 g after each dialysis session and then q 12 hours.

Patients on peritoneal dialysis should receive 3 g q 12 hours.

In hepatic dysfunction, reduce the dose by 50% or double the interval, as ordered.

CONTRAINDICATIONS & CAUTIONS

• Contraindicated in hypersensitivity to penicillins.
• Use cautiously in patients with other allergies, especially drug allergies.
• Also use cautiously in bleeding disorders because platelet dysfunction may result in hemorrhage; in GI disorders because drug may worsen them; and in hepatic or renal impairment because of an increased risk of toxicity.

PREPARATION & STORAGE

Available as a sterile powder in vials containing 1, 2, 3, or 4 g of drug or infusion bottles containing 2, 3, or 4 g of drug. Store vials and infusion bottles at or below 86° F. (30° C.). Reconstitute each gram of sterile powder with at least 10 ml of sterile water for injection, dextrose 5% injection, or 0.9% sodium chloride injection. Shake vigorously to dissolve drug. After reconstitution in solutions up to 100 mg/ml, mezlocillin may be frozen, remaining stable for 28 days.

For infusion, dilute further with 50 to 100 ml of sterile water for injection, 0.9% sodium chloride injection, dextrose 5% injection, dextrose 5% in 0.25% sodium chloride injection, Ringer's lactate injection, dextrose 5% in 0.45% sodium chloride injection, or Ringer's injection. Add daily dose of mezlocillin to amount of appropriate fluid to be administered over 24 hours.

At room temperature, solutions of 10 to 100 mg/ml are stable for 24 hours when diluted in Ringer's injection; for 48 hours when diluted in sterile water for injection, 0.9% sodium chloride, dextrose 5% in water, or dextrose 5% in 0.45% sodium chloride; and for 72 hours when diluted in Ringer's lactate or dextrose 5% in 0.25% sodium chloride.

Refrigerated solutions of 10 to 100 mg/ml are stable for 24 hours when diluted in Ringer's injection; for 48 hours when diluted in dextrose 5% in 0.45% sodium chloride; and for 7 days when diluted in sterile water for injection, 0.9% sodium chloride, dextrose 5% in water, dextrose 5% in 0.25% sodium chloride, or Ringer's lactate.

ADMINISTRATION

Direct injection: Inject reconstituted drug directly into vein or into I.V. tubing containing a free-flowing compatible solution over 3 to 5 minutes.
Intermittent infusion: Infuse diluted drug over 30 minutes. If infused by piggyback, temporarily discontinue the primary solution while drug infuses.
Continuous infusion: Adjust rate according to infusion volume.

INCOMPATIBILITY

Incompatible with aminoglycosides.

ADVERSE REACTIONS

Life-threatening: anaphylaxis, exfoliative dermatitis.
Other: abnormal platelet aggregation, abnormal taste sensation, acute interstitial nephritis, anemia, arthralgia, bacterial or fungal superinfection, chills, darkened or discolored tongue (fungal overgrowth), diarrhea, dizziness, eosinophilia, fatigue, fever, flatulence, giddiness, granulocytopenia, headache, hypernatremia, hypokalemia, leukopenia, malaise, muscle twitching, myalgia,

nausea, neutropenia, pain at infusion site, phlebitis, pruritus, rash, seizures, thrombocytopenia, thrombophlebitis, unusual bleeding or bruising, urticaria, vomiting.

INTERACTIONS

Aminoglycosides: possible synergistic activity against some organisms.
Anticoagulants, indanedione derivatives, NSAIDs, salicylates, sulfinpyrazone, thrombolytics: increased risk of bleeding.
Other hepatotoxic drugs: heightened risk of hepatotoxicity.
Probenecid (oral): increased or prolonged mezlocillin effects.

EFFECTS ON DIAGNOSTIC TESTS

Bleeding time: possibly prolonged.
BUN; serum alkaline phosphatase, bilirubin, creatinine, SGOT, SGPT: elevated levels.
Coombs' test: positive results.
Serum potassium: reduced levels.
Serum sodium: possible heightened levels.
Urine protein: false-positive results if using sulfosalicylic acid and boiling test, acetic acid test, biuret reaction, and nitric acid test.

SPECIAL CONSIDERATIONS

• Before giving drug, check for hypersensitivity to penicillins or cephalosporins. Negative history doesn't rule out future allergic reaction.
• Obtain specimens for culture and sensitivity tests before giving first dose. Therapy may begin before test results are available.
• In anaphylaxis, treatment is symptomatic and supportive. In toxicity, remove drug by hemodialysis.
• Check CBC frequently, and monitor serum potassium levels, especially in high-dose therapy or in fluid and electrolyte imbalance. Potassium supplements may be needed in hypokalemia.
• Monitor bleeding time and platelet count, especially in patients with renal impairment who are receiving maximum doses.
• Institute seizure precautions in patients receiving high drug doses.
• Change site every 48 hours to prevent vein irritation.
• When giving mezlocillin with an aminoglycoside, administer at separate sites.
• Monitor hepatic and renal function.
• If syphilis is suspected when treating gonorrhea, a darkfield examination and serology should be performed before therapy. Serologic studies should be repeated 3 months after mezlocillin therapy.
• Therapy for group A beta-hemolytic streptococcal infections lasts for at least 10 days to reduce the risk of rheumatic fever or glomerulonephritis. Other regimens last for 10 to 14 days or for at least 48 hours after eradication of infection is confirmed.
• Mezlocillin may be better suited to patients on salt-free diets than carbenicillin or ticarcillin because it contains 43 mg of sodium per gram of drug.
• Observe patient for fungal and bacterial superinfection with prolonged use.

miconazole
Monistat I.V.

Pregnancy Risk Category: C

PHARMACOKINETICS
Distribution: widely distributed in tissues and fluids, including inflamed joints, vitreous humor, and peritoneal cavity. Drug is poorly dis-

tributed in CSF, even if meninges are inflamed. It's 91% to 93% bound to plasma proteins. Not known if drug crosses the placenta. *Metabolism:* in the liver to inactive metabolites.
Excretion: in urine, with 14% to 22% excreted as inactive metabolites and less than 1% as unchanged drug. Not known if drug appears in breast milk. Triphasic half-life occurs in about 30 minutes, 2 hours, and 24 hours. Half-life isn't affected by dialysis or renal insufficiency.
Action: peak serum level, immediately after infusion.

MECHANISM OF ACTION
Miconazole is both fungistatic and fungicidal, depending on concentration. At fungistatic concentrations, miconazole causes cell wall thickening, altering wall permeability and inhibiting purine transport. At fungicidal concentrations, the cell wall remains intact and intracellular contents become necrotic. High concentrations interfere with peroxisomal enzymes, resulting in toxic intracellular peroxide concentrations and cell death.

Miconazole's spectrum of activity includes most pathogenic fungi, including *Coccidioides immitis, Candida albicans, C. tropicalis, C. parapsilosis, Cryptococcus neoformans, Histoplasma capsulatum, Paracoccidioides braziliensis, Sporothrix schenckii, Aspergillus flavus, A. ustus, Microsporum canis, Curvularia* species, *Drechslera hawaiiensis, Petriellidium boydii,* dermatophytes, and some gram-positive bacteria.

INDICATIONS & DOSAGE
• Coccidioidomycosis. *Adults:* 600 to 1,200 mg t.i.d. for 3 to 20 weeks (or longer). *Children:* 20 to 40 mg/kg daily, not to exceed 15 mg/kg per dose.

• Cryptococcosis. *Adults:* 400 to 800 mg t.i.d. for 1 to 20 weeks (or longer). *Children:* same dosage as for coccidioidomycosis.
• Paracoccidioidomycosis. *Adults:* 66 to 400 mg t.i.d. for 2 to 16 weeks (or longer). *Children:* same dosage as for coccidioidomycosis.
• Petriellidiosis. *Adults:* 200 to 1,000 mg t.i.d. for 5 to 20 weeks (or longer). *Children:* same dosage as for coccidioidomycosis.

CONTRAINDICATIONS & CAUTIONS
• Contraindicated in hypersensitivity to miconazole or to polyoxyl 35 castor oil.
• Use cautiously in hepatic impairment because decreased metabolism may increase risk of toxicity.

PREPARATION & STORAGE
Available in 20 ml ampules (10 mg/ml). Before infusion, dilute in at least 200 ml of 0.9% sodium chloride or dextrose 5% in water. If intact, ampules are stable for 24 months. Diluted solutions are stable for 48 hours. Avoid exposure to heat.

ADMINISTRATION
Direct injection: not recommended.
Intermittent infusion: Infuse through I.V. line containing compatible solution or through intermittent infusion device over 30 to 60 minutes. Use a central venous catheter or change infusion site every 48 to 72 hours to reduce risk of phlebitis.
Continuous infusion: not recommended.

INCOMPATIBILITY
None reported; however, manufacturer advises using only recommended I.V. solutions with drug.

ADVERSE REACTIONS

Life-threatening: anaphylaxis, cardiac arrest, respiratory arrest.
Other: anorexia, anxiety, bitter taste, blurred vision, diarrhea, drowsiness, dry eyes, dysrhythmias, fever, headache, hyponatremia, increased libido, macrocytic or normocytic anemia, nausea, phlebitis, pruritus, tachycardia, thrombocytopenia, thrombocytosis, vomiting.

INTERACTIONS

Amphotericin B: possible antagonized effect.
Coumarin, indanedione-derivative anticoagulants: enhanced anticoagulant effects.
Oral sulfonylurea agents: possible hypoglycemia.
Phenytoin: may increase serum levels with risk of phenytoin toxicity.

EFFECTS ON DIAGNOSTIC TESTS

Peripheral blood smear: moderate to marked erythrocyte aggregation and rouleau formation.
Serum lipoproteins: abnormal lipoprotein and immunoelectrophoretic patterns, probably caused by polyoxyl 35 castor oil in miconazole preparation.
Serum sodium: diminished levels.
Serum triglycerides: elevated levels.

SPECIAL CONSIDERATIONS

● Miconazole is highly toxic; it shouldn't be used to treat bacterial infections or trivial fungal infections.
● Insufficient dilution or overly rapid administration may cause anaphylactic reactions, transient tachycardia, dysrhythmias, or cardiac or respiratory arrest.
● Monitor blood pressure and heart rate every 30 minutes during initial therapy. Cardiac monitoring may be necessary if patient has a history of dysrhythmias.
● Help prevent nausea and vomiting by administering an antihistamine or antiemetic, by reducing dosage or slowing infusion rate, or by scheduling doses between meals.
● Monitor hemoglobin, hematocrit, serum electrolyte, and lipid levels.
● Give oral or I.V. diphenhydramine, as ordered, to reduce pruritus.
● Therapy may last up to 20 weeks.

Micrurus fulvius antivenin (Coral snake antivenin, North American coral snake antivenin)

Pregnancy Risk Category: D

PHARMACOKINETICS

Distribution: not known.
Metabolism: not well characterized.
Excretion: not known.
Action: peak serum level, immediately after administration.

MECHANISM OF ACTION

Antivenin contains globulins that neutralize and bind venom from the North American coral snake. Each vial (10 ml) of antivenin neutralizes at least 2 mg of coral snake venom.

INDICATIONS & DOSAGE

● North American coral snake bite.
Adults and children: 30 to 50 ml (3 to 5 vials). Initial dose reflects nature and severity of envenomation. Some clinicians advise giving 50 to 60 ml for pain or neurologic signs and 80 to 100 ml for signs of bulbar paralysis. Some patients may require a total dose of 100 ml or more.

Response to initial dose and continuing assessment determine need for additional antivenin doses.

CONTRAINDICATIONS & CAUTIONS

• Use cautiously in patients with asthma, other allergic manifestations, or allergies to horses or preparations containing equine serum.

PREPARATION & STORAGE

Available in package containing vials of drug (a light cream-colored solid) and 10 ml of diluent. To reconstitute, add diluent to vial of antivenin. Gently agitate vial; don't shake. For direct injection, dilute 10 ml of antivenin in 25 to 50 ml of 0.9% sodium chloride; for infusion, add reconstituted dose to 250 to 500 ml of 0.9% sodium chloride.

After reconstitution, antivenin solutions are opalescent, have a pH of 6.5 to 7.5, and should contain no more than 20% solids. Refrigerate antivenin. Avoid exposure to temperatures over 104° F. (40° C.); also avoid freezing diluent. Use reconstituted solutions within 48 hours and diluted solutions within 12 hours.

ADMINISTRATION

Direct injection: Using diluted dose, give test dose of 1 to 2 ml into vein over 3 to 5 minutes. Inject rest of dose at rate based on patient tolerance. If severe reaction occurs, stop immediately and treat symptomatically with an antihistamine, epinephrine, or both. Once reaction is controlled, continue infusion at slower rate.
Intermittent infusion: not recommended.
Continuous infusion: Using diluted dose, give test dose of 1 to 2 ml over 3 to 5 minutes. If no adverse reactions occur, infuse at a rate based on severity of envenomation and patient tolerance. If severe reaction occurs, treat symptomatically, then continue infusion at slower rate.

INCOMPATIBILITY

None reported.

ADVERSE REACTIONS

Life-threatening: anaphylaxis.
Other: flushing, pruritus, serum sickness (5 to 24 days after administration), urticaria, vomiting.

INTERACTIONS

Opiates: possible worsening of respiratory difficulty.
Sedatives: masked CNS signs.

EFFECTS ON DIAGNOSTIC TESTS

None reported.

SPECIAL CONSIDERATIONS

• If you're unfamiliar with snake bite management, consult a poison control center or a zoo.
• Because of the risk of severe systemic reaction, test for sensitivity with an intradermal skin test before giving antivenin. A negative allergy history and absence of skin test reaction don't rule out an immediate systemic reaction or serum sickness. A systemic reaction usually occurs within 30 minutes after skin test.
• In snake bite, immobilize the patient immediately, keep him warm, and remove constrictive jewelry. Keep oxygen, intubation equipment, an anaphylaxis kit, and ventilation equipment nearby. Give tetanus toxoid as ordered.
• When indicated, administer antivenin even before signs of envenomation develop. Such signs usually begin 1 to 7 hours after envenomation but may be delayed up to 18 hours. Once evident, they may progress rapidly; within 4 hours of a bite, respiratory paralysis may rapidly progress to death.
• Drug isn't effective against crotalid (pit viper) venom.

midazolam hydrochloride
Versed♦

Controlled Substance Schedule IV
Pregnancy Risk Category: D

PHARMACOKINETICS
Distribution: rapidly and widely distributed, with highest concentrations in the liver, kidneys, lungs, heart, and fat. This lipophilic drug is 93% to 97% protein bound. It crosses the blood-brain barrier and placenta.
Metabolism: in the liver. Drug undergoes rapid hydroxylation. Its metabolites are conjugated with glucuronic acid.
Excretion: in urine, primarily as metabolites. About 90% is excreted in 24 hours.
Action: onset, 1 to 5 minutes; duration, 1 to 6 hours.

MECHANISM OF ACTION
A short-acting benzodiazepine, midazolam depresses the CNS at the limbic and subcortical levels by potentiating gamma-aminobutyric acid.

INDICATIONS & DOSAGE
Dosages are highly individualized.
• Conscious sedation. *Adults:* initially, a maximum of 2.5 mg given over 2 to 3 minutes (some patients may respond to 1 mg), then increased in small increments at intervals of at least 2 minutes (to assess drug effect) until reaching desired effect. *Elderly or debilitated patients:* 1 to 1.5 mg initially, given over a longer duration.
• Induction of general anesthesia without premedication. *Adults age 55 and over:* 300 mcg/kg. *Adults under age 55:* 300 to 350 mcg/kg given over 20 to 30 seconds. *Adults with debilitation or severe systemic disease:* 150 to 250 mcg/kg. Increments

of 25% of initial dose may be needed to complete induction. Total dose shouldn't exceed 600 mcg/kg.
• Induction of anesthesia with premedication (opiate agonist). *Adults age 55 and over:* 200 mcg/kg. *Adults under age 55:* 250 mcg/kg. *Adults with debilitation or severe systemic disease:* 150 mcg/kg.

CONTRAINDICATIONS & CAUTIONS
• Contraindicated in hypersensitivity to midazolam or other benzodiazepines.
• Also contraindicated in severe shock, coma, or acute alcohol intoxication because midazolam potentiates existing hypotension.
• Because drug depresses the respiratory system, use cautiously in elderly or debilitated patients and in those with chronic obstructive pulmonary disease.
• Give cautiously in renal impairment because of more rapid induction and prolonged recovery.
• Also give cautiously in myasthenia gravis because drug can exacerbate this condition.
• In acute angle-closure glaucoma, drug may cause anticholinergic effect. Use with caution.
• Administer carefully in congestive heart failure and hepatic impairment because of the heightened risk of toxicity.
• Pediatric safety and efficacy haven't been established.

PREPARATION & STORAGE
Available in 1 mg/ml and 5 mg/ml ampules. Midazolam may be administered undiluted or diluted with dextrose 5% in water, 0.9% sodium chloride, or Ringer's lactate solution. Mixtures with dextrose 5% in water or 0.9% sodium chloride are stable

for 24 hours; those with Ringer's lactate, for 4 hours.

Store undiluted solution at room temperature and protect from light. Once diluted, solution no longer requires protection from light.

ADMINISTRATION
Only staff specially trained in administering anesthetics and managing their adverse reactions should give midazolam. Also, equipment for respiratory and cardiovascular support should be readily available.
Direct injection: Inject directly into vein or established I.V. line containing a compatible solution over 2 to 3 minutes for conscious sedation or over 20 to 30 seconds for anesthesia induction.
Intermittent infusion: not recommended.
Continuous infusion: not recommended.

INCOMPATIBILITY
Incompatible with dimenhydrate, pentobarbital sodium, perphenazine, prochlorperazine edisylate, and ranitidine hydrochloride.

ADVERSE REACTIONS
Life-threatening: airway obstruction, anaphylaxis, apnea, bronchospasm, cardiac arrest, hypoxia, laryngospasm, severe respiratory depression.
Other: agitation, anxiety, ataxia, confusion, constipation, decreased cardiac output, decreased systemic vascular resistance, dizziness, drowsiness, dry mouth, dysphonia, dyspnea, euphoria, headache, hiccups, hyperactivity, hyperventilation, involuntary muscle movement, lightheadedness, metallic taste, nausea, nightmares, nodal rhythms, oversedation, pain at injection site, paradoxical reactions, paresthesias, premature ventricular contractions,

prolonged emergence from anesthesia, retrograde amnesia, shallow respirations, slurred speech, tachycardia, tachypnea, vasovagal episodes, visual disturbances, vomiting, wheezing.

INTERACTIONS
Antihypertensives: worsened hypotension.
Fentanyl (high doses): severe hypotension.
H_2-receptor antagonists: severe CNS toxicity resulting from increased bioavailability of midazolam.
Hepatic enzyme inhibitors: heightened risk of toxicity.
Levodopa: diminished therapeutic effect.
Other CNS depressants: profound respiratory depression, hypoventilation, or apnea.
Parenteral anesthetics: additive depressant effects.

EFFECTS ON DIAGNOSTIC TESTS
None reported.

SPECIAL CONSIDERATIONS
• Give this potent drug slowly and in divided doses to titrate to effect. Rapid administration can lead to severe apnea, respiratory arrest, and hypotension, especially in elderly or debilitated patients.
• Elderly patients may experience prolonged recovery time.
• Monitor vital signs during administration.
• Warn patients not to drive or perform other tasks that require alertness until effects subside or until the day after drug administration, whichever is longer.
• Instruct patients to avoid alcohol or other CNS depressants for 24 hours after receiving drug unless the doctor tells them otherwise.

minocycline hydrochloride
Minocin♦

Pregnancy Risk Category: D

PHARMACOKINETICS
Distribution: widely distributed, with highest concentrations in saliva, sputum, and tears. Drug is more lipid-soluble than other tetracyclines. It's 55% to 88% bound to plasma proteins and readily crosses the placenta.
Metabolism: partially metabolized in the liver.
Excretion: mainly removed in feces, with 5% to 10% excreted unchanged. Half-life is 11 to 26 hours. Drug appears in breast milk.
Action: peak serum concentration, immediately after infusion.

MECHANISM OF ACTION
A bacteriostatic drug, minocycline may be bactericidal in high concentrations or with extremely susceptible organisms. Drug binds to 30S ribosomal subunits, inhibiting protein synthesis. It may also alter the cytoplasmic membrane, allowing leakage of intracellular components.

Minocycline acts against the gram-negative bacteria *Bartonella bacilliformis, Bordetella pertussis, Brucella, Calymmatobacterium granulomatis, Campylobacter fetus, Francisella tularensis, Haemophilus ducreyi, H. influenzae, Legionella pneumophilia, Leptotrichia buccalis, Neisseria gonorrhoeae, N. meningitidis, Pasteurella multocida, Pseudomonas pseudomallei, P. mallei, Shigella, Spirillum minor, Streptobacillus moniliformis, Vibrio cholerae, V. parahaemolyticus, Yersinia enterocolitica, Y. pestis,* and some strains of *Acinetobacter, Bacteroides, Enterobacter aerogenes, Escherichia coli* and *Klebsiella.*

The drug is also active against gram-positive bacteria, including *Bacillus anthracis, Actinomyces israelii, Arachnia propionica, Clostridium perfringens, C. tetani, Listeria monocytogenes, Nocardia, Propionibacterium acnes,* and some strains of staphylococci and streptococci. It's also active against *Rickettsia akari, R. prowazeki, R. rickettsii, R. tsutsugamushi, R. typhi, Coxiella burnetii, Chlamydia trachomatis, C. psittaci, Mycoplasma hominis, M. pneumoniae, Ureaplasma urealyticum, Borrelia recurrentis, Leptospira, Treponema pallidum,* and *T. pertenue.*

INDICATIONS & DOSAGE
• Severe infections caused by susceptible organisms. *Adults:* 200 mg initially, then 100 mg q 12 hours; or 100 to 200 mg initially, then 50 mg q 6 hours. *Children over age 8:* 4 mg/kg initially, then 2 mg/kg q 12 hours.

CONTRAINDICATIONS & CAUTIONS
• Contraindicated in hypersensitivity to tetracyclines.
• Contraindicated in children under age 8. Also contraindicated during the last half of pregnancy because of interference with fetal bone and tooth development and in breast-feeding mothers.
• Use with caution in hepatic impairment because of an increased risk of adverse reactions.

PREPARATION & STORAGE
Available in 100 mg vials. Reconstitute with 5 ml of sterile water for injection. Then dilute each 100 mg in 500 to 1,000 ml of compatible I.V. solution for infusion. Such solutions include dextrose 5% in 0.9%

sodium chloride, dextrose 5% in water, Ringer's injection, Ringer's lactate, and 0.9% sodium chloride. Store vials below 104° F. (40° C.) in light-resistant containers. Reconstituted solution is stable for 24 hours at room temperature.

ADMINISTRATION

Direct injection: not recommended.
Intermittent infusion: not recommended.
Continuous infusion: Infuse diluted drug over 6 to 12 hours, depending on ordered dose.

INCOMPATIBILITY

Incompatible with calcium-containing solutions.

ADVERSE REACTIONS

Life-threatening: anaphylaxis, exfoliative dermatitis, hepatotoxicity.
Other: abdominal discomfort; angioedema; anorexia; arthralgia; asthma; ataxia; bacterial and fungal superinfection; diarrhea; dizziness; drowsiness; eosinophilia; fatigue; fever; flatulence; headache; hyperpigmentation of skin and mucous membranes; Jarisch-Herxheimer reaction (in brucellosis or spirochetal infections); light-headedness; loose, bulky stools; nausea; pericarditis; photosensitivity; pruritus; pseudomembranous colitis; rash; thrombophlebitis; urticaria; vertigo; vestibular symptoms; vomiting.

INTERACTIONS

Aminoglycosides, penicillins: possible antagonized bactericidal activity.
Methoxyflurane: increased risk of nephrotoxicity.
Oral anticoagulants: potentiated effects.
Oral contraceptives: decreased effectiveness and breakthrough bleeding.

EFFECTS ON DIAGNOSTIC TESTS

Serum alkaline phosphatase, amylase, bilirubin, SGOT, SGPT: possible increased levels.
Serum creatinine: elevated levels.
Urine glucose: possible false-positive results with cupric sulfate method (Benedict's solution, Clinitest).
Urine nitrogen: increased levels.

SPECIAL CONSIDERATIONS

• Obtain specimens for culture and sensitivity tests before giving first dose. Therapy may begin before test results are available.
• Observe patient for fungal and bacterial superinfection with prolonged use.
• If diarrhea persists, collect stool specimen for culture to rule out pseudomembranous colitis.
• Use glucose oxidase method (Clinistix, Tes-Tape) to test for urine glucose.
• Dosage adjustments aren't necessary in renal impairment.
• Tetracyclines may cause permanent tooth discoloration, enamel hypoplasia, and decreased bone growth in children age 8 or younger and with maternal use during pregnancy.
• Switch to oral therapy with this drug as soon as possible.
• Observe I.V. site for signs of thrombophlebitis. Rotate I.V. site every 48 to 72 hours.
• Tell patient to use sunscreen and to wear protective clothing to avoid photosensitivity reactions.

mitomycin
Mutamycin♦

Pregnancy Risk Category: D

PHARMACOKINETICS
Distribution: throughout tissues with highest concentrations probably occurring in kidneys, muscles, eyes, lungs, intestines, stomach, and in cancer cells. Mitomycin crosses placenta but not blood-brain barrier.
Metabolism: primarily in liver, but also in kidneys, spleen, brain, and heart.
Excretion: in urine with 10% to 30% excreted unchanged. Less is excreted in feces. Plasma half-life is 17 minutes; elimination half-life, 50 minutes.
Action: peak plasma concentration, at end of infusion.

MECHANISM OF ACTION
An antineoplastic antibiotic, mitomycin is cell cycle nonspecific, although it's most active in G and S phases of cell division. Drug causes cross-linking of DNA and inhibits DNA synthesis. In high concentrations, it may also inhibit RNA and protein synthesis.

INDICATIONS & DOSAGE
• Neoplasms, including adenocarcinomas of the stomach, pancreas, and colon, head and neck cancers, chronic myelogenous leukemia, advanced biliary, ovarian, and lung cancers, cervical squamous cell carcinomas, and transitional cell carcinoma of the urinary bladder. *Adults:* Dosage based on clinical and hematologic response and on concurrent myelosuppressive therapy. Protocols vary. A common dosing schedule is 2 mg/m² daily for 5 days. Subsequently drug is stopped for 2 days, then dose is repeated for 5 more days. 12 day cycle repeated q 6 to 8 weeks. Or 20 mg/m² can be given in single dose and repeated q 6 to 8 weeks.

CONTRAINDICATIONS & CAUTIONS
• Contraindicated in existing or recent chicken pox or herpes zoster virus because of the risk of generalized disease.
• Also contraindicated if the patient's platelet count is less than 75,000/mm³, the WBC count is less than 3,000/mm³, or serum creatinine exceeds 1.7 mg/dl because of the enhanced risk of toxicity.
• Administer cautiously in mitomycin hypersensitivity.
• Because of an increased risk of bleeding, use with caution in coagulation disorders, prolonged prothrombin time or bleeding time, or increased bleeding from other causes.
• Also use with caution in renal impairment because of a heightened risk of toxicity, bone marrow depression because of increased myelosuppression, and in infection because of risk of generalized disease.

PREPARATION & STORAGE
Exercise extreme caution when preparing and administering mitomycin to avoid carcinogenic, teratogenic, and mutagenic risks. Use a biological containment cabinet, wear gloves and mask, and use syringes with Luer-lok fittings. Dispose of vials, needles, syringes, and unused drug carefully.

Mitomycin is supplied in 5 and 20 mg vials. Before reconstitution, store at room temperature. Reconstitute 5 mg vial with 10 ml and 20 mg vial with 40 ml of dextrose 5% and water, 0.9% sodium chloride, or sterile water for injection. Shake to dissolve; don't use until completely dissolved. For infusion, dilute further in 100 to 150 ml of dextrose 5% in water, 0.9% sodium chloride, or sodium lactate.

Reconstituted solutions remain stable for 7 days at room temperature or for 14 days if refrigerated. Solutions further diluted in dextrose 5% in water are stable for 3 hours at room temperature; in 0.9% sodium chloride, 12 hours; and in sodium lactate, 24 hours. If not used within 24 hours, protect from light.

ADMINISTRATION

Direct injection: Administer through a new I.V. site, preferably using a 23G or 25G winged-tip needle or an I.V. catheter. Use distal rather than major veins to allow for repeated venipunctures.
Intermittent infusion: Infuse diluted drug through a newly started I.V. line.
Continuous infusion: not recommended.

INCOMPATIBILITY

Incompatible with bleomycin sulfate.

ADVERSE REACTIONS

Life-threatening: acute bronchospasm, hemolytic uremic syndrome.
Other: alopecia, anorexia, blurred vision, cardiotoxicity, cellulitis or pain at infusion site, confusion, desquamation, diarrhea, drowsiness, dyspnea, edema, fatigue, fever, headache, hematemesis, malaise, mouth ulcers, myelosuppression, nausea, nonproductive cough, paresthesias, pruritus, pulmonary toxicity, purple bands on nail beds, renal toxicity, stomatitis, syncope, thrombophlebitis, vomiting.

INTERACTIONS

Doxorubicin: enhanced cardiotoxicity.

Live-virus vaccines: possible potentiated virus replication, resulting from immunosuppression.
Other bone marrow depressants: increased myelosuppression.

EFFECTS ON DIAGNOSTIC TESTS

BUN, serum creatinine: possible elevated levels.

SPECIAL CONSIDERATIONS

• Avoid extravasation because of the potential for severe ulceration and necrosis. If extravasation occurs, immediately stop infusion and restart at another site.
• Give drug only under constant supervision of a doctor experienced in use of chemotherapy.
• Expect toxic effects with therapeutic doses. Evaluate patient before each course of therapy.
• Because of cumulative myelosuppression, monitor hematologic studies weekly during treatment and for at least 7 weeks afterward.
• In leukopenia, nadir occurs in 6 weeks; in thrombocytopenia, in 4 to 6 weeks. Onset is 2 to 4 weeks.
• Adjust dosage in myelosuppression. Give 100% of previous dose when WBC count exceeds 3,000/mm³ and platelet count exceeds 75,000/mm³. Give 70% when WBC count is 2,000/mm³ to 3,000/mm³ and platelet count 25,000/mm³ to 75,000/mm³. Give 50% when WBC count is less than 2,000/mm³ and platelet count is less than 25,000/mm³.
• Administer antibiotics for infection during myelosuppression.
• Assess for renal dysfunction and tell patient to report hematuria, dysuria, or urinary frequency.
• Monitor pulmonary function during therapy.
• Inform the patient that drug-related alopecia is usually reversible.

- If no response after two courses of therapy, discontinue drug.
- Advise patient to avoid exposure to people with infections.

mitoxantrone
Novantrone♦

Pregnancy Risk Category: D

PHARMACOKINETICS
Distribution: rapid and extensive distribution to tissues; probably not well distributed into the cerebrospinal fluid. Mitoxantrone is 78% bound to plasma proteins.
Metabolism: in the liver to inactive metabolites and their glucuronide conjugates.
Elimination: 6% to 11% excreted through kidneys, with the remainder excreted through the liver. Of the renally excreted drug, 65% remains unchanged and 35% becomes metabolites. Not known if the drug appears in breast milk.

MECHANISM OF ACTION
Not fully understood. The drug reacts with DNA to produce cytotoxic effect and is probably cell cycle–nonspecific.

INDICATIONS & DOSAGE
- Combination therapy (with cytosine arabinoside) for acute nonlymphocytic leukemia. *Adults:* initial therapy, 12 mg/m^2 on days 1 and 3 (followed by 7 days of I.V. therapy with cytosine arabinoside); consolidation therapy, 12 mg/m^2 on days 1 and 2 (followed by 5 days of therapy with cytosine arabinoside).

CONTRAINDICATIONS & CAUTIONS
- Contraindicated in hypersensitivity to mitoxantrone.

- Also contraindicated in significant myelosuppression, unless benefits outweigh the risks.
- Use cautiously in patients with previous exposure to anthracyclines or other cardiotoxic drugs.
- Also use cautiously in patients with severe hepatic dysfunction because of possible decreased clearance of mitoxantrone.

PREPARATION & STORAGE
Exercise extreme caution when preparing or administering mitoxantrone to avoid mutagenic, teratogenic, and carcinogenic risks. Use a biological containment cabinet, wear gloves and mask, and use syringes with Luer-Lok fittings to prevent leakage of drug solution. Be careful to correctly dispose of needles, vials, and unused drug, and avoid contaminating work surfaces. Avoid inhalation of dust or vapors or contact with skin or mucous membranes.

Available as an aqueous solution of 2 mg/ml in volumes of 10, 12.5, and 15 ml. Store undiluted solution at room temperature. Avoid freezing.

Dilute dose in at least 50 ml of 0.9% sodium chloride injection or dextrose 5% injection. May be further diluted in dextrose 5% in water, 0.9% sodium chloride, or dextrose 5% and 0.9% sodium chloride. Once diluted, the mixture is stable for 48 hours at room temperature. Discard unused solution.

ADMINISTRATION
Direct injection: not recommended.
Intermittent infusion: Infuse diluted solution slowly into a free-flowing I.V. line of 0.9% sodium chloride or dextrose 5% in water over at least 3 minutes.
Continuous infusion: not recommended.

INCOMPATIBILITY
Incompatible with heparin sodium. Manufacturer recommends against mixing drug with any other drugs because not all incompatibilities are known.

ADVERSE REACTIONS
Life-threatening: allergic reaction, asymptomatic changes in left ventricular ejection fraction, congestive heart failure, dysrhythmias.
Other: abdominal pain, alopecia, anemia, chest pain, conjunctivitis, cough, diarrhea, dyspnea, EKG changes, hepatotoxicity, hypotension, jaundice, nausea, phlebitis, rashes, secondary infection, seizures, stomatitis, tachycardia, urticaria, vomiting.

INTERACTIONS
Myelosuppressive drugs: increased incidence of hematologic abnormalities.

EFFECTS ON DIAGNOSTIC TESTS
Serum uric acid: possible elevated levels.

SPECIAL CONSIDERATIONS
• Monitor hematology and chemistry laboratory parameters and liver function tests closely.
• Also monitor left ventricular ejection fraction during administration.
• Monitor serum uric acid levels during therapy. Keeping patient well hydrated, alkalinizing urine, and administering allopurinol may prevent uric acid nephropathy.
• Secondary infections should be treated with antibiotics, as ordered.
• If severe nonhematologic toxicity occurs during the first course of therapy, delay the second course until patient recovers.
• Inform patients that their urine may appear blue-green within 24 hours after administration. Tell them not to become alarmed by this. Some bluish discoloration of the sclera may also occur.
• Only doctors experienced with chemotherapy prescribe mitoxantrone.
• If contact with the eye occurs, irrigate with water or saline solution and contact an ophthalmologist.
• If the drug comes in contact with the skin, irrigate the area with water. It is not a vesicant.

morphine sulfate
Astramorph PF, Duramorph PF

Controlled Substance Schedule II
Pregnancy Risk Category: C

PHARMACOKINETICS
Distribution: rapidly distributed to kidneys, spleen, lungs, and liver. Minimal protein binding. Morphine readily crosses the placenta.
Metabolism: primarily in the liver.
Excretion: in urine, mainly as metabolites; 7% to 10% is excreted in feces. Elimination half-life is 2 to 3 hours. Drug appears in breast milk.
Action: peak effect, 20 minutes; duration, 4 to 5 hours.

MECHANISM OF ACTION
Morphine binds with stereospecific receptors in the CNS, altering the perception of pain and the emotional response to it.

INDICATIONS & DOSAGE
• Severe pain. *Adults:* 2.5 to 15 mg q 4 hours p.r.n. *Children:* 50 to 100 mcg/kg. Maximum single dose, 10 mg.
• Pain associated with MI. *Adults:* 8 to 15 mg, followed by smaller doses q 3 to 4 hours p.r.n.

• Severe chronic pain. *Adults:* 1 to 10 mg/hour by continuous infusion. Maintenance dosage, 20 to 150 mg/hour. *Children:* 0.025 to 2.6 mg/kg/hour.

CONTRAINDICATIONS & CAUTIONS

• Contraindicated in hypersensitivity to morphine and in acute respiratory depression because drug may exacerbate the condition.

• Also contraindicated in diarrhea resulting from pseudomembranous colitis or poisoning because morphine may slow the elimination of toxins.

• Use with caution in altered respiratory function because of an increased risk of respiratory depression; in dysrhythmias because drug can increase response through a vagolytic action.

• Administer carefully to patients with seizure disorders because the drug may induce or exacerbate seizures.

• Because of the potential for abuse, use cautiously in patients with a history of drug dependence or emotional instability or in those who show evidence of suicidal ideation.

• Administer carefully in acute abdominal conditions because morphine may mask symptoms; in gallbladder disease because drug may increase biliary contractions; in inflammatory bowel disease because toxic megacolon may develop; and after recent GI surgery because drug may alter GI motility.

• Because of the heightened risk of respiratory depression and prolonged CNS depression, use cautiously in hypothyroidism.

• Also use cautiously in head injury and increased intracranial pressure (from intracranial lesions) because morphine may mask clinical changes and elevate cerebrospinal fluid (CSF) pressure.

• Give cautiously to patients with hepatic or renal impairment because of an increased risk of toxicity.

• Also give cautiously in patients with prostatic hypertrophy, urethral stricture, or recent urinary tract surgery because morphine can cause urinary retention.

PREPARATION & STORAGE

Available in concentrations of 0.5, 1, 2, 4, 5, 8, 10, and 15 mg/ml in 1 ml ampules, vials, and disposable units, in 2 ml disposable units, in 10 ml ampules, and in 20 ml vials.

For direct injection, dilute with 4 or 5 ml of dextrose 5% in water. Dilute with larger volumes for slow infusion. Morphine is compatible with most common I.V. solutions. Store below 104° F. (40° C.), and protect from light and freezing.

ADMINISTRATION

Direct injection: Inject diluted drug over 4 to 5 minutes through I.V. tubing containing a free-flowing compatible solution. Monitor vital signs and respiratory status for at least 1 hour after injection.

Intermittent infusion: not recommended.

Continuous infusion: Infuse diluted drug at 1 to 10 mg/hour initially, increasing rate until reaching effective dosage. Monitor vital signs and respiratory status.

INCOMPATIBILITY

Incompatible with aminophylline, amobarbital sodium, soluble barbiturates, chlorothiazide, heparin sodium, meperidine, methicillin, phenobarbital sodium, phenytoin sodium, promethazine hydrochloride, sodium bicarbonate, sodium iodide, and thiopental sodium.

ADVERSE REACTIONS

Life-threatening: anaphylaxis, bradycardia, circulatory collapse, respiratory depression, tachycardia.

Other: agitation; coma; constipation; decreased mental acuity or depression; delirium; dizziness; dysphoria; euphoria; fainting; flushing; insomnia; nausea; nervousness; oliguria; pain at infusion site; pruritus; restlessness; sedation; seizures; sweating; urinary retention; urticaria; visual disturbances; vomiting; warmth of face, neck, and upper trunk; weakness.

INTERACTIONS

Antidiarrheals, antiperistaltics: enhanced risk of constipation and CNS depression.

Antihypertensives, diuretics: heightened risk of hypotension.

Antimuscarinics: increased risk of constipation, paralytic ileus, and urinary retention.

Buprenorphine: possible respiratory depression and reduced therapeutic morphine effect. May precipitate withdrawal symptoms in drug-dependent patients.

Hydroxyzine: enhanced analgesia, CNS depression, and hypotension.

MAO inhibitors: severe, unpredictable adverse reactions when given within 21 days of morphine. Reduce morphine dose.

Metoclopramide: antagonized effect on GI motility.

Naloxone: antagonized analgesic, CNS, and respiratory depressant effects.

Naltrexone: blocked therapeutic morphine effect and possible precipitation of withdrawal symptoms in drug-dependent patients.

Neuromuscular blockers: deepened respiratory depression.

Opioid-agonist analgesics: worsened CNS and respiratory depression, hypotension.

Other CNS depressants: deepened CNS depression and risk of habituation.

EFFECTS ON DIAGNOSTIC TESTS

Gastric emptying studies: possible delayed emptying.

Hepatobiliary imaging with technetium Tc 99m disofenin: delayed visualization, falsely resembling obstruction of common bile duct.

Lumbar puncture: elevated CSF pressure caused by respiratory depression–induced carbon dioxide retention.

Serum amylase, lipase: possible increased levels.

SPECIAL CONSIDERATIONS

• *Treatment of overdose:* Treat symptomatically and give naloxone, as ordered, to reverse respiratory depression.

• Keep emergency resuscitation equipment available.

• Monitor respirations frequently during infusion and every 15 minutes for 1 hour after infusion. If respirations fall below 8 breaths per minute, arouse patient to stimulate breathing. Notify doctor.

• Respiratory depression is more likely in elderly and pediatric patients.

• Administer drug with patient lying down to minimize hypotension. Tell him to get up slowly to lessen dizziness and faintness.

• Rapid infusion can cause life-threatening adverse reactions. Note that ambulatory patients and patients who aren't experiencing severe pain have a higher incidence of adverse reactions.

• Because opioid agonists stimulate vasopressin release, their use may heighten the risk of water intoxication in postoperative patients.

• Morphine shouldn't be used in pulmonary edema caused by a chemical respiratory irritant. The drug causes vasodilation and may produce adverse hemodynamic effects.

• With long-term use, habituation and physical dependence may develop. Withdrawal symptoms may begin in 24 hours and peak 36 to 72 hours after drug discontinuation. Most observable symptoms disappear in 5 to 14 days.

• May need to extend dose in patients with severe chronic pain who have become tolerant to analgesic effects of opiates.

• Assess bowel function frequently; a stool softener may be indicated.

• Morphine may be used in patient-controlled analgesia.

• Generic preparations may contain sulfites.

moxalactam disodium
Moxam♦

Pregnancy Risk Category: C

PHARMACOKINETICS
Distribution: widely, into body tissues and fluids, including aqueous humor, bronchial secretions, sputum, bone, bile, and ascitic, cerebrospinal, pleural, peritoneal, prostate, and synovial fluids. Moxalactam is 45% to 60% bound to plasma proteins and crosses the placenta.
Metabolism: not metabolized.
Excretion: in urine, with most excreted unchanged by glomerular filtration. A small amount is excreted in feces. Not known if drug appears in breast milk.
Action: peak serum concentration, 15 to 60 minutes.

MECHANISM OF ACTION
This semisynthetic 1-oxa-beta-lactam antibiotic is structurally related to third-generation cephalosporins, cephamycins, and penicillin. Moxalactam acts bactericidally by inhibiting mucopeptide synthesis in the bacterial cell wall, thus promoting osmotic instability.

The drug's spectrum of activity includes the gram-positive aerobic bacteria *Streptococcus pneumoniae,* most strains of groups A and B streptococci, and most strains of *Staphylococcus aureus.* The drug is also active against the gram-negative aerobic bacteria *Citrobacter freundii, C. diversus, Enterobacter aerogenes, E. cloacae, Escherichia coli, Klebsiella pneumoniae, K. oxytoca, Morganella morganii, Proteus mirabilis, P. rettgeri, P. vulgaris, Providencia, Salmonella, Serratia marcescens, Shigella,* and some strains of *Pseudomonas aeruginosa, Haemophilus influenzae, Neisseria meningitidis,* and *N. gonorrhoeae.*

Moxalactam also combats some anaerobic bacteria, including *Bacteroides, Eubacterium, Fusobacterium, Peptococcus, Peptostreptococcus, Propionibacterium, Veillonella,* and some strains of *Clostridium.*

INDICATIONS & DOSAGE
• Life-threatening infections caused by susceptible organisms or infections caused by less-susceptible organisms. *Adults:* up to 4 g q 8 hours for 5 to 14 days, then dosage gradually decreased. Maximum of 12 g daily. *Children age 1 to 14:* 50 mg/kg q 6 to 8 hours. *Infants age 1 month to 1 year:* 50 mg/kg q 6 hours. *Neonates age 1 to 4 weeks:* 50 mg/kg q 8 hours. *Neonates under 1 week:* 50 mg/kg q 12 hours. For all children and neonates, maximum daily dosage is 200 mg/kg divided q 12 hours.

• Severe infections caused by susceptible organisms. *Adults:* 2 to 4 g divided q 8 to 12 hours for 5 to 14 days.
• Moderate infections caused by susceptible organisms. *Adults:* 500 mg to 2 g divided q 8 to 12 hours.
Note: Adjust dosage in renal impairment. For adults, give 1 to 2 g initially, followed by maintenance dose based on creatinine clearance.

CONTRAINDICATIONS & CAUTIONS

• Contraindicated in hypersensitivity to cephalosporins, cephamycins, or penicillin.
• Use cautiously in hypoprothrombinemia and in bleeding, hepatic, renal, or intestinal disorders to avoid exacerbating these conditions.
• Also use cautiously in the elderly and in patients with prolonged parenteral or enteral nutrition, poor nutrition, malnutrition, or alcoholism because of the heightened risk of vitamin K deficiency.

PREPARATION & STORAGE

Available in 1 and 2 g vials. Reconstitute with 3 ml of sterile water for injection, 0.9% sodium chloride, or dextrose 5% in water. Shake well.

For direct injection, dilute to 10 ml/g. For infusion, dilute with 50 to 100 ml of a compatible solution. Moxalactam is compatible with most common I.V. solutions.

Reconstituted solutions remain stable for 24 hours at room temperature and for 4 days if refrigerated.

ADMINISTRATION

Direct injection: Inject over 3 to 5 minutes into vein or into I.V. tubing containing a free-flowing compatible solution.
Intermittent infusion: Using a Y set-up or a volume-control pump, infuse diluted drug over 15 to 30 minutes.

Continuous infusion: Over 24 hours, infuse daily dose diluted appropriately.

INCOMPATIBILITY

Incompatible with aminoglycosides.

ADVERSE REACTIONS

Life-threatening: anaphylaxis.
Other: abdominal cramps, anemia, angioedema, anorexia, bacterial and fungal superinfection, colitis, decreased platelet count, diarrhea, dizziness, dyspepsia, dyspnea, eosinophilia, fever, glossitis, granulocytopenia, headache, hematuria, hypoprothrombinemia, leukopenia, local burning and pain (for up to 20 minutes after injection), malaise, nausea, neutropenia, paresthesias, phlebitis, proteinuria, pruritus, pseudomembranous colitis, purpura, pyuria, rash, thrombocytopenia, thrombocytosis, thrombophlebitis, urticaria, vomiting.

INTERACTIONS

Alcohol: disulfiram-like reaction if ingested during or 48 hours after moxalactam therapy. Avoid using I.V. solutions containing alcohol.
Aminoglycosides: increased risk of nephrotoxicity.
Anticoagulants, NSAIDs, platelet aggregation inhibitors: enhanced risk of bleeding.
Penicillin: possible synergistic effects against some organisms.

EFFECTS ON DIAGNOSTIC TESTS

Activated partial thromboplastin time, prothrombin time (PT): prolonged.
CBC, platelet count: decreased.
Coombs' test: false-positive results.

SPECIAL CONSIDERATIONS

• Before first dose, note hypersensitivity to cephalosporins, cephamycins, or penicillin. Negative history doesn't rule out future allergic reaction.

• Obtain specimens for culture and sensitivity tests before first dose. Therapy may begin before receiving results.

• Monitor CBC, BUN and serum creatinine levels, PT, partial thromboplastin time, and urinalysis.

• If diarrhea persists during therapy, collect stool samples for culture to rule out pseudomembranous colitis.

• The doctor may order 10 mg of vitamin K weekly as prophylaxis against bleeding, or 5 to 10 mg to lengthen bleeding time.

• Before treating symptoms of bleeding, assess for malignancy or disseminated intravascular coagulation.

• Prolonged bleeding may necessitate administration of fresh frozen plasma, packed RBCs, and platelets.

• Encourage fluid intake, and monitor intake and output to assess renal function. In patients undergoing hemodialysis, give 50% to 100% of moxalactam dose at end of each session, as ordered. Drug is readily removed by hemodialysis.

• Advise home care patient to avoid alcohol during and up to 48 hours after moxalactam therapy.

• Observe for fungal and bacterial superinfection with prolonged use.

---

multivitamins
M.V.I.-12♦, M.V.I. Pediatric♦

Pregnancy Risk Category: A

PHARMACOKINETICS
Distribution: ascorbic acid (vitamin C), niacin (vitamin B_3), folic acid (vitamin B_9), and thiamine (vitamin B_1) are widely distributed in tissues. Dexpanthenol, also widely distributed, has highest concentrations in the liver, adrenal glands, heart, and kidneys. Pyridoxine (vitamin B_6) is mainly found in the liver, muscles, and brain. Riboflavin (vitamin B_2) has highest concentrations in GI mucosal cells, RBCs, and the liver, and cyanocobalamin (vitamin B_{12}) is found in the liver, bone marrow, and other tissues. Vitamin A is stored in the liver, vitamin D in fat and muscles. Vitamin E is distributed to all tissues; it's stored in fat. All vitamins cross the placenta.

Metabolism: in the liver. Vitamin D is also metabolized in the kidneys.

Excretion: Vitamins A, D, E, and cyanocobalamin are mainly eliminated in feces, with small amounts in urine; all other vitamins are removed in urine. Small amounts of dexpanthenol and folic acid are also excreted in feces.

Action: onset, duration: unknown.

MECHANISM OF ACTION
Vitamin C promotes collagen formation and tissue repair. *Niacin* is required for oxidation-reduction reactions and carbohydrate metabolism; *folic acid,* for nucleoprotein synthesis and erythropoiesis; *dexpanthenol,* for carbohydrate, protein, and lipid metabolism; and *pyridoxine,* for amino acid metabolism and carbohydrate and lipid metabolism. *Riboflavin* is necessary for energy and protein metabolism; *thiamine,* for carbohydrate metabolism; and *cyanocobalamin,* for nucleoprotein and myelin synthesis, cell reproduction, normal growth, and maintenance of erythropoiesis. *Vitamin D* helps to regulate serum calcium concentration. Though its function is unknown, *vitamin E* is thought to be an antioxidant. *Vitamin A* promotes growth, bone development, vision, reproduction, and integrity of mucosal and epithelial surfaces.

INDICATIONS & DOSAGE

• Maintenance vitamins during parenteral nutrition or in N.P.O. patients. *Adults and children age 11 and over:* Dosage varies. Maintenance nutrition requires one dose of multivitamin concentrate in I.V. infusion q 24 hours. *Children under age 11:* 1 vial of M.V.I. Pediatric daily in I.V. infusion. *Neonates weighing 1 to 3 kg:* 65% of M.V.I. Pediatric vial daily in I.V. infusion. *Neonates weighing less than 1 kg:* 30% of M.V.I. Pediatric vial daily.

CONTRAINDICATIONS & CAUTIONS

• Contraindicated in hypersensitivity to any vitamin and in hypervitaminosis.
• Use with caution in hereditary optic nerve atrophy (Leber's disease); cyanocobalamin may cause severe acute optic atrophy.

PREPARATION & STORAGE

M.V.I.-12 is available in a unit vial container with 5 ml of liquid in vial 1, 5 ml of liquid in vial 2, and 10 ml of lyophilized powder in vial 3. Mix contents of vials 1 and 2 by pressing down to force liquid from upper chamber into lower chamber. Or add 5 ml of sterile water for injection to the 10 ml vial of powder.

M.V.I. Pediatric is available in a 10 ml vial. Reconstitute by adding 5 ml of sterile water for injection, dextrose 5% in water, or 0.9% sodium chloride. Reconstituted solution is stable for 24 hours if refrigerated.

Dilute all prepared solutions in 500 to 1,000 ml of a compatible solution.

ADMINISTRATION

Direct injection: not recommended.
Intermittent infusion: Infuse diluted solution over ordered amount of time. Add to only one I.V. solution daily.
Continuous infusion: Infuse diluted solution over 24 hours.

INCOMPATIBILITY

Incompatible with acetazolamide, moderately alkaline solutions, amino acids (5.5%, 8.5%, or 10%), chlorothiazide sodium, dextrose 5% and Normosol-M, and tetracycline hydrochloride. Folic acid may be unstable in presence of calcium salts, and some vitamins, particularly thiamine, may be incompatible with sodium bisulfite. Manufacturer recommends against mixing M.V.I.-12 with fat emulsions.

ADVERSE REACTIONS

Life-threatening: anaphylaxis.
Other: allergic reactions (thiamine and folic acid), dizziness and faintness (with injection of undiluted drug), hepatotoxicity (vitamin A toxicity), tissue calcification (vitamin D toxicity).

INTERACTIONS

Levodopa: decreased effectiveness if given with pyridoxine.
Methotrexate: altered response (from interacting with folic acid).

EFFECTS ON DIAGNOSTIC TESTS

Serum calcium: elevated level in vitamin D toxicity.

SPECIAL CONSIDERATIONS

• M.V.I.-12 doesn't provide vitamin K_1 (give K_1 separately). M.V.I. Pediatric does contain vitamin K_1.
• Folic acid doses exceeding 0.1 mg/day may mask signs of pernicious anemia.
• Fat-soluble vitamins (A, D, E, and K) accumulate in the body. Hypervitaminosis of vitamins A and D can occur.

- Multivitamins shouldn't be used in severe vitamin deficiency.
- Megadoses of vitamins may be hazardous to fetus.

---

muromonab-CD3
Orthoclone OKT3♦

Pregnancy Risk Category: C

PHARMACOKINETICS
Distribution: widely distributed throughout the body.
Metabolism: not well characterized. Drug isn't metabolized but is thought to bind to circulating T cells.
Excretion: unknown.
Action: onset, within minutes; duration, 1 week.

MECHANISM OF ACTION
A murine monoclonal antibody, muromonab-CD3 reacts in the T-cell membrane with CD3, a molecule needed for antigen recognition. Drug blocks all known T-cell functions and reacts with most peripheral T cells in blood and body tissues to restore allograft function and reverse rejection.

INDICATIONS & DOSAGE
- Acute allograft rejection in kidney transplant. *Adults:* 5 mg daily for 10 to 14 days.

CONTRAINDICATIONS & CAUTIONS
- Contraindicated in existing or recent chicken pox and herpes zoster or if patient's temperature exceeds 100° F. (37.8° C.) because of the increased risk of severe generalized disease.
- Also contraindicated in patients with fluid overload (as evidenced by chest X-ray or weight gain greater than 3% within 1 week before treatment) because of a magnified risk of pulmonary edema.
- Use cautiously in infection because of the risk of severe adverse reactions and in patients with hypersensitivity to any murine product.
- Safe use in children hasn't been established.

PREPARATION & STORAGE
Available in 1 mg/ml ampules. Store in refrigerator unless otherwise specified by the manufacturer. Protect from freezing. Don't shake ampule. Draw solution into syringe through a low-protein-binding 0.2 or 0.22 micrometer filter, then discard filter and attach appropriate needle. Appearance of fine, translucent particles in solution does not indicate loss of potency.

ADMINISTRATION
Direct injection: Give dose by I.V. push directly into vein over less than 1 minute. Don't administer with I.V. fluids.
Intermittent infusion: not recommended.
Continuous infusion: not recommended.

INCOMPATIBILITY
No incompatibilities reported.

ADVERSE REACTIONS
Life-threatening: anaphylaxis, severe pulmonary edema.
Other: first-dose reaction (chest pain, chills, diarrhea, fever, nausea, shortness of breath, tremors, vomiting, wheezing), infection (within 45 days of treatment).
   First-dose reaction may occur 45 to 60 minutes after initial dose and may last for several hours. Monitor patient closely for 48 hours after initial dose. Symptoms are less com-

---

mon with second dose and rare thereafter.

INTERACTIONS
Live-virus vaccines: possible potentiated replication of virus, increased adverse effects, and diminished antibody response to vaccine.
Other immunosuppressants: enhanced risk of infection and lymphoproliferative disorders.

EFFECTS ON DIAGNOSTIC TESTS
None reported.

SPECIAL CONSIDERATIONS
• Reduce dosage of other immunosuppressants before giving drug.
• Chest X-ray taken 24 hours before initiation of treatment must be clear.
• As ordered, administer I.V. methylprednisolone sodium succinate before first dose, and give I.V. hydrocortisone sodium succinate 30 minutes later, to reduce incidence of first-dose reaction.
• Keep equipment and medication for advanced life support readily available during first dose.
• Give an antipyretic before therapy to reduce expected pyrexia and chills. Keep cooling blanket available. Reassure patient that adverse effects subside as treatment progresses.
• Monitor temperature, CBC, and tests for circulating T cells expressing the CD3 antigen.
• Instruct patient to avoid immunizations during therapy. Family members should also avoid immunization with oral polio vaccine and any contact with those vaccinated with it.
• Warn patient to avoid exposure to people with bacterial or viral infections. If infection develops, discontinue muromonab-CD3, as ordered.

• Usually, muromonab-CD3 is used with azathioprine, adrenocorticoids, or both.
• Aseptic meningitis has been reported in patients treated with this drug, although a direct causal relation hasn't been established.

nafcillin sodium
Nafcil, Nallpen, Unipen♦

Pregnancy Risk Category: B

PHARMACOKINETICS
Distribution: readily distributed to most body tissues and fluids, with highest concentration in the liver. Drug is 70% to 90% bound to plasma proteins, particularly albumin. Penetration in eye and cerebrospinal fluid is poor but increases with inflammation. Nafcillin crosses the placenta and appears in cord blood and amniotic fluid.
Metabolism: in the liver, with about 60% changed to inactive metabolites.
Excretion: occurs mainly in bile, with small amounts removed in urine by glomerular filtration. About 10% to 30% of the drug is excreted unchanged. Slight amounts probably appear in breast milk. In normal renal function, half-life averages 30 to 90 minutes; in renal or hepatic impairment, about 1 to 3 hours. It's also prolonged in neonates.
Action: peak serum concentrations, immediately after administration.

MECHANISM OF ACTION
A semisynthetic, penicillinase-resistant penicillin, nafcillin achieves its bactericidal effects by adhering to penicillin-binding proteins, inhibiting bacterial cell-wall synthesis. The drug acts against gram-positive aerobic bacteria, including *Staphylococ-*

cus aureus, S. epidermis, S. saprophyticus, groups A, B, C, and G streptococci, *Streptococcus pneumoniae,* and some strains of *S. viridans.* Susceptible gram-negative aerobic bacteria include some strains of *Neisseria meningitidis, N. gonorrhoeae, Haemophilus influenzae, Bordetella pertussis,* and *Pasteurella multocida.* Susceptible gram-positive anaerobic bacteria include some strains of *Actinomyces, Clostridium, Peptococcus, Peptostreptococcus,* and *Bacteroides.*

INDICATIONS & DOSAGE

• Severe systemic infections caused by susceptible organisms. *Adults:* 0.5 to 1 g q 4 hours (depending on severity of infection) for 14 days. *Children over age 1 month:* 50 to 100 mg/kg q 6 hours for 14 days.
• Osteomyelitis and endocarditis. *Adults:* 1 to 2 g q 4 hours for 4 to 8 weeks. *Children over age 1 month:* 100 to 200 mg/kg q 4 to 6 hours for 4 to 8 weeks.
• Meningitis. *Adults:* 100 to 200 mg/kg q 4 to 6 hours for at least 14 days.

CONTRAINDICATIONS & CAUTIONS

• Contraindicated in hypersensitivity to penicillins or cephalosporins.
• Use with caution in hepatic impairment because of an increased risk of adverse reactions; in eosinophilia or hemolytic anemia because of a heightened risk of adverse hematologic effects; and in GI disorders because of possible pseudomembranous colitis.
• Use cautiously in a patient on sodium restrictions.
• Also use cautiously in allergic patients because of predisposition to hypersensitivity reactions.

PREPARATION & STORAGE

Available as a white to yellow-white powder in vials of 500 mg and 1, 1.5, 2, 4, and 10 g. Store at room temperature. To reconstitute, add 1.7, 3.4, or 6.8 ml of sterile water for injection, bacteriostatic water for injection, or 0.9% sodium chloride to 500 mg, 1 g, or 2 g vials, respectively. For larger doses, follow manufacturer's directions.

For direct injection, further dilute with 15 to 30 ml of sterile water for injection or 0.45% or 0.9% sodium chloride for injection. For intermittent infusion, further dilute to a concentration of 2 to 40 mg/ml or according to manufacturer's directions (Nallpen). The drug is compatible with dextrose 5% in water, Ringer's lactate, or 0.9% sodium chloride.

After reconstitution with sterile water or 0.9% sodium chloride, solution of 250 mg/ml is stable for 3 days at 77° F. (25° C.), for 7 days if refrigerated, or for 3 months if frozen. At concentrations of 2 to 40 mg/ml, nafcillin begins to lose potency in 24 hours at room temperature or in 4 days if refrigerated.

ADMINISTRATION

Direct injection: Inject dose directly into vein or into I.V. line containing a free-flowing compatible solution. Administer over 5 to 10 minutes.
Intermittent infusion: Infuse dose over at least 30 to 60 minutes.
Continuous infusion: Add daily amount of nafcillin (only in concentrations of 2 to 40 mg/ml) to solution to be administered over 24 hours. Regulate accordingly.

INCOMPATIBILITY

Incompatible with aminoglycosides, aminophylline, ascorbic acid, beta-lactam antibacterials, bleomycin sulfate, droperidol, hydrocortisone so-

---

dium succinate, labetalol hydrochloride, methylprednisolone sodium succinate, nalbuphine hydrochloride, pentazocine lactate, promazine hydrochloride, verapamil hydrochloride, and vitamin B complex with C.

ADVERSE REACTIONS
Life-threatening: anaphylaxis.
Other: abdominal pain, acute interstitial nephritis, arthralgia, bacterial and fungal superinfection, diarrhea, dry mouth, eosinophilia, fever, hematuria, hypokalemia, nausea, neutropenia, pain at injection site, pruritus, pseudomembranous colitis, rash, stomatitis, thrombocytopenia, thrombophlebitis, unusual bleeding or bruising, urticaria, vomiting.

INTERACTIONS
Aminocaproic acid: potentiated nafcillin action.
Aminoglycosides: possible synergistic activity against some susceptible organisms.
Chloramphenicol, erythromycin, sulfonamides, tetracyclines: decreased nafcillin effects.
Heparin, oral anticoagulants: heightened risk of bleeding.
Oral contraceptives: possible decreased effectiveness.
Probenecid: slowed nafcillin excretion.

EFFECTS ON DIAGNOSTIC TESTS
Bleeding time: prolonged.
Serum aminoglycosides: possible falsely decreased levels.
Serum sodium: possible diminished levels.
Urine potassium: possible increased levels.
Urine protein: altered results using biuret or Coomassie brilliant blue method.

Urine or serum protein: possible false-positive results with turbidimetric methods using sulfosalicylic acid or trichloroacetic acid.

SPECIAL CONSIDERATIONS
● Before giving first dose, ask patient about previous allergic reactions to penicillins or cephalosporins. Negative history doesn't rule out future hypersensitivity reaction.
● Obtain specimens for culture and sensitivity tests before giving first dose. Therapy may begin before results are available.
● Obtain WBC count and differential before therapy and 1 to 3 times weekly during therapy.
● Also periodically obtain urinalysis, BUN, SGOT, and SGPT.
● Discontinue nafcillin, as ordered, if bone marrow toxicity, pseudomembranous colitis, or acute interstitial nephritis develops. Also expect to stop drug for eosinophilia, fever, arthralgia, hematuria, or elevated BUN or serum creatinine levels.
● If diarrhea persists during therapy, collect stool specimens for culture to rule out pseudomembranous colitis.
● Dialysis removes only slight amounts of drug.
● Observe patient for fungal and bacterial superinfection with prolonged use.

nalbuphine hydrochloride
Nubain

Pregnancy Risk Category: B
(D for prolonged use or in high doses given at term)

PHARMACOKINETICS
Distribution: not well bound to plasma proteins. Drug probably

crosses the placenta in small amounts.

Metabolism: in the liver.

Excretion: in feces and, to a lesser extent, in urine. Half-life is about 5 hours. Not known if drug appears in breast milk.

Action: onset, 2 to 3 minutes; duration, 3 to 4 hours.

MECHANISM OF ACTION

Nalbuphine binds with opiate receptors at many CNS sites, altering the perception of pain and the emotional response to it.

INDICATIONS & DOSAGE

• Moderate to severe pain and pre operative analgesia, as supplement to obstetric or surgical anesthesia.

Adults: 10 mg (or 0.14 mg/kg) q 3 to 6 hours. Maximum single dose, 20 mg. Maximum daily dose, 160 mg.

CONTRAINDICATIONS & CAUTIONS

• Contraindicated in sensitivity to nalbuphine.

• Also contraindicated in diarrhea associated with pseudomembranous colitis or poisoning because drug may delay removal of toxins from colon, thereby prolonging or worsening diarrhea.

• Avoid use in severely altered respiratory function because drug depresses respirations.

• Use with extreme caution in head injury and increased intracranial pressure because nalbuphine can raise CSF pressure.

• Use cautiously in patients with nausea and vomiting from MI because drug may exacerbate these effects.

• Use cautiously in patients receiving chronic opiate therapy. High doses of nalbuphine may precipitate

withdrawal, but low doses do not suppress the abstinence syndrome.

• Administer carefully to patients about to undergo biliary tract surgery or to patients with gallbladder disease because nalbuphine may induce spasm in the sphincter of Oddi; to patients with acute abdominal conditions because drug may mask diagnosis; after recent GI surgery because drug may alter GI motility; and in inflammatory bowel disease because of potential for toxic megacolon.

• Also administer carefully to patients with sulfite sensitivity because sulfite preservatives in injection may cause allergic reactions.

• In asthma or chronic respiratory disease, give nalbuphine carefully because the drug may decrease respiratory drive and increase airway resistance.

• In hypothyroidism, also give carefully because of an increased risk of respiratory and CNS depression.

• Use carefully in patients with a history of seizures because the drug's metabolite may induce or exacerbate seizures.

• In prostatic hypertrophy, obstruction, urethral stricture, recent urinary tract surgery, or renal dysfunction, use cautiously because the drug may cause urinary retention.

• Also use cautiously in hepatic or renal impairment because of slowed drug clearance and heightened risk of toxicity, and in elderly patients because of increased sensitivity to drug effects.

PREPARATION & STORAGE

Supplied in 1 and 2 ml ampules, 10 ml vials, and 1 ml disposable syringes in 10 mg/ml or 20 mg/ml concentrations. Protect from freezing, excessive light, and heat. Store at room temperature. Nalbuphine is compatible with dextrose 5% in water, Ringer's lactate, and 0.9% sodium chloride.

ADMINISTRATION
Direct injection: Inject drug directly into vein or into an I.V. line containing a compatible free-flowing I.V. solution over 2 to 3 minutes. Avoid rapid injection, which can precipitate anaphylaxis, peripheral circulatory collapse, or cardiac arrest.
Intermittent infusion: not recommended.
Continuous infusion: not recommended.

INCOMPATIBILITY
Incompatible with diazepam, nafcillin sodium, pentobarbital sodium, and thiethylperazine maleate.

ADVERSE REACTIONS
Life-threatening: anaphylaxis, apnea, severe bradycardia or tachycardia, severe respiratory depression, shock.
Other: abdominal pain, anorexia, blurred or double vision, confusion, constipation, depression, dizziness, drowsiness, dry mouth, facial flushing, faintness, fatigue, fever, headache, hypertension, hypotension, malaise, nausea, nervousness, nightmares, paresthesias, restlessness, seizures, speech difficulties, sweating, trembling, unusual dreams, urinary retention, urticaria, vomiting, weakness.

INTERACTIONS
Alcohol, general anesthetics, hypnotics, neuromuscular blockers, phenothiazines and other tranquilizers, sedatives: possible deepened respiratory depression.
Antihypertensives, diuretics: potentiated hypotensive effects.

Antimuscarinics: heightened potential for constipation, paralytic ileus, and urinary retention.
Antiperistaltic antidiarrheals: increased risk of constipation and CNS depression.
Buprenorphine: possible additive respiratory depression and reduced therapeutic effects of nalbuphine.
Hydroxyzine: intensified analgesia, CNS depression, and hypotension.
MAO inhibitors: unpredictable, severe adverse reactions if given within days of nalbuphine.
Metoclopramide: decreased effect on GI motility.
Naloxone: antagonized analgesic, CNS, and respiratory depressant effects.
Naltrexone: possible blocked analgesic effects.
Opioid-agonist analgesics: possible partially antagonized analgesic and CNS depressant effects, resulting in additive side effects or precipitation of withdrawal symptoms if patient is dependent on opioid-agonist drugs.
Other opioid analgesics: possible deepened CNS and respiratory depression, hypotension, and heightened risk of habituation.

EFFECTS ON DIAGNOSTIC TESTS
Gastric emptying studies: possible delayed emptying.
Hepatobiliary imaging: possible cause of constriction in the sphincter of Oddi and increased biliary tract pressure. Both resemble bile duct obstruction.
Lumbar puncture: elevated cerebrospinal fluid (CSF) pressure.
Serum amylase, lipase: unreliable results for up to 24 hours after nalbuphine administration.

SPECIAL CONSIDERATIONS
• *Treatment of overdose:* Provide airway and respiratory support. Give

naloxone, as needed, to reverse respiratory depression. Also administer I.V. fluids and vasopressors to maintain blood pressure.

• Administer drug with patient lying down to minimize hypotensive effects. Tell patient to get up slowly to reduce dizziness and faintness.

• Monitor respiratory status for at least 1 hour after administration. Keep resuscitation equipment available. If respirations drop below 8 breaths/minute, arouse patient to stimulate breathing. Notify doctor; he may order naloxone or respiratory support.

• Habituation and psychological dependence may occur with long-term use. Drug's abuse potential equals that of pentazocine but is less than that of codeine or propoxyphene.

• In long-term use of other opiate agonists, give only 25% of initial nalbuphine dose, as ordered. Monitor for withdrawal symptoms. If necessary, give slowly in small increments. If withdrawal symptoms fail to occur, increase dose progressively until reaching desired level of analgesia.

• Reduce dosage for the elderly.

• May contain sulfites.

---

naloxone hydrochloride
Narcan♦

Pregnancy Risk Category: B

PHARMACOKINETICS
Distribution: widely distributed to all body fluids and tissues, with highest concentrations in skeletal muscle, kidneys, liver, brain, lungs, and heart. Naloxone readily crosses the blood-brain barrier and placenta.
Metabolism: mainly metabolized in the liver, but also in the CNS, kidneys, lungs, and placenta.

Excretion: principally removed in urine, as unchanged drug or metabolites, with small amounts excreted in feces; 25% to 40% is excreted as metabolites in 6 hours, 50% in 24 hours, and 60% to 70% in 72 hours. Estimated half-life is 60 to 90 minutes; in neonates, about 3 hours. Not known if drug appears in breast milk.
Action: onset, 2 minutes; duration (dose-dependent), about 45 minutes for a 0.4 mg dose.

MECHANISM OF ACTION
Antagonizes opiate effects by competing for the same CNS receptor sites. Drug possesses no agonist activity of its own.

INDICATIONS & DOSAGE
• Opioid toxicity. *Adults:* 0.01 mg/kg initially, repeated q 2 to 3 minutes p.r.n.; or 0.4 mg followed by continuous infusion of 0.4 mg/hr. *Children:* 0.01 mg/kg initially, repeated q 2 to 3 minutes for up to two more doses; or 0.4 mg/hr by continuous infusion. *Neonates:* 0.01 mg/kg initially, repeated q 2 to 3 minutes until desired response is obtained.

• Postoperative opioid depression. *Adults:* 0.1 to 0.2 mg q 2 to 3 minutes until ventilation is adequate; may be repeated at 1- to 2-hour intervals. *Children:* 0.005 to 0.01 mg q 2 to 3 minutes until ventilation is adequate and child is alert; may be repeated at 1- to 2-hour intervals.

CONTRAINDICATIONS & CAUTIONS
• Contraindicated in hypersensitivity to naloxone.
• Use cautiously in patients who are physically dependent on opioids. A sudden reversal of narcotic effect could cause acute abstinence syndrome.

• Also use cautiously in postoperative patients with cardiac dysfunction or in those receiving cardiotoxic drugs because cardiac collapse may occur.

PREPARATION & STORAGE
Available in 0.02, 0.4, and 1 mg vials, ampules, and syringes. Store at 59° to 86° F. (15° to 30° C.) and protect from light. Avoid freezing. For a concentration of 0.004 mg/ml, mix 2 mg of drug in 500 ml of dextrose 5% in water or 0.9% sodium chloride. Solution is stable for 24 hours. Discard unused portion after 24 hours. For a concentration of 0.02 mg/ml, dilute 0.5 ml of adult dose (0.4 mg) with 9.5 ml of sterile water or 0.9% sodium chloride for injection.

ADMINISTRATION
Direct injection: Inject drug directly into vein or into an established I.V. line containing a free-flowing compatible solution.
Intermittent infusion: not recommended.
Continuous infusion: Infuse at rate titrated to patient's needs. Pediatric rate may range from 0.024 to 0.16 mg/kg/hour.

INCOMPATIBILITY
No incompatibilities reported. However, manufacturer recommends that naloxone not be mixed with any other drug, especially preparations containing bisulfite, metabisulfite, long-chain or high-molecular-weight anions, or alkaline solutions.

ADVERSE REACTIONS
Life-threatening: anaphylaxis.
Other: blood pressure changes, diaphoresis, dysrhythmias, irritability, nausea, pain, pulmonary edema, seizures, tremors, ventricular tachycardia, vomiting, withdrawal symptoms (diarrhea, fever, hyperactive reflexes and seizures in neonates, irritability, restlessness, rhinorrhea, sneezing, sweating, tachycardia, tremors, weakness, yawning).

INTERACTIONS
Butorphanol, nalbuphine, opioid-agonist analgesics, pentazocine: reversal of analgesic effects, possible precipitation of withdrawal symptoms.

EFFECTS ON DIAGNOSTIC TESTS
None reported.

SPECIAL CONSIDERATIONS
• To reverse effects of opioid agonists used during anesthesia without inhibiting pain control, carefully titrate naloxone dosage, as ordered.
• In the detoxified opioid addict, give naloxone challenge test, as ordered, before therapy. Administer 25% of initial dose, then observe for 30 seconds. If patient develops no withdrawal symptoms, give rest of dose and continue monitoring.
• Closely monitor respiratory, cardiac, and hemodynamic status for at least 24 hours. Duration of action of some narcotics may be longer than that of naloxone. Also, respiratory rate may suddenly exceed patient's normal rate.
• Because naloxone's action may be shorter than that of the opioid, continuous infusion may be necessary.
• Monitor for signs of withdrawal.
• Lack of response indicates condition is not caused by opioid CNS depressant.
• Naloxone has been used investigationally to treat senile dementia in Alzheimer's disease, to improve circulation in refractory shock, and to relieve constipation.

neostigmine methylsulfate
Prostigmin♦

Pregnancy Risk Category: C

PHARMACOKINETICS

Distribution: throughout most tissues, with highest concentrations in the liver and heart; 15% to 25% of drug is bound to serum albumin. Only high doses cross the blood-brain barrier. Drug may cross the placenta.

Metabolism: hydrolyzed by cholinesterases at neuromuscular junction. Also metabolized by hepatic microsomal enzymes.

Excretion: in urine, by renal tubular secretion, as unchanged drug and inactive metabolites. Half-life ranges from 47 to 60 minutes. Drug doesn't appear in breast milk.

Action: onset, within 5 minutes; peak effect, in 20 to 30 minutes.

MECHANISM OF ACTION

An anticholinesterase agent, neostigmine blocks effects of acetylcholinesterase at the neuromuscular junction, allowing accumulation of acetylcholine. This results in prolonged increase in skeletal muscle strength and intestinal muscle tone, bradycardia, ureteral constriction, bronchial and pupillary constriction, and salivary and sweat gland secretion.

INDICATIONS & DOSAGE

● Myasthenia gravis. Dosage varies widely, depending on patient needs and response. *Adults:* 0.5 to 2.5 mg p.r.n. *Children:* 0.01 to 0.04 mg/kg q 2 to 3 hours p.r.n.

● Antidote for nondepolarizing neuromuscular blocking agents. *Adults:* 0.5 to 2.5 mg, repeated p.r.n. to maximum total dose of 5 mg. *Children:* 0.04 mg/kg of body weight.

CONTRAINDICATIONS & CAUTIONS

● Contraindicated in hypersensitivity to neostigmine.

● Also contraindicated in mechanical obstruction of intestinal or urinary tract because drug increases intestinal and urinary muscle tone and activity.

● In patients with asthma, bradycardia, or dysrhythmias, use cautiously because drug may worsen these conditions.

● Also use cautiously in patients with peptic ulcer, epilepsy, and hyperthyroidism.

● Give carefully after surgery because respiratory difficulty may be aggravated by postoperative pain, sedation, secretions, or atelectasis.

PREPARATION & STORAGE

Available in 1 ml ampules of 1:2,000 (0.5 mg/ml) and 1:4,000 (0.25 mg/ml). Also available in multidose vials of 1:1,000 (1 mg/ml) and 1:2,000 (0.5 mg/ml). Protect solution from light and avoid freezing. Neostigmine needs no further dilution.

ADMINISTRATION

Direct injection: Inject drug slowly into tubing of patent, free-flowing I.V. line containing dextrose 5% in water, 0.9% sodium chloride, or another compatible I.V. solution.

Intermittent infusion: not recommended.

Continuous infusion: not recommended.

INCOMPATIBILITY

No incompatibilities reported.

ADVERSE REACTIONS

Life-threatening: anaphylaxis, aspiration of excessive oral secretions, severe bradycardia, severe bronchospasm, respiratory paralysis.

Other: clumsiness; confusion; dyspnea; fasciculations; fatigue; irritability; muscarinic effects (abdominal cramps, blurred vision, diaphoresis, diarrhea, excessive salivation, increased bronchial secretions, lacrimation); muscle cramps, twitching, or weakness; nausea; pupillary constriction; rash; thrombophlebitis; vomiting; wheezing.

INTERACTIONS

Aminoglycosides: possible reversed neuromuscular blockade.

Antimuscarinic agents (especially atropine): antagonized muscarinic effects of neostigmine.

Cholinesterase inhibitors: possible additive toxicity.

Depolarizing neuromuscular blocking agents (such as decamethonium and succinylcholine): prolonged neuromuscular blockade.

Edrophonium: increased risk of cholinergic crisis.

Guanadrel, guanethidine, mecamylamine, trimethaphan: antagonized effects of neostigmine.

Local ester-derivative anesthetics: increased risk of toxicity resulting from reduced metabolism.

Magnesium: possible antagonized neostigmine effects.

Nondepolarizing neuromuscular blocking agents (such as gallamine, metocurine, pancuronium, and tubocurarine): antagonized effects.

Procainamide, quinidine: possible antagonized neostigmine action.

EFFECTS ON DIAGNOSTIC TESTS

None reported.

SPECIAL CONSIDERATIONS

● Administer atropine or glycopyrrolate, as ordered, as antidote for adverse muscarinic effects. When giving I.V. neostigmine, always keep an anticholinergic, such as atropine, available and drawn into a separate syringe.

● Establish baseline respiratory rate, and maintain a patent airway, using suctioning, oxygen, and assisted ventilation as necessary.

● When drug is used to reverse the effects of nondepolarizing neuromuscular blockers, keep patient on assisted ventilation. Drug works best if patient is hyperventilated to lower his PCO_2 level.

● Also establish baseline heart rate and blood pressure. If heart rate is below 80 beats/minute, give atropine, as ordered, before neostigmine. Some clinicians recommend giving adults 0.6 to 1.2 mg of atropine I.V. or 0.2 to 0.6 mg glycopyrrolate I.V. before or with high doses of neostigmine.

● Measure vital capacity and muscle strength periodically to assess myasthenic patient's response to neostigmine.

● Be alert for cholinergic crisis in patients with myasthenia gravis. In cholinergic crisis, muscle weakness results from excessive cholinergic stimulation and usually occurs 1 hour after last dose of neostigmine. It's accompanied by adverse muscarinic effects and fasciculations. Stop drug.

● Resistance to neostigmine may develop.

● I.V. dose will be about 3% the size of an oral dose.

netilmicin sulfate
Netromycin♦

Pregnancy Risk Category: D

PHARMACOKINETICS
Distribution: principally dispersed into extracellular fluid with rapid distribution into tissues, including renal cortex, liver, gallbladder, stomach, and appendix; urine and sputum; and pericardial, synovial, peritoneal, and blister fluids. Drug diffuses poorly into cerebrospinal fluid and ocular tissue but crosses the placenta; fetal levels are 16% to 50% of maternal levels. Drug is minimally bound to protein.
Metabolism: not metabolized.
Excretion: removed unchanged in urine by glomerular filtration. In normal renal function, 74% of dose is excreted in 24 hours, but drug may persist for 10 to 20 days because of tissue accumulation. Small amounts appear in breast milk.
Action: peak serum level, at end of infusion.

MECHANISM OF ACTION
A semisynthetic aminoglycoside, netilmicin achieves its bactericidal effects by binding directly to the 30S ribosomal subunit of sensitive microorganisms. Its spectrum of activity includes the gram-negative bacteria *Citrobacter diversus, C. freundii, Enterobacter aerogenes, E. cloacae, Escherichia coli, Klebsiella, Morganella morganii, Proteus* (including *P. mirabilis* and *P. vulgaris), Providencia* (including *P. rettgeri), Salmonella, Serratia,* and *Shigella;* most strains of *Haemophilus influenzae, Neisseria gonorrhoeae, N. meningitidis,* and *Pseudomonas* (including *P. aeruginosa);* and some strains of *Acinetobacter, Alcaligenes, Bordetella, Moraxella,* and *Yersinia.* Susceptible gram-positive bacteria include *Staphylococcus aureus, S. epidermidis,* and most streptococci.

INDICATIONS & DOSAGE
• Severe systemic infections. *Adults and children over age 13:* 1.3 to 2.2 mg/kg q 8 hours or 2 to 3.25 mg/kg q 12 hours for 7 to 14 days. *Children 6 weeks to 13 years:* 1.83 to 2.67 mg/kg q 8 hours or 2.75 to 4 mg/kg q 12 hours for 7 to 14 days. *Neonates under 6 weeks:* 2 to 3.25 mg/kg q 12 hours for 7 to 14 days. *Adults with renal impairment:* Dosage reflects serum concentration. Initially, give 1.3 to 3.25 mg/kg, then 1.3 to 2.2 mg/kg q 24 hours (calculated by multiplying serum creatine level by 8) or in equally divided doses q 8 to 12 hours. Supplemental dose of 2 mg/kg is given after each dialysis session.

CONTRAINDICATIONS & CAUTIONS
• Contraindicated in aminoglycoside hypersensitivity.
• Use cautiously in neuromuscular disease, such as myasthenia gravis, parkinsonism, or infant botulism because netilmicin may cause neuromuscular blockade, thus worsening weakness.
• Also use cautiously in patients with renal dysfunction or cystic fibrosis because of a heightened risk of toxicity, and in eighth cranial nerve impairment because of possible ototoxicity.
• Because of the increased risk of severe dehydration and nephrotoxicity, give carefully to febrile, dehydrated, or severely burned patients.

PREPARATION & STORAGE
Available in 1.5 ml vials of 100 mg/ml concentrations in clear, colorless,

or pale solutions. Store at room temperature and avoid freezing.

Dilute appropriate dose with 50 to 200 ml of any of these compatible solutions: sterile water for injection; 0.9% sodium chloride; dextrose 5% in 0.9% sodium chloride; dextrose 5% or 10% in water; Ringer's injection; dextrose 5% in Ringer's lactate; Ringer's lactate; Isolyte E, M, or P and dextrose 5%; Plasma-Lyte M 56 or 148 and dextrose 5%; dextrose 5% and electrolyte #48; Ionosol B with dextrose 5%; dextrose 5% with Polysal; 10% Travert with Electrolyte #2 or #3; Normosol-R; 10% fructose; or Polysal.

Diluted solutions of 2.1 to 3 mg/ml retain potency in glass containers for 72 hours at room temperature or for 7 days when refrigerated at 39° F.(4° C.).

ADMINISTRATION
Direct injection: not recommended.
Intermittent infusion: Administer diluted solution over 30 minutes to 2 hours into an intermittent infusion device or through tubing containing a free-flowing compatible solution. After infusion, flush line with 0.9% sodium chloride or dextrose 5% in water.
Continuous infusion: not recommended.

INCOMPATIBILITY
Incompatible with cephalosporins, furosemide, and penicillins. Manufacturer recommends mixing no other drugs with netilmicin.

ADVERSE REACTIONS
Life-threatening: anaphylaxis, apnea.
Other: anemia, arthalgia, bacterial and fungal superinfection, blurred vision, disorientation, eighth cranial nerve damage (tinnitus, vertigo), eosinophilia, fever, granulocytopenia,

headache, hematuria, hypotension, leukopenia, muscle twitching, nausea, nystagmus, oliguria, palpitations, paralysis, pruritus, rash, seizures, thrombocytopenia, tubular necrosis, urticaria, vomiting.

INTERACTIONS
Amphotericin B, bacitracin, bumetanide, carmustine, cephalothin, cisplatin, cyclosporine, gentamicin, kanamycin, streptomycin, streptozocin, tobramycin: increased risk of nephrotoxicity or ototoxicity.
Antihistamines, dimenhydrinate, loxapine, phenothiazines, thioxanthines, trimethobenzamide: possible masked signs of ototoxicity.
Antimyasthenics: possible antagonized effects.
Beta-lactam antibiotics: possible synergistic effects against some organisms.
Diuretics: increased ototoxicity.
Halogenated hydrocarbon inhalation anesthetics, massive transfusion of citrated blood, neuromuscular blockers: possible potentiation of neuromuscular blockade and respiratory failure.
Indomethacin (I.V.): decreased renal clearance of netilmicin in neonates.
Methoxyflurane (parenteral), polymyxin: increased risk of nephrotoxicity or neuromuscular blockade.
Opioid analgesics: deepened respiratory depression.
Vancomycin: heightened risk of nephrotoxicity or ototoxicity and possible synergistic effects against some organisms.

EFFECTS ON DIAGNOSTIC TESTS
BUN, serum creatinine: increased levels.
Serum alkaline phosphatase, bilirubin, LDH; SGOT; SGPT: possible elevated levels.

Serum calcium, magnesium, potassium, sodium: possible diminished levels.
Urinalysis: increased excretion of protein, cells, and casts.

SPECIAL CONSIDERATIONS
• Obtain specimens for culture and sensitivity tests before first dose. Therapy may begin before test results are available.
• Calculate dose in terms of ideal body weight.
• Monitor respiratory effort, and make sure ventilator is available; neuromuscular blockade may cause respiratory depression. Netilmicin is the most potent neuromuscular blocker of all aminoglycosides.
• Monitor BUN and creatinine levels. Also monitor cranial nerve VIII function and for bacterial and fungal superinfection. Keep patient well hydrated to minimize chemical irritation of renal tubules.
• Obtain periodic peak and trough levels. Coordinate collection times with the laboratory. Desired peak level is 6 to 10 mcg/ml; trough level, 0.5 to 2 mcg/ml. Peak levels are lower in patients with edema, ascites, fever, and severe burns because of altered extracellular fluid volume; they're 2 to 3 times higher after rapid infusion.
• If no response occurs in 3 to 5 days, stop therapy, as ordered, and obtain new specimens for culture and sensitivity tests.
• If a cephalosporin or penicillin is ordered concurrently, administer at different sites.
• Dialysis may remove drug; patients undergoing hemodialysis or peritoneal dialysis may need dosage adjustment.
• May contain sulfites or benzyl alcohol.

niacinamide (nicotinamide)

Pregnancy Risk Category: A
(C if greater than RDA)

PHARMACOKINETICS
Distribution: widely dispersed into body tissues. Drug crosses the placenta.
Metabolism: in the liver to N-methylated derivative and its glycine conjugate, nicotinuric acid.
Excretion: in urine as metabolites and small amounts of unchanged drug. With higher doses, larger amounts of unchanged drug are removed in urine. Some drug appears in breast milk. Half-life is about 45 minutes.
Action: onset, unknown; duration, unknown.

MECHANISM OF ACTION
A component of the water-soluble vitamin B_3 complex, niacinamide is essential for lipid metabolism, tissue respiration, and glycogenolysis.

INDICATIONS & DOSAGE
• Pellagra. *Adults:* 25 to 100 mg two or more times daily. Dosage schedule reflects patient needs. *Children:* up to 100 mg daily.

CONTRAINDICATIONS & CAUTIONS
• Contraindicated in hypersensitivity to niacinamide.
• Use cautiously in diabetes mellitus because large doses may impair glucose tolerance; in gout because of the risk of hyperuricemia; in hepatic disease because drug may further damage the liver; and in peptic ulcer because drug may reactivate ulcer.

Unmarked trade names available in the United States only.
♦ Also available in Canada.   ♦ ♦ Available in Canada only.

• Also use cautiously in hemorrhage because drug activates the fibrinolytic system.

PREPARATION & STORAGE

Available in 30 ml vials containing 100 mg/ml. Drug is stable at room temperature. Avoid freezing.

For intermittent infusion, dilute 50 to 100 mg of drug in 50 ml of 0.9% sodium chloride. Concentration shouldn't exceed 10 mg/ml. For continuous infusion, dilute dose in ordered volume (500 to 1,000 ml) of IVH or other common solution.

ADMINISTRATION

Direct injection: Slowly inject dose directly into vein or add to free-flowing compatible I.V. solution.
Intermittent infusion: Infuse diluted dose through established I.V. line; maximum rate, 2 mg/minute.
Continuous infusion: Administer diluted daily dose over 24 hours; maximum rate, 2 mg/minute.

INCOMPATIBILITY

Incompatible with alkaline solutions, kanamycin, or streptomycin.

ADVERSE REACTIONS

Life-threatening: anaphylaxis.
Other: diarrhea, dizziness, dry skin, flushing, headache, hepatic dysfunction, hyperglycemia, hyperuricemia, nausea, orthostatic hypotension, pruritus, urticaria, vomiting.

INTERACTIONS

Sympathetic blockers: additive vasodilation and orthostatic hypotension.

EFFECTS ON DIAGNOSTIC TESTS

Urine catecholamines: elevated levels with fluorimetric methods.
Urine glucose: false-positive results, using cupric sulfate method (Benedict's solution, Clinitest).

SPECIAL CONSIDERATIONS

• Monitor hepatic function and blood glucose early in therapy.
• Warn patient taking an antihypertensive drug about orthostatic hypotension.
• May need to adjust dosages of antidiabetic agents.
• Use glucose oxidase methods (Clinistix, Tes-tape) to determine urine glucose level.

---

nitroglycerin

Nitro-Bid♦, Nitrol♦, Nitrostat♦, Tridil♦

Pregnancy Risk Category: C

PHARMACOKINETICS

Distribution: widely distributed throughout the body. Not known if drug crosses the placenta.
Metabolism: in the liver, rapidly and nearly complete.
Excretion: in urine, as metabolites. Half-life is 1 to 4 minutes. Not known if drug appears in breast milk.
Action: onset, immediate; peak effect, 1 to 2 minutes; duration (dose-related), several minutes.

MECHANISM OF ACTION

Nitroglycerine's specific mechanism of action is unknown. Drug relaxes vascular smooth muscle, causing vasodilation and reducing myocardial oxygen requirements. Subsequent improvement in myocardial blood flow to ischemic areas relieves angina, decreases peripheral venous stasis, and reduces venous ventricular volume and myocardial tension (preload). At higher doses, drug decreases peripheral vascular resistance moderately, thus reducing

---

arterial pressure and ventricular outflow resistance (afterload).

INDICATIONS & DOSAGE

• Congestive heart failure and chest pain associated with myocardial infarction; acute angina pectoris; blood pressure reduction during surgery. *Adults:* 5 mcg/minute initially, then increased by 5 mcg/minute q 3 to 5 minutes until desired response is achieved. If response is inadequate at 20 mcg/minute, increase dose by as much as 20 mcg/minute and give q 3 to 5 minutes if necessary. Once partial response is obtained, increase interval between doses and reduce dose. Maximum dose isn't established.

CONTRAINDICATIONS & CAUTIONS

• Contraindicated in hypersensitivity to nitroglycerin or nitrates.
• Also contraindicated in increased intracranial pressure because drug may raise cerebrospinal fluid pressure, and in hypotension or uncorrected hypovolemia because of the risk of severe hypotension or shock.
• Avoid use in constrictive pericarditis or pericardial tamponade because drug may further impair coronary circulation, and in hypertrophic cardiomyopathy because drug may intensify angina.
• Use cautiously in glaucoma because drug may briefly increase intraocular pressure; in hyperthyroidism because tachycardia may aggravate ischemia; and in recent MI, hypotension, and tachycardia because drug may aggravate ischemia.
• In severe hepatic impairment, administer carefully because drug increases the risk of methemoglobinemia, and in severe renal impairment because of reduced drug excretion.

PREPARATION & STORAGE

Several preparations of nitroglycerin for I.V. injection are available in various concentrations. Each comes with diluent instruction and dosage.

Nitro-Bid is supplied in 1, 5, and 10 ml vials of 5 mg/ml. Dilute with dextrose 5% in water or 0.9% sodium chloride. For a concentration of 50 mcg/ml, mix 1 ml of drug in 100 ml of solution; for 100 mcg/ml, mix 1 ml of drug in 50 ml of solution; for 200 mcg/ml, mix 2 ml of drug in 50 ml of solution.

Nitrol is available in a 10 ml ampule containing 5 mg/ml. Dilute initially by adding one 10 ml ampule (50 mg) to 500 ml of dextrose 5% in water or 0.9% sodium chloride to yield 100 mcg/ml. For maintenance infusion, dilute two ampules in 500 ml of solution for a concentration of 200 mcg/ml, or four ampules in 500 ml of solution for 400 mcg/ml.

Nitrostat I.V. comes in a kit with a 10 ml ampule containing 0.8 mg/ml and a disposable I.V. infusion set. Mix contents of ampule with 250 ml of dextrose 5% in water or 0.9% sodium chloride for 30 mcg/ml.

Tridil I.V. is supplied in ampules of 5 mg/10 ml, 25 mg/5 ml, 25 mg/5 ml for single use, and 50 mg/10 ml. Mix a 25 or 50 mg ampule with 500 ml of dextrose 5% in water or 0.9% sodium chloride for 50 or 100 mcg/ml, respectively. Diluting 5 mg of drug in 100 ml of solution yields 50 mcg/ml.

Store nitroglycerin preparations at room temperature and protect from light. Avoid freezing. After reconstitution, drug is stable for 48 hours at room temperature. Mix and store in glass bottle, which is usually supplied (along with tubing) with most products.

Keep in mind that the type of infusion set affects the amount of drug delivered. Use only nonabsorbent tubing; PVC tubing may absorb up to 80% of diluted drug from solution. Using PVC extension tubing for the infusion pump may negate advantages of the non-PVC set supplied with the drug.

ADMINISTRATION

Direct injection: not recommended.
Intermittent infusion: not recommended.
Continuous infusion: Infuse diluted drug at the rate required for therapeutic effect. Always use a volume-control device and a microdrip regulator. Closely monitor the patient's response to nitroglycerin.

INCOMPATIBILITY

Avoid mixing with any other drug because of possible incompatibility.

ADVERSE REACTIONS

Life-threatening: reflex tachycardia, severe hypotension.
Other: dizziness, flushing, headache, intoxication (alcohol in diluent), nausea, orthostatic hypotension, syncope, vomiting, weakness.

INTERACTIONS

Acetylcholine, histamine, norepinephrine: possible decreased effects.
Antihypertensives, ethanol (alcohol), opioid analgesics, other vasodilators: possible profound hypotension from additive vasodilation.
Beta blockers, calcium channel blockers, tricyclic antidepressants: enhanced hypotension.
Ergot alkaloids: possible precipitation of angina and reversal of nitroglycerin's antianginal effects.
Sympathomimetics: reduced antianginal effects and worsened hypotension.

EFFECTS ON DIAGNOSTIC TESTS

Serum cholesterol: decreased levels with Zlatkis-Zak color reaction method.
Serum methemoglobin: elevated levels with excessive doses.
Urine catecholamine, vanillylmandelic acid: markedly increased levels.

SPECIAL CONSIDERATIONS

• *Treatment of overdose:* Elevate the legs and reduce the infusion rate or temporarily stop the infusion. If severe hypotension persists, give an alpha-adrenergic agonist (methoxamine or phenylephrine) I.V., as ordered.
• During therapy, monitor blood pressure and heart rate and rhythm continuously; response to nitroglycerin varies greatly.
• If patient has a pulmonary artery catheter in place, frequently monitor pulmonary capillary wedge pressure.
• Assist patient with sitting up and standing until he can tolerate orthostatic hypotension.
• Give an analgesic for headache, if ordered.

---

nitroprusside sodium
Nipride♦, Nitropress

Pregnancy Risk Category: C

PHARMACOKINETICS

Distribution: unknown.
Metabolism: rapidly converted to cyanogen (cyanide radical), probably by interaction with sulfhydryl groups in erythrocytes and tissues, and then converted to thiocyanate in liver.
Excretion: entirely eliminated as metabolites. Half-life of thiocyanate is 3 to 7 days in patients with normal renal function.

Action: onset, immediate; duration, 1 to 10 minutes.

MECHANISM OF ACTION
Nitroprusside directly dilates vascular smooth muscle, producing peripheral vasodilation and hypotensive action. This effect isn't hindered by adrenergic blocking agents or vagotomy. Drug also reduces peripheral resistance and cardiac output.

INDICATIONS & DOSAGE
• Rapid blood pressure reduction in hypertensive emergencies, control of hypotension during anesthesia, reduction of preload and afterload in cardiac pump failure or cardiogenic shock. *Adults and children who aren't receiving other hypotensive drugs:* 0.5 to 10 mcg/kg/minute; average dose, 3 mcg/kg/minute.

CONTRAINDICATIONS & CAUTIONS
• Contraindicated in inadequate cerebral circulation or coronary artery insufficiency because of reduced tolerance to hypotension; in compensatory hypertension, as in an atrioventricular shunt or coarctation of the aorta, because hypotension may be life-threatening; and during emergency surgery for patients near death.
• Use with extreme caution in patients who are poor surgical risks; hypotension may be life-threatening.
• Use with caution in severe renal impairment because of reduced thiocyanate excretion; in hepatic insufficiency because of decreased drug metabolism; and in hypothyroidism because thiocyanate inhibits iodine uptake and binding.
• Give drug cautiously in anemia or hypovolemia (correct these before treatment) because nitroprusside decreases tolerance to these conditions, and in Leber's hereditary optic atrophy or tobacco amblyopia because affected patients lack the enzyme needed for nitroprusside metabolism.
• Also give cautiously in pulmonary impairment because drug may aggravate hypovolemia, and in low serum vitamin B_{12} levels because drug interferes with vitamin B_{12} metabolism and distribution, exacerbating the condition.
• In the elderly, use nitroprusside carefully because of heightened sensitivity to the drug's effects.

PREPARATION & STORAGE
Available as a powder in 50 mg vial. Reconstitute with 2 to 3 ml of dextrose 5% in water or sterile water for injection *without* preservatives. Then dilute in 250 to 1,000 ml of dextrose 5% in water to desired concentration. Store at room temperature, and protect from light, heat, and moisture. Reconstituted solution is stable for 24 hours. Discard solution if discolored (blue, green, or dark red), which indicates a reaction with another substance. After reconstitution, cover with aluminum foil or other opaque material.

ADMINISTRATION
Use nitroprusside only if adequate staff and equipment are available for arterial blood pressure monitoring.
Direct injection: not recommended.
Intermittent infusion: not recommended.
Continuous infusion: Using an infusion pump, administer diluted solution at a rate that maintains desired hypotensive effect.

INCOMPATIBILITY
Incompatible with bacteriostatic water for injection. Don't add any other drug or preservative to nitroprusside solution.

ADVERSE REACTIONS

Life-threatening: cyanide toxicity (absent reflexes, coma, widely dilated pupils, distant heart sounds, hypotension, imperceptible pulse, pink skin, extremely shallow breathing), excessive hypotension, thiocyanate intoxication (anorexia, blurred vision, confusion, delirium, dizziness, dyspnea, fatigue, loss of consciousness, metabolic acidosis, rash, tinnitus, weakness).

Other: abdominal pain, anxiety, apprehension, diaphoresis, dizziness, headache, muscle twitching, nasal stuffiness, nausea, palpitations, reflex tachycardia, restlessness, retrosternal discomfort, vomiting.

Adverse effects seldom occur at recommended dosage in short-term therapy.

INTERACTIONS

Dobutamine: increased cardiac output and decreased pulmonary wedge pressure.

Estrogens, sympathomimetics: diminished hypotensive effect.

Ganglionic blocking agents, general anesthetics (halothane), other antihypertensive drugs: additive hypotensive effect.

EFFECTS ON DIAGNOSTIC TESTS

Plasma cyanide, cyanocobalamin, thiocyanate: possible elevated levels.

Serum bicarbonate, PCO_2, pH: possible decreased levels.

Serum creatinine: elevated levels.

Serum lactate: possible increased levels.

SPECIAL CONSIDERATIONS

• *Treatment of overdose:* Give nitrites to prevent methemoglobin formation. In massive overdose, administer amyl nitrate by inhalation q 15 to 30 seconds/minute until a 3% sodium nitrite solution can be pre-

pared. Administer this solution at a maximum rate of 5 ml/minute, up to a total dose of 15 ml. Monitor blood pressure closely. Then give I.V. sodium thiosulfate solution of 12.5 g/ 50 ml of dextrose 5% in water over 10 minutes. Monitor carefully; thiocyanate levels may rise rapidly in patients with renal impairment. Hemodialysis or peritoneal dialysis can remove excess thiocyanate.

• In patients with low serum vitamin B_{12} levels or Leber's optic atrophy, hydroxocobalamin is an antidote for cyanogen and may be given before and during nitroprusside administration.

• Avoid extravasation.

• In patients with hepatic impairment, monitor plasma cyanogen concentrations daily after 1 or 2 days.

• Slowing infusion rate or temporarily discontinuing drug may alleviate adverse reactions.

• If metabolic acidosis occurs, discontinue drug and expect to try alternative therapy.

norepinephrine bitartrate
Levophed♦

Pregnancy Risk Category: D

PHARMACOKINETICS

Distribution: primarily localized to sympathetic nervous tissue. Drug crosses the placenta but not the blood-brain barrier.

Metabolism: in the liver and other tissues by enzymes catechol-*O*-methyltransferase and monoamine oxidase.

Excretion: in urine, primarily as metabolites. Small amounts (4% to 16%) excreted unchanged. Not known if drug appears in breast milk.

Action: onset, immediate; duration, 1 to 2 minutes after stopping infusion.

MECHANISM OF ACTION

A naturally occurring catecholamine, norepinephrine stimulates alpha-adrenergic receptors to produce vasoconstriction, increasing coronary artery blood flow and blood pressure. Drug also stimulates beta-adrenergic receptors to stimulate myocardium and increase cardiac output.

INDICATIONS & DOSAGE

• Advanced cardiac life support during CPR. *Adults:* 8 to 12 mcg/minute initially, then adjusted to maintain desired blood pressure range, usually 2 to 4 mcg/minute. *Children:* 0.1 mcg/kg/minute initially, then adjusted to maintain desired blood pressure range, usually 2 mcg/minute.

CONTRAINDICATIONS & CAUTIONS

• Contraindicated in hypersensitivity to norepinephrine, other sympathomimetics, or sulfite content in preparation.
• Also contraindicated in patients with hypotension from blood loss because of the risk of tissue hypoxia, lactic acidosis, low urine output, and severe vasoconstriction.
• Avoid use in mesenteric or peripheral vascular thrombosis or other occlusive vascular disorders (such as arteriosclerosis, Buerger's disease, diabetes mellitus) because norepinephrine may precipitate or aggravate ischemia.
• Also avoid use in patients receiving cyclopropane or halothane anesthetics or in hypoxia or hypercapnia because norepinephrine produces ventricular tachycardia or fibrillation.

• Give drug cautiously to patients with hyperthyroidism, hypertension, or severe cardiac disease and to the elderly because of an increased risk of adverse reactions.

PREPARATION & STORAGE

Available in 4 ml ampules containing 1 mg/ml. Store ampules at room temperature. For infusion, mix 1 ampule (4 mg) of norepinephrine in 1,000 ml of dextrose 5% in water or dextrose 5% in 0.9% sodium chloride for a concentration of 4 mcg/ml. Alter concentration, as necessary, to reflect patient's drug and fluid volume requirements. Discard diluted solution after 24 hours. Also discard if solution contains particulate matter or if it's brown, pink, or yellow.

ADMINISTRATION

Direct injection: not recommended.
Intermittent infusion: not recommended.
Continuous infusion: Insert a plastic I.V. catheter deeply into large vein. Don't use leg veins in the elderly or in patients with peripheral vascular disease. Use microdrip tubing and an infusion pump to carefully regulate flow rate. Infuse drug at a rate that maintains blood pressure at a low normal, usually 80 to 100 mm Hg systolic or, for previously hypertensive patients, a maximum of 40 mm Hg below previous systolic pressure.

INCOMPATIBILITY

Incompatible with aminophylline, amobarbital sodium, cephalothin, cephapirin, chlorothiazide, chlorpheniramine maleate, lidocaine hydrochloride, pentobarbital sodium, phenobarbital sodium, secobarbital sodium, sodium bicarbonate, sodium iodide, streptomycin sulfate, thiopental sodium, and whole blood.

Also, manufacturer recommends that drug not be mixed in 0.9% sodium chloride.

ADVERSE REACTIONS

Life-threatening: apnea, bradycardia, cerebral hemorrhage, fibrillation, hypertension (severe), increased peripheral vascular resistance, low cardiac output, seizures, ventricular tachycardia.

Other: angina, anxiety, atrioventricular dissociation, bigeminy, dizziness, fever, headache, insomnia, junctional rhythm, low urine output, metabolic acidosis, pallor, precordial pain, restlessness, thyroid swelling, tissue necrosis and sloughing with extravasation, tremors, weakness.

Early signs of overdose include intense sweating, pharyngeal or retrosternal pain, photophobia, and vomiting.

INTERACTIONS

Amphetamines, doxapram, mazindol, methylphenidate: enhanced CNS stimulation and pressor effect.
Antihypertensives: possible reduced pressor response.
Atropine sulfate: increased pressor response.
Cardiac glycosides, levodopa: heightened risk of dysrhythmias.
CNS stimulants: potentiated effects.
Desmopressin, lypressin, vasopressin: decreased antidiuretic effect.
Dihydroergotamine, ergonovine, methylergonovine, methysergide: enhanced vasoconstriction.
Ergoloid mesylates, ergotamine: risk of peripheral vascular ischemia and gangrene.
Ergonovine, ergotamine, methylergonovine, oxytocin: potentiated pressor effect.
Guanadrel, guanethidine, mecamylamine, methyldopa: diminished hypotensive effect of these drugs and enhanced pressor effect of norepinephrine.
Hydrocarbon inhalation anesthetics: ventricular tachycardia or fibrillation.
Lithium: decreased pressor response.
Maprotiline, tricyclic antidepressants: potentiated cardiovascular effects.
Other sympathomimetics: augmented CNS stimulation and cardiovascular effects.
Rauwolfia alkaloids: decreased hypotensive effect of these drugs and prolonged action of norepinephrine.
Thyroid hormones: increased effects of these hormones and norepinephrine.

EFFECTS ON DIAGNOSTIC TESTS

EKG: possible atrioventricular dissociation, bigeminy, bradycardia, junctional rhythm, ventricular fibrillation or tachycardia.
Serum glucose: possible increased levels.

SPECIAL CONSIDERATIONS

• Inclusion of 5 to 10 mg of phentolamine in norepinephrine infusion may prevent sloughing if extravasation occurs. Also, inclusion of 10 mg of heparin in each 500 ml of norepinephrine infusion may reduce the incidence of venous thrombosis.
• When treating shock, drug shouldn't be used as replacement for blood, plasma, fluids, or electrolytes.
• During infusion, check blood pressure every 2 minutes until stable, then every 5 to 15 minutes, using intra-arterial monitoring.
• Also monitor the patient's mental status and skin temperature and color of extremities (especially earlobes, lips, and nail beds).
• Avoid extravasation, which may cause local necrosis. Monitor infusion site every 2 minutes until blood

pressure stabilizes, then every 5 minutes. If extravasation occurs (infusion site will be blanched and cold), stop infusion immediately, and infiltrate area with 5 to 10 mg of phentolamine in 5 to 10 ml of 0.9% sodium chloride, using a 25G needle. Then remove the I.V. line and protect the area from further trauma. During prolonged infusion, rotate I.V. sites to prevent blanching.
• Continuously monitor EKG. Notify doctor of dysrhythmias. Check heart rate every 5 to 15 minutes.
• Insert an indwelling urinary catheter and monitor hourly urine output. If less than 30 ml/hour, notify doctor.
• Withdraw drug slowly; sudden cessation may cause severe hypotension. Monitor vital signs hourly until stable after stopping infusion. If systolic pressure drops below 70 mm Hg, restart infusion, as ordered.
• Avoid prolonged use when possible, to prevent ischemia of vital organs.
• May contain sulfites.

---

normal serum albumin (normal human serum albumin)
Albuconn 5% and 25%, Albuminar 5% and 25%, Albutein 5% and 25%, Buminate 5% and 25%, Plasbumin 5% and 25%

Pregnancy Risk Category: C

COMPOSITION
Consisting of at least 96% albumin, normal serum albumin is a solution made from pooled human blood, plasma, serum, or placentas obtained from healthy donors. Clear to yellow-brown, virtually odorless, and moderately viscous, albumin solutions have a pH between 6.4 and 7.4, adjusted with sodium carbonate, sodium bicarbonate, or acetic acid. Solutions contain sodium caprylate and sodium acetyltryptophanate as stabilizers but have no preservatives or antimicrobials.

Both 5% and 25% solutions contain 130 to 160 mEq/liter of sodium; 5% albumin is isotonic and 25% albumin is hypertonic, equivalent to five times the normal oncotic pressure.

Normal serum albumin includes no clotting factors, is nonreactive to hepatitis B surface antigen (HB$_s$Ag), and contains no significant isoagglutinins or other antibodies. It may be administered regardless of blood type or Rh factor. Albumin has been pasteurized at 140° F. (60° C.) for 10 hours.

INDICATIONS & DOSAGE
• Shock. *Adults:* 25 g given over 15 to 30 minutes. If no response, dose may be repeated. Thereafter, dosage reflects patient condition. Maximum dosage, 125 g/day for up to 2 days (5 liters of 5% solution or 1 liter of 25% solution). *Children:* 25 g over 15 to 30 minutes. *Premature infants:* 1 g/kg. *Adults with nephrosis:* 25 to 50 g repeated q 1 to 2 days.
• Hypoproteinemia. *Adults:* 1,000 to 1,500 ml of 5% solution daily or 25 to 100 g of 25% solution daily. *Children:* 25% to 50% of adult dose.
• Burns. Dosage reflects extent of burn, protein loss, denuded skin areas, and decreased albumin synthesis (which may persist for up to 60 days). *Adults:* dose sufficient to maintain serum albumin at 2 to 3 g/dl.
• Preoperative adjunct in cardiopulmonary bypass procedures. *Adults:* dose sufficient to maintain serum albumin at 2 to 3 g/dl.
• Hyperbilirubinemia. *Premature infants:* 4 ml/kg (1 g of albumin) or 120 ml/m^2 (30 g of albumin) of 25% solution given 1 to 2 hours before transfusion. *Premature infants with*

---

low serum protein levels: 1.4 to 1.8 ml/kg of 25% solution.

CONTRAINDICATIONS & CAUTIONS
• Contraindicated in albumin hypersensitivity; in severe anemia because volume expansion may worsen disorder; and in severe cardiac failure because of the risk of circulatory overload.
• Also contraindicated in patients with normal or increased intravascular volume because of the risk of hypertension.
• Use with caution in patients with low cardiac reserve without albumin deficiency because circulatory overload and pulmonary edema may occur.

PREPARATION & STORAGE
Available in sterile, nonpyrogenic vials packed with infusion kits; 5% solution supplied in 50, 250, 500, and 1,000 ml vials and 25% solution in 20, 50 and 100 ml vials. Store below 99° F. (37° C.), but don't freeze. Discard unused portion after 4 hours. For continuous infusion, add 25% solution to 500 to 1,000 ml of dextrose 5% in water or 0.9% sodium chloride. To obtain a 10% solution, dilute 25% solution in a 1 to 1.5 ratio in dextrose 10% in water.

ADMINISTRATION
Direct injection: not recommended.
Intermittent infusion: Infuse at rate appropriate to patient's condition, usually over 15 to 30 minutes. When albumin is used for plasma volume expansion, don't exceed rate of 2 to 4 ml/minute with 5% solution and 1 ml/minute with 25% solution. In hypoproteinemia, don't exceed 5 to 10 ml/minute of 5% solution or 2 to 3 ml/minute of 25% solution. In hypertension or mild to moderate car-

diac failure, infuse 10% solution slowly.
Continuous infusion: Infuse diluted solution slowly; adjust according to patient response and changes in blood pressure.

INCOMPATIBILITY
No incompatibilities reported.

ADVERSE REACTIONS
Life-threatening: anaphylaxis, fluid overload.
Other: chills, fever, hypotension, nausea, rash, tachycardia.

INTERACTIONS
None reported.

EFFECTS ON DIAGNOSTIC TESTS
Serum alkaline phosphatase: possible elevated levels.

SPECIAL CONSIDERATIONS
• Minimize allergic reactions by giving antihistamines, as ordered, before infusion and by slowing infusion rate.
• Monitor vital signs before, during, and after infusion. Also monitor serum albumin, total protein, hemoglobin, hematocrit, and electrolyte levels.
• Watch closely for signs of circulatory overload or pulmonary edema. If signs occur, discontinue infusion, keep vein open with ordered solution, and notify the doctor.
• Check intake and output, and report changes in output. Increased colloid pressure mobilizes extracellular fluid, causing diuresis for 3 to 20 hours.
• Monitor patients with cerebral edema. Withhold fluids for 8 hours after infusion to avoid fluid overload.

Unmarked trade names available in the United States only.
♦Also available in Canada.   ♦ ♦ Available in Canada only.

• In surgical or trauma patients, watch for possible bleeding points undetected at lower blood pressures.
• One volume of 25% albumin is equivalent to 5 volumes of 5% albumin in producing hemodilution and relative anemia.
• Sodium content (130 to 160 mEq/liter) may necessitate reduced albumin dose in patients with sodium restriction.

---

ondansetron hydrochloride
Zofran

Pregnancy Risk Category: B

PHARMACOKINETICS
Distribution: about 70% to 76% protein bound. Also distributes into erythrocytes.
Metabolism: exclusively in liver; 95% by hydroxylation, glucuronide formation, and *N*-demethylation; about 5% appears in the urine as the unchanged drug.
Excretion: in the urine. Most of the drug (95%) is excreted as metabolites. The elimination half-life is about 3.5 hours; half-life increases to 7.9 hours in elderly patients. Not known if the drug appears in breast milk.
Action: The drug's antiemetic effect varies considerably. Peak level, 6 to 20 minutes after infusion. Optimal dosage interval appears to be 2 to 8 hours.

MECHANISM OF ACTION
Ondansetron is a potent member of a new class of antiemetic agents known as serotonin type 3 (5-hydroxytryptamine type 3; 5-HT$_3$)-receptor antagonists. It blocks serotonin type 3 receptors in the CNS (in the medulla at the chemoreceptor trigger zone) to prevent activation of the vomiting center. In the peripheral nervous system, it acts at the vagal nerve terminals to block visceral afferents in the GI tract and prevent muscular movements of the abdomen and diaphragm associated with vomiting.

INDICATIONS & DOSAGE
• Prevention of nausea and vomiting associated with single-day courses of emetogenic chemotherapy (including cisplatin). *Adults and children over age 4:* Drug is given in three doses of 0.15 mg/kg. Give first dose 30 minutes before chemotherapy; subsequent doses at 4 and 8 hours after first dose. Do not give drug bolus (push) or I.M.

CONTRAINDICATIONS & CAUTIONS
• Contraindicated in patients sensitive to the drug.
• Use cautiously in patients with compromised liver function because ondansetron is extensively metabolized.

PREPARATION & STORAGE
Available in 20 ml multiple-dose vials containing 2 mg/ml. Solution has pH of 3.3 to 4.0. Before administration, dilute drug in 50 ml of compatible solution (such as dextrose 5% in water for injection, 0.9% sodium chloride for injection, dextrose 5% in 0.9% sodium chloride for injection, dextrose 5% in 0.45% sodium chloride for injection, and 3% sodium chloride for injection). Drug is stable for up to 48 hours in PVC bags after dilution when refrigerated at 39° F. (4° C.) or kept at room temperature 77° F. (25° C.). Store at room temperature and protect from light. Not necessary to protect from light during administration.

ADMINISTRATION

Direct injection: not recommended.
Intermittent infusion: Dilute drug in 50 ml of compatible solution and infuse over 15 minutes.
Continuous infusion: may be given concurrently with compatible drugs when administered through the Y-site of the infusion set.

INCOMPATIBILITY

Limited data indicate that ondansetron is incompatible with acyclovir sodium, aminophylline, amphotericin B, ampicillin sodium, ampicillin sodium-sulbactam sodium, amsacrine, cefoperazone sodium, fluorouracil, furosemide, ganciclovir sodium, lorazepam, methylprednisolone sodium succinate, mezlocillin disodium, and piperacillin sodium.

ADVERSE REACTIONS

Life-threatening: bronchospasm (rare).
Other: constipation, diarrhea, headache, rash, sedation, transient elevations of SGOT and SGPT levels.

INTERACTIONS

Drugs that alter hepatic drug metabolizing enzymes (such as cimetidine or phenobarbital): may alter ondansetron's pharmacokinetics. However, no dosage adjustment appears necessary.

EFFECTS ON DIAGNOSTIC TESTS

SGOT, SGPT: possible altered levels.

SPECIAL CONSIDERATIONS

• Treat overdose with appropriate supportive therapy.
• Clinical trials show ondansetron provides substantially better control of emesis than metoclopramide with fewer adverse effects (such as acute dystonic reactions or akathisia).

However, standard course of ondansetron costs about 50% more than similar course of high-dose metoclopramide. Benefits of ondansetron must be weighed against added cost to the patient and hospital.
• Drug is not currently indicated for use in patients receiving multiple-day courses of antineoplastic therapy or for prophylaxis of delayed nausea and vomiting.
• Although decreased clearance and increased half-life occur in elderly patients, there are no recommendations for reducing dosage because these changes have not been linked to reduced safety or efficacy.
• In clinical trials, the use of dexamethasone combined with ondansetron provided significantly better control of emesis than the use of ondansetron alone.
• Several studies have shown that ondansetron helps control nausea and vomiting caused by anthracyclines, cisplatin, cyclophosphamide, ifosfamide, and melphalan.
• Drug may control emesis caused by radiation therapy.
• Drug contains methylparaben and propylparaben preservatives.
• Inspect solutions for particulate matter or discoloration before giving drug.
• Little information is available regarding drug's use in patients with hepatic or renal failure.

orphenadrine citrate
Banflex, Flexoject, Flexon, K-Flex, Marflex, Myolin, Neocyten, Norflex♦, O-Flex, Orphenate

Pregnancy Risk Category: C

PHARMACOKINETICS

Distribution: not well characterized, but probably widespread, especially to organs with greatest perfusion, such as the lungs. Orphenadrine may cross the placenta. Drug has low protein-binding capability.

Metabolism: in the liver, but not completely understood. Drug is almost totally metabolized to at least eight metabolites.

Excretion: principally eliminated in urine as metabolites and small amounts of unchanged drug. Small amounts are also excreted in feces. Not known if drug appears in breast milk. Half-life is about 14 hours.

Action: onset, immediate; duration, 12 hours.

MECHANISM OF ACTION

Precise mechanism unknown. Drug reduces postsynaptic reflexes, thereby inhibiting transmission of spinal cord impulses to skeletal muscle.

INDICATIONS & DOSAGE

• Acute pain in musculoskeletal disorders. *Adults:* 60 mg q 12 hours.

CONTRAINDICATIONS & CAUTIONS

• Contraindicated in orphenadrine hypersensitivity.

• Also contraindicated in glaucoma, myasthenia gravis, prostatic hypertrophy, bladder neck obstruction, duodenal or pyloric obstruction, achalasia, and tachydysrhythmias because drug's antimuscarinic action may aggravate these disorders.

• Use cautiously in fever because of the risk of hyperthermia; in CNS depression because drug may exacerbate symptoms; in renal or hepatic impairment because of the increased risk of toxicity; in gastric ulcer because drug may delay gastric emptying with possible antral stasis; and in GI infections because drug may slow GI motility, resulting in reten-

tion of the causative organism or toxin.

• Also use orphenadrine cautiously in the elderly because they may be more sensitive to the drug's effects.

• Pediatric safety hasn't been established.

PREPARATION & STORAGE

Available in 2 ml ampules and 10 and 30 ml vials with a concentration of 30 mg/ml. Store at room temperature; protect ampules from light. Drug needs no further dilution for injection.

ADMINISTRATION

Direct injection: Inject drug directly into a vein or into an I.V. line containing a free-flowing compatible solution. Administer over 5 to 10 minutes with the patient supine.

Intermittent infusion: not recommended.

Continuous infusion: not recommended.

INCOMPATIBILITY

No incompatibilities reported.

ADVERSE REACTIONS

Life-threatening: anaphylaxis, aplastic anemia, ventricular dysrhythmias.

Other: abdominal cramps, bradycardia (transient), confusion, constipation, depression, difficult urination, dizziness, drowsiness, dry mouth, fatigue, headache, insomnia, irritability, nausea, palpitations, rash, restlessness, tachycardia, trembling, visual disturbances, vomiting.

INTERACTIONS

Alcohol, CNS depressants: deepened CNS depression.

Amitriptyline, prochlorperazine, thioridazine: possible potentiation of orphenadrine's cholinergic action.

OXACILLIN SODIUM 395

Antimuscarinic drugs: intensified effects.
Propoxyphene: possible additive CNS effects and precipitation of hypoglycemia.

EFFECTS ON DIAGNOSTIC TESTS
Serum alkaline phosphatase, SGOT, SGPT: possible elevated levels.

SPECIAL CONSIDERATIONS
• Carefully check all dosages. Even a slight overdose can cause toxicity.
• Monitor vital signs and input and output.
• Support renal function. Dialysis may be helpful in serum concentrations above 4 mcg/ml.
• Keep patient recumbent for 10 minutes after injection. Then help him to sit up slowly.
• Relieve dry mouth with cool drinks and sugarless gum or candy.
• Orphenadrine may be used alone or in combination with aspirin as an adjunct to rest, physical therapy, and other comfort measures.
• Replace parenteral therapy with oral therapy as soon as possible.
• During long-term therapy, monitor liver function and CBC.

oxacillin sodium
Bactocill, Prostaphlin

Pregnancy Risk Category: B

PHARMACOKINETICS
Distribution: into synovial, pleural, pericardial, and ascitic fluids, and bone, bile, lungs, and sputum. Concentration in cerebrospinal fluid is low but rises with inflamed meninges. Drug is 89% to 94% protein-bound. It crosses the placenta.

Metabolism: partially altered to active and inactive metabolites in the liver.
Excretion: rapidly removed in urine as unchanged drug and metabolites by renal tubular secretion and glomerular filtration. Drug appears in breast milk. Half-life is 30 minutes to 2 hours.
Action: peak plasma level, at end of infusion.

MECHANISM OF ACTION
A semisynthetic penicillinase-resistant penicillin that adheres to penicillin-binding proteins (PBP-1 and PBP-3), inhibiting bacterial cell-wall synthesis. Its spectrum of activity includes most gram-positive and gram-negative aerobic cocci, including *Staphylococcus aureus, S. epidermidis, S. saprophyticus;* groups A, B, C, and G streptococci; *Streptococcus pneumoniae;* and some strains of viridans streptococci. It's also active against a few gram-positive aerobic and anaerobic bacilli, including *Corynebacterium diphtheriae, Erysipelothrix rhusiopathiae, Neisseria gonorrhoeae, Pasteurella multocida, Clostridium, Peptococcus,* and *Peptostreptococcus,* and some strains of *Neisseria meningitidis* and *Actinomyces.*

INDICATIONS & DOSAGE
• Severe infections caused by susceptible organisms. *Adults:* 1 g q 4 to 6 hours. *Children weighing less than 40 kg:* 100 to 200 mg/kg in equal doses q 6 hours.
• Mild to moderate infections caused by susceptible organisms. *Adults:* 250 to 500 mg q 4 to 6 hours. *Children weighing less than 40 kg:* 50 mg/kg in equal doses q 6 hours.
• Endocarditis or chronic osteomyelitis caused by susceptible organisms. *Adults:* 1.5 to 2 g q 4 hours.

Note: Adjust dosage in renal impairment. For adults, dosage reflects creatinine clearance. If clearance is less than 10 ml/minute, dosage is 1 g q 4 to 6 hours.

CONTRAINDICATIONS & CAUTIONS
• Contraindicated in penicillin hypersensitivity.
• Use with caution in hypersensitivity to cephalosporins or other drugs.
• Also use with caution in interstitial nephritis because drug may exacerbate disorder, and in patients with a history of GI disease, such as ulcerative colitis, regional enteritis, or antibiotic-associated colitis.

PREPARATION & STORAGE
Available in powder form in 250 and 500 mg and 1, 2, and 4 g vials. Reconstitute with sterile water for injection or 0.9% sodium chloride. For direct injection, add 5 ml of sterile water for injection or 0.9% sodium chloride to 250 or 500 mg vial; 10 ml to 1 g vial; 20 ml to 2 g vial; and 40 ml to 4 g vial. For intermittent infusion, mix 50 to 100 ml of diluent with 1 or 2 g vial and 98 ml with 4 g vial. Solutions are stable for 3 days at room temperature and for 1 week if refrigerated. Compatible solutions include dextrose 5% in Ringer's lactate, dextrose 5% in 0.9% sodium chloride, dextrose 5% or 10% in water, Ringer's lactate, and 0.9% sodium chloride.

ADMINISTRATION
Direct injection: Inject drug over 10 minutes through an intermittent infusion device or into an I.V. line containing a free-flowing compatible solution.
Intermittent infusion: Infuse diluted solution through an intermittent infusion device or using an I.V. line containing a free-flowing compatible solution over the ordered duration.
Continuous infusion: not recommended.

INCOMPATIBILITY
Incompatible with aminoglycosides and tetracyclines. May be incompatible with verapamil.

ADVERSE REACTIONS
Life-threatening: anaphylaxis, pseudomembranous colitis.
Other: agranulocytosis, bacterial and fungal superinfection, eosinophilia, hepatotoxicity, leukopenia, neurotoxicity, neutropenia, phlebitis, thrombophlebitis. *In neonates receiving 150 to 175 mg/kg daily:* transient albuminuria, azotemia, hematuria.

INTERACTIONS
Aminoglycosides: synergistic effects against some organisms. However, drugs are physically and chemically incompatible. Don't mix together or administer simultaneously.
Chloramphenicol, erythromycin, sulfonamides, tetracyclines: possible reduced bactericidal effect.
Probenecid: increased serum concentration, resulting from inhibited renal tubular secretion.
Rifampin: possible prevention or delay in emergence of rifampin-resistant strains of *S. aureus*.

EFFECTS ON DIAGNOSTIC TESTS
Serum, urine protein: possible misleading results when using sulfosalicylic acid or trichloracetic acid.
SGOT, SGPT: possible increased levels, resulting from hepatotoxicity.

SPECIAL CONSIDERATIONS
• Before giving drug, ask about previous reactions to penicillin or cephalosporins; negative history doesn't rule out future hypersensitivity.

• Obtain specimens for culture and sensitivity tests before first dose. Therapy may start immediately.
• Monitor WBC before therapy and 1 to 3 times weekly during therapy.
• Assess renal and hepatic function before therapy and periodically during therapy. Closely monitor neonates for hepatotoxicity and nephrotoxicity.
• Discontinue drug if signs of hypersensitivity, pseudomembranous colitis, hepatotoxicity, or bacterial or fungal superinfection occur; institute appropriate therapy, as ordered.
• If diarrhea persists during therapy, obtain stool specimen for culture.
• Dialysis removes only minimal amounts of oxacillin.
• Drug contains about 2.5 mEq of sodium per gram.

---

oxymorphone hydrochloride
Numorphan♦

Pregnancy Risk Category: B (D for prolonged use or use at term)

PHARMACOKINETICS
Distribution: throughout body tissues. Drug crosses the placenta and blood-brain barrier.
Metabolism: in liver.
Excretion: in urine. Small amounts appear in breast milk.
Action: onset, 5 to 10 minutes; duration, 3 to 4 hours.

MECHANISM OF ACTION
Drug produces analgesia by binding with CNS opiate receptors, altering pain perception and emotional response to it.

INDICATIONS & DOSAGE
• Moderate to severe pain. *Adults:* Initially, 0.5 mg q 3 to 4 hours.

Dose may be increased cautiously up to 1 mg in nondebilitated patients.

CONTRAINDICATIONS & CAUTIONS
• Contraindicated in oxymorphone sensitivity and in children under age 12.
• Also contraindicated in patients with diarrhea related to pseudomembranous colitis or poisoning because drug may slow elimination of toxins from the GI tract.
• Avoid use in acute respiratory depression because drug may exacerbate the condition.
• Use with extreme caution in altered respiratory function because of possible respiratory depression, and in head injury and increased intracranial pressure because drug may mask changes in level of consciousness, impair CNS function, and elevate CSF pressure.
• In hepatic or renal impairment, use cautiously and in lower doses because drug clearance may be slowed.
• In elderly or debilitated patients, administer carefully because of increased sensitivity to drug effects.
• Use cautiously in patients with a history of dysrhythmias or seizures because drug may exacerbate symptoms, and in hypothyroidism because drug may heighten the risk of respiratory and CNS depression.
• Also use cautiously in acute abdominal conditions because drug may mask signs; in gallbladder disease because drug may precipitate biliary contractions; in recent GI surgery because drug may alter GI motility; and in inflammatory bowel disease because of an increased risk of toxic megacolon.
• In prostatic hypertrophy or obstruction, urethral stricture, or recent urinary tract surgery, give

---

oxymorphone cautiously because of the enhanced risk of urine retention.
• Also administer cautiously to patients with a history of substance abuse, emotional instability, or suicidal ideation because of possible abuse.

PREPARATION & STORAGE
Supplied in 1 and 1.5 mg/ml ampules and in 1.5 mg/ml vials. Protect from freezing, light, and excessive heat. Store between 59° and 86° F. (15° and 30° C.). No further dilution is needed for direct injection. Compatible solutions include dextrose 5% in water, dextrose 5% in 0.9% sodium chloride, and Ringer's lactate.

ADMINISTRATION
Direct injection: Inject dose directly into a vein or into an I.V. line containing a free-flowing compatible solution. Administer over 2 to 3 minutes.
Intermittent infusion: not recommended.
Continuous infusion: not recommended.

INCOMPATIBILITY
No incompatibilities reported.

ADVERSE REACTIONS
Life-threatening: anaphylaxis, bradycardia, respiratory depression, tachycardia.
Other: abdominal pain, blurred or double vision, cold clammy skin, confusion, constipation, decreased salivation, dizziness, drowsiness, dry mouth, facial redness or flushing, faintness, false sense of well-being, headache, increased gallbladder pain, malaise, nightmares or unusual dreams, pinpoint pupils, seizures, severe weakness, sweating, trembling, unusual nervousness or fatigue, urine retention.

Withdrawal symptoms include abdominal cramps, aching, anorexia, diarrhea, fever, gooseflesh, increased sweating, insomnia, nausea, rhinorrhea, shivering, sneezing, vomiting, and yawning.

INTERACTIONS
Alcohol, general anesthetics, hypnotics, neuromuscular blockers, sedatives: deepened respiratory depression. Reduce oxymorphone dose.
Antidiarrheals, antiperistaltics: heightened risk of severe constipation and CNS depression.
Antihypertensives, diuretics, hydroxyzine: potentiated hypotension.
Antimuscarinics: severe constipation, paralytic ileus, and urine retention.
Buprenorphine: reduced oxymorphone effects; withdrawal symptoms in physically dependent patients.
Hydroxyzine: potentiated analgesia, CNS depression, and hypotension.
Magnesium sulfate: deepened CNS depression.
MAO inhibitors: severe, unpredictable reactions. Reduce oxymorphone dose.
Metoclopromide: antagonized effects.
Naloxone: antagonized analgesic, CNS, and respiratory depressant effects.
Naltrexone: blocked analgesic effects of oxymorphone; withdrawal symptoms in physically dependent patients.
Other opioid analgesics: potentiated CNS and respiratory depression and hypotension in non-opioid–dependent patients.
Phenothiazines: deepened respiratory depression and increased risk of habituation.

EFFECTS ON DIAGNOSTIC TESTS

CSF analysis: increased CSF pressure.

Gastric emptying studies: delayed emptying.

Hepatobiliary imaging: delayed visualization when using technetium Tc 99m disofenin.

Serum alkaline phosphate, bilirubin, LDH, SGOT, SGPT: increased levels.

Serum amylase, lipase: elevated levels.

SPECIAL CONSIDERATIONS

• *Treatment of overdose:* Support airway and respirations. As ordered, give naloxone, repeating as needed to reverse respiratory depression. Administer I.V. fluids and vasopressors to maintain blood pressure.

• For improved analgesia, give before patient has intense pain. Drug isn't intended for mild pain.

• Don't administer drug if respirations are below 12 breaths/minute.

• Monitor respirations for at least 1 hour after giving dose. Keep resuscitation equipment available. If respirations fall below 8 breaths/minute, arouse patient to stimulate breathing. Notify the doctor; he may order naloxone or respiratory support.

• To minimize hypotension, administer with patient supine. Instruct him to rise slowly to reduce dizziness and faintness.

• Decreased salivation may contribute to candidiasis, dental caries, and discomfort.

• Dependence can develop with long-term use.

• Assess patient's bowel function, and administer a stool softener if needed.

oxytetracycline hydrochloride
Terramycin

Pregnancy Risk Category: D

PHARMACOKINETICS

Distribution: readily distributed to most body tissues and fluids, including synovial, pleural, ascitic, prostatic, seminal, and gingival fluids; sinus secretions; aqueous and vitreous humor; and bile. Drug localizes in bone, liver, spleen, tumors, and teeth. Small amounts penetrate the blood-brain barrier, but concentrations vary. Drug readily crosses the placenta. Protein binding is low (10% to 40%).

Metabolism: not metabolized.

Excretion: in urine by glomerular filtration and in feces in small amounts. About 70% is excreted unchanged in 72 hours. Usual half-life is 6 to 10 hours; in renal impairment, it's 47 to 66 hours. Drug appears in breast milk.

Action: onset, immediately upon administration.

MECHANISM OF ACTION

A broad-spectrum, bacteriostatic antibiotic and antiprotozoal agent, oxytetracycline inhibits protein synthesis of sensitive microorganisms by binding to the 30S ribosomal subunit. Susceptible gram-negative bacteria include *Bartonella bacilliformis, Bordetella pertussis, Brucella, Campylobacter fetus, Calymmatobacterium granulomatis, Francisella tularensis, Haemophilus ducreyi, H. influenzae, Legionella pneumophilia, Leptotrichia buccalis, Neisseria gonorrhoeae, N. meningitidis, Pasteurella multocida, Pseudomonas mallei, P. pseudomallei, Shigella, Spirillum minus, Streptobacillus mon-*

---

iliformis, Vibrio cholerae, V. para-haemolyticus, Yersinia enterocolitica, Y. pestis, and some strains of *Acinetobacter, Bacteroides, Enterobacter aerogenes, Escherichia coli,* and *Klebsiella.*

Susceptible gram-positive bacteria include *Actinomyces israelii, Arachnia propionica, Bacillus anthracis, Clostridium perfringens, C. tetani, Listeria monocytogenes, Nocardia,* and *Propionibacterium acnes.* Drug is also active against *Borrelia recurrentis, Chlamydia psittaci, C. trachomatis, Coxiella burnetii, Leptospira, Mycoplasma hominis, M. pneumoniae, Rickettsia akari, R. prowazekii, R. rickettsii, R. tsutsugamushi, R. typhi, Treponema pallidum, T. pertenue,* and *Ureaplasma urealyticum.*

INDICATIONS & DOSAGE
● Infections caused by susceptible organisms. *Adults:* 250 to 500 mg q 12 hours. Maximum dosage, 2 g daily. *Children age 8 and older:* 6 mg/kg q 12 hours or 5 to 10 mg/kg q 12 hours, depending on severity of infection.
Note: Adjust dosage in renal failure. For adults, dosage may be reduced, or interval between doses may be lengthened as needed.

CONTRAINDICATIONS & CAUTIONS
● Contraindicated in hypersensitivity to tetracyclines.
● Also contraindicated during second half of pregnancy, in breast-feeding women, and in children under age 8 (unless other drugs are ineffective or contraindicated) because drug may permanently discolor teeth, cause enamel hypoplasia, and inhibit fetal skeletal growth.
● Use cautiously in renal or hepatic impairment because of risk of toxic-ity, and in myasthenia gravis because weakness may worsen.

PREPARATION & STORAGE
Supplied as a yellow crystalline powder in 250 and 500 mg vials. Reconstitute each vial with 10 ml of sterile water for injection or dextrose 5% injection. For intermittent infusion, dilute to a final volume of 100 ml with dextrose 5% injection, 0.9% sodium chloride injection, or Ringer's injection. For continuous infusion, dilute with 1,000 ml of compatible solution.

Use Ringer's injection with caution because it contains calcium. However, the calcium in this diluent usually doesn't precipitate oxytetracycline in an acid medium. Solution is stable in most I.V. fluids that have a pH less than 6.0. Dilution in multielectrolyte solutions may cause discoloration but no significant loss of potency.

Before reconstitution, store at 59° to 86° F. (15° to 30° C.), and protect from light. After reconstitution, solutions with a concentration of 25 or 50 mg/ml remain potent for 48 hours if refrigerated at 41° F. (5° C.). After final dilution, administer immediately. Store carefully and discard outdated drug; nephrotoxicity has been associated with improperly stored or expired drug.

ADMINISTRATION
Direct injection: contraindicated.
Intermittent infusion: Infuse slowly over 20 to 30 minutes into established I.V. line containing a free-flowing compatible solution. Avoid extravasation.
Continuous infusion: Infuse diluted solution over 8 to 12 hours.

INCOMPATIBILITY
Incompatible with aminophylline, amphotericin B, ampicillin sodium,

---

calcium chloride, calcium gluconate, carbenicillin disodium, cephapirin, chloramphenicol sodium succinate, erythromycin gluceptate, hydrocortisone sodium succinate, Ionosol D-CM, Ionosol B with dextrose 5%, Ionosol PSL, Ionosol T with dextrose 5%, iron dextran, magnesium, meperidine, methicillin, methohexital, oxacillin, penicillin G potassium, penicillin G sodium, pentobarbital sodium, phenobarbital sodium, sodium bicarbonate, and vitamin B with C.

ADVERSE REACTIONS
Life-threatening: anaphylaxis, exfoliative dermatitis.
Other: anogenital lesions, anorexia, bacterial and fungal superinfection, bulging fontanelles (reversible), diarrhea, discolored teeth or tongue, dizziness, dysphagia, enamel hypoplasia, enterocolitis, eosinophilia, fatty infiltration of liver (at high doses in pregnant women), hemolytic anemia, hepatotoxicity (at high doses), hyperpigmentation, hypersensitivity reaction (anaphylactoid purpura, angioedema, exacerbation of systemic lupus erythematosus, pericarditis, urticaria), liver failure, meningeal irritation, nausea, neutropenia, photosensitivity, pseudomembranous colitis, rash, thrombocytopenia, thrombophlebitis, vomiting.

INTERACTIONS
Lithium carbonate: heightened risk of toxicity.
Methoxyflurane: increased risk of nephrotoxicity.
Oral anticoagulants: potentiated effects.
Oral contraceptives: diminished effects.
Penicillin: impaired bactericidal action.

EFFECTS ON DIAGNOSTIC TESTS
BUN: elevated levels.
CBC: reduced RBC, eosinophil, neutrophil, and platelet counts.
Prothrombin time: prolonged.
Serum alkaline phosphatase, amylase, SGOT, SGPT: increased levels.
Urine catecholamines: falsely elevated levels.
Urine glucose: false-positive results when using cupric sulfate method (Benedict's solution or Clinitest); false-negative results when using glucose oxidase method (Clinistix or Tes-Tape).

SPECIAL CONSIDERATIONS
• Check for tetracycline hypersensitivity before therapy.
• Obtain specimens for culture and sensitivity tests before therapy. Begin therapy before results are available.
• Slow infusion if venous irritation occurs.
• Closely monitor for overgrowth of nonsusceptible organisms, including fungi. If superinfection occurs, discontinue drug, as ordered, and initiate appropriate therapy.
• If diarrhea persists, collect stool specimens for culture to rule out pseudomembranous colitis.
• Discontinue drug if photosensitivity occurs. Instruct patient to avoid direct sunlight, to use sunscreens, and to wear protective clothing.
• Group A beta-hemolytic streptococcal infections require treatment for at least 10 days.
• During prolonged therapy, monitor serum drug levels and kidney, liver, and hematopoietic function.
• In postpartum patients with pyelonephritis, serum levels mustn't exceed 15 mcg/ml.

Unmarked trade names available in the United States only.
♦ Also available in Canada.   ♦ ♦ Available in Canada only.

- Liver failure is fatal in pregnant patients with renal dysfunction and at daily dosages exceeding 2 g.
- Use parenteral route only when oral administration is not feasible. Switch to oral route as soon as possible.
- Oxytetracycline may be used when penicillin is contraindicated.
- Drug may be used as adjuvant therapy in intestinal amebiasis.
- Dialysis removes moderate amount of drug.

oxytocin, synthetic injection
Pitocin, Syntocinon♦

Pregnancy Risk Category: not applicable

PHARMACOKINETICS
Distribution: throughout extracellular fluid. Drug probably crosses the placenta.
Metabolism: in the liver and kidneys. Drug also is destroyed by oxytocinase, an enzyme produced in early pregnancy.
Excretion: in urine, with small amounts excreted unchanged. Drug appears in breast milk. Half-life is 3 to 5 minutes.
Action: onset, immediate; duration, 20 to 40 minutes.

MECHANISM OF ACTION
Oxytocin acts selectively on uterine and mammary gland smooth muscle, increasing uterine tone and frequency of established contractions. Drug also facilitates lactation.

INDICATIONS & DOSAGE
- Induction and stimulation of labor. *Adults:* usually 1 to 2 milliunits/minute. Dosage is determined by uterine response. May be increased q 15 to 30 minutes in increments of 1 to 2 milliunits/minute until contraction pattern simulates that of normal labor. Maximum dosage, 20 milliunits/minute.
- Incomplete or inevitable abortion. *Adults:* 10 to 20 milliunits/minute. After abortion, 20 to 100 milliunits/minute.
- Control of postpartum uterine bleeding. *Adults:* 20 to 40 milliunits/minute.
- Evaluation of fetal distress after 31 weeks. *Adults:* initially, 0.5 milliunits/minute, increased q 15 minutes to a maximum dosage of 20 milliunits/minute. Stop infusion when three moderate contractions occur within 10 minutes.

CONTRAINDICATIONS & CAUTIONS
- Contraindicated in oxytocin hypersensitivity.
- Also contraindicated during labor in significant cephalopelvic disproportion, cord presentation or prolapse, total placenta previa, uterine inertia, severe toxemia, hypertonic uterine contractions, and fetal distress when delivery isn't imminent.
- Avoid use when vaginal delivery is contraindicated, as in patients with cervical carcinoma.
- Use cautiously in abortion using hypertonic saline because of the increased risk of water intoxication, and in patients with cardiac disease because of the heightened risk of fluid overload, dysrhythmias, hypotension, and reflex tachycardia.
- Because of possible uterine rupture, also use cautiously in patients who have had cervical or uterine surgery.
- Administer carefully in abruptio placentae, borderline cephalopelvic disproportion, grand multiparity, patients over age 35 or those who have a history of sepsis or difficult or

traumatic delivery, partial placenta previa, unengaged fetal head, and unfavorable fetal positions that require predelivery rotation.

PREPARATION & STORAGE
Available in a concentration of 10 units/ml in 10 ml vials, in 0.5 and 1 ml ampules, and in 1 ml disposable syringes. Store below 77° F. (25° C.). If stored correctly, drug reportedly remains stable for 5 years.

For infusion to initiate labor, add 1 ml drug to 1,000 ml of dextrose 5% in water, 0.9% sodium chloride, or Ringer's lactate. For infusion to control postpartum bleeding, add 1 to 4 ml to 1,000 ml of dextrose 5% in water or 0.9% sodium chloride. For use after abortion, thoroughly mix 1 ml of drug with 500 ml of dextrose 5% in 0.9% sodium chloride or with 0.9% sodium chloride. For evaluation of fetal distress, dilute 0.5 to 1 ml in 1,000 ml of dextrose 5% in water.

ADMINISTRATION
Oxytocin should be given only by qualified staff in a hospital with intensive care and surgical facilities.
Direct injection: not recommended.
Intermittent infusion: not recommended.
Continuous infusion: Use an infusion pump. Start I.V. line with 0.9% sodium chloride, adding oxytocin-containing solution as a secondary line to port as close to infusion needle as possible. Discontinue infusion at the first sign of uterine hyperactivity or fetal distress. Don't administer drug for more than 8 hours.

INCOMPATIBILITY
Incompatible with dextran, fibrinolysin, Normosol-M with dextrose 5%, or warfarin sodium.

ADVERSE REACTIONS
Life-threatening: dysrhythmias, fetal intracranial hemorrhage, hypotension, hypertension, increased cardiac output, increased venous return, tachycardia, uterine hyperstimulation (resulting in abruptio placentae, amniotic fluid embolism, impaired uterine blood flow, tetanic contractions, and uterine rupture), water intoxication.
Other: fetal bradycardia, hemorrhage, increased postpartum bleeding (because of oxytocin-induced afibrinogenemia, hypoprothrombinemia, and thrombocytopenia), infection, nausea, neonatal jaundice, paradoxical inhibition of expulsion of placenta, pelvic hematoma, premature ventricular contractions, vomiting.

INTERACTIONS
Caudal block anesthetics with vasoconstrictors: possible severe hypertension.
Cyclopropane, enflurane, halothane, isoflurane: altered cardiovascular effects (decreased tachycardia, worsened hypotension, abnormal atrioventricular rhythms).
Other oxytocics: possible uterine hypertonicity.
Sympathomimetic pressor amines: severe, persistent hypertension and postpartum rupture of cerebral vessels.
Thiopental anesthetics: delayed induction of labor.

EFFECTS ON DIAGNOSTIC TESTS
Serum bilirubin: possible elevated neonatal levels.
Serum chloride, sodium: possible decreased maternal levels.

SPECIAL CONSIDERATIONS

• Keep magnesium sulfate (20% solution) available to relax myometrium.

• Continuously monitor frequency, duration, and force of uterine contractions; resting uterine tone; fetal heart rate; fetal and maternal blood pressure; and intrauterine pressure.

• Stop infusion if contractions occur less than 2 minutes apart, exceed 50 mm Hg, or last longer than 90 seconds. Turn patient on her side, and notify the doctor.

• To avoid antidiuretic effects, restrict fluid intake, avoid prolonged infusion of low-sodium fluids and high oxytocin doses, and monitor intake and output.

• Don't administer simultaneously by more than one route.

pancuronium bromide
Pavulon♦

Pregnancy Risk Category: C

PHARMACOKINETICS

Distribution: widely dispersed in extracellular fluid. Small amounts cross the placenta, especially in the first trimester.

Metabolism: in the liver.

Excretion: about 80% removed in urine and up to 10% in feces as unchanged drug or metabolites. Not known if drug appears in breast milk.

Action: onset, 30 to 45 seconds; duration, 60 to 90 minutes. Because of drug accumulation, duration increases in elderly and debilitated patients and with prolonged administration.

MECHANISM OF ACTION

Drug produces skeletal muscle relaxation. It inhibits neuromuscular transmission by competing with acetylcholine for cholinergic receptors on the motor end plate.

INDICATIONS AND DOSAGE

• Adjunct to anesthesia. *Adults and children over 1 month:* 0.04 to 0.1 mg/kg. Additional doses of 0.01 mg/kg may be given at 25- to 60-minute intervals. *Neonates:* individualized.

• Controlled assisted ventilation. *Adults and children over age 1 month:* 0.015 mg/kg. *Neonates:* individualized.

Note: Large doses may increase frequency and severity of tachycardia.

CONTRAINDICATIONS & CAUTIONS

• Contraindicated in hypersensitivity to pancuronium or bromides, in patients with tachycardia, and in those for whom an increase in heart rate is undesirable.

• Use cautiously in bronchogenic carcinoma, myasthenia gravis, or Eaton-Lambert syndrome because of the risk of increased neuromuscular blockade; in renal impairment because of possible prolonged neuromuscular blockade; and in patients with electrolyte imbalance because of possible altered neuromuscular blocking effects.

• Also use cautiously in hepatic impairment or hyperthermia because of possible diminished intensity or duration of drug effect; and in pulmonary impairment or respiratory depression because of possible worsened respiratory depression.

• Also use cautiously in severe obesity or neuromuscular disease because of possible airway or ventilatory problems.

• Also use cautiously in breast-feeding women.

• In neonates, use cautiously because of increased sensitivity.

PREPARATION & STORAGE
Available in 2 and 5 ml ampules containing 2 mg/ml and in 10 ml vials containing 1 mg/ml. Store at 36° to 46° F. (2° to 8° C.). Drug remains potent for 6 months at room temperature. Don't store in plastic containers. (However, you may give drug in plastic syringes.) For infusion, dilute pancuronium with ordered amount of dextrose 5% in water, 0.9% sodium chloride, or Ringer's lactate.

ADMINISTRATION
Drug should be given only by staff trained in giving I.V. anesthetics and managing adverse reactions.
Direct injection: Slowly inject into an established I.V. line containing a compatible free-flowing solution.
Intermittent infusion: Infuse diluted drug at ordered rate.
Continuous infusion: not recommended.

INCOMPATIBILITY
Incompatible with barbiturates.

ADVERSE REACTIONS
Life-threatening: apnea, bronchospasm.
Other: excessive sweating and salivation (particularly in children), hypersensitivity reactions, hypotension, tachycardia.

INTERACTIONS
Aminoglycosides, capreomycin, citrated blood (massive transfusions), clindamycin, inhalation anesthetics, lincomycin, polymyxin, procaine (I.V.), trimethaphan: enhanced neuromuscular blockade.
Anticholinesterase-like drugs, calcium salts: reversal of neuromuscular blockade.
Antimyasthenics: possible antagonized pancuronium effects.

Beta-adrenergic blockers: possible prolonged effects of pancuronium.
Cardiac glycosides: possible increased effects.
Lidocaine: enhanced neuromuscular blockade and possible potentiated pancuronium blockade.
Lithium, magnesium, potassium-depleting drugs, procainamide, quinidine: possible potentiated pancuronium blockade.
Opioid analgesics: deepened respiratory depression, decreased risk of bradycardia and hypotension, prevention or reversal of opioid-induced muscle rigidity.
Other neuromuscular blocking agents: enhanced neuromuscular blockade.
Succinylcholine: increased intensity and duration of neuromuscular blockade.

EFFECTS ON DIAGNOSTIC TESTS
Neuromuscular tests: unreliable results.

SPECIAL CONSIDERATIONS
• Be prepared to give mechanical ventilation or airway support since apnea will follow administration. Keep antagonists, such as neostigmine and edrophonium, and resuscitation equipment available.
• Closely monitor vital signs. Also monitor serum electrolytes and intake and output.
• Adequate anesthesia is necessary when using pancuronium; drug has no effect on consciousness, pain threshold, or cerebration.
• Keep in mind that the patient may be conscious. Continue to give him explanations and encouragement, reassuring him that drug effects are temporary.
• When moving the patient in bed, protect him from injury. Take special

care with his eyes because of absent blink reflex.
• May contain benzyl alcohol.

---

papaverine hydrochloride

Pregnancy Risk Category: C

PHARMACOKINETICS
Distribution: throughout the body, concentrating in adipose tissue and the liver. About 90% of drug is protein-bound. Not known if drug crosses the placenta.
Metabolism: in the liver.
Excretion: in urine as inactive metabolites. Half-life varies from 30 minutes to 2 hours.

MECHANISM OF ACTION
Drug relaxes vascular and other smooth muscle via phosphodiesterase inhibition, resulting in increased concentrations of cyclic AMP.

INDICATIONS & DOSAGE
• Cerebral and peripheral ischemia associated with arterial spasm and myocardial ischemia; smooth-muscle spasm (coronary occlusion, sequelae of peripheral and pulmonary embolism); and visceral spasm. *Adults:* 30 to 120 mg q 3 hours. *Children:* 1.5 mg/kg q 6 hours.

CONTRAINDICATIONS & CAUTIONS
• Contraindicated in atrioventricular heart block because drug may depress atrioventricular nodal and intraventricular conduction, producing ventricular dysrhythmias.
• Use cautiously in angina or recent cerebrovascular accident because drug further decreases blood flow to ischemic areas, and in depressed myocardial function because large doses may cause exacerbation.

• In glaucoma, administer cautiously because drug may increase intraocular pressure. Also give cautiously in hepatic dysfunction.

PREPARATION AND STORAGE
Available in 30 mg/ml ready-to-use 2 ml ampules and 10 ml vials. Give drug undiluted, or dilute in equal amount of sterile water for injection. Store at 59° to 86° F. (15° to 30° C.).

ADMINISTRATION
Direct injection: Inject directly into vein over 1 to 2 minutes.
Intermittent infusion: not recommended.
Continuous infusion: not recommended.

INCOMPATIBILITY
Incompatible with alkaline solutions, aminophylline with trimecaine hydrochloride, and Ringer's lactate.

ADVERSE REACTIONS
Life-threatening: apnea, dysrhythmias.
Other: blurred vision, diaphoresis, dizziness, drowsiness, flushing, hypertension, hypotension, increased respiratory depth, sedation, tachycardia, thrombosis at injection site.

INTERACTIONS
CNS depressants: increased CNS depression.
Levodopa: decreased effects.
Morphine: increased vasodilation.
Tobacco use (smoking): interference with therapeutic effects.

EFFECTS ON DIAGNOSTIC TESTS
CBC: increased eosinophils.
Serum alkaline phosphatase, bilirubin, SGOT: possible elevated levels.

Unmarked trade names available in the United States only.
♦Also available in Canada.   ♦♦Available in Canada only.

SPECIAL CONSIDERATIONS
• *Treatment of overdose:* Hemodialysis may be useful.
• Monitor liver function tests, and check skin and eye color for signs of jaundice. Discontinue drug if patient has hepatic dysfunction.
• Monitor blood pressure and heart rate and rhythm, especially in patients with coronary artery disease.
• FDA states that papaverine may not be effective for diseases indicated.
• I.V. route is used only when immediate effect is desired.

---

paraldehyde♦♦

Controlled Substance Schedule IV
Pregnancy Risk Category: C

PHARMACOKINETICS
Distribution: widely distributed. Concentration in cerebrospinal fluid is 25% to 30% lower than that in serum. Drug crosses the placenta.
Metabolism: about 80% to 90% metabolized in the liver.
Excretion: through the lungs across the alveolar membrane, with 11% to 28% removed unchanged. Trace amounts excreted in urine. Not known if drug appears in breast milk. Half-life is about 7 hours.
Action: onset, 10 to 15 minutes; duration, about 8 hours.

MECHANISM OF ACTION
Unknown, but drug is thought to depress the reticular activating system.

INDICATIONS & DOSAGE
• Sedation. *Adults:* 5 ml.
• Tetanic seizures. *Adults:* 4 to 5 ml q 4 hours as needed.
• Status epilepticus. *Adults:* 0.2 to 0.4 ml/kg. *Children:* 0.1 to 0.15 ml/kg.

• Insomnia. *Adults:* 10 ml.

CONTRAINDICATIONS & CAUTIONS
• Contraindicated for obstetric anesthesia because of marked fetal respiratory depression.
• Use cautiously in pulmonary disease because of possible respiratory depression and increased bronchial secretions, and in hepatic dysfunction because of risk of toxicity.

PREPARATION & STORAGE
Supplied in 5 and 30 ml vials as a clear, colorless liquid with a strong characteristic odor. Store in well-filled, tightly sealed light-resistant glass container below 77° F. (25° C.). Drug solidifies at about 54° F. (12° C.). Protect from heat, open flame, and sparks. Discard unused contents of container if open more than 24 hours or if solution turns brown or smells like acetic acid. Dilute for infusion by adding ordered dose to 200 ml of 0.9% sodium chloride. Use only glass syringes and infusion containers.

ADMINISTRATION
Direct injection: not recommended.
Intermittent infusion: Infuse diluted dose into established open I.V. line at maximum rate of 1 ml/minute.
Continuous infusion: not recommended.

INCOMPATIBILITY
Incompatible with plastic; drug decomposes.

ADVERSE REACTIONS
Life-threatening: cardiomegaly, circulatory collapse, coma, hypotension, metabolic acidosis, pulmonary edema, pulmonary hemorrhage, respiratory depression, toxic hepatitis.
Other: abdominal cramps, cloudy urine, confusion, decreased urina-

tion, dyspnea, halitosis, muscle twitching, nausea, nephrosis, rash, respiratory distress, severe weakness, tachypnea, thrombophlebitis, vomiting.

INTERACTIONS
Alcohol, antihypertensives with CNS depressant effects, barbiturates, general anesthetics, magnesium sulfate, MAO inhibitors, tricyclic antidepressants, other CNS depressants: deepened CNS depression.
Disulfiram: slowed metabolism of paraldehyde.

EFFECTS ON DIAGNOSTIC TESTS
Phentolamine test, serum and urine ketones: possible false-positive results.
Urine 17-hydroxycorticosteroids: unreliable results using modified Reddy-Jenkins-Thorn procedure.

SPECIAL CONSIDERATIONS
• *Treatment of overdose:* Maintain a patent airway, control respirations, and give oxygen. To treat metabolic acidosis, give sodium bicarbonate or sodium lactate, as ordered.
• Monitor vital signs, especially respirations, during and after administration. Keep suction equipment available to remove excessive bronchial secretions.
• Keep room well ventilated to control odor of exhaled medication.
• Avoid long-term use of larger than therapeutic doses because of potential for tolerance and dependence. After long-term use, taper slowly to avoid withdrawal syndrome. Rapid withdrawal may produce delirium tremens and hallucinations.
• I.V. use recommended for emergencies only because of an increased risk of circulatory collapse and pulmonary edema.

• I.V. form has been largely replaced by less hazardous sedative hypnotics.

---

penicillin G potassium
Pfizerpen

penicillin G sodium
Crystapen♦♦

Pregnancy Risk Category: B

PHARMACOKINETICS
Distribution: widely distributed to most body fluids and bone. Usually poor cerebrospinal fluid (CSF) penetration improves in meningeal inflammation. Drug crosses the placenta and is 45% to 68% protein-bound.
Metabolism: by hydrolysis of beta-lactam ring to inactive penicilloic acid.
Excretion: in urine (10% by glomerular filtration, 90% by renal tubular secretion). About 60% is excreted unchanged in 6 hours. Half-life is 30 minutes to 1 hour. In renal impairment, excretion rate increases twofold to threefold. Drug appears in breast milk.
Action: peak serum level, unknown.

MECHANISM OF ACTION
Both drugs join with penicillin-binding proteins to inhibit bacterial cell-wall synthesis. They act against susceptible gram-positive aerobic bacteria, including non-penicillinase-producing *Staphylococcus aureus; S. epidermidis; Streptococcus pneumoniae;* groups A, B, C, G, H, K, L, and M streptococci; *Streptococcus viridans;* and nonenterococcal group D streptococci. They're also effective against most strains of *Corynebacterium diphtheriae;* many strains of *Bacillus anthracis, Erysipelothrix*

---

*rhusiopathiae,*and *Listeria monocytogenes;* and some strains of enterococci.

Susceptible gram-negative bacteria include *Neisseria meningitidis, Eikenella corrodens, Haemophilus ducreyi, H. influenzae, H. parainfluenzae, Pasteurella multocida, Spirillum minus,* and *Streptobacillus moniliformis;* most strains of non-penicillinase-producing *Neisseria gonorrhoeae;* and some strains of *Bordetella pertussis.*

Both drugs are also active against the anaerobic bacteria *Actinomyces israelii, Arachnia, Bifidobacterium, Clostridium tetani, C. botulinum, C. perfringens, Eubacterium, Lactobacillus, Peptococcus, Peptostreptococcus,* and *Propionibacterium;* and some spirochetes, including *Borrelia recurrentis, Leptospira, Treponema pallidum,* and *T. pertenue.*

INDICATIONS & DOSAGE

Both drugs are given in the same dosages.

• Anthrax. *Adults and children over age 12:* 5 to 20 million units daily in equally divided doses until cured.

• *Clostridium* infection. *Adults and children over age 12:* 20 million units daily.

• Disseminated gonorrhea. *Adults and children weighing at least 45 kg:* 10 million units daily for 3 days. *Children weighing under 45 kg:* 100,000 to 150,000 units/kg daily for 7 days. *Children with meningitis weighing under 45 kg:* 250,000 units/kg daily in six divided doses for 10 days. *Neonates:* 25,000 units/ kg b.i.d. for week 1, then 75,000 units/kg daily in three to four divided doses for weeks 2 to 4. *Neonates with meningitis:* 100,000 units/ kg daily in three to four divided doses for 10 days.

• Endocarditis from enterococci. *Adults and children over age 12:* 20 to 40 million units daily in equally divided doses q 4 hours or by continuous infusion for 4 to 6 weeks.

• Endocarditis from *S. viridans* nonenterococcal group D streptococci. *Adults and children over age 12:* 10 to 20 million units daily in equally divided doses q 4 hours or by continuous infusion for 2 to 4 weeks.

• *Erysipelothrix* endocarditis. *Adults and children over age 12:* 2 to 20 million units daily for 4 to 6 weeks.

• *Fusobacterium* infection. *Adults and children over age 12:* 400,000 to 500,000 units q 6 to 8 hours.

• Gonococcal arthritis and septicemia. *Neonates:* 75,000 to 100,000 units/kg daily in four divided doses for 7 days.

• Gonococcal ophthalmia. *Adults and children over age 12:* 10 million units daily for 5 days. *Neonates:* 100,000 units/kg daily in four divided doses for 7 days.

• *Listeria* infection. *Adults and children over age 12:* 15 to 20 million units daily in equally divided doses for 2 to 4 weeks. *Neonates:* 500,000 to 1 million units daily.

• *N. meningitidis* infection. *Adults and children over age 12:* 20 to 30 million units daily by continuous infusion.

• Prophylaxis for bacterial endocarditis. *Adults and children over age 12:* 2 million units 30 minutes to 1 hour before surgery, then 1 million units 6 hours after surgery.

• *P. multocida* infection. *Adults and children over age 12:* 4 to 6 million units daily for 2 weeks.

• Pulmonary or abdominal actinomycosis. *Adults and children over age 12:* 10 to 20 million units daily for 4 to 6 weeks followed by oral penicillin or tetracycline for an additional 6 to 12 months.

• Rat-bite fever. *Adults and children over age 12:* 12 to 15 million units daily for 3 to 4 weeks.

• Severe infections caused by susceptible streptococci or non-penicillinase-producing staphylococci. *Adults and children over age 12:* 5 to 14 million units daily in equally divided doses q 4 hours.

• Syphilis. *Adults and children over age 12:* 2 to 4 million units q 4 hours for 10 days, then given I.M.

In adults with renal or hepatic impairment, dosage reflects degree of impairment, severity of infection, and susceptible causative organism.

CONTRAINDICATIONS & CAUTIONS

• Contraindicated in hypersensitivity to penicillin and cephalosporins.

• Use cautiously in allergies because of the enhanced risk of hypersensitivity, in GI disorders because of the increased risk of pseudomembranous colitis, and in renal impairment because of reduced drug elimination.

PREPARATION & STORAGE

Available in a variety of vial sizes containing 200,000 or 500,000 units and 1, 5, 10, or 20 million units of penicillin G potassium and 5 million units of penicillin G sodium. Reconstitute with sterile water for injection, 0.9% sodium chloride, or dextrose 5% in water, as manufacturer directs. For intermittent infusion, dilute in 50 to 100 ml of 0.9% sodium chloride or dextrose 5% in water. For continuous infusion, dilute daily dose in 1 to 2 liters of compatible I.V. solution.

To prepare, first loosen powder in vial, then hold vial horizontally while rotating it and slowly directing stream of diluent against vial wall. Shake vigorously. Diluted solution is stable for 24 hours at room temperature and for 7 days at 36° to 46° F. (2° to 8° C.).

ADMINISTRATION

Direct injection: not recommended.
Intermittent infusion: Infuse diluted drug over 1 to 2 hours. For children or neonates, infuse over 15 to 30 minutes.
Continuous infusion: Infuse diluted solution over 24 hours.

INCOMPATIBILITY

Penicillin G potassium is incompatible with amikacin, aminophylline, amphotericin B, cephalothin, chlorpromazine, dextran, dopamine, heparin sodium, hydroxyzine hydrochloride, lincomycin, metaraminol bitartrate, metoclopramide, oxytetracycline, pentobarbital sodium, phenytoin sodium, prochlorperazine mesylate, promazine, promethazine hydrochloride, sodium bicarbonate, tetracycline hydrochloride, thiopental, vancomycin, and vitamin B complex with C.

Penicillin G sodium is incompatible with 10% fat emulsions, 10% invert sugar, amphotericin B, bleomycin, cephalothin sodium, chlorpromazine, heparin sodium, hydroxyzine hydrochloride, lincomycin, methylprednisolone sodium succinate, oxytetracycline, potassium chloride, prochlorperazine mesylate, promethazine hydrochloride, and tetracycline hydrochloride.

ADVERSE REACTIONS

Life-threatening: acute interstitial nephritis, anaphylaxis, coma, congestive heart failure, encephalopathy, hepatotoxicity, hyperkalemia.
Other: arthralgia, asterixis, bacterial and fungal superinfection, coagulation disorders, confusion, dysphagia, eosinophilia, hallucinations, hemolytic anemia, hypernatremia, hyperreflexia, hypotension, Jarisch-Herxheimer reaction (in treatment of syphilis), lethargy, leukopenia, lymphadenopathy, metabolic alka-

losis, myoclonus, neutropenia, phlebitis, pruritus, rash, seizures, thrombocytopenia, thrombocytopenic purpura, thrombophlebitis, twitching, urticaria.

INTERACTIONS

Aminoglycosides: additive or synergistic effect against some organisms.
Chloramphenicol, erythromycin, sulfonamides, tetracycline: possible antagonism of penicillin's bactericidal activity.
Oral contraceptives: decreased efficacy with breakthrough bleeding.
Potassium-sparing diuretics: heightened risk of hyperkalemia with penicillin G potassium.
Probenecid, sulfinpyrazone: increased or prolonged serum penicillin concentrations.
Salicylates: displacement of penicillin from binding sites.

EFFECTS ON DIAGNOSTIC TESTS

Urine delta-aminolevulinic acid (ALA): increased levels, when using Mauzerall and Granick methods.
Cerebrospinal fluid protein: positive results with Folin-Ciocalteau method.
Coombs' test: positive.
Human leukocyte antigen testing: possible interference with results.
Phenolsulfonphthalein and aminohippurate sodium test: depressed excretion.
Phenylketonuria test: unreliable results in neonates.
Serum albumin: possible diminished levels.
Serum potassium, sodium: possible elevated levels.
Serum uric acid: elevated levels.
Urinalysis: possible rise in specific gravity in patients with dehydration or decreased urine output.

Urine glucose: false-positive findings with cupric sulfate tests (Clinitest, Benedict's solution).
Urine protein: false-positive results if biuret reagent is used.
Urine 17-ketogenic steroids and 17-ketosteroids: elevated levels with Norymberski or Zimmerman method.

SPECIAL CONSIDERATIONS

• *Treatment of anaphylaxis:* Discontinue drug and treat symptoms. Anaphylaxis may occur within 30 minutes of infusion. As ordered, administer antihistamines, epinephrine, or corticosteroids. Further treatment may include intubation and cardiopulmonary resuscitation.
• Ask patient about penicillin or cephalosporin allergy before first dose. Negative history doesn't rule out future allergic reaction.
• Obtain specimens for culture and sensitivity tests before first dose. Start therapy immediately.
• Administer penicillin and aminoglycosides separately at different sites.
• Take special care to prevent infusion near major peripheral nerves or blood vessels; severe or permanent neurovascular damage may occur.
• Change I.V. site every 48 hours.
• Monitor vital signs, CBC, prothrombin and partial thromboplastin times, BUN, SGOT, and serum electrolyte and creatinine levels. Monitor intake and output and give fluids.
• Watch for signs of bleeding or hypersensitivity. Monitor for bacterial or fungal superinfection, especially when using indwelling I.V. catheters.
• Use Clinistix or Tes-Tape for urine glucose tests.
• Patients undergoing dialysis may need dosage adjustment. Patients with poor renal function are also at risk of seizures because of high serum concentration of drug.

• Penicillin can be removed by hemodialysis but is minimally removed by peritoneal dialysis.

• Penicillin G potassium and penicillin G sodium differ only in potassium and sodium content: penicillin G potassium contains 1.7 mEq (66 mg) of potassium and 0.3 mEq (7 mg) of sodium per 1 million units; penicillin G sodium contains 2 mEq (46 mg) of sodium per 1 million units.

---

pentamidine isethionate
Pentam

Pregnancy Risk Category: C

PHARMACOKINETICS
Distribution: probably extensive and highly protein-bound. CNS penetration is poor. Not known if drug crosses the placenta.
Metabolism: not known.
Excretion: probably removed in urine unchanged. Half-life is 6.2 to 6.5 hours, longer in renal impairment. Not known if drug appears in breast milk.

MECHANISM OF ACTION
Not fully understood. Drug may inhibit synthesis of DNA, RNA, phospholipids, and protein and interfere with folate transformation. Drug acts against many protozoa, including *Leishmania, Pneumocystis carinii,* and some strains of *Trypanosoma.*

INDICATIONS & DOSAGE
• *P. carinii* pneumonia. *Adults and children:* 4 mg/kg once daily for 14 days. *Alternative children's dosage:* 150 mg/m² once daily for 5 days followed by 100 mg/m² once daily for 9 days. Adults and children with AIDS who don't respond in 14 days may receive drug for 7 more days.

• Leishmaniasis (visceral) caused by *Leishmania donovani. Adults and children:* 2 to 4 mg/kg once daily or every other day up to 15 doses, or 4 mg/kg 3 times weekly for 5 to 25 weeks or longer, depending on response.

• Trypanosomiasis. *Adults and children:* 4 mg/kg once daily for 10 days, or 3 to 4 mg/kg once daily or every other day for 7 to 10 doses.
Note: Adjust dosage in renal impairment. Dosage for adults reflects creatinine clearance. If clearance is less than 10 ml/minute, give usual dose q 48 hours.

CONTRAINDICATIONS & CAUTIONS
• Use cautiously in patients with anemia or a history of bleeding disorders because of the increased risk of blood dyscrasias. Also use cautiously in patients with cardiac disease because of possible cardiotoxicity.
• Because of the increased risk of toxicity, administer the drug cautiously in hepatic or renal impairment.
• Also administer cautiously in diabetes mellitus, hypoglycemia, or hypotension to avoid exacerbation.

PREPARATION & STORAGE
Available as a powder in 300 mg vials. Before reconstituting, store at 36° to 46° F. (2° to 8° C.). Protect both dry powder and reconstituted solution from light. Drug contains no preservatives.

Reconstitute with 3 to 5 ml of sterile water for injection or dextrose 5% in water. For infusion, dilute further in 50 to 250 ml of dextrose 5% in water.

Solutions of 1 to 2.5 mg/ml remain potent for up to 24 hours at room temperature. Discard any unused portion. Reportedly, reconsti-

---

tuted solutions in dilution of 1 to 2 mg/ml remain stable for 48 hours if stored in PVC bags at 72° to 79° F. (22° to 26° C.) in normal fluorescent light. However, small amounts may be absorbed into PVC infusion sets.

ADMINISTRATION
Direct injection: not recommended.
Intermittent infusion: Infuse diluted drug over 60 minutes.
Continuous infusion: not recommended.

INCOMPATIBILITY
No incompatibilities reported.

ADVERSE REACTIONS
Life-threatening: anaphylaxis, bronchospasm, dysrhythmias, hypoglycemia, hypotension, Stevens-Johnson syndrome.
Other: abdominal pain; acute pancreatitis; anemia; anorexia; anxiety; blurred vision; chills; cold, pale skin; cold sweats; confusion; diabetes mellitus; diarrhea; dizziness; drowsiness; fainting; fatigue; fever; flushed, red, dry skin; fruity breath odor; hallucinations; headache; hyperglycemia; hyperkalemia; hypocalcemia; Jarisch-Herxheimer reaction (in patients with *P. carinii* pneumonia); leukopenia; light-headedness; metallic taste; nausea; nephrotoxicity; neuralgia; phlebitis; pruritus; rapid or irregular pulse; rash; shakiness; thrombocytopenia; toxic epidermal necrolysis; unusual hunger or thirst; vomiting; weakness.

INTERACTIONS
Other nephrotoxic drugs: possible worsened nephrotoxicity.

EFFECTS ON DIAGNOSTIC TESTS
BUN, serum creatinine, potassium: possible increased levels.
Platelet count: reduced.

Serum alkaline phosphatase, bilirubin, SGOT, SGPT: possible elevated levels.
Serum calcium: possible diminished levels.
Serum glucose: possible elevated or reduced levels.

SPECIAL CONSIDERATIONS
• Because drug may cause severe hypotension, keep patient supine during administration and for several hours afterward. Closely monitor blood pressure, and keep resuscitation equipment available.
• Because of possible severe adverse reactions, give drug only to patients who test positive for susceptible organisms.
• Monitor fluid status (especially in AIDS patients because they're at risk for dehydration) to ensure adequate hydration and minimize possible nephrotoxicity.
• Before, during, and after therapy, monitor CBC, platelets, and EKG. Also monitor SGOT, SGPT, BUN and serum alkaline phosphatase, bilirubin, calcium, creatinine, and glucose levels.
• Severe hypoglycemia (serum glucose less than 25 mg/dl) may occur in up to 10% of patients. Have 50% dextrose available for I.V. use. Monitor blood glucose levels carefully.

pentazocine lactate
Talwin♦

Controlled Substance Schedule IV
Pregnancy Risk Category: B
(D with prolonged use or with high doses at term)

PHARMACOKINETICS
Distribution: widely dispersed to all tissues. Drug is 60% bound to

plasma proteins. It crosses the placenta.

Metabolism: in the liver.

Excretion: in urine; small amount in feces. Drug appears in breast milk.

Action: onset, 2 to 3 minutes; peak effect, 15 to 30 minutes; duration, 2 to 3 hours.

MECHANISM OF ACTION

A partial opiate agonist, pentazocine binds with opiate receptors at many CNS sites, thus altering the perception of pain and the emotional response to it. As a weak antagonist, pentazocine doesn't reverse opiate-induced respiratory depression, but may precipitate withdrawal in opiate-dependent patients. Its exact mechanism of action is unknown.

INDICATIONS & DOSAGE

• Pain. *Adults and children over age 12:* 30 mg (maximum single dose) q 3 to 4 hours as needed. Maximum daily dose, 360 mg.

• Obstetric pain. *Adults:* 20 mg when contractions become regular, then 20 mg q 2 to 3 hours as needed for 2 or 3 doses.

CONTRAINDICATIONS & CAUTIONS

• Contraindicated in hypersensitivity to drug, in diarrhea associated with pseudomembranous colitis or poisoning because of delayed elimination of toxins, and in acute respiratory depression because drug may exacerbate the condition.

• Use cautiously in chronic respiratory impairment or during acute asthma attack because drug decreases respiratory drive and increases airway resistance; in patients with head injury, elevated intracranial pressure, or intracranial lesions because deepened respiratory depression raises intracranial pressure and drug may mask symptoms; and

in hypothyroidism because of possible worsened respiratory depression and prolonged CNS depression.

• Also use cautiously in acute abdominal conditions because drug may mask symptoms, in gallbladder disease because of possible biliary contraction, in recent GI surgery because GI motility may slow, in inflammatory bowel disease because of the heightened risk of toxic megacolon, and in hepatic impairment because of diminished drug metabolism.

• In obstructive urinary disease, prostatic hypertrophy, and recent urinary tract surgery, give drug cautiously because of possible urine retention.

• In renal impairment, also give cautiously because of possible increased toxicity.

• Administer pentazocine carefully in patients with seizures or dysrhythmias because of possible precipitation or exacerbation, and in patients with acute MI because drug increases arterial pressure and systemic vascular resistance.

• Patients with a history of substance abuse or emotional instability face a greater risk of habituation. Those with opioid-agonist dependence may develop withdrawal symptoms. Use appropriate caution.

• Safety in children under age 12 hasn't been established.

PREPARATION AND STORAGE

Available in concentrations of 30 mg/ml in 1, 1.5, and 2 ml ampules; in 1, 1.5, and 2 ml disposable syringes; and in 10 ml multidose vials. Store below 104° F. (40° C.), preferably at room temperature. Protect from freezing. No dilution necessary.

ADMINISTRATION

Direct injection: Inject drug slowly into I.V. tubing containing a compatible free-flowing solution. Monitor patient tolerance. Rapid injection may lead to anaphylaxis, peripheral circulatory collapse, or cardiac arrest.

Intermittent infusion: not recommended.

Continuous infusion: not recommended.

INCOMPATIBILITY
Incompatible with aminophylline, amobarbital sodium, glycopyrrolate, pentobarbital sodium, phenobarbital sodium, secobarbital sodium, and sodium bicarbonate.

ADVERSE REACTIONS
Life-threatening: respiratory depression.

Other: abdominal pain, altered taste, anorexia, blurred vision, chills, circulatory depression, confusion, constipation, diaphoresis, diarrhea, diplopia, disorientation, dizziness, drowsiness, dry mouth, dysuria, edema, euphoria, excitement, faintness, flushed skin, hallucinations, headache, hypertension, insomnia, irritability, leukopenia, light-headedness, miosis, muscle tremors, nausea, nystagmus, paresthesias, pruritus, rash, sclerosis at injection site (if I.V. line is infiltrated), sedation, seizures, syncope, tachycardia, tinnitus, toxic epidermal necrolysis, unusual dreams, urine retention, urticaria, vertigo, vomiting.

INTERACTIONS
Antihypertensives, diuretics: potentiated hypotensive effect.

Antimuscarinics: heightened risk of severe constipation, paralytic ileus, and urine retention.

Antiperistaltic antidiarrheals: increased risk of severe constipation and deepened CNS depression.

Buprenorphine: possible reduced therapeutic effect of pentazocine.

CNS depressants: enhanced risk of CNS and respiratory depression, hypotension, and habituation.

MAO inhibitors: magnified risk of adverse reactions, necessitating lower pentazocine doses.

Naloxone: antagonized CNS and respiratory depressant effects.

Naltrexone: antagonized therapeutic effects and possible precipitation of withdrawal symptoms in physically dependent patients.

Neuromuscular blocking agents: deepened or prolonged respiratory depression.

Opioid agonist analgesics: additive CNS and respiratory depression and hypotension.

EFFECTS ON DIAGNOSTIC TESTS
Cerebrospinal fluid (CSF) analysis: possible elevated CSF pressure.

Gastric emptying: delayed.

Hepatic imaging: with technetium Tc 99m disofenin, delayed visualization.

Serum amylase, lipase: possible elevated levels.

SPECIAL CONSIDERATIONS
• *Treatment of overdose:* Reverse severe respiratory depression with naloxone, as ordered. Then treat supportively.

• During administration, closely monitor respiratory status.

• Keep patient supine during administration to minimize hypotension. Advise him to rise slowly to reduce faintness and dizziness.

• In patients on long-term therapy with other opiate agonists, give only 25% of initial pentazocine dose and monitor for withdrawal symptoms. If necessary, give dose slowly in small increments. If no adverse reactions occur, increase dose progressively to desired level of analgesia.

- Elderly patients may require lower doses.
- Dependence can occur with long-term use.
- May contain sulfites.

---

pentobarbital sodium
Nembutal♦

Controlled Substance Schedule II
Pregnancy Risk Category: D

PHARMACOKINETICS
Distribution: widely distributed with highest concentrations in the brain, liver, and kidneys. Drug is 35% to 40% bound to plasma proteins. It readily crosses the placenta.
Metabolism: by hepatic microsomal enzymes.
Excretion: in urine, with less than 1% removed unchanged. Drug appears in breast milk.
Action: onset, within 1 minute; duration, 15 minutes.

MECHANISM OF ACTION
Essentially unknown. Pentobarbital depresses the CNS, interfering with transmission of impulses to cortex.

INDICATIONS & DOSAGE
- Insomnia, anesthesia (adjunct), and seizures. *Adults:* 100 mg initially, then smaller doses as needed at 1-minute intervals, to a maximum of 500 mg. Dose is lower in elderly. *Children:* 50 mg initially, then smaller doses at 1-minute intervals until desired effect is reached.
- Cerebral ischemia or cerebral edema following stroke, head trauma, or Reye's syndrome (barbiturate coma). *Adults:* 1 to 3 mg/kg/hour I.V. after initial loading dose sufficient to produce burst suppression of electroencephalogram, or EEG (5 to 34 mg/kg).

CONTRAINDICATIONS & CAUTIONS
- Contraindicated in hypersensitivity to barbiturates and in patients with intermittent or variegate porphyria because the drug may aggravate symptoms.
- Use cautiously in severe anemia, hyperkinesis, and hyperthyroidism because drug may aggravate these conditions; in asthma because of increased risk of hypersensitivity reactions, such as bronchospasm; and in respiratory dysfunction because of possible additive respiratory depression.
- Also administer cautiously in borderline hyperadrenalism because pentobarbital diminishes the effects of exogenous hydrocortisone and endogenous cortisol; in pain because drug may cause paradoxical excitement or mask symptoms; in hepatic impairment because of decreased drug metabolism; and in renal impairment because of reduced drug excretion.
- Because of the risk of habituation, administer carefully to patients with a history of substance abuse or emotional instability.
- Also administer cautiously to depressed patients because pentobarbital may worsen suicidal tendencies.

PREPARATION & STORAGE
Available in concentrations of 50 mg/ml in 2 ml vials, in 1 and 2 ml prefilled syringes, and in 20 and 50 ml multidose vials. Store at room temperature. Drug is compatible with most common solutions, such as dextrose 5% in water and 0.9% sodium chloride.

ADMINISTRATION
Direct injection: Inject drug into I.V. tubing of free-flowing compatible solution at a rate not exceeding 50 ml/minute. Avoid extravasation;

---

solution is alkaline and may cause local tissue damage and necrosis. Guard against inadvertent intra-arterial injection, which may cause arterial spasm, severe pain, and possibly gangrene.
Intermittent infusion: not recommended.
Continuous infusion: not recommended.

INCOMPATIBILITY
Incompatible with benzquinamide, butorphanol, chlorpheniramine, chlorpromazine, cimetidine, codeine phosphate, dimenhydrinate, diphenhydramine, droperidol, ephedrine, fentanyl citrate, glycopyrrolate, hydrocortisone sodium succinate, hydroxyzine hydrochloride, insulin (regular), meperidine, methadone hydrochloride, midazolam hydrochloride, morphine, nalbuphine, norepinephrine, opium alkaloids, oxytetracycline, penicillin G potassium, pentazocine lactate, perphenazine, phenytoin sodium, prochlorperazine edisylate, promazine, promethazine hydrochloride, ranitidine hydrochloride, sodium bicarbonate, streptomycin, succinylcholine, tetracycline hydrochloride, triflupromazine, and vancomycin.

ADVERSE REACTIONS
Life-threatening: apnea, bronchospasm, coma, exfoliative dermatitis, laryngospasm, respiratory depression, severe bradycardia and junctional rhythms, Stevens-Johnson syndrome.
Other: angioedema, agranulocytosis, arthralgia, CNS depression, constipation, cough, delirium, depression, diarrhea, drowsiness, euphoria, fever, hangover, headache, hypotension, impaired judgment, impaired motor skills, insomnia, lethargy, megaloblastic anemia, mood distortion, myalgia, nausea, neuralgia, nightmares, pain at injection site, paradoxical excitement, photosensitivity, rash, restlessness, serum sickness, thrombocytopenic purpura, thrombophlebitis, urticaria, vasodilation, vertigo, vomiting.

INTERACTIONS
Ascorbic acid: increased excretion.
Calcium channel blockers: excessive hypotension during titration.
Carbamazepine: increased metabolism and decreased serum concentrations of either drug.
Carbonic anhydrase inhibitors: enhanced risk of osteopenia.
Cardiac glycosides, corticosteroids, cyclosporine, dacarbazine, levothyroxine, oral anticoagulants, quinidine: enhanced metabolism and decreased efficacy.
CNS depressants: additive CNS depression and heightened risk of habituation.
Cyclophosphamide: intensified leukopenia.
Disopyramide, griseofulvin: reduced serum levels, resulting in ineffective disopyramide response (effect on griseofulvin response unknown).
Divalproex sodium, valproic acid: deepened CNS depression and neurologic toxicity.
Doxycycline: shortened half-life.
Guanadrel, guanethidine, loop diuretics: increased orthostatic hypotension.
Halogenated hydrocarbon anesthetics: magnified risk of hepatotoxicity.
Haloperidol: altered pattern and frequency of seizures.
Hydantoin anticonvulsants: unpredictable effects.
Hypothermia-producing drugs: enhanced risk of hypothermia.
Ketamine: heightened risk of hypotension or respiratory depression.
Leucovorin: antagonized anticonvulsant effects of pentobarbital.

Loxapine, phenothiazines, thioxan-thines: lowered seizure threshold. Expect to adjust dosage.

MAO inhibitors: pro longed CNS depression and possible alteration of seizure pattern.

Maprotiline: enhanced CNS depressant effects and diminished anticonvulsant effects.

Methylphenidate: increased risk of pentobarbital toxicity.

Mexiletine: accelerated metabolism, decreasing plasma concentration.

Posterior pituitary hormones: heightened risk of dysrhythmias and coronary insufficiency.

Primidone: altered seizure pattern.

Tricyclic antidepressants: decreased efficacy and enhanced CNS depression.

Vitamin D: reduced efficacy.

Xanthines: increased theophylline clearance, resulting in subtherapeutic serum levels.

EFFECTS ON DIAGNOSTIC TESTS

Cyanocobalamin ^{57}Co: impaired absorption.

Phentolamine test: false-positive results.

Serum bilirubin: possible decreased levels.

Sulfobromophthalein test: increased retention, causing elevated results.

SPECIAL CONSIDERATIONS

• For seizures, use minimum doses to avoid augmented postseizure CNS and respiratory depression.

• Keep emergency resuscitation equipment available.

• Monitor vital signs, blood pressure, and cardiac function.

• Monitor EEG and blood levels when used for barbiturate coma. Patient will require mechanical ventilation.

---

perphenazine
Trilafon♦

Pregnancy Risk Category: C

PHARMACOKINETICS

Distribution: to most fluids and tissues with high concentrations in the brain, lungs, liver, kidneys, and spleen. Drug is highly bound to plasma proteins. It crosses the placenta.

Metabolism: in the liver.

Excretion: primarily eliminated in urine, mostly as metabolites, with some drug excreted in feces. Drug probably appears in breast milk.

Action: onset, unknown; duration, unknown.

MECHANISM OF ACTION

Controls severe nausea and vomiting by inhibiting the medullary chemoreceptor trigger zone.

INDICATIONS & DOSAGE

• Severe vomiting, intractable hiccups, violent retching during surgery. *Adults:* 1 mg at no less than 1- to 2-minute intervals for 5 mg total, or maximum dose of 5 mg by infusion.

CONTRAINDICATIONS & CAUTIONS

• Contraindicated in hypersensitivity to perphenazine and related compounds.

• Also contraindicated in severe CNS depression, coma, severe cardiovascular disease, bone marrow depression or blood dyscrasias.

• Use cautiously in alcoholism because drug may enhance CNS depression; in glaucoma, peptic ulcers, or urine retention because drug may exacerbate these disorders; and in symptomatic prostatic hypertrophy

---

because drug may increase urinary retention.
• Also use cautiously in seizure disorders because of lowered seizure threshold, and in Reye's syndrome, encephalitis, encephalopathy, intestinal obstruction, brain tumor, meningitis, or tetanus because drug may mask signs.
• Elderly or debilitated patients are especially sensitive to the drug's antimuscarinic or sedative effects. Use with caution.
• Administer carefully in hepatic impairment because decreased drug metabolism enhances CNS effects, in patients with history of hepatic encephalopathy secondary to cirrhosis because of heightened sensitivity to CNS effects, and in renal impairment because of reduced drug excretion.
• Also administer cautiously in chronic respiratory disorders or acute respiratory infections because respiratory depression may worsen, and in hypocalcemia because dystonic reactions are more likely.

PREPARATION & STORAGE
Available in 1 ml ampules containing 5 mg/ml. Dilute to 0.5 mg/ml by adding 1 ml of drug to 10 ml of 0.9% sodium chloride for direct injection or to an ordered amount for infusion. Store at 59° to 86° F. (15° to 30° C.). Slight yellow discoloration won't affect potency or efficacy, but discard if markedly discolored or if a precipitate forms.

ADMINISTRATION
Direct injection: Inject into an I.V. line containing a free-flowing compatible solution at 1- to 2-minute intervals.
Intermittent infusion: Infuse drug slowly into an I.V. line containing a free-flowing compatible solution.
Continuous infusion: not recommended.

INCOMPATIBILITY
Incompatible with aminophylline, cefoperazone sodium, opium alkaloids hydrochloride, midazolam, oxytocin, pentobarbital sodium, and thiethylperazine maleate.

ADVERSE REACTIONS
Life-threatening: anaphylaxis, bronchospasm, cardiac arrest, laryngeal edema.
Other: angioedema, anorexia, constipation, contact dermatitis, diarrhea, dizziness, dyspepsia, hypotension, paralytic ileus, syncope, tachycardia.

INTERACTIONS
Amantadine, antidyskinetics, antihistamines, antimuscarinics: potentiated antimuscarinic effects.
Amphetamines: diminished effects.
Beta-adrenergic blockers: elevated levels of these drugs and perphenazine.
CNS depressants: additive CNS and respiratory depression and hypotension.
Dopamine: antagonized peripheral vasoconstriction.
Ephedrine, mephentermine, metaraminol, methoxamine, phenylephrine: reduced pressor response of these drugs; also, shortened duration of methoxamine and phenylephrine.
Epinephrine: possible severe hypotension and tachycardia, resulting from alpha-adrenergic blockade.
Extrapyramidal reaction–causing drugs: enhanced severity and frequency of reactions.
Levodopa: reduced effectiveness.
MAO inhibitors, tricyclic antidepressants: prolonged and intensified sedative and antimuscarinic effects.
Metrizamide: possible lowered seizure threshold.
Quinidine: additive cardiac effects.

EFFECTS ON DIAGNOSTIC TESTS

EKG: Q- and T-wave changes.
Gonadorelin test: blunted response, resulting from increased serum prolactin.
Metyrapone test: reduced corticotropin secretion.
Urine amylase, bilirubin, 5-hydroxyindolacetic acid, porphobilinogens, urobilinogen, uroporphyrins: possible false-positive results.

SPECIAL CONSIDERATIONS

• Keep patient supine during and for 30 to 60 minutes after administration. Monitor blood pressure before and after administration.
• For severe hypotension requiring a vasopressor, use norepinephrine or phenylephrine. Do not give epinephrine.

---

phenobarbital sodium
Luminal♦

Controlled Substance Schedule IV
Pregnancy Risk Category: D

PHARMACOKINETICS

Distribution: widely distributed to all tissues. Drug crosses the blood-brain barrier and the placenta.
Metabolism: in the liver.
Excretion: primarily in urine. Small amounts are removed in feces. Drug appears in breast milk. Half-life ranges from 2 to 5 days.
Action: onset, 5 minutes; duration, 4 to 6 hours, but sedative effect may persist for up to 10 hours.

MECHANISM OF ACTION

Not fully understood. Drug probably decreases nerve cell excitability in the cerebral cortex and reticular formation. Anticonvulsant effect may result from gamma-aminobutyric acid–like activity in the motor cortex.

INDICATIONS & DOSAGE

• Status epilepticus and acute seizure disorders. *Adults:* 200 to 600 mg, or 40 to 120 mg at 5- to 10-minute intervals. Don't exceed 20 mg/kg total dosage. *Children:* 100 to 400 mg, or 20 to 80 mg at 5- to 10-minute intervals. Don't exceed 20 mg/kg total dosage.

CONTRAINDICATIONS & CAUTIONS

• Contraindicated in hypersensitivity to barbiturates.
• Also contraindicated in severe pulmonary disease because drug-induced respiratory depression further compromises ventilation, and in patients with a history of acute intermittent or variegate porphyria because the drug exacerbates these disorders.
• Use cautiously in hepatic or renal impairment because of slowed drug metabolism and excretion; in patients with elevated serum ammonia because the drug impairs the liver's ability to metabolize ammonia; in patients with cardiovascular disease or unstable blood pressure because of increased adverse cardiovascular effects or hypotension; and in patients with acute or chronic pain, in the elderly, and in children because these groups are more susceptible to paradoxical CNS excitement.
• In diabetes mellitus, hyperthyroidism, and hypothyroidism, give carefully because symptoms may worsen.
• Be cautious when giving drug to patients with a history of drug abuse, depression, or suicidal tendencies because of potential for sedative effects and abuse.

PREPARATION & STORAGE

Available in single-dose vials, ampules, and prefilled syringes in concentrations of 30, 60, 65, 120, and 130 mg/ml. Discard if solution contains precipitate. Drug is compatible with commonly used I.V. solutions.

ADMINISTRATION

Direct injection: Inject dose slowly, not exceeding 60 mg/minute, into vein or I.V. tubing containing a freely flowing compatible solution. Observe injection site for signs of thrombophlebitis. If patient reports local pain, stop injection and check cannula placement. Avoid extravasation; high alkalinity of drug causes tissue necrosis.

Intermittent infusion: not recommended.

Continuous infusion: not recommended.

INCOMPATIBILITY

Incompatible with alcohol–dextrose solutions, cephalothin sodium, chlorpromazine hydrochloride, codeine phosphate, ephedrine hydrochloride, hydralazine, hydrocortisone sodium succinate, insulin (regular), levorphanol, meperidine, morphine, norepinephrine, oxytetracycline, pentazocine lactate, prochlorperazine mesylate, promazine, promethazine hydrochloride, ranitidine hydrochloride, streptomycin, tetracycline hydrochloride, and vancomycin.

ADVERSE REACTIONS

Life-threatening: overly rapid injection can cause apnea, bronchospasm, hypotension, and laryngospasm.

Other: agranulocytosis, ataxia, bradycardia, coma, confusion, delirium, depression, drowsiness, diarrhea, epigastric pain, euphoria, fever, headache, hypoventilation, impaired judgment, joint or muscle pain, lethargy, megaloblastic anemia, nausea, nightmares, pain or thrombophlebitis at injection site, paradoxical excitement, rash, restlessness, rhinitis, severe subcutaneous necrosis, thrombocytopenic purpura, urticaria, vertigo.

INTERACTIONS

CNS depressants: deepened CNS depression.

Ascorbic acid, chlorpromazine: increased excretion.

Calcium channel blockers: excessive hypotension.

Carbamazepine: decreased serum concentration and reduced half-life of both drugs.

Carbonic anhydrase inhibitors: possible enhanced osteopenia.

Cardiac glycosides, corticosteroids, fenoprofen, levothyroxine, quinidine, tricyclic antidepressants, xanthines: diminished effects, resulting from increased hepatic metabolism.

Coumarin or indanedione-derivative anticoagulants: reduced prothrombin time and anticoagulant effects.

Cyclophosphamide: increased leukopenia, resulting from reduced half-life.

Disopyramide, griseofulvin, mexiletine: lowered serum concentrations. Disopyramide loses efficacy.

Disulfiram, MAO inhibitors: reduced phenobarbital metabolism, prolonging drug's effect.

Divalproex sodium, valproic acid: possible enhanced CNS toxicity.

Doxycycline: depressed antibiotic activity.

Estrogens: reduced efficacy.

Guanadrel, guanethidine, loop diuretics: enhanced risk of orthostatic hypotension.

Halogenated inhalation anesthetics: increased risk of hepatotoxicity or nephrotoxicity.

Haloperidol, loxapine, maprotiline, phenothizines, primidone, thioxanthines: possible lowered seizure threshhold.

Hydantoin anticonvulsants: variable and unpredictable metabolism.
Hypothermia-producing drugs: heightened risk of hypothermia.
Ketamine: augmented risk of hypotension and respiratory depression.
Leucovorin: antagonized anticonvulsant effect.
Phenytoin: possible increased or decreased levels.
Vitamin D: reduced efficacy.

EFFECTS ON DIAGNOSTIC TESTS

Cyanocobalamin ^{57}Co: impaired absorption.
Phentolamine test: false-positive results.
Serum bilirubin: possible decreased levels.

SPECIAL CONSIDERATIONS

• *Treatment of overdose:* Signs include clammy skin, coma, cyanosis, hypotension, and pupillary constriction. Treatment is chiefly supportive. Maintain a patent airway, using oxygen and assisted ventilation as necessary. Keep patient well hydrated with I.V. fluids, and give sodium bicarbonate to alkalinize urine and increase drug excretion. In severe overdose, peritoneal dialysis and hemodialysis are helpful. Keep resuscitation equipment readily available.
• Establish baseline blood pressure and continuously monitor for hypotension.
• Obtain baseline respiratory rate, and continuously monitor. If rate falls below 12 breaths/minute, notify the doctor. If below 8 breaths/minute, rouse the patient and encourage him to breathe more deeply (to rate of at least 12 breaths/minute). If patient can't be aroused, manually ventilate him at 12 to 16 breaths/minute with hand-held respirator. Notify doctor immediately, and prepare for possible intubation.

• Discontinue drug immediately if a skin reaction occurs; it may indicate a possibly fatal reaction.
• For full anticonvulsant effect, wait 30 minutes after initial dose before giving additional doses. Maintain serum level at 15 to 40 mcg/ml. Halt injections when seizures stop or when total dosage is reached.
• Tolerance may develop after about 2 weeks of therapy.
• In patients receiving anticoagulants, closely monitor prothrombin time; adjust anticoagulant dosage as needed.
• Don't give drug within 24 hours of liver function tests.
• Drug dependence and severe withdrawal symptoms may follow long-term therapy. When discontinuing drug, withdraw single dose over 5 to 6 days to prevent withdrawal symptoms and rebound rapid-eye-movment stage of sleep.
• Diazepam is the drug of choice for status epilepticus. Because of slow onset time, phenobarbital's usefulness is limited.

phentolamine mesylate
Regitine, Rogitine♦♦

Pregnancy Risk Category: C

PHARMACOKINETICS

Distribution: not well characterized. Not known if drug crosses the blood-brain barrier or the placenta.
Metabolism: not known.
Excretion: in urine. About 10% is excreted unchanged. Fate of remainder isn't known. Not known if drug appears in breast milk.
Action: onset, 2 minutes; duration, 15 to 30 minutes.

MECHANISM OF ACTION

Phentolamine produces alpha-adrenergic blockade, thereby inhibiting response to adrenergic stimuli. Drug also antagonizes effects of circulating epinephrine and norepinephrine, causing vasodilation and reducing peripheral vascular resistance. In CHF, phentolamine reduces preload and pulmonary artery pressure, increases cardiac output, and exerts a positive inotropic effect.

INDICATIONS & DOSAGE

• Diagnosis of pheochromocytoma. *Adults:* 5 mg. *Children:* 1 mg or 0.1 mg/kg.
• Hypertension in pheochromocytoma before surgical removal of tumor. *Adults:* 5 mg 1 to 2 hours before surgery. *Children:* 1 mg or 0.1 mg/kg 1 to 2 hours before surgery, repeated if needed.
• Left ventricular failure secondary to acute MI. *Adults:* 0.17 to 0.4 mg/minute by continuous infusion.
• Norepinephrine extravasation. *Adults:* 10 mg in 10 ml of 0.9% sodium chloride into affected tissues within 12 hours of extravasation.
• Prevention of severe tissue sloughing in norepinephrine infusion. *Adults:* 10 mg added to each 1,000 ml norepinephrine infusion.
• Hypertensive crisis from interaction between MAO inhibitor and sympathomimetic amines. *Adults:* 5 to 10 mg.

CONTRAINDICATIONS & CAUTIONS

• Contraindicated in sensitivity to phentolamine or related drugs and possibly in acute MI.
• Use cautiously in coronary artery disease, angina, or past MI because reflex tachycardia may precipitate angina or CHF; also in gastritis or peptic ulcer to avoid exacerbating these disorders.

PREPARATION & STORAGE

Supplied in 5 mg vials with 1 ml ampule of sterile water for injection as diluent. Store unreconstituted powder at room temperature. Reconstitute with diluent to 5 mg/ml. Reconstituted product remains stable for 48 hours at room temperature or for 7 days at 36° to 46° F. (2° to 8° C.). Manufacturer recommends that solution be used immediately after reconstitution. For infusion, dilute 5 to 10 mg of drug in 500 ml of 0.9% sodium chloride.

ADMINISTRATION

Direct injection: Delay injection until venipuncture effect subsides, then rapidly inject 5 mg.
Intermittent infusion: not recommended.
Continuous infusion: Infuse at rate ordered for norepinephrine solution; to treat left ventricular failure, infuse at rate necessary to control symptoms, using infusion pump.

INCOMPATIBILITY

None known.

ADVERSE REACTIONS

Life-threatening: anaphylaxis, cerebral vascular spasm or occlusion, MI.
Other: abdominal pain, acute and prolonged or orthostatic hypotension, angina, confusion, diarrhea, dizziness, dyspnea, dysrhythmias, exacerbation of peptic ulcer, flushing, incoordination, nasal congestion, nausea, severe or sudden headache, slurred speech, tachycardia, vomiting, weakness.

INTERACTIONS

Diazoxide: diminished effects.
Dopamine: antagonized peripheral vasoconstriction.
Ephedrine, metaraminol, phenylephrine: decreased pressor response.

Epinephrine: possible severe hypotension and tachycardia.
Guanadrel, guanethidine: increased incidence of bradycardia or orthostatic hypotension.
Methoxamine (preceded by phentolamine): possible blocked pressor response with severe hypotension.

EFFECTS ON DIAGNOSTIC TESTS
Phentolamine test: false-positive results in uremic patients or patients who receive sedatives, opiates, or antihypertensive drugs.

SPECIAL CONSIDERATIONS
• In severe hypotension or other signs of shock, treat with norepinephrine and supportive measures. For dysrhythmias, administer cardiac glycosides. Don't use epinephrine.
• When treating left ventricular failure, continuously monitor EKG and left ventricular function.
• Don't give sedatives or narcotics in the 24 hours before pheochromocytoma test. Halt rauwolfia alkaloids at least 4 weeks before.
• Before performing pheochromocytoma test, make sure that patient's blood pressure has returned to pretreatment level. Give drug rapidly, recording blood pressure immediately after injection, every 30 seconds for 3 minutes, then every 60 seconds for 7 more minutes. Severe hypotension after test dose indicates pheochromocytoma.

---

phenylephrine hydrochloride
Neo-Synephrine Injection♦

Pregnancy Risk Category: C

PHARMACOKINETICS
Distribution: in plasma.

Metabolism: in the liver and intestines by monoamine oxidase.
Excretion: in urine. Not known if drug appears in breast milk.
Action: onset, immediate; duration, 15 to 20 minutes.

MECHANISM OF ACTION
This drug stimulates alpha-adrenergic receptors (with little, if any, effect on beta-adrenergic receptors), causing vasoconstriction and increasing blood pressure.

INDICATIONS & DOSAGE
• Shock or severe hypotension.
Adults: initially, 0.1 to 0.18 mg/minute; then, after blood pressure stabilizes, 0.04 to 0.06 mg/minute.
• Mild to moderate hypotension.
Adults: 0.1 to 0.5 mg (usual dose, 0.2 mg). Subsequent doses given at intervals of at least 10 minutes.
• Paroxysmal atrial tachycardia.
Adults: initial dose, 0.5 mg. Administer subsequent doses in increments of 0.1 to 0.2 mg, depending on blood pressure (systolic not to exceed 160 mm Hg), with no single dose exceeding 1 mg.
• Hypotensive emergencies during spinal anesthesia. *Adults:* initial dose, 0.2 mg. Give later doses in increments of 0.1 to 0.2 mg, with no single dose exceeding 0.5 mg.

CONTRAINDICATIONS & CAUTIONS
• Contraindicated in ventricular tachycardia because of arrhythmogenic effects; in severe hypertension because of possible exacerbation; in MI because of possible increased cardiac work and ischemia; and in hypersensitivity to phenylephrine or sulfites.
• Also contraindicated in mesenteric or peripheral vascular thrombosis, acute pancreatitis, or hepatitis because drug may precipitate or ag-

gravate ischemia or infarction in affected organ.
• Give cautiously in hyperthyroidism because of the increased risk of bradycardia; in incomplete heart block because of possible exacerbation; in severe arteriosclerosis because of possible ischemia; and in myocardial disease because of increased cardiac work and possible exacerbation of heart failure.
• In the elderly, use drug with caution because of diminished cerebral and coronary circulation.
• I.V. use isn't recommended in children.

PREPARATION & STORAGE
Available in 1 ml ampules and disposable cartridge units (10 mg/ml or 1% solution). Store at room temperature. Discard brown or particulate-containing solutions. For infusion, dilute 10 mg in 500 ml of dextrose 5% in water or 0.9% sodium chloride. Discard diluted solutions after 48 hours. Drug is compatible with most I.V. solutions.

ADMINISTRATION
Direct injection: Inject dose over 1 minute to treat mild to moderate hypotension or hypotensive emergencies during spinal anesthesia. Inject dose over 20 to 30 seconds for paroxysmal atrial tachycardia; rapid injection may cause short paroxysms of ventricular tachycardia, ventricular extrasystoles, or a sensation of fullness in the head.
Intermittent infusion: not recommended.
Continuous infusion: Infuse diluted drug at rate required to maintain adequate blood pressure and tissue perfusion. Regulate rate with microdrip tubing and infusion pump. Administer through a patent I.V. line into large vein in the antecubital fossa to prevent extravasation. Closely monitor infusion site.

INCOMPATIBILITY
Incompatible with alkaline solutions and iron salts.

ADVERSE REACTIONS
Life-threatening: cerebral hemorrhage, decreased cardiac output, hypertension, respiratory distress, severe bradycardia, ventricular tachycardia.
Other: angina, anxiety, blurred vision, decreased renal perfusion, decreased urine output, dizziness, headache, light-headedness, metabolic acidosis, necrosis or tissue sloughing (with extravasation), pallor, palpitations, paresthesias in extremity after injection, pilomotor response, restlessness, seizures, sweating, tremors, ventricular extrasystoles, vomiting, weakness.

INTERACTIONS
Alpha-adrenergic blockers: decreased phenylephrine duration of action and pressor effect.
Antihypertensives, diuretics: possible diminished pressor response.
Atropine sulfate, mazindol, methylphenidate, oxytocin: potentiated pressor response, increasing risk of severe hypertension and cerebral hemorrhage.
Beta-adrenergic blockers: partial blockade of phenylephrine-induced myocardial stimulation. May be used to block phenylephrine-induced ventricular dysrhythmias.
Diatrizoates, iothalamate, ioxaglate: intensified neurologic effects.
Digitalis, hydrocarbon inhalation anesthetics, sympathomimetics: possible increased myocardial irritability and serious dysrhythmias.
Dihydroergotamine, ergonovine, ergotamine, methylergonovine, methysergide: enhanced vasoconstriction.
Doxapram, thyroid hormones: increased pressor effects.
Guanadrel, guanethidine, MAO inhibitors, maprotiline, tricyclic antidepressants: possible prolonged hypertension.

Levodopa: heightened risk of dysrhythmias.

Mecamylamine, methyldopa, trimethaphan: diminished hypotensive effects.

Nitrates: reduced antianginal effect.

Rauwolfia alkaloids: diminished hypotensive effects and possible prolonged phenylephrine action.

EFFECTS ON DIAGNOSTIC TESTS

EKG: possible bradycardia, ventricular tachycardia or fibrillation.

SPECIAL CONSIDERATIONS

• *Treatment of overdose:* Treat hypertension with phentolamine and cardiac dysrhythmias with propranolol, as ordered.

• If extravasation occurs, discontinue infusion and restart at another site. Infiltrate area with 5 to 10 mg of phentolamine in 10 to 15 ml of 0.9% sodium chloride, using syringe with a fine needle. For best results, treat within 12 hours.

• During infusion, check blood pressure every 2 minutes until stable, then every 5 to 15 minutes via intra-arterial monitoring. Discontinue slowly to avoid severe hypotension.

• Correct hypovolemia either before or during phenylephrine administration; hypovolemic patients are more susceptible to effects of severe vasoconstriction. Monitor central venous pressure or left ventricular filling pressure to help detect hypovolemia. Keep in mind that phenylephrine isn't a substitute for blood, plasma, fluid, or electrolytes.

• Continuously monitor EKG. Note heart rate every 5 to 15 minutes. Notify doctor of dysrhythmias.

• Insert indwelling urinary catheter and monitor urine output hourly. Inform doctor if urine output falls below 30 ml/hour.

• Monitor vital signs hourly until stable after stopping infusion. Watch for severe hypotension. Restart infusion if systolic pressure drops below 70 mm Hg. Maintain blood pressure slightly below patient's usual blood pressure.

• Hypoxia and acidosis reduce drug's effectiveness.

• May contain sulfites.

phenytoin sodium
Dilantin♦

Pregnancy Risk Category: D

PHARMACOKINETICS

Distribution: throughout tissues, with highest concentrations in the liver and adipose tissue; 70% to 95% of drug is protein-bound (less in patients with renal or hepatic dysfunction). Drug crosses the placenta.

Metabolism: in the liver, to inactive metabolites. With small dose increases, serum levels are substantially higher; however, they're lower in renal dysfunction. Rate of metabolism is accelerated in children.

Excretion: in urine by glomerular filtration as glucuronides, with 1% excreted unchanged. Small amounts are also excreted in feces. Within 24 hours, 60% to 75% of dose is excreted. Excretion may be enhanced by alkaline urine. Drug appears in breast milk. Average half-life is 14 hours.

Action: onset, 3 to 5 minutes; peak serum levels, 1 to 2 hours.

MECHANISM OF ACTION

Precise mechanism of anticonvulsant action is unknown. Phenytoin reduces voltage and spread of electrical stimulation within the motor cortex by stabilizing neuronal membranes and by either increasing efflux or decreasing influx of sodium ions across cell membranes. Antiarrhythmic effect in digitalis-induced dysrhythmias follows normalization of sodium influx to Purkinje fibers.

INDICATIONS & DOSAGE

• Status epilepticus. *Adults:* initially, 150 to 250 mg by direct injection; then 100 to 150 mg after 30 minutes if necessary, or 8 to 18 mg/kg, not to exceed 50 mg/minute. Maximum total daily dosage, 1.5 g. *Children:* 10 to 15 mg/kg at 0.5 to 1.5 mg/kg/minute. Maximum total daily dosage, 20 mg/kg.

• Ventricular tachycardia, paroxysmal atrial tachycardia, or dysrhythmias caused by digitalis toxicity. *Adults:* 100 mg by direct injection q 5 minutes until dysrhythmias disappear or 1 g maximum reached.

CONTRAINDICATIONS & CAUTIONS

• Contraindicated in hypersensitivity to hydantoins.

• Because phenytoin delays conduction in cardiac muscle, avoid use in sinus bradycardia, sinoatrial block or second- or third-degree atrioventricular (AV) block, and Adams-Stokes syndrome.

• Use cautiously in bradycardia, myocardial insufficiency, heart failure, and first-degree AV block because phenytoin depresses pacemaker action and force of myocardial contractility.

• Also use cautiously in respiratory depression because drug may exacerbate symptoms; in hepatic impairment or renal disease because of altered metabolism; in hypoglycemia-induced seizures because phenytoin may worsen hypoglycemia; and in patients with diabetes mellitus or other hyperglycemic states because drug may worsen hyperglycemia.

• Administer carefully in hypotension because of possible exacerbation; in impaired thyroid function because drug decreases serum T_4; in blood dyscrasias because of heightened risk of serious infection; and in fever lasting for more than 24 hours because fever reduces phenytoin levels.

PREPARATION & STORAGE

Available in 100 and 250 mg ampules containing 50 mg/ml. Store at room temperature; avoid freezing. Solution should be clear. If it's refrigerated, discard if slight yellowing doesn't clear after slow warming.

ADMINISTRATION

Direct injection: To prevent skin discoloration, avoid injecting drug into dorsal hand veins. Inject dose directly into vein using a 0.22 μm in-line filter. Alternately, inject into I.V. line containing a compatible solution infusing at a rate of less than 50 mg/minute. In elderly or debilitated patients, give at rate of 17 to 25 mg/minute.

Intermittent infusion: Infuse prescribed dose at ordered rate.

Continuous infusion: not recommended.

INCOMPATIBILITY

Incompatible with amikacin, aminophylline, bretylium, cephapirin, clindamycin phosphate, codeine phosphate, dextrose 5% in water, dobutamine, fat emulsions, insulin (regular), lactated Ringer's, levorphanol, lidocaine hydrochloride, lincomycin, meperidine, metaraminol, methadone hydrochloride, morphine, norepinephrine, nitroglycerin, pentobarbital, procaine, secobarbital sodium, 0.45% sodium chloride, 0.9% sodium chloride, and streptomycin.

ADVERSE REACTIONS

Life-threatening: cardiovascular collapse, exfoliative dermatitis, severe CNS depression, ventricular fibrillation.

Other: anorexia, ataxia, blood dyscrasias, blurred vision, bullous or purpuric dermatitis, clumsiness, confusion, constipation, diplopia, dizziness, drowsiness, dysphagia, epigastric pain, fever, gingival hyperplasia, hypertrichosis, hypotension, insomnia, irritability, loss of taste, lupus erythematosus, lymph-adenopathy, muscle weakness, nausea, nystagmus, osteomalacia, rash, seizures, slurred speech, toxic amblyopia, twitching, unusual excitement.

INTERACTIONS

Adrenocorticoids, carbamazepine, cardiac glycosides, corticotropin, cyclosporine, dacarbazine, disopyramide, doxycycline, estrogen-containing contraceptives, levodopa, quinidine: decreased effectiveness, resulting from increased metabolism.

Alcohol (acute ingestion), amiodarone, anticoagulants, anticonvulsants, benzodiazepines, chloramphenicol, cimetidine, disulfiram, haloperidol, inhalation anesthetics: enhanced phenytoin effects, resulting from increased serum levels and toxicity.

Alcohol (chronic use), antacids, barbiturates, calcium sulfate, carbamazepine, CNS depressants, folic acid, primidone, rifampin, xanthines: possible decreased phenytoin levels.

Dopamine: possible potentiated hypotension.

Isoniazid, loxapine, MAO inhibitors, maprotiline, phenothiazines, phenylbutazone, pimozide, sulfinpyrazone, sulfonamides, trazodone: heightened phenytoin effects, resulting from increased serum levels and toxicity.

Ketoconazole, miconazole: altered metabolism and delayed peak serum levels.

Leucovorin: antagonized anticonvulsant effects.

Levothyroxine: reduced serum T_4 levels.

Lidocaine, propranolol: additive myocardial depression.

Mexiletine: possible lowered serum levels.

Nifedipine, verapamil: possible significant alteration of serum levels.

Streptozocin: possible diminished therapeutic effects.

Valproic acid: seizures, resulting from interference with phenytoin protein binding.

Vitamin D: possible reduced efficacy.

EFFECTS ON DIAGNOSTIC TESTS

Dexamethasone, metyrapone tests: possible decreased levels.

Protein-bound iodine: reduced levels.

Resin or red blood cell T_3 uptake: possible increased uptake.

Serum alkaline phosphatase, gamma glutamyl transpeptidase, glucose: possible elevated levels.

SPECIAL CONSIDERATIONS

• *Treatment of overdose:* Immediately discontinue drug. Therapeutic serum level is 10 to 20 mcg/ml; toxic level, above 20 mcg/ml; lethal level, 100 mcg/ml. Phenytoin has no known antidote.

• Monitor EKG, blood pressure, and respiratory status.

• Frequently check I.V. site because phenytoin extravasation causes severe tissue damage.

• Closely monitor serum levels.

• Dosage requirements usually increase during pregnancy.

• Flush I.V. tubing before and after use with 0.9% saline solution, to remove drug and reduce venous irritation.

• Closely monitor for seizures. Keep intubation and aspiration equipment and padded side rails available.

• If measles-like rash appears, immediately discontinue drug.

• Monitor intake and output; hydration affects seizure threshold.

• In diabetic patients, monitor serum glucose levels. If serum glucose level increases, adjust insulin dosage, as ordered.

• Drug may turn urine pink or red to reddish brown.

Unmarked trade names available in the United States only.
♦ Also available in Canada.   ♦♦ Available in Canada only.

- Phenytoin is also used to treat neuralgia and migraine headache.
- Each milliliter of phenytoin for injection contains 0.2 mEq of sodium.

physostigmine salicylate
Antilirium♦

Pregnancy Risk Category: C

PHARMACOKINETICS
Distribution: throughout the body. Drug easily crosses the blood-brain barrier and probably crosses the placenta.
Metabolism: hydrolyzed by cholinesterases at neuromuscular junction.
Excretion: not fully understood. Small quantities are excreted in urine. Estimated half-life is 15 to 40 minutes. Not known if drug appears in breast milk.
Action: onset, 3 to 5 minutes; duration, 1 to 2 hours.

MECHANISM OF ACTION
Physostigmine blocks cholinesterase destruction of acetylcholine at central and peripheral cholinergic sites of neurotransmission, thus increasing available acetylcholine. Accumulated acetylcholine promotes increased receptor stimulation.

INDICATIONS & DOSAGE
- Reversal of anticholinergic drug effects (except those of atropine or scopolamine) or sedative effects of benzodiazepines. *Adults:* 0.5 to 2 mg initially, then repeated q 20 minutes to desired effect or until adverse cholinergic effects occur. With recurrence of life-threatening signs, such as dysrhythmias or coma, give 1 to 4 mg at 30- to 60-minute intervals as needed. *Children:* 0.02 mg/kg initially, then repeated at 5- to 10-minute intervals to desired effect

or until adverse cholinergic effects occur. Maximum total dose, 2 mg.
- Reversal of anticholinergic effects of atropine sulfate or scopolamine hydrobromide as preanesthetics.
Adults: Dose is twice that of anticholinergic drug, depending on weight. For example, to reverse effects of 0.5 mg of atropine, give 1 mg of physostigmine.
- Postoperative intestinal atony.
Adults: 0.5 to 2 mg.

CONTRAINDICATIONS & CAUTIONS
- Contraindicated in asthma, cardiovascular disease, diabetes mellitus, or gangrene because drug may aggravate the condition, and in mechanical obstruction of the intestinal or urinary tract or in vagotonia because drug may worsen the obstruction by increasing muscle tone.
- Use cautiously in patients with a history of seizures because of the risk of increased seizures, and in patients with bradycardia or parkinsonian syndrome because symptoms may worsen.
- Also use cautiously in physostigmine hypersensitivity.

PREPARATION & STORAGE
Available in concentration of 1 mg/ml in 2 ml ampules and 1 ml syringes. Parenteral solution may be slightly discolored (tinted red, blue, or brown). Discard solution if discoloration is marked. Store in light-resistant containers at room temperature. Avoid freezing.

ADMINISTRATION
Direct injection: Slowly inject drug into large vein or into I.V. tubing containing free-flowing compatible solution. Don't exceed 1 mg/minute for adults or 0.5 mg/minute for children. Rapid injection can cause bra-

---

dycardia, breathing difficulty, hypersalivation, and seizures.
Intermittent infusion: not recommended.
Continuous infusion: not recommended.

INCOMPATIBILITY
No incompatibilities reported.

ADVERSE REACTIONS
Life-threatening: asystole, bronchospasm, cholinergic crisis, respiratory paralysis.
Other: abdominal cramps, blurred vision, bradycardia, diarrhea, dyspnea, dysrhythmias, excessive salivation, hallucinations, headache, hypotension, increased bronchial secretions, lacrimation, miosis, muscle cramps, nausea, palpitations, restlessness, seizures, sweating, thrombophlebitis, twitching, urinary frequency, vomiting, weakness.

INTERACTIONS
Acetylcholine, bethanechol, carbachol, methacholine: enhanced effects of physostigmine.
Benzodiazepines: possible diminished effects.
Procainamide, quinidine: possible reversed cholinergic effects on muscle.
Succinylcholine: additive depolarizing neuromuscular blockade.

EFFECTS ON DIAGNOSTIC TESTS
None reported.

SPECIAL CONSIDERATIONS
• *Treatment of overdose:* Administer 2 to 4 mg of atropine by direct injection at 3- to 10-minute intervals. Use 1 mg for children. Counteract ganglionic and skeletal muscle effects with pralidoxime chloride, given 50 to 100 mg/minute. Institute

mechanical ventilation and suction secretions frequently.
• Always keep suction and cardiopulmonary resuscitation equipment and atropine sulfate available. Draw physostigmine and atropine into separate syringes.
• Remember that physostigmine should be reserved for life-threatening situations, when diagnosis of anticholinergic overdose is well established and possibility of mixed drug ingestion has been ruled out.
• Establish baseline heart rate and blood pressure. During administration, continue to monitor for tachycardia, bradycardia, dysrhythmias, and hypotension. Report significant changes to doctor immediately.
• Monitor for signs of cholinergic crisis. Reduce dosage, as ordered, if sweating or nausea occurs. If excessive salivation, vomiting, urination, cramping, or diarrhea occurs, discontinue drug and notify doctor.
• Closely monitor patient for changes in level of consciousness. Because physostigmine's action lasts for only 1 to 2 hours, the patient may relapse into coma, necessitating administration of additional doses of physostigmine.

phytonadione (vitamin K₁)
AquaMEPHYTON

Pregnancy Risk Category: C

PHARMACOKINETICS
Distribution: briefly concentrated in the liver. Small amounts accumulate in tissues but are subsequently destroyed. Body stores only minimal amount. Vitamin K crosses the placenta.
Metabolism: rapidly metabolized in the liver.

Excretion: in urine and feces.
Action: onset, 1 to 2 hours; duration, 12 to 14 hours.

MECHANISM OF ACTION
Promotes hepatic formation of active prothrombin (Factor II), proconvertin (Factor VII), plasma thromboplastin component or Christmas factor (Factor IX), and Stuart factor (Factor X).

INDICATIONS & DOSAGE
• Drug-induced hypoprothrombinemia with existing or imminent bleeding. *Adults:* 10 to 50 mg q 4 hours as needed. Dosage guided by coagulation studies.

CONTRAINDICATIONS & CAUTIONS
• Contraindicated in hypersensitivity to vitamin K₁ or any ingredient in the preparation.
• Use cautiously in hepatic impairment because drug may exacerbate the condition.

PREPARATION & STORAGE
Available in 0.5 and 1 ml ampules and 2.5 and 5 ml multidose vials containing 2 and 10 mg/ml. Protect drug from light, even after dilution. For direct injection, dilute with 10 ml of preservative-free dextrose 5% in water, 0.9% sodium chloride, or dextrose 5% in 0.9% sodium chloride. For infusion, dilute with 50 to 100 ml of any of these solutions. Administer immediately after dilution. Discard unused drug.

ADMINISTRATION
Direct injection: Using a 21G or 23G needle, inject diluted drug directly into vein or into I.V. tubing containing a free-flowing compatible solution at a maximum rate of 1 mg/minute.

Intermittent infusion: Infuse diluted drug at a maximum rate of 1 mg/minute.
Continuous infusion: not recommended.

INCOMPATIBILITY
Incompatible with phenytoin sodium.

ADVERSE REACTIONS
Life-threatening: anaphylaxis, bronchospasm, cardiac arrest, circulatory collapse, respiratory arrest, shock.
Other: cardiac irregularities, chest pain or tightness, convulsive movements, cyanosis, dizziness, dulled consciousness, dyspnea, facial flushing, hyperhidrosis, transient hypotension, unusual taste.

INTERACTIONS
Anticoagulants (oral): decreased effect.
Dactinomycin: diminished phytonadione effects.
Primaquine: enhanced potential for adverse phytonadione reactions.

EFFECTS ON DIAGNOSTIC TESTS
None reported.

SPECIAL CONSIDERATIONS
• I.V. use is restricted to emergencies because of possible severe reactions. Whenever possible, administer S.C. or I.M.
• Never give drug undiluted by I.V. push. Even dilution and slow infusion may not prevent severe reactions. To reverse vitamin K effects, administer heparin or warfarin, as ordered.
• Monitor coagulation studies 12 hours after administration and repeat as needed.
• Vitamin K₁ is used in hypoprothrombinemia caused by vitamin K deficiency or in moderate to severe

bleeding caused by coumadin or in-dandione derivatives. It won't antag-onize the action of heparin.
• May contain benzyl alcohol.

pipecuronium bromide
Arduan

Pregnancy Risk Category: C

PHARMACOKINETICS
Distribution: Limited data available. Drug distributes rapidly through plasma; distribution half-life is about 6 minutes.
Metabolism: Several metabolites have been identified in animal stud-ies; limited human data have re-vealed a 3-desacetyl metabolite, which is pharmacologically active. However, no active metabolites have been found in plasma.
Excretion: About 56% of a dose is recovered from the urine; 41% is ex-creted unchanged and 15% is ex-creted as the 3-desacetyl metabolite.
Action: onset, approximately 5 min-utes. Duration, dose dependent; pa-ralysis can last for 1 to 2 hours.

MECHANISM OF ACTION
A nondepolarizing muscle relaxant, pipecuronium competes with acetyl-choline for receptor sites at the mo-tor end plate. Because this action may be antagonized by cholinester-ase inhibitors, it is considered a competitive antagonist.

INDICATIONS & DOSAGE
• Induction of skeletal muscle relax-ation during surgery as an adjunct to general anesthesia. *Adults and chil-dren:* Dosage is highly individual-ized. The following doses may serve as a guide, assuming that the patient is not obese and has normal renal function. Initially, 70 to 85 mcg/kg

may be used for endotracheal intu-bation and to maintain paralysis for 1 to 2 hours. If succinylcholine is used for endotracheal intubation, ini-tial doses of 50 mcg/kg will provide good relaxation for 45 minutes or more. Maintenance doses of 10 to 15 mcg/kg may be used to provide relaxation for about 50 minutes.

CONTRAINDICATIONS & CAUTIONS
• There are no known contraindica-tions. Use only under direct medical supervision by personnel familiar with the use of neuromuscular blocking agents and techniques in-volved in maintaining a patent air-way.
• Because of the lack of safety data, this drug is not recommended for use in patients requiring prolonged mechanical ventilation in the ICU. It is not recommended before or after other nondepolarizing neuromuscular blocking agents. It is also not recom-mended for use during cesarean sec-tion because safety to the neonate has not been established.
• Because drug is excreted by kid-neys, use with caution in patients with renal failure. Data are lacking on use of drug in liver disease.
• Use cautiously in patients with myasthenia gravis or myasthenic syndrome (Eaton-Lambert syn-drome). Such patients are sensitive to nondepolarizing relaxants; shorter-acting agents are recom-mended.

PREPARATION & STORAGE
Supplied in vials containing 10 mg. Store powder at room temperature or in the refrigerator at 36° to 86° F. (2° to 30° C.). Reconstitute with 10 ml solution before use to yield a so-lution of 1 mg/ml. Large volumes of diluent or addition of the drug to a

hanging I.V. solution is not recommended.

If refrigerated, drug is stable for 24 hours when reconstituted with sterile water for injection, 0.9% sodium chloride injection, dextrose 5% in water, lactated Ringer's injection, or dextrose 5% in saline.

When reconstituted with bacteriostatic water for injection, the drug is stable for 5 days at room temperature or in the refrigerator. Note that bacteriostatic water contains benzyl alcohol and is not intended for use in neonates.

If reconstituted with any solution other than bacteriostatic water for injection, unused portions of the drug should be discarded.

ADMINISTRATION
Direct injection: Inject into tubing of a free flowing I.V. solution.
Intermittent infusion: not recommended.
Continuous infusion: not recommended.

INCOMPATIBILITY
Limited data available. Do not mix with other drugs or administer from a large volume I.V.

ADVERSE REACTIONS
Life-threatening: prolonged muscle weakness, respiratory insufficiency or apnea.
Other: anuria, atrial fibrillation, bradycardia, cerebrovascular accident, dyspnea, hypertension, hypotension, increased creatinine, myocardial ischemia, respiratory depression, thrombosis, ventricular extrasystole.

INTERACTIONS
Aminoglycosides (dihydrostreptomycin, gentamicin, kanamycin, neomycin, and streptomycin); bacitracin; colistin; polymyxin B;

sodium colistimethate; and tetracyclines: increased muscle weakness. Use together cautiously.
Inhalational anesthetics, quinidine: may enhance the activity of nondepolarizing blockers.
Magnesium salts: may enhance neuromuscular blockade.

EFFECTS ON DIAGNOSTIC TESTS
Serum creatinine: possible elevated levels.

SPECIAL CONSIDERATIONS
• Because the drug has minimal vagolytic action, bradycardia during anesthesia is likely.
• A nerve stimulator and train-of-four (T_4) monitoring are recommended to assess recovery of muscle strength. Before attempting pharmacologic reversal with neostigmine, some evidence of spontaneous recovery should appear.
• Because of its prolonged duration of action, pipecuronium bromide is recommended only for procedures that take 90 minutes or longer.
• Dosage should be adjusted to ideal body weight in obese patients.
• Experimental evidence suggests that alkalosis may counteract paralysis and acidosis may enhance it. Electrolyte disturbances may also influence response.
• Pipecuronium may be administered after succinylcholine when the latter is used to facilitate intubation; however, there is no evidence to support the safe use of pipecuronium before succinylcholine to decrease side effects of the latter drug.
• Not recommended for use in children younger than 3 months of age. Limited evidence suggests that children (age 1 to 14 years) under balanced anesthesia or halothane anesthesia may be less sensitive to the drug.

piperacillin sodium
Pipracil♦

Pregnancy Risk Category: B

PHARMACOKINETICS
Distribution: diffuses readily into most tissues, including the kidneys, liver, lungs, heart, and skin, and into bile, peritoneal fluid, bronchial secretions, and wound drainage. Usually low cerebrospinal fluid concentration increases in meningeal inflammation. Drug readily crosses the placenta. It's 16% to 22% protein-bound, primarily to albumin and globulin.
Metabolism: minimal.
Excretion: largely unchanged. Most of dose is excreted in urine by glomerular filtration and renal tubular secretion—49% to 90% in first 24 hours. About 10% to 20% is excreted in feces. Usual half-life is 30 to 90 minutes. Excretion may be prolonged in neonates, infants, and patients with renal or hepatic impairment. Small amounts appear in breast milk.
Action: onset, immediate; duration 3 to 5 hours.

MECHANISM OF ACTION
An extended-spectrum, bactericidal penicillin, piperacillin inhibits synthesis of cell wall mucopeptide, rendering the wall unstable. Drug is most effective during active cell multiplication. Inadequate dosage may result in only bacteriostatic action.

Susceptible gram-positive aerobic bacteria include non-penicillinase-producing strains of *Staphylococcus aureus* and *S. epidermidis;* groups A, B, C, and G streptococci; *Streptococcus pneumoniae;* and viridans streptococci.

Susceptible gram-negative aerobic bacteria include *Eikenella corrodens, Escherichia coli, Haemophilus influenzae, H. parainfluenzae, Morganella morganii, Neisseria meningitidis, N. gonorrhoeae, Proteus mirabilis, P. vulgaris, Providencia rettgeri, Pseudomonas aeruginosa, Salmonella, Shigella,* and some strains of *Acinetobacter, Citrobacter, Enterobacter, Flavobacterium, Klebsiella, Moraxella,* and *Serratia.* Susceptible anaerobes include some strains of *Actinomyces, Bifidobacterium, Clostridium* (including *C. perfringens), Eubacterium, Lactobacillus, Peptococcus, Peptostreptococcus,* and *Propionibacterium acnes.*

INDICATIONS & DOSAGE
● Severe systemic infections caused by susceptible organisms. *Adults:* 200 to 300 mg/kg or 12 to 18 g in divided doses four to six times daily. *Children age 1 month to 12 years:* 50 mg/kg q 4 hours.
● Complicated urinary tract infections. *Adults:* 125 to 200 mg/kg or 8 to 16 g in divided doses q 6 to 8 hours.
● Uncomplicated urinary tract infections. *Adults:* 100 to 125 mg/kg or 6 to 8 g in divided doses q 6 to 12 hours.
● Acute *P. aeruginosa* infection in cystic fibrosis (in conjunction with aminoglycosides). *Adults:* 300 to 600 mg/kg daily.
● Prophylaxis for abdominal surgery. *Adults:* 2 g before surgery, during surgery, and q 6 hours after surgery for up to 24 hours.
● Maximum daily adult dosage for any indication, 24 g.
Note: Adjust dosage in renal failure. For adults, dosage reflects creatinine clearance. In uncomplicated urinary tract infections, give 3 g q 12 hours if clearance is less than 20 ml/min; if clearance is more than 20 ml/min,

give usual adult dose. In complicated urinary tract infections, give 3 g q 12 hours if clearance is less than 20 ml/min; if clearance is 20 to 40 ml/min, give 3 g q 8 hours; if clearance is more than 40 ml/min, give usual adult dose. In serious systemic infections, give 4 g q 12 hours if clearance is less than 20 ml/min; if clearance is 20 to 40 ml/min, give 4 g q 8 hours; if clearance is more than 40 ml/min, give usual adult dose.

CONTRAINDICATIONS & CAUTIONS

• Contraindicated in hypersensitivity to penicillins or cephalosporins.
• Also contraindicated in children under age 12 because safe use hasn't been established.
• Because of the increased risk of toxicity, drug requires cautious use in hepatic or renal dysfunction.
• Drug also must be used cautiously in patients with sodium-restricted diets. Each gram of piperacillin sodium provides 42.5 mg (1.85 mEq) of sodium.
• Use cautiously in patients with ulcerative colitis because of possible exacerbation.

PREPARATION & STORAGE

Available in powder form in 2, 3, and 4 g vials. Store at room temperature. Reconstitute each gram of drug with 5 ml of sterile bacteriostatic water for injection or bacteriostatic sodium chloride injection. Shake vigorously to dissolve. For infusion, dilute reconstituted solution with at least 50 ml of dextrose 5% in water, 0.9% sodium chloride, dextrose 5% in 0.9% sodium chloride, or Ringer's lactate. After reconstitution, drug remains stable for 24 hours at room temperature or for 7 days when refrigerated at 36° to 46° F. (2° to 8° C.).

ADMINISTRATION

Direct injection: Inject reconstituted drug directly into vein over 3 to 5 minutes.
Intermittent infusion: Infuse reconstituted and diluted solution into a patent I.V. line containing a free-flowing compatible solution over 30 minutes.
Continuous infusion: Inject reconstituted 24-hour dose into required daily I.V. volume. Infuse at rate needed for delivery of required fluid volume.

INCOMPATIBILITY

No incompatibilities reported.

ADVERSE REACTIONS

Life-threatening: anaphylaxis.
Other: abnormal platelet aggregation, anemia, granulocytopenia, headache, hypersensitivity (arthralgia, chills, eosinophilia, fever, malaise, myalgia, pruritus, rash), hypokalemia, leukopenia, neuromuscular irritability, neutropenia, overgrowth of nonsusceptible organisms, phlebitis, prolonged bleeding times (3 to 12 days after start of therapy), pseudomembranous colitis, thrombocytopenia, vein irritation.

INTERACTIONS

Anticoagulants: enhanced bleeding tendency from inhibition of platelet aggregation.
Anturane, probenecid: increased penicillin serum levels and possible toxicity from decreased renal excretion.

EFFECTS ON DIAGNOSTIC TESTS

Bleeding time, platelet aggregation, prothrombin time: in high doses, interference with test results.
BUN, serum creatinine, sodium: increased levels.
Coombs' test: positive.

Serum bilirubin, LDH, SGOT,
SGPT: elevated levels.

SPECIAL CONSIDERATIONS
• Treat anaphylaxis symptomatically. Keep emergency equipment available.
• Obtain specimens for culture and sensitivity tests before first dose. Therapy may start before test results are available.
• Before giving piperacillin, ask patient if he's had allergic reactions to penicillin. A negative history of penicillin allergy doesn't rule out future allergic reaction.
• Closely monitor for possible hypersensitivity for at least 30 minutes after administration.
• Check CBC frequently and monitor serum potassium level. Monitor prothrombin and bleeding times. Assess patient for possible bleeding.
• Change I.V. site every 48 hours to avoid vein irritation.
• Duration of therapy depends on type of infection but usually continues for at least 48 to 72 hours after patient is asymptomatic. Periodically monitor renal, hepatic, and cardiovascular status in patients on prolonged therapy.
• Piperacillin is nearly always given with another antibiotic. Give at least 1 hour before bacteriostatic antibiotics.
• Observe patient for fungal and bacterial superinfection with prolonged use.
• Hemodialysis removes drug, but peritoneal dialysis does not.

plasma
(fresh frozen plasma, liquid plasma)

Pregnancy Risk Category: Not applicable

COMPOSITION
Fresh frozen plasma and liquid plasma each contain 91% water, 2% carbohydrate, and 7% proteins, specifically globulins, antibodies, and clotting factors. Freezing within 6 hours of collection preserves all clotting factors (about 1 unit/ml). Storage in liquid state results in loss of clotting Factors V and VIII. One unit of plasma has a volume of 200 to 250 ml.

INDICATIONS & DOSAGE
• Coagulation disorders related to liver disease, disseminated intravascular coagulation, congenital clotting factor deficiencies, and dilutional coagulopathy after massive blood replacement. *Adults:* Dose reflects disorder and patient's condition.
Children: 15 to 30 ml/kg for acute hemorrhage and 10 to 15 ml/kg for clotting factor deficiency. Repeat as needed.

CONTRAINDICATIONS & CAUTIONS
• Contraindicated for use as a volume expander because of the risk of transmitting blood-borne viral disease, which doesn't occur with crystalloid or colloid solution.
• Also contraindicated as a protein source for nutritionally deficient patients.
• Avoid giving liquid plasma to replace clotting Factors V and VIII because these factors degenerate rapidly in a liquid state.

PREPARATION & STORAGE

Before administration, thaw fresh frozen plasma at 99° F. (37° C.). Thawing takes 45 to 60 minutes. Then refrigerate at 39° F. (4° C.) for maximum of 24 hours, pending transfusion.

Liquid plasma may be refrigerated at 39° F. for a maximum of 47 days or frozen at 0° F. (– 18° C.) for a maximum of 5 years.

ADMINISTRATION

Direct injection: not recommended.
Intermittent infusion: not recommended.
Continuous infusion: Give over 1 to 2 hours through a transfusion set containing a 170-micron filter. Begin transfusion slowly, following institutional guidelines. Take vital signs. If patient shows no evidence of a reaction, adjust flow to prescribed rate. Closely monitor patient throughout transfusion.

INCOMPATIBILITY

Incompatible with all drugs and solutions except 0.9% sodium chloride.

ADVERSE REACTIONS

Life-threatening: acquired immune deficiency syndrome; anaphylaxis; cytomegalovirus; hepatitis B; non-A, non-B hepatitis.
Other: flushing, itching, urticaria, volume overload (cough, crackles at lung base, distended neck veins, dyspnea).

INTERACTIONS

None reported.

EFFECTS ON DIAGNOSTIC TESTS

Bleeding time, partial prothrombin time, prothrombin time: correction of abnormal values after effective dosage.

Clotting Factors V and VIII: increased levels after administration of significant amounts of fresh frozen plasma.

SPECIAL CONSIDERATIONS

• *Treatment of anaphylaxis:* Acute onset is accompanied by anxiety, urticaria, and wheezing, progressing to cyanosis, shock, and cardiac arrest. Stop transfusion immediately at the hub of the needle, and keep vein open with 0.9% sodium chloride. Notify the doctor. Support blood pressure, prepare 0.4 ml of 1:1,000 epinephrine for injection, and treat symptomatically.
• If flushing, itching, or urticaria occurs, slow the transfusion until symptoms resolve. Give antihistamines, as ordered.
• If volume overload occurs, stop the transfusion and keep vein open with a slow drip of 0.9% sodium chloride. Place the patient's feet in a dependent position, and notify the doctor. Treat symptomatically and administer a diuretic, as ordered.
• To reduce the risk of volume overload, use clotting factor concentrates (cryoprecipitate, lyophilized Factor VIII and IX) if available.
• Before requesting the release of plasma from the blood bank, record vital signs and establish a patent venous catheter.
• Plasma contains virtually no RBCs, making RBC crossmatch unnecessary. Plasma should be ABO compatible with recipient RBCs: Recipient type A is compatible with plasma type A or AB; type B, with B or AB; type AB, with AB; and type O, with O, A, B, or AB.
• Rh type isn't significant. Patient can receive either Rh positive or Rh negative plasma.
• Tell patient to report any unusual symptoms immediately.

---

plasma protein fraction 5%
Plasmanate, Plasma-Plex,
Plasmatein 5%, Protenate 5%

Pregnancy Risk Category: C

COMPOSITION
Plasma protein fraction (PPF) is a
5% solution of proteins derived from
pooled human blood, serum, or
plasma containing about 83% to
90% albumin and no more than 17%
globulin and other proteins. Each
milliliter of PPF contains 4.4 g of
albumin. The solution is isotonic
and equivalent to normal plasma
both osmotically and oncotically. Because blood group isoagglutinins
have been removed, PPF may be administered without regard to the patient's blood group. Its sodium
content is 130 to 160 mEq/liter.

INDICATIONS & DOSAGE
• Hypovolemic shock in hypoprotein-
emic patients (total protein <5.2 g/
dl). *Adults:* initially, 250 to 500 ml.
Children: initially, 6.6 to 33 ml/kg.
Rate and volume reflect patient's
condition and response. Dose may be
repeated after 15 to 30 minutes if
response is inadequate.
• Hypoproteinemia in burn patients,
after first 24 hours. *Adults:* 1,000 to
1,500 ml daily. Larger doses may be
necessary in severe hypoproteinemia
with continuing loss of plasma proteins. Maximum total daily dosage,
44 ml/kg.

CONTRAINDICATIONS & CAUTIONS
• Contraindicated in allergic reactions to albumin or other plasma-
containing products; in nutritional
deficiencies because product isn't
therapeutic and exposes patient to
viral infection; in severe anemia because increased blood volume significantly reduces hemoglobin; and in
cardiac failure because of increased
risk of pulmonary edema.
• Also contraindicated in first 24
hours after burn injury because of
rapid protein loss, and in cardiopulmonary bypass surgery because
rapid infusion may cause hypotension.
• Use cautiously in hepatic or renal
failure because of added protein,
fluid, and sodium, and in hypertension, cardiac disease, and severe
pulmonary infection because of increased blood volume and blood
pressure after infusion.

PREPARATION & STORAGE
PPF is ready for use. Solution varies
from near colorless to straw to dark
brown. Store at room temperature—
not over 86° F. (30° C.). Don't use
if solution is cloudy, has been frozen, or contains sediment. Administer within 4 hours of opening
container. Use bottle only once; it
contains no preservatives. Discard
unused portion.

ADMINISTRATION
Direct injection: not recommended.
Intermittent infusion: not recommended.
Continuous infusion: Infuse undiluted or in combination with other
parenteral solutions, such as whole
blood, plasma, 0.9% sodium chloride, glucose, or sodium lactate.
Don't administer near site of infection or trauma. Infusion rate depends on response but shouldn't
exceed 10 ml/minute. Faster rates
may result in sudden hypotension.
As volume approaches normal, reduce rate to 5 to 8 ml/minute. In
children, infuse at 5 to 10 ml/min-
ute. Make sure administration set
has adequate filter (provided by
manufacturer).

INCOMPATIBILITY
Incompatible with alcohol-containing solutions, norepinephrine, and protein hydrolysates.

ADVERSE REACTIONS
Life-threatening: acquired immune deficiency syndrome; anaphylaxis; cytomegalovirus; hepatitis B; non-A, non-B hepatitis.
Other: back pain, chest pain, chills, erythema, fever, flushing, hypersalivation, nausea, urticaria, vomiting.

INTERACTIONS
None reported.

EFFECTS ON DIAGNOSTIC TESTS
Alkaline phosphatase: possible elevated levels.

SPECIAL CONSIDERATIONS
• Although PPF is a pooled human plasma derivative, crossmatching is unnecessary.
• Frequently monitor blood pressure in shock patients; widening pulse pressure correlates with increased stroke volume or cardiac output.
• Stop infusion if blood pressure suddenly falls. Correct with vasopressors.
• If allergic reaction occurs, discontinue and give antihistamines.
• Monitor hemoglobin; increased blood volume may cause significant fall. Transfusion of whole blood or packed RBCs may be necessary.
• Monitor serum albumin levels in patients with hypoproteinemia. Treating the underlying disorder and replacing amino acids and proteins restore albumin levels more effectively than PPF or albumin infusions.
• After PPF infusion, closely observe injured or postoperative patients; elevated blood pressure may cause bleeding from severed blood

vessels that may not have bled at lower blood pressure.
• PPF isn't normally used for temporary albumin redistribution associated with major surgery.

platelets (thrombocytes)
Platelet Concentrate

Pregnancy Risk Category: not applicable

COMPOSITION
Platelets are irregularly shaped disks about half the size of RBCs. They migrate and adhere to damaged blood vessels to stop bleeding. Normal platelet count is 150,000 to 400,000/mm^3. Random-donor platelets are derived from 1 unit of whole blood containing at least 5.5×10^{10} platelets and a variable number of lymphocytes suspended in 50 to 70 ml of plasma. With single-donor platelets, 1 unit contains at least 3×10^{11} platelets (equivalent to 6 random units) and a variable number of lymphocytes suspended in 200 to 400 ml of plasma.

INDICATIONS & DOSAGE
• Treatment or prevention of hemorrhage in thrombocytopenia or platelet dysfunction. *Adults:* 4 to 10 units, depending on patient's condition. *Children:* 1 unit/7 to 10 kg.

CONTRAINDICATIONS & CAUTIONS
• Contraindicated in bleeding caused by abnormal clotting factors; in rapid platelet destruction (as in idiopathic thrombocytopenic purpura or untreated disseminated intravascular coagulation); and in thrombocytopenia caused by septicemia or hyper-

splenism because platelets wouldn't be effective.

• Human leukocyte antigen (HLA)-matched platelets are unnecessary in patients in whom HLA antibodies have not been documented.

PREPARATION & STORAGE

Random-donor platelets are separated from 1 unit of whole blood within 6 hours of collection. Usually, multiple units are pooled into a single container to provide the required dose. Single-donor platelets are prepared by platelet pheresis. Store at room temperature in the blood bank for a maximum of 5 days. After the sterile seal is broken, administer within 4 hours.

ADMINISTRATION

Direct injection: Draw prefiltered platelet concentrate into a syringe, and inject slowly through a 19G to 23G catheter. Direct injection is primarily used in neonatal transfusion.
Intermittent infusion: not recommended.
Continuous infusion: Infuse through blood component recipient set with a 170-micron filter via a 19G to 21G needle. Begin infusion slowly, according to hospital guidelines. Take vital signs. Adjust flow gradually to prescribed rate and closely monitor the patient. Infuse as rapidly as patient can tolerate, within 4 hours or less. Blood bank can reduce volume if circulatory overload is a risk.
Caution: Avoid passing platelet concentrates through depth-type filters. Also, don't use recipient sets with rubber connections, to which platelets can adhere.

INCOMPATIBILITY

Combine only with 0.9% sodium chloride.

ADVERSE REACTIONS

Life-threatening: acquired immune deficiency syndrome; anaphylaxis; cytomegalovirus infection; hepatitis B; non-A, non-B hepatitis.
Other: alloimmunization; febrile, nonhemolytic reactions (anxiety, headache, myalgia, sudden chills, temperature above 100.4° F. [38° C.]); flushing; pruritus; urticaria.

INTERACTIONS

None reported.

EFFECTS ON DIAGNOSTIC TESTS

Direct Coombs' test: may detect erythrocyte-bound antibody if large volume of incompatible platelet-rich plasma has been transfused.
Platelet count: increased by 5,000 to 10,000/mm^3 per unit in adults and 50,000/mm^3 per unit in children if therapy has resolved or controlled the cause of thrombocytopenia.

SPECIAL CONSIDERATIONS

• *Treatment of anaphylaxis:* Stop transfusion at the hub of the needle and keep vein open with 0.9% sodium chloride. Notify the doctor. Treat symptomatically. Prepare 0.4 ml of 1:1,000 epinephrine for injection.

• Thrombocytopenia or platelet dysfunction should be documented before administering platelets.

• Platelets contain minimal RBCs, so RBC crossmatching is unnecessary. However, platelet-rich plasma should be ABO compatible with recipient RBCs if volume exceeds 120 ml for adults or 1 to 2 ml/kg for infants and children.

• Describe procedure to patient. Also instruct him to immediately report any unusual symptoms.

• Record vital signs and establish a patent venous catheter before requesting the release of platelets from the blood bank. Allow 15 to 30 minutes for the blood bank to prepare and label platelets.

• If flushing, itching, or urticaria occurs, slow transfusion until symptoms resolve. The doctor may prescribe antihistamines.

• Alloimmunization occurs in many previously transfused or pregnant patients. It may inhibit platelet survival and cause febrile, nonhemolytic reactions. Administering HLA-matched platelets may prevent premature platelet destruction if anti-HLA antibodies have formed.

• If patient develops febrile, nonhemolytic reaction, stop the transfusion. Keep vein open with 0.9% sodium chloride, and treat symptomatically. Administer an antipyretic. Use of leukocyte-poor platelets prepared by resedimentation may prevent recurrence.

• Because of increased risk of hemorrhage, nonbleeding patients with a platelet level below 20,000/mm³ and surgical patients with a level of less than 100,000/mm³ may require platelet therapy. Platelets may also be used to treat hemorrhage if platelet count is less than 50,000/mm³.

• Single-donor platelet transfusion lessens the risk of disease transmission and HLA antibody formation.

---

plicamycin (mithramycin)
Mithracin

Pregnancy Risk Category: D

PHARMACOKINETICS
Distribution: highest concentrations in Kupffer's cells of the liver, in renal tubular cells, and along formed bone surfaces. Plicamycin crosses the blood-brain barrier, where concentrations are low but persist longer than elsewhere. Drug probably crosses the placenta.
Metabolism: unknown.
Excretion: primarily eliminated in urine within 4 hours.

MECHANISM OF ACTION
Drug inhibits RNA synthesis and also lowers serum calcium levels.

INDICATIONS & DOSAGE
• Testicular cancer. *Adults:* 25 to 30 mcg/kg daily for 8 to 10 days or until toxicity occurs. Maximum dosage, 10 doses daily or a total of 30 mcg/kg daily. May repeat monthly.
• Hypercalcemia and hypercalciuria (related to cancer). *Adults:* 25 mcg/kg daily for 3 or 4 days. May repeat at intervals of 1 week or more.

CONTRAINDICATIONS & CAUTIONS
• Contraindicated in blood dyscrasias, impaired bone marrow function, coagulation disorders, thrombocytopathy, or thrombocytopenia because of the increased risk of hemorrhage.
• Administer cautiously in severe renal or hepatic impairment because of possible irreversible toxicity.
• Use with caution in electrolyte imbalance, especially hypocalcemia, hypokalemia, and hypophosphatemia to avoid exacerbation.

PREPARATION & STORAGE
Use extreme caution when preparing or administering plicamycin to avoid mutagenic, teratogenic, and carcinogenic risks. Use a biological containment cabinet, wear gloves and masks, and use syringes with Luer-Lok tips to prevent drug leakage. Correctly dispose of vials, needles, syringes, and unused drug.

Plicamycin is available in 2,500-mcg vials. Refrigerate unreconstituted vials. Reconstitute drug with 4.9 ml of sterile water for injection for a concentration of 500 mcg/ml. For infusion, dilute appropriate dose in 1,000 ml of dextrose 5% in water or 0.9% sodium chloride. Discard unused solution. Reconstituted solution remains stable for 24 hours at room temperature and for 48 hours when refrigerated.

ADMINISTRATION
Direct injection: not recommended.
Intermittent infusion: Infuse diluted drug over 4 to 6 hours. (Rapid infusion increases incidence and severity of GI disease.)
Continuous infusion: not recommended.

INCOMPATIBILITY
None reported. However, drug may form a complex with metal ions such as iron and readily hydrolyzes in acidic solutions (pH less than 4).

ADVERSE REACTIONS
Life-threatening: hemorrhagic diathesis, pancytopenia.
Other: anorexia, depression, diarrhea, dizziness, drowsiness, fatigue, fever, flushing, headache, impaired liver function, irritability, irritation and cellulitis at injection site, lethargy, malaise, nausea, nervousness, phlebitis, rash, stomatitis, toxic epidermal necrolysis, vomiting, weakness.

INTERACTIONS
Aspirin, dextran, dipyridamole, sulfinpyrazone, valproic acid: increased risk of hemorrhage.
Estrogens, oral contraceptives: heightened risk of hepatotoxicity.
Heparin, oral anticoagulants, thrombolytic agents: increased platelet aggregation and risk of hemorrhage.

Live-virus vaccines: potentiated virus replication.

EFFECTS ON DIAGNOSTIC TESTS
BUN, serum creatinine: elevated levels.
Clotting time: increased.
Hemoglobin, platelet count, WBC count: decreased.
Serum alkaline phosphatase, bilirubin, isocitrate dehydrogenase, LDH, ornithine carbamoyltransferase, sorbitol dehydrogenase, SGOT, SGPT: elevated levels.
Serum calcium, phosphorus, potassium: reduced levels.
Sulfobromophthalein test: enhanced retention.
Urine protein: possible elevated levels.

SPECIAL CONSIDERATIONS
• *Treatment of hemorrhage:* Administer blood transfusions, vitamin K, and corticosteroids, as ordered. Use aminocaproic acid to counteract increased fibrinolytic activity, if indicated.
• If plicamycin extravasation occurs, stop the infusion and restart it in another area. Apply cold to reduce pain and prevent swelling. However, if the patient develops swelling, apply moderate heat to reduce discomfort and irritation.
• Administer antiemetics before and during treatment to help reduce nausea.
• Correct dehydration, volume depletion, or electrolyte imbalance before plicamycin therapy.
• Therapeutic effects are unlikely without toxic effects.
• Frequently obtain platelet counts and prothrombin and bleeding times during therapy and for several days after last dose.

Unmarked trade names available in the United States only.
♦ Also available in Canada.   ♦ ♦ Available in Canada only.

• Monitor liver and kidney function daily in patients with preexisting impairment.
• Therapy may be interrupted if bleeding occurs, SGOT level exceeds 600 units/ml, LDH level exceeds 2,000 units/ml, or BUN level exceeds 25 mg/dl.

polymyxin B sulfate
Aerosporin♦

Pregnancy Risk Category: B

PHARMACOKINETICS
Distribution: widely distributed to tissues, with about 50% reversibly bound to cell membrane phospholipids. Drug doesn't cross the placenta or appear in cerebrospinal fluid (even with inflamed meninges), synovial fluid, or aqueous humor.
Metabolism: unknown.
Excretion: primarily excreted by glomerular filtration, with about 60% removed unchanged in urine. Half-life is about 4 to 6 hours in adults (2 to 3 days if creatinine clearance is less than 10 ml/minute); 8 hours in infants. Not known if drug appears in breast milk.
Action: peak serum level, unknown.

MECHANISM OF ACTION
This bactericidal drug alters permeability of bacterial cell-wall membrane, resulting in cell leakage. It's active against most aerobic gram-negative bacilli, except for most species of *Proteus* and *Neisseria.*

INDICATIONS & DOSAGE
• Acute urinary tract infection or septicemia caused by sensitive organisms. *Adults and children age 2 and over:* 15,000 to 25,000 U/kg daily (less than 15,000 U/kg daily in renal impairment) divided q 12

hours. *Children under age 2:* up to 40,000 U/kg daily divided q 12 hours.

CONTRAINDICATIONS & CAUTIONS
• Contraindicated in polymyxin hypersensitivity.
• Use cautiously in renal impairment or nitrogen retention because of possible nephrotoxicity and neurotoxicity.
• Use only if less toxic antibiotics are ineffective.

PREPARATION & STORAGE
Available as powder in 500,000 unit glass vials. Protect from light and store below 86° F. (30° C.). Reconstitute in 2 ml of sterile water for injection or 0.9% sodium chloride. Then dilute in 300 to 500 ml of dextrose 5% in water. Store solution in refrigerator, and use within 72 hours.

ADMINISTRATION
Direct injection: not recommended.
Intermittent infusion: Infuse diluted drug over 60 to 90 minutes.
Continuous infusion: Add daily dose to total fluids scheduled for infusion over 24 hours. Rate depends on volume.

INCOMPATIBILITY
Incompatible with amphotericin B, cefazolin sodium, cephalothin sodium, chloramphenicol sodium succinate, chlorothiazide sodium, heparin sodium, penicillins, prednisolone sodium phosphate, tetracycline hydrochloride. Also incompatible with cobalt, iron, manganese salts, and magnesium.

ADVERSE REACTIONS
Life-threatening: anaphylaxis, nephrotoxicity, neurotoxicity (respiratory paralysis).

Other: albuminuria, ataxia, azotemia, bacterial and fungal superinfection, blurred vision, coma, confusion, cylindruria, dizziness, drowsiness, eosinophilia, fever, flushing, nystagmus, paresthesias (circumoral and peripheral), seizures, slurred speech, thrombophlebitis, urticaria, weakness.

INTERACTIONS
Anesthetics, neuromuscular blockers: possible respiratory paralysis because of increased or prolonged skeletal muscle relaxation.
Nephrotoxic drugs: additive nephrotoxicity and neurotoxicity.

EFFECTS ON DIAGNOSTIC TESTS
None reported.

SPECIAL CONSIDERATIONS
• Administer only to hospitalized patients who've had baseline renal function tests performed.
• Obtain specimens for culture and sensitivity tests before starting therapy.
• During therapy, monitor renal function, intake and output, and serum drug levels, especially in patients with renal impairment. Adjust dosage, as ordered.
• Discontinue drug if urine output declines, serum creatinine or BUN levels rise, or patient develops respiratory paralysis.
• Watch for signs of bacterial or fungal superinfection and treat appropriately if superinfection occurs.
• Keep ventilatory support equipment available if drug is used with anesthetics or neuromuscular blockers.
• Dialysis doesn't remove appreciable amounts of drug.

---

potassium chloride
Potassium Chloride Injection

Pregnancy Risk Category: A

PHARMACOKINETICS
Distribution: in extracellular fluid and cells, where concentration may reach 40 times that outside cells.
Metabolism: not metabolized.
Excretion: in urine, primarily by glomerular filtration and renal tubular secretion. Small amounts excreted in sweat and feces. Drug appears in breast milk.
Action: onset, immediate; duration, unknown.

MECHANISM OF ACTION
The predominant cation in cells, potassium is essential for enzymatic reactions and nerve impulse transmission in the heart, brain, and skeletal muscle. It's also necessary for maintaining normal renal function, acid-base balance, and many cellular metabolic processes.

INDICATIONS & DOSAGE
• Hypokalemia. Dosage reflects patient needs and response. *Adults:* 150 mEq daily. If serum potassium exceeds 2.5 mEq/liter, up to 200 mEq daily (concentration less than 40 mEq/liter), not to exceed 10 mEq/hour. If serum potassium is less than 2 mEq/liter, up to 400 mEq daily, not to exceed 40 mEq/hour. *Children:* 2 to 3 mEq/kg or 40 mEq/m² daily. Maximum daily dose, 3 mEq/kg.

CONTRAINDICATIONS & CAUTIONS
• Contraindicated in severe renal impairment, untreated Addison's disease, hyperkalemia, acute dehydration, heat cramps, and burns because

elevated serum potassium levels can exacerbate these conditions.

• Use cautiously in patients with cardiac disorders because potassium may trigger conduction disturbances.

• In patients who require digitalis and in those with renal impairment, use cautiously because of the heightened risk of hyperkalemia.

• Also use cautiously in myotonia congenita; potassium may worsen symptoms.

• Use cautiously in breastfeeding women.

PREPARATION & STORAGE

Supplied in 5, 10, 15, 20, 30, and 60 ml ampules and vials containing 10, 20, 30, 40, 60, 90, and 120 mEq potassium. Store at room temperature. Always dilute before use. Dilution varies widely, but potassium concentration usually shouldn't exceed 40 mEq/liter. In emergencies, maximum concentration of 80 mEq/liter may be temporarily exceeded.

ADMINISTRATION

Direct injection: not used.
Intermittent infusion: not used.
Continuous infusion: Infuse diluted solution slowly, not to exceed 20 mEq/hour. Overly rapid infusion can cause fatal hyperkalemia. Infusion rate shouldn't exceed 1 mEq/minute for adults or 0.02 mEq/kg/minute for children.

INCOMPATIBILITY

Incompatible with amikacin, amphotericin B, diazepam, ergotamine, fat emulsion (10%), mannitol (20% or 25%), penicillin G sodium, phenytoin sodium, promethazine hydrochloride, streptomycin.

ADVERSE REACTIONS

Life-threatening: cardiac arrest, cardiac depression, dysrhythmias.

Other: anxiety, confusion, dyspnea, fatigue, leg heaviness or weakness, pain and phlebitis at injection site, paresthesias, weakness.

INTERACTIONS

Calcium salts (parenteral): antagonized cardiotoxicity of potassium.
Captopril, enalapril: possible hyperkalemia because of reduced aldosterone production.
Corticosteroids: possible decreased effectiveness of potassium supplements.
Potassium-sparing diuretics: possible severe hyperkalemia.
Quinidine: usually enhanced antiarrhythmic effects.

EFFECTS ON DIAGNOSTIC TESTS

Serum potassium: increased levels.

SPECIAL CONSIDERATIONS

• *Treatment of overdose:* Discontinue potassium-containing foods and drugs. Give insulin I.V., as ordered, in 10% to 25% dextrose solution (10 units insulin/20 g dextrose) at 300 to 500 ml/hour. Also give sodium bicarbonate I.V. to correct acidosis. May use exchange resins, hemodialysis, or peritoneal dialysis.

• Adding concentrated potassium chloride solutions to a hanging flexible plastic container can cause hyperkalemia because of inadequate mixing. When adding potassium solutions, invert the plastic container to avoid pooling of concentrated potassium at its base. Then knead the container to mix contents.

• Review renal function tests before giving potassium. Adequate renal function is essential to prevent hyperkalemia.

• In dehydrated patients, administer 1 liter of potassium-free fluid before potassium therapy.

- Monitor EKG, serum potassium BUN, and serum creatinine, pH, and intake and output.
- Discontinue infusion if patient develops signs of renal dysfunction, especially oliguria and elevated serum creatinine levels.
- Don't administer potassium chloride postoperatively until urine flow is established.
- In digitalized patients, treat hyperkalemia with caution; rapid reduction of serum potassium levels may result in digitalis toxicity.
- Potassium chloride is usually the salt of choice in treating hypokalemia; the chloride ion corrects hypochloremia, which often accompanies hypokalemia.

---

potassium phosphate
Potassium Phosphate Injection

Pregnancy Risk Category: C

PHARMACOKINETICS
Distribution: into extracellular fluid and cells, where potassium concentration may reach 40 times that outside cells. Phosphate remains in extracellular fluid.
Metabolism: not metabolized.
Excretion: about 90% in urine by glomerular filtration and remaining 10% in feces. Not known if drug appears in breast milk.
Action: onset, immediate; duration, unknown.

MECHANISM OF ACTION
By replacing phosphate, a buffer, potassium phosphate helps to maintain acid-base equilibrium of renal tubular fluids and regulate renal excretion of hydrogen ions. Drug also contributes to urine acidification, which maintains calcium solubility and reduces the possibility of calcium urolithiasis.

INDICATIONS & DOSAGE
- Electrolyte imbalance. *Adults:* equivalent of 10 millimoles (mM) or 310 mg of phosphorus daily. *Children:* equivalent of 1.5 to 2 mM or 46.5 to 62 mg of phosphorus daily. Dose must be individualized.

CONTRAINDICATIONS & CAUTIONS
- Contraindicated in hyperkalemia, hyperphosphatemia, infected urolithiasis caused by magnesium ammonium phosphate stones, and severe renal dysfunction (less than 30% of normal function) because of the increased risk of toxicity.
- Use cautiously in hypoparathyroidism because of possible hyperphosphatemia, and in osteomalacia, acute pancreatitis, chronic renal disease, and vitamin D deficiency because of the heightened risk of hypocalcemia.
- Because elevated potassium levels can cause conduction disturbances, use cautiously in patients with cardiac disorders, especially those taking digitalis.
- Also give carefully in severe Addison's disease, acute dehydration, myotonia congenita, severe renal insufficiency, and extensive tissue necrosis resulting from severe burns because of possible hyperkalemia.

PREPARATION & STORAGE
Supplied in 5 and 15 ml flip-top vials, 5 ml pin-top vial, and 50 ml bulk additive vial. Available strength is equivalent to 3 mM or 93 mg/ml of phosphorus. For infusion, dilute and thoroughly mix in a larger volume of compatible fluid. Store at room temperature.

ADMINISTRATION
Direct injection: not recommended.

Intermittent infusion: not recommended.

Continuous infusion: Infuse diluted solution slowly over the ordered time to avoid phosphate intoxication and severe hyperkalemia. Rate must be individualized.

INCOMPATIBILITY

Incompatible with dobutamine and solutions that contain calcium and magnesium, such as Ringer's lactate, Ringer's injection, dextrose and Ringer's injection, dextrose 10% in 0.9% sodium chloride, and Ionosol solutions.

ADVERSE REACTIONS

Life-threatening: hypocalcemic tetany, hyperkalemia, hyperphosphatemia.

Other: arm and leg pain, bone and joint pain, confusion, dizziness, dyspnea, edema of hands and feet, fatigue, headache, heaviness of legs, irregular heartbeat, muscle cramps, oliguria, pain at injection site, paresthesias, phlebitis, seizures, weakness.

INTERACTIONS

Captopril, enalapril, potassium-containing drugs, potassium-sparing diuretics: possible hyperkalemia.

Cardiac glycosides: increased risk of dysrhythmias if hyperkalemia occurs.

Mexiletine: possible accelerated excretion.

Quinidine: enhanced effects.

Salicylates: risk of toxicity.

Vitamin D (including calcifediol and calcitriol): possible heightened risk of hyperphosphatemia.

EFFECTS ON DIAGNOSTIC TESTS

Radionuclide bone imaging: decreased bone uptake of technetium Tc 99m.

SPECIAL CONSIDERATIONS

• *Treatment of overdose:* Discontinue potassium phosphate and correct serum electrolyte levels.

• Don't administer postoperatively until urine flow is established.

• Frequently monitor serum electrolyte levels (calcium, phosphorus, potassium, and sodium) and renal function (BUN and serum creatinine levels). Also monitor EKG for signs of conduction disturbances.

• I.V. infusion of phosphates in high concentrations can cause hypocalcemia.

---

pralidoxime chloride
Protopam Chloride♦

Pregnancy Risk Category: C

PHARMACOKINETICS

Distribution: dispersed throughout extracellular fluid, with poor binding to plasma protein. Drug penetrates the CNS.

Metabolism: exact process unknown; may occur in liver.

Excretion: 80% to 90% rapidly eliminated unchanged and as metabolite in urine within 12 hours, possibly by renal tubular secretion. Half-life ranges from 1 to 3 hours. Not known if drug appears in breast milk.

Action: onset, 5 to 15 minutes after injection; duration, unknown.

MECHANISM OF ACTION

Pralidoxime reactivates phosphorylated and carbamylated cholinesterase at neuromuscular junctions and autonomic effector sites and, to a lesser degree, within the CNS. Cholinesterase reactivation reverses anticholinesterase-induced paralysis of respiratory and skeletal muscles.

INDICATIONS & DOSAGE

• Poisoning by organophosphate cholinesterase inhibitors. *Adults:* 1 to 2 g. *Children:* 20 to 40 mg/kg. May be repeated in 1 hour if weakness persists.
• Overdose of anticholinesterase drugs (ambenonium, neostigmine, pyridostigmine) used in myasthenia gravis. *Adults:* 1 to 2 g, then 250 mg q 5 minutes.
Note: Reduce dosage in patient with renal impairment.

CONTRAINDICATIONS & CAUTIONS

• Contraindicated in hypersensitivity to any component of pralidoxime chloride.
• Also contraindicated in carbaril exposure because pralidoxime may increase carbaril toxicity.
• Use cautiously in patients receiving anticholinesterase drugs for myasthenia gravis because pralidoxime may precipitate myasthenic crisis.

PREPARATION & STORAGE

Supplied in a 20 ml vial containing 1 g of drug in white to off-white porous cake. Store vial at room temperature. Reconstitute with 20 ml of sterile water for injection (without preservatives) for a concentration of 50 mg/ml. For infusion, dilute reconstituted drug with 100 ml of 0.9% sodium chloride. Use solution within a few hours.

ADMINISTRATION

Direct injection: Inject dose over at least 5 minutes directly into vein or into I.V. tubing containing a free-flowing compatible solution.
Intermittent infusion: Infuse diluted drug over 15 to 30 minutes.
Continuous infusion: not recommended.

INCOMPATIBILITY

No incompatibilities reported.

ADVERSE REACTIONS

Life-threatening: laryngospasm.
Other: blurred vision, diplopia, dizziness, drowsiness, headache, hypertension, hyperventilation, maculopapular rash, muscle rigidity, nausea, tachycardia, weakness.

INTERACTIONS

Anticholinergic drugs: possible risk of myasthenic crisis in patients with myasthenia gravis.

EFFECTS ON DIAGNOSTIC TESTS

SGOT, SGPT: elevated levels for about 2 weeks after drug administration.

SPECIAL CONSIDERATIONS

• During administration, keep oxygen available as well as equipment for suctioning, emergency tracheostomy, and gastric lavage.
• Monitor vital signs and intake and output.
• Reduce administration rate or discontinue drug if patient develops hypertension. As ordered, give 5 mg of phentolamine I.V.
• If patient has ingested poison, carefully monitor him for 48 to 72 hours because of possible delayed intestinal absorption.
• Administer atropine concomitantly to treat poisoning with organophosphate cholinesterese inhibitors. Watch closely for signs of atropine toxicity (such as blurred vision, delirium, dry mouth, excitement, hallucinations, and tachycardia). Concurrent administration speeds onset of toxicity.
• Observe for rapid weakening in myasthenia gravis patients treated for overdose of carbamate anticholinesterase agents. Patients can pass

quickly from cholinergic crisis to myasthenic crisis. Keep edrophonium available to establish differential diagnosis and help reverse myasthenic crisis.

• Treatment is most effective when started within 24 hours of poisoning or overdose. It's usually of no benefit after 36 hours.

• Not effective in poisoning resulting from phosphorus, inorganic phosphates, or organophosphates with no anticholinesterase activity.

prednisolone sodium phosphate
Hydeltrasol, Key-Pred-SP, Predate-S

Pregnancy Risk Category: C

PHARMACOKINETICS
Distribution: rapidly dispersed to muscles, liver, skin, intestines, and kidneys. May bind to plasma protein transcortin; only unbound drug is active. Drug crosses the placenta.
Metabolism: primarily in the liver; some in most other tissues.
Excretion: in urine as inactive metabolites and small amounts of unchanged drug. Negligible amounts appear in bile. Half-life is about 2 to 3½ hours. Drug appears in breast milk.
Action: onset, rapid; duration, short but variable, depending on dose, frequency and time of administration, and length of therapy. Peak serum level, in 1 to 2 hours.

MECHANISM OF ACTION
A synthetic glucocorticoid, prednisolone decreases or prevents inflammation by inhibiting phagocytosis, lysosomal enzyme release, and synthesis and release of several chemical mediators of inflammation.

Drug suppresses the immune response, presumably by preventing or suppressing cell-mediated immune reactions (delayed hypersensitivity). It also stimulates protein catabolism, increases glucose availability, enhances lipolysis and mobilization of fatty acids from adipose tissues, decreases bone formation and increases bone resorption, and suppresses pituitary release of corticotropin.

INDICATIONS & DOSAGE
• Severe inflammation, immunosuppression. *Adults:* depending on disorder, 4 to 60 mg, then 10 to 400 mg daily. *Children:* suggested dosage 0.04 to 0.25 mg/kg or 1.5 to 7.5 mg/m^2 daily in a single dose or b.i.d. Dosage reflects severity of disorder and response to drug.

CONTRAINDICATIONS & CAUTIONS
• Contraindicated in hypersensitivity to corticosteroids or to any component of the drug.
• Also contraindicated in sepsis or septic shock because of anti-inflammatory and immunosuppressive effects.
• Give cautiously in acquired immunodeficiency syndrome (AIDS) or predisposition to AIDS because of the increased risk of severe, uncontrollable infections and neoplasms, and in systemic fungal infections and uncontrolled viral or bacterial infections because drug may exacerbate these conditions.
• In cardiac disease, congestive heart failure, or hypertension, give cautiously because fluid retention may be hazardous.
• Use cautiously in open-angle glaucoma because drug may raise intraocular pressure, and in ocular herpes

simplex infections because of possible corneal perforation.

• Administer cautiously in hepatic impairment because of the increased risk of toxicity and in renal impairment or calculi because drug may exacerbate fluid retention.

• Because prednisolone may further increase fatty acid or cholesterol levels, use it cautiously in hyperlipidemia.

• In hypoalbuminemia or conditions predisposing to this disorder (such as cirrhosis or nephrotic syndrome), give carefully because of the increased risk of toxicity.

• Use cautiously in hyperthyroidism because accelerated metabolism may reduce drug effects; in hypothyroidism because decreased metabolism may enhance drug effects; in myasthenia gravis because the drug may worsen weakness initially and produce respiratory distress; in osteoporosis because the drug may exacerbate bone loss; and in diabetes mellitus and latent or active tuberculosis (or a positive skin test) because the drug may exacerbate or activate these disorders.

• Also use cautiously in children and the elderly. Children may develop increased intracranial pressure (pseudotumor cerebri), causing papilledema, oculomotor or abducens nerve paralysis, vision loss, and headache. Elderly patients may develop hypertension.

PREPARATION & STORAGE
Available in 2, 5, and 10 ml vials containing 20 mg/ml. For infusion, dilute with dextrose 5% in water, 0.9% sodium chloride, or dextrose 5% in 0.9% sodium chloride. Store between 59° and 86° F. (15° and 30° C.). Protect from freezing and light.

ADMINISTRATION
Direct injection: Inject undiluted drug over 1 minute.
Intermittent infusion: Infuse ordered dose over prescribed duration.
Continuous infusion: Infuse ordered dose over prescribed duration.

INCOMPATIBILITY
Incompatible with calcium gluceptate or gluconate, dimenhydrinate, metaraminol, methotrexate sodium, polymyxin B, prochlorperazine edisylate, promazine, promethazine hydrochloride.

ADVERSE REACTIONS
Most adverse reactions are dose- or duration-dependent.
Life-threatening: anaphylaxis, dysrhythmias (after rapid, high-dose infusion).
Other: anxiety; blurred or decreased vision; burning, numbness, pain, or tingling at injection site; chest tightness; depression or other mood changes; dyspnea; facial flushing; false sense of well-being; frequent urination; GI upset; growth suppression in infants (when drug is taken by breast-feeding mother); hallucinations; hypertension; hypotension; increased appetite; increased thirst; infection; insomnia; irregular or bounding heartbeat; rash; restlessness; seizures; urticaria; wheezing.

INTERACTIONS
Acetaminophen: heightened risk of hepatotoxicity.
Aminoglutethimide: adrenal suppression.
Anabolic steroids, androgens: increased risk of edema.
Anticholinesterase drugs: severe weakness in myasthenia gravis patients.
Anticoagulants: usually, decreased effects; rarely, increased effects.

Barbiturates, ephedrine, phenytoin, rifampin: enhanced prednisolone metabolism.

Cardiac glycosides: increased risk of dysrhythmias or digitalis toxicity.

Isoniazid: enhanced metabolism and excretion.

Mexiletine: augmented metabolism.

Mitotane: suppressed adrenocorticoid effects.

Nondepolarizing neuromuscular blockers: increased or prolonged respiratory depression or paralysis.

Oral contraceptives: altered metabolism and protein binding of prednisolone.

Other immunosuppressive drugs: increased risk of infection, lymphomas, and lymphoproliferative disorders.

Potassium-depleting drugs: enhanced potassium-wasting effects of prednisolone.

Potassium supplements: reduced effects.

Ritodrine: risk of pulmonary edema or even death.

Salicylates: increased excretion.

Sodium-containing drugs: risk of edema and elevated blood pressure.

Somatotropin, somatrem: diminished growth response.

Streptozocin: heightened risk of hyperglycemia.

Thyroid hormones: decreased prednisolone metabolism.

Toxoids, vaccines: diminished response.

Troleandomycin: reduced prednisolone metabolism.

Ulcerogenic drugs: magnified risk of GI ulcers.

EFFECTS ON DIAGNOSTIC TESTS

ACTH stimulation test, plasma cortisol: possible decreased levels.

Basophil, eosinophil, lymphocyte, monocyte counts: possible decline.

Gonadorelin test: altered results.

Nitroblue tetrazolium test: possible false-negative results.

Platelet count: increased or decreased.

Polymorphonuclear leukocyte count: possible rise.

Protein-bound iodine, serum thyroxine: possible reduced levels.

Protirelin test: reduced response.

Radioactive iodine test: possible diminished uptake of ^{123}I or ^{131}I.

Radionuclide brain imaging: with high doses, decreased uptake of sodium pertechnetate Tc 99m or technetium 99m–labeled radionuclides in cerebral tumors.

Serum calcium, potassium: reduced levels.

Serum cholesterol, sodium: possible increased levels.

Serum glucose, urine glucose: possible elevated levels.

Serum uric acid: possible heightened levels in acute leukemia; reduced levels otherwise.

Urine 17-hydroxycorticosteroids and urine 17-ketosteroids: possible diminished levels.

SPECIAL CONSIDERATIONS

• Because of the risk of anaphylactoid reactions, keep emergency resuscitation equipment nearby.

• Monitor EKG for dysrhythmias, observe for signs of infection, and watch for depression or psychotic episodes, especially with high-dose therapy.

• In patients with diabetes, monitor urine and serum glucose levels. Increase insulin dose, as ordered.

• In acute adrenal insufficiency, expect to begin therapy by direct injection, then continue with slow I.V. infusion or I.M. administration.

• Monitor drug effect. Gradually titrate drug to lowest effective dose and administer for shortest possible time. Reduce dose gradually when discontinuing drug.

• In severe or life-threatening conditions (such as organ transplant rejection, acute nephritis associated with systemic lupus erythematosus, or acute respiratory distress syndrome), single-dose or short-term therapy with exceedingly high doses (pulse therapy) may be effective.
• After discontinuation of short-term (up to 5 days), high-dose therapy, adrenal recovery may take 1 week; after prolonged high-dose therapy, recovery may take up to 1 year or may never occur.
• May contain sulfites.

procainamide hydrochloride
Pronestyl♦

Pregnancy Risk Category: C

PHARMACOKINETICS
Distribution: rapidly dispersed into the liver, spleen, kidneys, lungs, heart, muscles, cerebrospinal fluid, and brain; 14% to 23% bound to plasma proteins. Drug crosses the placenta.
Metabolism: in the liver, where 25% is converted to the active metabolite *N*-acetylprocainamide (NAPA). About 40% of drug is converted in patients with rapid acetylation or renal impairment.
Excretion: in urine by tubular secretion and glomerular filtration; 40% to 70% is excreted unchanged. Procainamide and NAPA appear in breast milk. Procainamide half-life is 2½ to 5 hours; NAPA, about 7 hours. In renal impairment or congestive heart failure, NAPA accumulates to toxic levels in serum; procainamide levels remain normal.
Action: peak serum level, immediately after infusion.

MECHANISM OF ACTION
A Class I antiarrhythmic, procainamide decreases myocardial automaticity, excitability, and conduction velocity.

INDICATIONS & DOSAGE
• Dysrhythmias (paroxysmal atrial tachycardia, premature ventricular contractions, ventricular tachycardia, and, in some cases, atrial fibrillation). *Adults:* initially, 100 mg given slowly (not exceeding 50 mg/minute), then repeated to control dysrhythmias. Maximum dosage, 1 g, or 500 to 600 mg by infusion over 25 to 30 minutes at 2 to 6 mg/minute. Maintenance dosage, 1 to 6 mg/minute titrated to maintain control of dysrhythmias. Maximum dose, 1 g. *Children:* dosage not established. Recommendations include 3 to 6 mg/kg (not exceeding 100 mg) repeated p.r.n. at 10- to 30-minute intervals (not exceeding 30 mg/kg in 24 hours), or 3 to 6 mg/kg over 5 minutes, followed by maintenance infusion of 0.02 to 0.08 mg/kg/minute.
• Malignant hyperthermia. *Adults:* 200 to 900 mg, then maintenance infusion of 0.02 to 0.08 mg/kg/minute.
Note: In all indications, lowered doses may be required in congestive heart failure or renal impairment.

CONTRAINDICATIONS & CAUTIONS
• Contraindicated in hypersensitivity to procaine or other local anesthetics.
• Also contraindicated in second- or third-degree or complete AV heart block because of possible additive myocardial depression, and in atypical ventricular tachycardia because drug may cause exacerbation.
• Use cautiously in cardiac glycoside toxicity, severe first-degree AV block, or bundle branch block be-

cause of the risk of enhanced myocardial depression with ventricular tachycardia or asystole.

• Also use cautiously in congestive heart failure or hepatic or renal impairment because of possible drug accumulation and toxicity; in bronchial asthma because of possible hypersensitivity; in myasthenia gravis because drug may worsen weakness; and in systemic lupus erythematosus (SLE) because drug may cause exacerbations.

PREPARATION & STORAGE
Supplied in 10 ml (100 mg/ml) and 2 ml (500 mg/ml) vials. Store at room temperature. Protect from light and freezing. Don't use if markedly discolored or if precipitate has formed. For injection or loading infusion, dilute 1 g with 50 ml of dextrose 5% in water to yield 20 mg/ml. For continuous infusion, dilute 1 g with 500 ml of dextrose 5% in water to yield 2 mg/ml. In patients with fluid restrictions, dilute 1 g with 250 ml of dextrose 5% in water to yield 4 mg/ml. Note that drug may form a complex with dextrose, causing gradual loss of potency.

ADMINISTRATION
Direct injection: Inject dose over 2 minutes or longer directly into vein or into I.V. tubing containing a free-flowing compatible solution.
Intermittent infusion: Give loading infusion at 1 ml/minute for 25 to 30 minutes. Therapeutic effects usually occur after infusion of 100 to 200 mg. If no effect occurs after infusing 500 mg, wait at least 10 minutes to allow for drug distribution, then continue administration.
Continuous infusion: Using an infusion pump, give diluted solution at ordered rate, usually 2 to 6 mg/minute.

Patients receiving infusions should be attended at all times.

INCOMPATIBILITY
Incompatible with bretylium, ethacrynate, and phenytoin sodium.

ADVERSE REACTIONS
Life-threatening: severe hypotension, tachycardia (sympathetic response to hypotension), ventricular asystole or fibrillation with overly rapid administration.
Other: agranulocytosis, anorexia, bleeding or bruising, chills, confusion, depression, diarrhea, dizziness, drowsiness, fatigue, fever, flushing, hallucinations, joint swelling or pain, light-headedness, nausea, pruritus, rash, vomiting, weakness.

INTERACTIONS
Antiarrhythmics: possible additive or antagonized effects.
Antidyskinetics, antihistamines, antimuscarinics (especially atropine and related drugs): possible intensified atropine-like effects.
Antihypertensives: possible additive hypotension.
Antimyasthenics: possible decreased effects.
Bethanechol: antagonized cholinergic effects.
Bone marrow depressants: increased leukopenia and thrombocytopenia.
Bretylium: diminished inotropic effects and potentiated hypotension.
Cimetidine: elevated serum procainamide levels.
Lidocaine: additive CNS effects.
Neuromuscular blockers: prolonged or enhanced effects.
Pimozide: possible dysrhythmias.

EFFECTS ON DIAGNOSTIC TESTS
Coombs' test: possible false-positive result.

EKG: widened QRS complex, prolonged PR and QT intervals, and reduced QRS and T-wave voltage.
Platelet count: possible decline.
Serum alkaline phosphatase, bilirubin, LDH, SGPT: possible increased levels.
WBC count: possible drop.

SPECIAL CONSIDERATIONS

• *Treatment of overdose:* Signs include severe hypotension, confusion, dizziness or fainting, drowsiness, nausea and vomiting, oliguria, and unusually rapid or irregular heartbeat. If patient develops these signs, stop drug immediately. Replace fluids, then give norepinephrine or phenylephrine, as ordered. Maintain airway patency and ventilate the patient as necessary. Infusion of ⅙ M sodium lactate injection may reverse procainamide's cardiotoxic effects. Hemodialysis reduces serum half-life of procainamide, removing both procainamide and NAPA.
• Keep phenylephrine or norepinephrine available to treat severe hypotension.
• During administration, continuously monitor blood pressure and cardiac function (including EKG). Place the patient in a supine position for blood pressure monitoring. Discontinue drug if patient develops excessive hypotension, widened QRS complexes, or signs of impending myocardial infarction.
• In ventricular tachycardia, discontinue infusion if ventricular rate declines significantly without attaining regular AV conduction.
• Discontinue drug if signs of SLE or hemolytic anemia appear.
• Monitor response to drug and adjust dosage, as ordered.
• May contain benzyl alcohol and sulfites.

prochlorperazine edisylate
Compazine

Pregnancy Risk Category: C

PHARMACOKINETICS
Distribution: widespread, with high concentrations in the brain, lungs, liver, kidney, and spleen. Drug is highly bound to plasma proteins and readily crosses the placenta and blood-brain barrier.
Metabolism: principally occurs in the liver. Most metabolites are inactive; a few may contribute to drug action.
Excretion: in feces principally as metabolites and in urine as metabolites and unchanged drug. Small amounts appear in breast milk.
Action: onset, almost immediate; duration, varied, up to 12 hours.

MECHANISM OF ACTION
Not fully understood; thought to directly affect the medullary chemoreceptor trigger zone, apparently by blocking dopamine receptors.

INDICATIONS & DOSAGE
Dosage reflects patient's needs and response to drug.
• Severe nausea and vomiting resulting from surgery or toxins, radiation, or cytotoxic drugs. *Adults:* 5 to 10 mg (1 to 2 ml). May repeat every 3 to 4 hours.
• Prevention of nausea and vomiting during surgery. *Adults:* 5 to 10 mg by direct injection 15 to 30 minutes before induction of anesthesia. Repeat once before surgery, if necessary. Or 20 mg/liter by infusion 15 to 30 minutes before induction of anesthesia. Maximum dosage, 40 mg daily.

CONTRAINDICATIONS & CAUTIONS

• Contraindicated in hypersensitivity to prochlorperazine or other phenothiazines.
• Also contraindicated in severe CNS depression, coma, and severe cardiovascular disease because the drug may worsen these conditions.
• I.V. prochlorperazine isn't recommended for children.
• Use cautiously in Parkinson's disease because of the risk of enhanced extrapyramidal effects; in myelosuppression because of the increased risk of bone marrow toxicity; in cardiovascular disease because of the heightened risk of transient hypotension; in hepatic impairment because of possible altered drug metabolism and increased sensitivity to CNS effects; in seizure disorders because the drug may precipitate seizures; and in alcoholism because of possible deepened CNS depression.
• In patients with peptic ulcer, chronic respiratory disorders, or urine retention, administer prochlorperazine cautiously because of possible exacerbation.
• Also administer cautiously to patients exposed to extreme heat because the drug can disrupt the thermoregulatory mechanism; to patients with glaucoma or a predisposition to glaucoma because drug may potentiate the disorder; and to debilitated patients. Such patients usually require lowered doses.
• In symptomatic prostatic hypertrophy, use cautiously because of the enhanced risk of urine retention.
• Use cautiously in breastfeeding women.

PREPARATION & STORAGE

Available as a 5 mg/ml concentration in 2 ml ampules, 10 ml vials, 2 ml disposable syringes, and 1 and 2 ml prefilled cartridges. Store at room temperature and protect from light and freezing. Don't use if markedly discolored or a precipitate is present. Dilute for continuous infusion with at least 1 liter of a compatible isotonic solution, such as 0.9% sodium chloride, to yield 20 mg/liter.

ADMINISTRATION

Direct injection: Slowly inject undiluted drug at a rate of 5 mg/ml/minute. Never give as bolus injection.
Intermittent infusion: not recommended.
Continuous infusion: Infuse diluted drug at ordered rate over prescribed duration.

INCOMPATIBILITY

Incompatible with aminophylline, amphotericin B, ampicillin sodium, calcium gluceptate and gluconate, cephalothin sodium, chloramphenicol sodium succinate, chlorothiazide, dexamethasone sodium phosphate, dimenhydrinate, heparin sodium, hydrocortisone sodium succinate, hydromorphone, methicillin, methotrexate sodium, midazolam hydrochloride, penicillin G potassium and sodium, phenobarbital sodium, phenytoin sodium, prednisolone sodium phosphate, thiopental, vitamin B complex with C. Also incompatible with solutions containing methylparaben or propylparaben.

Don't mix prochlorperazine in the same syringe with any other drug.

ADVERSE REACTIONS

Life-threatening: anaphylaxis, bronchospasm, cardiac arrest, dysrhythmias, hypotension.
Other: akathisia, blood pressure changes, blurred vision or any visual change, breast pain or swelling, chewing movements, constipation, difficulty speaking, discolored skin and eyes (yellow-brown to grayish purple), dizziness, drowsiness, dry

---

Unmarked trade names available in the United States only.
♦Also available in Canada.   ♦♦Available in Canada only.

mouth, dysphagia, dyspnea, dystonic reactions, fainting, fatigue, fever, hyperpnea, irregular or rapid pulse, lip smacking, masklike facies, menstrual irregularities, muscle spasms (especially of face, neck, and back), nasal congestion, pale skin, photosensitivity, rapid or wormlike tongue movements, rash, restlessness, seizures, shuffling gait, sore throat, stiffness, sweating increase or decrease, trembling of hands and fingers, unusual breast milk secretion, urinary difficulty or incontinence, weakness, weight gain.

INTERACTIONS

Alcohol: possible deepened CNS and respiratory depression, hypotension, potentiated CNS excitation.

Amantadine, antidyskinetics, antihistamines, antimuscarinics (such as atropine): possible intensified adverse effects, especially confusion, hallucinations, and nightmares.

Amphetamines: reduced effects.

Anticonvulsants (including barbiturates): lowered seizure threshold; inhibited phenytoin metabolism.

Antithyroid agents: heightened risk of agranulocytosis.

Barbiturate anesthetics: possible CNS excitation.

Beta-adrenergic blockers: elevated serum levels of both interacting drugs.

Bone marrow depressants: worsened leukopenia or thrombocytopenia.

Bromocriptine: inhibited effects resulting from increased serum prolactin levels.

CNS depressants: possible deepened CNS and respiratory depression, hypotension.

Dopamine: possible antagonism of peripheral vasoconstriction.

Ephedrine, metaraminol: reduced pressor response.

Epinephrine: severe hypotension and tachycardia, resulting from antagonized alpha-adrenergic effects.

Guanadrel or guanethidine: decreased hypotensive effects.

Levodopa: inhibited effects.

MAO inhibitors, tricyclic antidepressants: possible prolonged and intensified sedative and antimuscarinic effects.

Mephentermine: antagonized antipsychotic effects of prochlorperazine or pressor effects of mephentermine.

Methoxamine, phenylephrine: diminished pressor effects and shortened duration of action.

Metrizamide: lowered seizure threshold.

Other photosensitizing drugs: possible additive effects.

Ototoxic drugs: possible masked symptoms of ototoxicity. Use together cautiously.

Quinidine: increased cardiac effects.

EFFECTS ON DIAGNOSTIC TESTS

EKG: possible Q- and T-wave changes.

Gonadorelin test: blunted response.

Metyrapone stimulation: reduced ACTH secretion.

Urine bilirubin: possible false-negative results.

Urine pregnancy tests: possible false-positive or false-negative results, depending on test used.

Urine amylase, 5-hydroxyindoleacetic acid, porphobilinogens, urobilinogen, uroporphyrins: possible false-positive results.

SPECIAL CONSIDERATIONS

• *Treatment of overdose:* Anticholinergic antiparkinson drugs may help to control extrapyramidal reactions.

• Because of the risk of hypotension, use I.V. route only for closely monitored patients.

- Initially administer low doses to the elderly. Increase gradually.
- Antiemetic effect may mask signs of drug toxicity or obscure diagnosis of conditions having nausea as a primary symptom.
- Skin contact with drug can cause contact dermatitis.
- May contain benzyl alcohol and sulfites.

promazine hydrochloride
Sparine♦

Pregnancy Risk Category: C

PHARMACOKINETICS
Distribution: widespread, with high concentrations in the brain, lungs, liver, kidneys, and spleen. Drug is highly bound to plasma proteins. It readily crosses the placenta and blood-brain barrier.
Metabolism: exact process unknown, but drug is extensively metabolized in the liver. Most metabolites are inactive, but some (such as 7-hydroxychlorpromazine, mesoridazine) may contribute to drug action.
Excretion: primarily in urine, with minute amounts excreted in feces, mostly as metabolites. Drug may appear in breast milk.
Action: peak effect in 2 to 4 hours.

MECHANISM OF ACTION
Promazine is thought to block postsynaptic dopamine receptors in the brain. Drug also produces alpha-adrenergic blocking effects and inhibits release of hypothalamic, pituitary, and hypophyseal hormones.

INDICATIONS & DOSAGE
- Severe agitation. *Adults:* 50 to 150 mg, then additional doses at 30-minute intervals (maximum daily dos-

age, 300 mg). Use lowest possible effective dose.

CONTRAINDICATIONS & CAUTIONS
- Contraindicated in phenothiazine hypersensitivity.
- Also contraindicated in severe CNS depression, coma, and severe cardiovascular disease because drug may worsen these conditions.
- Use cautiously in alcoholism because of possible worsened CNS depression; in Parkinson's disease because of the risk of enhanced extrapyramidal effects; and in hepatic impairment because of possible altered drug metabolism and enhanced sensitivity to CNS effects.
- Drug may potentiate glaucoma; use cautiously.
- In patients with peptic ulcer, chronic respiratory disorders, or urine retention, administer promazine cautiously because of the risk of exacerbating these conditions.
- Administer cautiously in symptomatic prostatic hypertrophy because of the increased risk of urine retention and in seizure disorders because promazine may trigger seizures.
- Safety and efficacy haven't been established in children younger than age 12.

PREPARATION & STORAGE
Available as a 25 mg/ml concentration in 10 ml vials and 1 ml prefilled cartridges. Also supplied as a 50 mg/ml concentration in 2 and 10 ml vials and 1 and 2 ml prefilled cartridges. Store at room temperature, and protect from light and freezing. Don't use if markedly discolored or if a precipitate is present. Dilute with 0.9% sodium chloride or dextrose 5% in water to yield a concentration of 25 mg/ml or less.

ADMINISTRATION

Direct injection: Slowly inject diluted solution into vein or into an I.V. line containing a free-flowing compatible solution. Avoid extravasation.

Intermittent infusion: not recommended.

Continuous infusion: not used.

INCOMPATIBILITY

Incompatible with aminophylline, chloramphenicol sodium succinate, chlorothiazide, dimenhydrinate, fibrinogen, fibrinolysin (human), heparin sodium, hydrocortisone sodium succinate, methohexital, nafcillin, penicillin G potassium, pentobarbital sodium, phenobarbital sodium, phenytoin sodium, prednisolone sodium phosphate, sodium bicarbonate, thiopental, vitamin B complex with C, warfarin.

ADVERSE REACTIONS

Life-threatening: anaphylaxis, bronchospasm, dysrhythmias, laryngospasm.

Other: akathisia, blood pressure changes, blurred vision or any visual change, breast pain or swelling, chewing movements, constipation, difficulty speaking, dizziness, drowsiness, dry mouth, dysphagia, dyspnea, dystonic reactions, fainting, fatigue, fever, hyperpnea, irregular or rapid pulse, lip smacking, mask-like facies, menstrual irregularities, muscle spasms (especially of face, neck, and back), nasal congestion, pale skin, photosensitivity, rapid or wormlike tongue movements, rash, restlessness, seizures, shuffling gait, sore throat, stiffness, sweating increase or decrease, trembling of hands and fingers, unusual breast milk secretion, urinary difficulty or incontinence, weakness, yellow eyes or skin.

INTERACTIONS

Alcohol: possible deepened CNS and respiratory depression, hypotension, potentiated CNS excitation.

Amantadine, antidyskinetics, antihistamines, antimuscarinics (such as atropine): possible intensified adverse effects, especially confusion, hallucinations, and nightmares.

Amphetamines: reduced effects.

Anticonvulsants (including barbiturates): lowered seizure threshold; inhibited phenytoin metabolism.

Antithyroid agents: heightened risk of agranulocytosis.

Barbiturate anesthetics: possible CNS excitation.

Beta-adrenergic blockers: elevated serum levels of both interacting drugs.

Bone marrow depressants: worsened leukopenia or thrombocytopenia.

Bromocriptine: inhibited effects resulting from increased serum prolactin levels.

CNS depressants: possible deepened CNS and respiratory depression, hypotension.

Dopamine: possible antagonism of peripheral vasoconstriction.

Ephedrine, metaraminol: reduced pressor response.

Epinephrine: severe hypotension and tachycardia, resulting from antagonized alpha-adrenergic effects.

Guanadrel or guanethidine: decreased hypotensive effects.

Levodopa: inhibited effects.

Lithium: extrapyramidal symptoms and possible accelerated rate of renal excretion.

MAO inhibitors, tricyclic antidepressants: possible prolonged and intensified sedative and antimuscarinic effects.

Mephentermine: antagonized antipsychotic effects of promazine or pressor effects of mephentermine.

Methoxamine, phenylephrine: diminished pressor effects and shortened duration of action.
Metrizamide: lowered seizure threshold.
Other photosensitizing drugs: possible additive effects.
Ototoxic drugs: possible masked symptoms of ototoxicity. Use together cautiously.
Quinidine: increased cardiac effects.
Riboflavin: possible increased requirements.

EFFECTS ON DIAGNOSTIC TESTS
EKG: possible Q- and T-wave changes.
Gonadorelin test: blunted response.
Metyrapone stimulation test: possible reduced ACTH secretion.
Urine bilirubin: possible false-negative results.
Urine pregnancy tests: possible false-positive or false-negative results, depending on test used.

SPECIAL CONSIDERATIONS
• *Treatment of overdose:* Maintain respiratory function and body temperature. Control dysrhythmias with I.V. phenytoin, as ordered. Give digitalis for cardiac failure and vasopressors, such as norepinephrine, for hypotension. Don't use epinephrine, which may result in severe hypotension. Control seizures with diazepam, followed by phenytoin, while monitoring EKG. For acute parkinson-like symptoms, administer benztropine or diphenhydramine, as ordered.
• Administer promazine I.V. only to hospitalized patients, and change to oral therapy as soon as possible.
• Administer drug promptly. Solutions prepared with 0.9% sodium chloride and left to sit at room temperature in daylight lost 15% of potency in 24 hours.

• Monitor blood pressure, EKG, and blood studies throughout therapy.
• Keep patient supine for 1 hour after administration because drug may cause orthostatic hypotension. Advise him to change position slowly.
• Skin contact with promazine injection may cause contact dermatitis.
• Carefully monitor elderly patients. They have a higher incidence of adverse reactions.
• Debilitated patients may require lower doses.

promethazine hydrochloride
Anergan, Pentazine, Phenazine, Phenergan♦, Prometh, Prorex, V-Gan

Pregnancy Risk Category: C

PHARMACOKINETICS
Distribution: widely dispersed in tissues. In organs, lowest concentrations occur in the brain, but these are higher than plasma concentrations. Drug is 76% to 90% bound to plasma proteins. Readily crosses the placenta.
Metabolism: in the liver.
Excretion: eliminated slowly in urine and feces. Not known if drug appears in breast milk.
Action: onset, 3 to 5 minutes; duration, 6 to 12 hours as antihistamine, 2 to 8 hours as sedative.

MECHANISM OF ACTION
This drug competes with histamine for H_1-receptor sites on effector cells, preventing (but not reversing) histamine-mediated spasmodic and congestive responses. The drug also has antiemetic effects, probably through inhibition of the medullary chemoreceptor trigger zone, as well as antivertigo effects resulting from

central antimuscarinic action on this trigger zone, the vestibular apparatus, and the vomiting center. It also acts as a sedative-hypnotic, possibly by indirectly reducing stimulation to the brain stem reticular system.

INDICATIONS & DOSAGE
• Allergic reactions. *Adults:* 25 mg, repeated in 2 hours if necessary.
• Nausea and vomiting. *Adults:* 12.5 to 25 mg q 4 hours p.r.n. *Children:* 0.25 to 0.5 mg/kg four to six times daily.
• Obstetric sedation. *Adults:* 50 mg during early labor stage; then 25 to 75 mg in established labor (given with an opiate agonist). If necessary, 25 to 50 mg dose may be repeated once or twice at 4-hour intervals. Maximum dosage, 100 mg in 24 hours.
• Sedation and relief of apprehension, postoperative pain (anesthesia and analgesia adjunct). *Adults:* 25 to 50 mg p.r.n. Maximum dosage, 150 mg daily.

CONTRAINDICATIONS & CAUTIONS
• Contraindicated in promethazine hypersensitivity and in breastfeeding women.
• Avoid use in coma because high doses may cause exacerbation.
• Use cautiously in acute asthma or respiratory disorders because antimuscarinic drying effects may thicken secretions, impairing expectoration. The drug may also suppress the cough reflex.
• In severe obesity or neuromuscular disease, also use cautiously because of possible airway or ventilation problems.
• In bladder neck obstruction, symptomatic prostatic hypertrophy, or predisposition to urine retention, use cautiously because the drug may

precipitate or aggravate urine retention.
• Give cautiously in hepatic impairment because of decreased drug metabolism; in jaundice because drug may aggravate disorder; in myelosuppression because of an increased risk of leukopenia and agranulocytosis; in cardiovascular disease because of possible transient hypotension; and in hypertension because drug may worsen the disorder.
• Administer cautiously to patients with angle-closure glaucoma or predisposition to this condition because increased intraocular pressure may precipitate an acute attack.
• Because drug may reduce GI motility and tone, resulting in obstruction and gastric retention, give drug cautiously in patients with stenosis caused by peptic ulcer or with a history of peptic ulcer.
• Also give cautiously to patients with epilepsy because drug may intensify seizures; and to elderly patients, who are more susceptible to dizziness, sedation, confusion, and hypotension.

PREPARATION & STORAGE
Available as a 25 mg/ml concentration in 1 and 10 ml ampules, 1 and 10 ml vials, and 1 ml prefilled cartridges. Store at room temperature, and protect from light and freezing. Don't use if solution is discolored or if a precipitate is present.

ADMINISTRATION
Direct injection: Inject at a rate not exceeding 25 mg/minute into an I.V. line containing a free-flowing compatible solution. Rapid administration may reduce blood pressure temporarily.
Concentration shouldn't exceed 25 mg/ml. Be sure I.V. line is patent before injection, and avoid extravasation or inadvertent intraarterial in-

jection because of possible gangrene or severe arteriospasm.
Intermittent infusion: not recommended.
Continuous infusion: not recommended.

INCOMPATIBILITY
Incompatible with aminophylline, carbenicillin disodium, chloramphenicol sodium succinate, chlorothiazide, diatrizoate meglumine (34.3%) and diatrizoate sodium (35%), diatrizoate meglumine (52%) and diatrizoate sodium (8%), diatrizoate sodium (75%), dimenhydrinate, heparin sodium, hydrocortisone sodium succinate, iodipamide meglumine (52%), iothalamate meglumine (60%), iothalamate sodium (80%), methicillin, methohexital, morphine, penicillin G potassium and sodium, pentobarbital sodium, phenobarbital sodium, phenytoin sodium, prednisolone sodium phosphate, thiopental, vitamin B complex.

ADVERSE REACTIONS
Life-threatening: anaphylaxis, bronchospasm, laryngospasm.
Other: agranulocytosis; blurred vision; clumsiness; decreased alertness; dizziness; drowsiness; dry mouth, nose, and throat; dyspnea; excitement; fever; flushing; GI upset; hypotension; irritability; leukopenia; muscle spasms, especially of the neck or back; nausea; nervousness; nightmares; obstructive jaundice; photosensitivity; rash; restlessness; sore throat; tachycardia; ticlike movements of head and face; tinnitus; trembling of hands; unsteadiness; vomiting.

INTERACTIONS
Alcohol: possible potentiated effects.

Alphaprodine: increased analgesia, CNS and respiratory depression, and hypotensive effects.
Amantadine, antidyskinetics, antihistamines, antimuscarinics (especially atropine): potentiated antimuscarinic effects.
Amphetamines: diminished effects.
Anticonvulsants, including barbiturates, metrizamide (intrathecal): possible lowered seizure thresholds.
Antithyroid agents: heightened risk of agranulocytosis.
Apomorphine: reduced emetic response; deepened CNS depression.
Beta-adrenergic blockers: elevated serum levels of interacting drugs.
Bromocriptine: hindered effects, resulting from possible increased serum prolactin levels.
Dopamine: possible antagonized peripheral vasoconstriction.
Ephedrine: possible reduced alpha-adrenergic blocking action of promethazine.
Epinephrine: possible severe hypotension and tachycardia, resulting from antagonized alpha-adrenergic action of promethazine.
Guanadrel, guanethidine: decreased effects.
Hepatotoxic drugs: enhanced risk of hepatotoxicity.
Levodopa: possible diminished effects.
MAO inhibitors, tricyclic antidepressants: potentiated effects.
Metaraminol: usually decreased pressor response.
Methoxamine: possible diminished pressor effects and shortened duration of action.
Other CNS depressants (especially anesthetics, barbiturates, opioids): potentiated effects.
Ototoxic drugs: possible masked symptoms of ototoxicity.
Photosensitizing drugs: possible heightened effects.

Quinidine: possible additive cardiac effects.

Riboflavin: possible increased requirements.

EFFECTS ON DIAGNOSTIC TESTS

Skin tests using allergen extracts: possible inhibition of cutaneous histamine response, producing false-negative results.

Glucose tolerance: increased level.

Urine pregnancy tests: false-positive or false-negative results.

SPECIAL CONSIDERATIONS

• *Treatment of overdose:* Give oxygen and I.V. fluids as needed to maintain cardiopulmonary function. Give phenylephrine or norepinephrine to treat hypotension. Don't use epinephrine, which may further lower blood pressure. Also administer anticholinergic antiparkinson drugs, diphenhydramine, or barbiturates, as ordered, to treat extrapyramidal symptoms.

• When giving barbiturates with promethazine, decrease barbiturate dosage by at least one-half, as ordered. When giving narcotics with drug, reduce narcotic dosage by one-fourth to one-half.

• Reduce dosage, as ordered, in dehydrated patients or those with oliguria because diminished urine excretion may potentiate toxicity.

• Watch for extrapyramidal reactions, especially in the elderly.

• Be aware that antiemetic effects may obscure signs of intestinal obstruction, brain tumor, or promethazine overdose.

• May contain sulfites. Prorex also contains benzyl alcohol.

propofol
Diprivan

Pregnancy Risk Category: B

PHARMACOKINETICS

Distribution: highly lipophilic, propofol distributes rapidly to well-perfused tissues. Like thiobarbiturate compounds, it subsequently redistributes to lean muscle and fat. Cessation of drug effects results partly from this rapid redistribution.

Metabolism: not fully characterized. Drug is principally conjugated within the liver.

Excretion: primarily renal; 70% of the drug is excreted in urine within 24 hours and 90% within 5 days.

MECHANISM OF ACTION

Propofol produces a dose-dependent CNS depression similar to benzodiazepines and barbiturates. It causes hypnosis rapidly with minimal excitation.

INDICATIONS & DOSAGE

• Induction of anesthesia. *Adults:* Doses must be individualized according to patient's condition and age. Most patients classified as American Society of Anesthesiologists (ASA) Physical Status category (PS) I or II under age 55 require 2 to 2.5 mg/kg. The drug is usually administered in 40 mg boluses q 10 seconds until the desired response is obtained.

Elderly, debilitated, or hypovolemic patients, or patients in ASA PS III or IV should receive half of the usual induction dose (20 mg boluses q 10 seconds).

• Maintenance of anesthesia. *Adults:* Propofol may be given as a variable rate infusion, titrated to clinical effect. Most patients may be maintained with 0.1 to 0.2 mg/kg/minute

(6 to 12 mg/kg/hour). Elderly, debilitated, or hypovolemic patients, or patients in ASA PS III or IV should receive half of the usual maintenance dose (0.05 to 0.1 mg/kg/minute or 3 to 6 mg/kg/hour).

CONTRAINDICATIONS & CAUTIONS

• Contraindicated in patients hypersensitive to propofol or any components of the emulsion, including soybean oil, egg lecithin, and glycerol.
• Avoid using propofol for obstetrical anesthesia (safety to the fetus hasn't been established). Also avoid using in increased intracranial pressure or impaired cerebral circulation (hypotension may substantially reduce cerebral perfusion).
• Because the drug is given as an emulsion, give cautiously to patients with diabetic hyperlipidemia or with a history of lipid metabolism disorders, such as pancreatitis or primary hyperlipoproteinemia.
• Use cautiously in elderly or debilitated patients and in those with circulatory disorders. Although the drug's hemodynamic effects can vary, the major effect in patients maintaining spontaneous ventilation is hypotension with little or no change in heart rate and cardiac output. Blood pressures can decrease by as much as 30%. However, the incidence and degree of diminished cardiac output increases in patients undergoing assisted or controlled positive-pressure ventilation.

PREPARATION & STORAGE

Supplied in 20 ml ampules containing 10 mg/ml. If drug is to be diluted before infusion, use only dextrose 5% in water, and do not dilute to a concentration less than 2 mg/ml. After dilution, drug is probably more stable in glass containers than in plastic ones.

When administered into a running I.V., propofol emulsion is compatible with dextrose 5% in water, lactated Ringer's injection, lactated Ringer's and 5% dextrose injection, 5% dextrose and 0.45% sodium chloride injection, and 5% dextrose and 0.2% sodium chloride injection. Store unopened ampules above 40° F. (4° C.) and below 72° F. (22° C.). Do not refrigerate.

ADMINISTRATION

Direct injection: For induction in an adult, administer 40 mg q 10 seconds until desired response is obtained.
Intermittent infusion: For maintenance of anesthesia in an adult, give 0.1 to 0.2 mg/kg/minute.
Continuous infusion: not recommended.

INCOMPATIBILITY

Do not mix with other drugs.

ADVERSE REACTIONS

Life-threatening: none reported.
Other: abdominal cramping, apnea, bradycardia, clonic-myoclonic movement, cough, dizziness, fever, flushing, headache, hiccups, hypertension, hypotension, local effects at injection site (burning, coldness, numbness, pain, stinging, or tingling), nausea, twitching, vomiting.

INTERACTIONS

Potent inhalational anesthetics (such as enflurane, halothane, and isoflurane), or supplemental anesthetics (such as nitrous oxide and opiates): possible enhanced anesthetic and cardiovascular actions of propofol.
Premedication with opiates or opiates with sedatives: may enhance reduction of systolic, diastolic, and mean arterial pressure, as well as cause a more pronounced decrease

in cardiac output. Induction dose requirements may also be decreased.

EFFECTS ON DIAGNOSTIC TESTS
None reported.

SPECIAL CONSIDERATIONS
• Propofol should be given only by staff familiar with airway management and administration of I.V. anesthetics.
• Propofol pharmacokinetics aren't altered by hepatic cirrhosis, chronic renal failure, or sex of patient.
• Propofol has no vagolytic activity. Premedication with anticholinergics, such as glycopyrrolate or atropine, may help manage potential increases in vagal tone caused by other drugs or surgery.
• Treatment for significant hypotension or bradycardia includes increased rate of fluid administration, pressor agents, elevation of lower extremities, or atropine. Apnea often occurs during induction and may persist for longer than 60 seconds. Ventilatory support may be required.
• Not recommended for use in children because safety and efficacy haven't been established.
• Not recommended for breastfeeding mothers. Propofol is excreted in breast milk.

---

propranolol hydrochloride
Inderal♦

Pregnancy Risk Category: C

PHARMACOKINETICS
Distribution: widely dispersed throughout tissues, including the lungs, liver, kidneys, and heart, with more than 90% bound to plasma proteins. Drug crosses the blood-brain barrier and placenta.

Metabolism: in the liver.
Excretion: primarily in urine, with only 1% to 4% removed in feces; fecal excretion rises in severe renal impairment. Small amounts of drug appear in breast milk. Half-life varies from 10 minutes to 6 hours and may decrease in renal impairment.
Action: onset, immediate; duration, 3½ to 6 hours.

MECHANISM OF ACTION
Propranolol competitively blocks beta-adrenergic receptors in the myocardium and in bronchial and vascular smooth muscle, reducing heart rate, decreasing myocardial contractility and cardiac output, and increasing systolic ejection time and cardiac volume. Propranolol also reduces conduction velocity and myocardial automaticity. The drug's hypotensive effects stem from its ability to block peripheral adrenergic receptors, decreasing sympathetic outflow from the CNS and suppressing renin release.

INDICATIONS & DOSAGE
• Life-threatening dysrhythmias or those occurring under anesthesia.
Adults: 0.5 to 3 mg repeated after 2 minutes and again after 4 hours if necessary. *Children:* 0.01 to 0.1 mg/kg (up to a maximum of 1 mg per dose) q 6 to 8 hours.
• Substitute for oral administration during surgery. *Adults:* 10% of oral dose.

CONTRAINDICATIONS & CAUTIONS
• Contraindicated in Raynaud's syndrome and malignant hypertension because of possible peripheral arterial insufficiency, and in bronchial asthma because beta-adrenergic blockade may lead to increased airway resistance and bronchospasm.

• Also contraindicated in sinus bradycardia, heart block greater than first degree, myocardial infarction (systolic pressure below 100 mm Hg), congestive heart failure (unless caused by tachydysrhythmia treatable with propranolol), and usually cardiogenic shock. Further myocardial depression can occur with these conditions.

• Avoid use in myasthenia gravis because the drug may exacerbate symptoms.

• Use cautiously in cardiac impairment because drug may precipitate congestive heart failure, and in hyperthyroidism because drug may mask tachycardia.

• Give carefully to patients with nonallergic bronchospastic disease because drug may increase airway resistance and bronchospasm.

• Give cautiously to patients with depression because of possible exacerbation.

• In patients with hepatic or renal failure, give cautiously because of risk of adverse reactions.

• In patients with diabetes mellitus who receive oral hypoglycemic drugs, propranolol may trigger hyperglycemic reactions or hypoglycemia and may inhibit pancreatic insulin release. Use cautiously.

• Use cautiously in breastfeeding women.

• Pediatric safety and efficacy haven't been established.

PREPARATION & STORAGE

Available in 1 ml ampules containing 1 mg/ml. Drug is compatible with 0.9% sodium chloride solution and dextrose 5% in water. Store at room temperature and protect from light and freezing.

ADMINISTRATION

Direct injection: Inject drug at a maximum rate of 1 mg/minute through an I.V. line containing a free-flowing compatible solution.
Intermittent infusion: not recommended.
Continuous infusion: not recommended.

INCOMPATIBILITY

No incompatibilities reported.

ADVERSE REACTIONS

Life-threatening: AV dissociation, cardiac arrest, complete heart block, intensified AV block, pulmonary edema, ventricular fibrillation.
Other: alopecia (reversible), bradycardia, confusion, constipation, diarrhea, dizziness, dry mouth, eosinophilia (transient), flatulence, fluid retention, hallucinations, hypotension, irritability, laryngospasm, light-headedness, lupuslike reactions, migraine, nausea, partial heart block, peripheral arterial insufficiency, peripheral neuropathy, pharyngitis, respiratory distress, rhinitis, vomiting.

INTERACTIONS

Antiarrhythmic drugs (such as lidocaine, phenytoin, procainamide, or quinidine): possible additive or antagonistic cardiac effects and magnified toxic effects.
Atropine, other antimuscarinics: possible reversal of propranolol-induced bradycardia.
Cimetidine: reduced propranolol clearance, resulting from inhibited hepatic metabolism.
Diuretics, other antihypertensives: potentiated hypotension.
Levodopa: antagonized hypotensive and positive inotropic effects.
Neuromuscular blockers: possible potentiated effects.
Phenothiazines: enhanced hypotensive effects, especially with high phenothiazine doses.

Sympathomimetics (such as isoproterenol and epinephrine): antagonized beta-adrenergic effects.
Tricyclic antidepressants: antagonized cardiac effects.

EFFECTS ON DIAGNOSTIC TESTS

Antinuclear antibody titers: possible dose-related increases.
BUN, serum creatinine: possible elevated levels.
Intraocular pressure: reduced.
Radionuclide cardiac scan: possible decreased myocardial uptake of thallous chloride.
Serum alkaline phosphatase, LDH; SGOT, SGPT: possible increased levels.
Serum lipoproteins, triglycerides: possible elevated levels.
Serum potassium, uric acid: possible increased levels.

SPECIAL CONSIDERATIONS

• *Treatment of overdose:* If patient is hypotensive, correct severe bradycardia with atropine I.V. and, if necessary, give isoproterenol, dobutamine, or epinephrine. For premature ventricular contractions, administer I.V. lidocaine or phenytoin. For cardiac failure, give oxygen, diuretics, and digitalis. A transvenous pacemaker may be used if drug therapy is unsuccessful.

For hypotension, place patient in Trendelenburg position and administer I.V. fluids (unless pulmonary edema is present) and an I.V. vasopressor. If seizures occur, give I.V. diazepam (or, if necessary, phenytoin). For bronchospasm, give isoproterenol or a theophylline derivative. Glucagon may be used to counter cardiovascular effects of propranolol overdose.
• Carefully monitor EKG, blood pressure, and central venous pressure during administration.

• Stay alert for adverse reactions; they're more frequent and severe with I.V. administration than with oral administration.
• Change to oral propranolol as soon as possible. Keep in mind that I.V. doses are appreciably smaller than oral ones.
• Adjust dosage, as ordered, in elderly patients to reflect their response to drug.
• Give lower doses in hepatic impairment.

---

protamine sulfate

Pregnancy Risk Category: C

PHARMACOKINETICS

Distribution: not well characterized. However, drug is known to combine with heparin in the bloodstream. Not known if it crosses the placenta.
Metabolism: as protamine-heparin complex, may be partly metabolized or degraded, thus freeing heparin.
Excretion: not well characterized. Not known if drug appears in breast milk.
Action: onset, 30 to 60 seconds; duration, about 2 hours, depending on body temperature.

MECHANISM OF ACTION

When administered after heparin, protamine forms a stable complex with strongly acidic heparin sodium or heparin calcium. This complex possesses no anticoagulant activity. When administered in the absence of heparin, protamine has weak anticoagulant effects, probably because it inhibits thrombin generation.

INDICATIONS & DOSAGE

• Severe heparin overdose. *Adults:* Dosage reflects heparin dose, route, and time elapsed since administra-

tion. Typically, 1 mg of protamine sulfate neutralizes about 90 units of heparin sodium derived from bovine lung tissue, 100 units of heparin calcium derived from porcine intestinal mucosa, or 115 units of heparin sodium derived from porcine intestinal mucosa. Dosage guidelines: 1 to 1.5 mg/100 units heparin when given a few minutes after I.V. heparin injection; 0.5 to 0.75 mg/100 units heparin when given 30 to 60 minutes after I.V. heparin injection; 0.25 to 0.375 mg/100 units heparin when given more than 2 hours after I.V. heparin injection; 25 to 50 mg after continuous infusion of heparin; 1 to 1.5 mg/100 units heparin after deep S.C. heparin injection, or 25 to 50 mg by continuous infusion over 8 to 16 hours or expected duration of heparin absorption.
• Neutralization of heparin administered during extracorporeal circulation in arterial and cardiac surgery or dialysis procedures. *Adults and children:* usually 1.5 mg/100 units heparin.

CONTRAINDICATIONS & CAUTIONS
• Contraindicated in protamine hypersensitivity. Also contraindicated in neonates if drug is reconstituted with bacteriostatic water containing benzyl alcohol.
• Use cautiously in patients with allergies to fish; protamine is derived from fish sperm.
• Use cautiously in patients with diabetes who receive protamine zinc insulin and in infertile or vasectomized men because of increased risk of protamine sensitivity. Also use cautiously in patients who have received high doses of protamine in the past.

PREPARATION & STORAGE
Available in a concentration of 10 mg/ml as liquid in 5 and 25 ml vials or supplied as powder in 50 and 250 mg vials. Store liquid in refrigerator and powder at room temperature. Avoid freezing.
Reconstitute powder with sterile water for injection or bacteriostatic water for injection containing 0.9% benzyl alcohol (5 ml for 50 mg vial or 25 ml for 250 mg vial) to yield 10 mg/ml. Shake vigorously. If reconstituted with sterile water, use immediately and discard unused portions. If reconstituted with bacteriostatic water and benzyl alcohol, solution remains stable for 72 hours at room temperature.
Reconstituted solutions aren't intended for further dilution, but if desired, may be diluted in dextrose 5% in water or 0.9% sodium chloride. Don't store diluted solutions; they contain no preservatives.

ADMINISTRATION
Direct injection: Inject reconstituted drug slowly over 1 to 3 minutes. Don't give more than 50 mg in 10 minutes. Overly rapid administration can cause severe hypotension and anaphylactoid reactions.
Intermittent infusion: not recommended.
Continuous infusion: not recommended.

INCOMPATIBILITY
Incompatible with cephalosporins and penicillins.

ADVERSE REACTIONS
Life-threatening: anaphylaxis, hypotension.
Other: bradycardia, coughing, dyspnea, flushing, heparin rebound, hypersensitivity reactions (angioedema, urticaria), malaise, nausea, vomit-

ing, warm sensation, weakness, wheezing.

INTERACTIONS
None reported.

EFFECTS ON DIAGNOSTIC TESTS
Coagulation tests: normal levels after neutralization of heparin by protamine.

SPECIAL CONSIDERATIONS
• *Treatment of overdose:* Monitor coagulation tests and provide symptomatic care if necessary.
• Before giving protamine, ensure adequate blood volume. Correct hypovolemia with I.V. fluids or with blood transfusions if patient hemorrhaged from heparin overdose.
• Monitor patient continuously throughout therapy. Check vital signs frequently.
• Keep epinephrine 1:1,000 available to treat hypersensitivity.
• Monitor coagulation studies, such as activated clotting time, activated partial thromboplastin time, or thrombin time. These should be performed 5 to 15 minutes after therapy and repeated as necessary.
• Carefully titrate protamine dose, especially if the patient received a large heparin dose.
• Don't give more than 100 mg over 2 hours (protamine's duration of action) unless coagulation studies indicate need for higher dosage.
• Closely observe patients who've undergone extracorporeal circulation during arterial and cardiac surgery or hemodialysis. Heparin rebound with bleeding can occur 30 minutes to 18 hours later despite heparin neutralization by protamine sulfate.
• Drug is used to treat severe heparin overdose only. Mild overdose can be corrected by discontinuing heparin.

• Advise patient that he may experience transitory flushing after administration.

---

pyridostigmine bromide
Mestinon, Regonol

Pregnancy Risk Category: C

PHARMACOKINETICS
Distribution: widespread. Drug crosses the blood-brain barrier only with high doses. It also crosses the placenta.
Metabolism: hydrolyzed by cholinesterases and metabolized by liver enzymes.
Excretion: in urine. Half-life is about 90 minutes. Drug appears in breast milk.
Action: onset, 2 to 5 minutes; duration, 2 to 3 hours.

MECHANISM OF ACTION
Drug blocks the effects of acetylcholinesterase at the neuromuscular junction, allowing accumulation of acetylcholine. This results in prolonged and enhanced effects, including miosis, bradycardia, increased intestinal and skeletal muscle tone, constriction of bronchi and ureters, and increased salivary and sweat gland secretion. Accumulation at the motor end plate increases muscle strength and response to repetitive nerve stimulation. Accumulation at receptor sites reverses muscle paralysis induced by nondepolarizing neuromuscular blockers.

INDICATIONS & DOSAGE
• Myasthenia gravis. Dosage varies widely. *Adults:* 2 mg q 2 to 3 hours or about 1/30 of patient's oral maintenance dose.
• Antidote for nondepolarizing neuromuscular blockers (such as tubocu

---

rarine, metocurine, gallamine, pancuronium). *Adults:* 10 to 20 mg or 0.1 to 0.25 mg/kg, given with or shortly after 0.6 to 1.2 mg of atropine sulfate I.V. or 0.2 to 0.6 mg of glycopyrrolate I.V. (about 0.2 mg of glycopyrrolate for each 5 mg of pyridostigmine bromide).

CONTRAINDICATIONS & CAUTIONS

• Contraindicated in hypersensitivity to anticholinesterase drugs or bromides, and in breastfeeding women.
• Also contraindicated in mechanical obstruction of the intestinal or urinary tract because drug increases smooth muscle tone and activity.
• Use with caution in asthma, pneumonia, postoperative atelectasis, urinary tract infections, and dysrhythmias (especially bradycardia, atrioventricular block, and recent coronary occlusion). Drug may exacerbate these conditions.
• Also use with caution in epilepsy, hyperthyroidism, peptic ulcer, and vagotonia because drug may mask their signs.
• After surgery, administer carefully because drug may exacerbate breathing difficulty caused by pain, sedation, secretions, or atelectasis.

PREPARATION & STORAGE

Available in a concentration of 5 mg/ml in 2 ml ampules and 5 ml vials. Store at room temperature. Protect from light and freezing.

ADMINISTRATION

Direct injection: Inject undiluted drug slowly into an I.V. line containing a compatible free-flowing solution. Observe for thrombophlebitis at I.V. site.
Intermittent infusion: not recommended.
Continuous infusion: not recommended.

INCOMPATIBILITY

Unstable in alkaline solutions.

ADVERSE REACTIONS

Life-threatening: bradycardia, bronchospasm, excessive salivation leading to possible aspiration, hypotension, respiratory paralysis.
Other: abdominal cramps, acne, agitation, anxiety, blurred vision, clumsiness, confusion, diaphoresis, diarrhea (severe), fasciculations, headache, increased bronchial secretions, increased weakness (especially in arms, neck, shoulders, and tongue), irritability, lacrimation, nausea, pupillary constriction, restlessness, seizures, slurred speech, thrombophlebitis at injection site, twitching, unsteadiness, vomiting.

INTERACTIONS

Aminoglycosides, capreomycin, hydrocarbon inhalation anesthetics (such as halothane), lincomycin, polymyxins, quinine: possible antagonized antimyasthenic effects.
Antimuscarinic agents (especially atropine): antagonized muscarinic effects of pyridostigmine and reduced GI motility.
Depolarizing neuromuscular blockers (such as succinylcholine): prolonged neuromuscular blockade.
Edrophonium: possible cholinergic crisis (overdose) with symptoms similar to those of myasthenic crisis (underdose); also worsening of patient's condition.
Guanadrel, guanethidine, mecamylamine, procainamide, quinidine, trimethaphan: possible antagonized antimyasthenic effects.
Local ester-derivative anesthetics: increased risk of toxicity.
Nondepolarizing neuromuscular blockers: antagonized effects.
Other cholinesterase inhibitors (such as demecarium, echothio-

phate, and possibly topical mala-thion): possible additive toxicity. *Parenteral local anesthetics:* antagonized antimyasthenic effects.

EFFECTS ON DIAGNOSTIC TESTS
None reported.

SPECIAL CONSIDERATIONS
• *Treatment of overdose:* Signs of pyridostigmine's muscarinic effects include abdominal cramps, diaphoresis, diarrhea, excessive bronchial and salivary secretions, lacrimation, nausea, and vomiting. If these signs occur, promptly discontinue drug. Give atropine sulfate I.V., 1 to 4 mg, then additional doses q 5 to 30 minutes, as needed. Maintain airway and adequate ventilation.
• Always keep atropine sulfate available in a separate syringe when giving pyridostigmine. Give 0.6 to 1.2 mg of atropine, as ordered, before or with high doses of pyridostigmine.
• Stop all other cholinergic drugs during pyridostigmine therapy to avoid toxicity.
• Establish baseline respiratory rate, heart rate, and blood pressure.
• If heart rate is below 80 beats/minute, give atropine before pyridostigmine.
• Maintain a patent airway, using suctioning, oxygen, and assisted ventilation as necessary.
• When giving pyridostigmine to reverse effects of nondepolarizing neuromuscular blockers, keep patient on ventilator. Wait 15 to 30 minutes for full effects. Observe closely for possible recurrence of respiratory depression. Delayed recovery is associated with hypokalemia, debilitation, carcinomatosis, aminoglycoside antibiotic therapy, and use of anesthetics (such as ether).

• Be alert for cholinergic crisis, which can occur with overdose. Discontinue anticholinesterase therapy. In cholinergic crisis, muscle weakness usually occurs 1 hour after last pyridostigmine dose. It's accompanied by adverse muscarinic effects and fasciculations. Weakness that occurs 3 or more hours after the last pyridostigmine dose may indicate myasthenic crisis and the need for more drug. An edrophonium chloride (Tensilon) test may also be used to differentiate cholinergic crisis from myasthenic crisis.
• Periodically measure vital capacity and muscle strength to assess myasthenic patient's response to drug, especially with increasing doses.
• Severe myasthenia gravis is associated with accelerated pyridostigmine metabolism and excretion. This results in resistance to drug effects.
• In myasthenia gravis, muscle groups may respond differently to the same drug. No response and persistent weakness may occur in one muscle group, increased strength in another.

---

pyridoxine hydrochloride (vitamin B$_6$)
Beesix, Hexa-Betalin♦, Pyroxine

Pregnancy Risk Category: A
(C if greater than RDA)

PHARMACOKINETICS
Distribution: in the liver and, to a lesser extent, in muscle and the brain. Although pyridoxine isn't bound to plasma proteins, pyridoxal and pyridoxal phosphate, the principal forms found in blood, are highly protein-bound. Drug crosses the placenta.

Metabolism: converted to pyridoxal phosphate in RBCs. Pyridoxine also metabolized in the liver.
Excretion: in urine. Excessive amounts excreted largely unchanged. Half-life may be 15 to 20 days. Drug appears in breast milk.
Action: unknown.

MECHANISM OF ACTION

After conversion to pyridoxal phosphate, pyridoxine hydrochloride acts as a coenzyme in protein, carbohydrate, and fat metabolism. It's also involved in conversion of tryptophan to niacin or serotonin.

INDICATIONS & DOSAGE

• Vitamin B_6 deficiency. *Adults:* 4.0 to 6.3 mg I.V. daily.
• Pyridoxine dependency syndrome. *Adults:* 30 to 600 mg daily. *Infants with seizures:* 10 to 100 mg during seizure.
• Drug-induced pyridoxine deficiency. *Adults:* 50 to 200 mg daily for 3 weeks, then 25 to 100 mg daily p.r.n.
• Cycloserine poisoning. *Adults:* 300 mg or more daily.
• Isoniazid poisoning. *Adults:* dose equal to amount of isoniazid ingested, usually 1 to 4 g, followed by 1 g I.M. q 30 minutes until entire dose is given. Usually given with anticonvulsants p.r.n.
• Hydrazine poisoning. *Adults:* 25 mg/kg. One-third given I.M. and remainder by I.V. infusion over 3 hours.
• Mushroom poisoning (genus *Gyromitra*). *Adults:* 25 mg infused over 15 to 30 minutes repeated p.r.n. Maximum dosage, 15 to 20 g daily.

CONTRAINDICATIONS & CAUTIONS

• Contraindicated in pyridoxine sensitivity.

PREPARATION & STORAGE

Available in 1, 10, and 30 ml vials, each containing a concentration of 100 mg/ml. Store at room temperature, and protect from light and freezing. For intermittent infusion, dilute with recommended solutions to ordered concentrations.

ADMINISTRATION

Direct injection: Inject undiluted drug into I.V. line containing a free-flowing compatible solution.
Intermittent infusion: Infuse diluted drug over prescribed duration.
Continuous infusion: not used.

INCOMPATIBILITY

Incompatible with alkaline solutions, erythromycin estolate, iron salts, kanamycin, oxidizing agents, riboflavin, sodium phosphate, and streptomycin.

ADVERSE REACTIONS

Life-threatening: none reported.
Other: drowsiness, headache, nausea, paresthesias, seizures (after high I.V. doses).

INTERACTIONS

Chloramphenicol, cycloserine, ethionamide, hydralazine, immunosuppressants, isoniazid, penicillamine: possible anemia or peripheral neuritis because of antagonized pyridoxine effects or increased excretion. May require increased pyridoxine dosage.
Estrogens: possible increased pyridoxine requirements.
Levodopa: may reverse antiparkinsonian effects (but not with levodopa-carbidopa combinations).

EFFECTS ON DIAGNOSTIC TESTS

Serum folic acid: decreased levels.
SGOT: increased levels.
Urine urobilinogen: possible false-positive results.

SPECIAL CONSIDERATIONS
• Give pyridoxine I.V. when oral route is unsuitable (in nausea, vomiting, and preoperative and postoperative conditions) or impossible (in malabsorption syndrome, after gastric resection).
• Signs and symptoms of vitamin B_6 deficiency include personality changes, stomatitis, and heightened risk of GU infections.
• Be alert for symptoms of overdose (ataxia and severe neuropathy) in patients receiving high doses for several weeks or months.
• Dosages of 200 mg daily for more than 30 days may cause pyridoxine-dependency syndrome.
• Increase dosage, as ordered, in hemodialysis patients.
• Use of high-dose pyridoxine during pregnancy may cause pyridoxine-dependency seizures in neonates.
• Infants with hereditary pyridoxine-dependency syndrome require high-dose pyridoxine in the first week of life to prevent seizures and mental retardation. Drug usually stops seizures within 3 minutes.

---

quinidine gluconate

Pregnancy Risk Category: C

PHARMACOKINETICS
Distribution: to all tissues except brain, with 80% to 90% bound to plasma proteins (primarily albumin). Highest concentrations appear in the heart, liver, kidneys, and skeletal muscles. Drug also binds to hemoglobin. It crosses the placenta.
Metabolism: in the liver.
Excretion: probably by glomerular filtration, with 10% to 20% excreted unchanged in urine in 24 hours. Excretion increases with acidic urine and decreases in alkaline urine.

Plasma half-life is normally 6 to 8 hours but may range from 3 to 16 hours or longer. Small quantities of drug appear in breast milk.
Action: peaks in 3 to 4 hours.

MECHANISM OF ACTION
Quinidine exerts direct and indirect antimuscarinic effects on cardiac tissue.

INDICATIONS & DOSAGE
• Dysrhythmias (atrial fibrillation or flutter, paroxysmal atrial or junctional tachycardia, ventricular or atrial premature contractions, ventricular tachycardia). *Adults:* initially, 16 mg/minute (1 ml/minute), then adjusted to control dysrhythmias. Usual dose required to control ventricular dysrhythmias is 300 mg or less. Maximum dosage, 4 g daily. Dosage may need to be reduced in patients with congestive heart failure or hepatic disease. *Children:* 30 mg/kg daily or 900 mg/m² daily in five divided doses.
• Severe malaria caused by *Plasmodium falciparum* (when I.V. quinine dihydrochloride isn't available). *Adults:* initially, 24 mg/kg over 4 hours, then maintenance dosage of 12 mg/kg q 8 hours for 7 days. *Note:* Dosage may need adjustment in hemodialysis patients.

CONTRAINDICATIONS & CAUTIONS
• Contraindicated in hypersensitivity to quinidine or cinchona derivatives and in myasthenia gravis because drug may worsen weakness.
• Also contraindicated in digitalis-induced AV conduction disorders, complete AV block, severe intraventricular conduction defects associated with a widened QRS complex, or escape junctional or ventricular

---

rhythms because of additive cardiac depression.

• Use cautiously in the elderly and in patients with hepatic or renal impairment because of decreased quinidine metabolism and risk of toxicity.

• Because symptoms can mask those of quinidine hypersensitivity, administer cautiously to patients with asthma, emphysema, weakness, or febrile infection.

• Use cautiously in incomplete AV block because of potential for complete block, and in congestive heart failure or hypotension because quinidine may decrease myocardial contractility or blood pressure and aggravate these conditions.

• Administer carefully in cardiac glycoside intoxication because drug may intensify cardiac depression and inhibit intracardial conduction; in hypokalemia because of possible reduced drug effect; and in psoriasis or in a patient with a history of thrombocytopenia because drug may worsen these disorders.

• Pediatric safety and efficacy haven't been determined.

PREPARATION & STORAGE

Available in 10 ml vials (80 mg/ml). Store at room temperature, and protect from light and freezing. For intermittent infusion, dilute with dextrose 5% in water to ordered concentration. For continuous infusion, dilute 800 mg (one vial) with 40 ml of dextrose 5% in water to yield 16 mg/ml. Don't use solution if brown. Discard diluted solutions after 24 hours.

ADMINISTRATION

Direct injection: not recommended.
Intermittent infusion: Infuse solution through I.V. line over prescribed duration.
Continuous infusion: Infuse solution through I.V. line initially at 1 ml/

minute, then adjust rate to control dysrhythmias.

INCOMPATIBILITY

Incompatible with alkalies, amiodarone, and iodides.

ADVERSE REACTIONS

Life-threatening: agranulocytosis, anaphylaxis, hemolytic anemia, hemorrhage, hepatotoxicity, hypoglycemia (severe), respiratory arrest, thrombocytopenia, torsades de pointes (usually self-limiting polymorphic ventricular tachycardia), ventricular fibrillation.
Other: angioedema, bleeding or bruising, blurred vision or other vision changes, cinchonism, confusion, diarrhea, dyspnea, EKG changes, fainting, fatigue, fever, headache (severe), jaundice, light-headedness, nausea, pallor, photosensitivity, pleuritic chest pain, polyarthritis, premature ventricular contractions, pruritus, rash, tachycardia, tinnitus, vertigo, weakness, wheezing.

INTERACTIONS

Antiarrhythmics (lidocaine, phenytoin, procainamide, propranolol): possible additive cardiac effects.
Anticholinergic drugs: potentiated effects.
Antihypertensives: possible potentiated hypotension because quinidine may lower blood pressure.
Antimuscarinic drugs: possible intensified atropine-like effects.
Bethanechol: possible antagonized cholinergic effects.
Bretylium: possible diminished inotropic effects and potentiated hypotension.
Cardiac glycosides: possible increased serum levels.
Cholinergic drugs: reduced effectiveness in terminating paroxysmal atrial tachycardia.

Cimetidine and drugs that alkalinize urine (acetazolamide, sodium bicarbonate, some antacids, thiazide diuretics): increased serum levels of quinidine, resulting from decreased metabolism.

Hepatic enzyme inducers: possible reduced serum levels of quinidine because of enhanced hepatic metabolism.

Neuromuscular blockers (gallamine, metocurine, pancuronium, succinylcholine, tubocurarine): potentiated effects.

Nifedipine: possible decreased serum levels of quinidine; possible increase with discontinuation of nifedipinc.

Pimozide: possible dysrhythmias (prolonged Q-T interval).

Potassium-containing drugs: usually, heightened quinidine effects.

Quinine: increased risk of cinchonism.

Verapamil: possible hypotension in patients with hypertrophic cardiomyopathy.

Warfarin: heightened effects.

EFFECTS ON DIAGNOSTIC TESTS

EKG: widened QRS complex, prolonged QT interval, T-wave flattening.

Serum alkaline phosphatase, SGOT, SGPT: possible elevated levels.

Serum glucose: possible decreased levels.

SPECIAL CONSIDERATIONS

• *Treatment of overdose:* Signs of overdose include absence of P waves and widening of QRS complex and PR and QT intervals, anuria, apnea, ataxia, extrasystoles, hallucinations, hypotension, irritability, lethargy, respiratory distress, seizures, thrashing, twitching, and ventricular dysrhythmias. If these signs develop, promptly discontinue drug and give oxygen and ventilatory support. Also assist with cardiac pacing and administer hypertensives, urine acidifiers, and I.V. fluids as necessary. Replace fluids, then give metaraminol or norepinephrine, as ordered, to treat hypotension. Infuse ⅙ M sodium lactate to reduce quinidine's cardiotoxic effects.

• During infusion, continuously monitor blood pressure and cardiac function (including EKG). Rapid infusion of as little as 200 mg may drop blood pressure by 40 to 50 mm Hg.

• Monitor serum quinidinc and potassium levels; quinidine levels above 8 mcg/ml are toxic.

• In patients with dysrhythmias, discontinue quinidine in excessive widening of the QRS complex (25% greater than before infusion), disappearance of P wave, decline of a rapid heart rate (to 120 beats/minute), or restoration of normal sinus rhythm.

• I.V. quinidine is used to treat acute dysrhythmias; oral or I.M. administration is preferred for maintenance therapy.

• GI adverse effects, especially diarrhea, are signs of toxicity.

ranitidine
Zantac

Pregnancy Risk Category: B

PHARMACOKINETICS

Distribution: widespread, with 10% to 19% bound to plasma proteins. Drug probably enters cerebrospinal fluid. Not known if it crosses the placenta.

Metabolism: in the liver.

Excretion: primarily in urine, with about 70% removed unchanged.

Half-life is 2 to 2½ hours. Drug appears in breast milk.
Action: peaks in 15 minutes.

MECHANISM OF ACTION

This H_2-receptor antagonist inhibits histamine's action on gastric parietal cells, thus reducing basal and nocturnal gastric acid secretion. It also inhibits stimulation of gastric acid secretion by food, betazole, pentagastrin, insulin, and vagal reflex. Other effects include increased gastric nitrate-reducing organisms; a small, transient, dose-related increase in serum prolactin; and possibly impaired vasopressin release.

INDICATIONS & DOSAGE

• Active duodenal ulcer and pathologic hypersecretory conditions, such as Zollinger-Ellison syndrome and multiple endocrine adenomas, in hospitalized N.P.O. patients. *Adults:* 50 mg q 6 to 8 hours. Maximum dosage, 400 mg daily.
Note: Adjust dosage in renal impairment. For adults with creatinine clearance less than 50 ml/minute, dosage is 50 mg q 18 to 24 hours, increasing to q 12 hours or more often, if needed.

CONTRAINDICATIONS & CAUTIONS

• Contraindicated in ranitidine hypersensitivity.
• Use cautiously in breastfeeding women and in renal or hepatic impairment because of possible increased serum levels.

PREPARATION & STORAGE

Available in 2 and 10 ml vials containing 25 mg/ml. Store at room temperature. Protect from light and freezing. For direct injection, dilute 50 mg dose with compatible I.V. solution (such as 0.9% sodium chloride, dextrose 5% or 10% in water, lactated Ringer's, sodium bicarbonate 5%) to a total volume of 20 ml. For intermittent infusion, dilute 50 mg dose with 100 ml of a compatible I.V. solution. Solutions remain stable for 48 hours at room temperature. Don't use if discolored or if a precipitate is present.

ADMINISTRATION

Direct injection: Inject drug into a patent I.V. line over at least 5 minutes.
Intermittent infusion: Infuse diluted drug into a patent I.V. line through a piggyback set over 15 to 20 minutes.
Continuous infusion: Infuse 150 mg in 1,000 ml of a compatible solution over 24 hours at a rate of 6.25 mg/hour. No loading dose required.

INCOMPATIBILITY

Incompatible with amphotericin B, chlorpromazine hydrochloride, clindamycin phosphate, methotrimeprazine, midazolam hydrochloride, opium alkaloids hydrochloride, and pentobarbital sodium.

ADVERSE REACTIONS

Life-threatening: anaphylaxis (rare).
Other: agitation; alopecia; arthralgias; bradycardia; bronchospasm; confusion; constipation; depression; diarrhea; dizziness; drowsiness; eosinophilia; fever; granulocytopenia; hallucinations; headache; hepatitis; insomnia; leukopenia; malaise; nausea; pancytopenia; premature ventricular contractions; rash; tachycardia; thrombocytopenia; transient pain, burning, or itching at I.V. site; vertigo; vomiting.

INTERACTIONS

Acetaminophen: inhibited metabolism (dose-dependent).
Metoprolol: altered pharmacokinetics and lengthened half-life.

Procainamide, theophyllines: decreased clearance.
Tobacco: possible impairment of ranitidine's suppression of nocturnal gastric acid secretion.
Warfarin: possible diminished clearance.

EFFECTS ON DIAGNOSTIC TESTS
Gastric acid secretion: reduced response to pentagastrin. Don't give drug for 24 hours before the test.
Serum gamma-glutamyl transpeptidase, SGOT, SGPT: possible increased levels.
Skin tests: using allergen extracts, possible false-negative results because of inhibited cutaneous histamine response.
Urine protein: possible false-positive results of Multistix test. Use sulfosalicylic acid instead.

SPECIAL CONSIDERATIONS
• Malignant GI neoplasm should be ruled out before ranitidine therapy.
• Monitor SGPT levels if patient receives 400 mg daily for 5 days or longer. Begin on fifth day of therapy and check daily until discontinuation.
• Reduce dose, as ordered, in patients with hepatic or renal impairment.
• Hemodialysis removes drug.

red blood cells, packed

Pregnancy Risk Category: Not applicable

COMPOSITION
Derived from whole blood after sedimentation or centrifugation, packed red cells are suspended in about 50 ml of plasma or 100 ml of an additive nutrient solution. This product and whole blood have equal oxygen-carrying capacity because they contain equal numbers of RBCs. However, packed red cells contain less sodium and potassium than whole blood. The volume of each unit of packed red cells is 250 to 350 ml; the hematocrit is 65% to 80%.

INDICATIONS & DOSAGE
• Restoration or maintenance of adequate oxygenation with minimal expansion of blood volume, especially in severe symptomatic anemia, slow blood loss, or congestive heart failure. *Adults:* number of units determined by clinical status. *Children:* 10 ml/kg (not to exceed 15 ml/kg).

CONTRAINDICATIONS & CAUTIONS
• Contraindicated in asymptomatic anemia or conditions that may be managed effectively with crystalloid or colloid solutions.
• Give large amounts of packed red cells cautiously because of the risk of hypervolemia.

PREPARATION & STORAGE
Store packed red cells at 34° to 43° F. (1° to 6° C.) in a continuously monitored refrigerator. If temperature goes beyond this range, the risk increases for reduced viability, hemolysis, and bacterial proliferation. Maximum storage is 35 to 42 days, depending on the preservative or anticoagulant used. Preservatives, such as adenine, saline, and dextrose, are removed before transfusion if the patient's at risk for circulatory overload.

For rapid infusion, dilute with 50 to 100 ml of 0.9% sodium chloride. Add the 0.9% sodium chloride via a closed sterile system using a Y-type infusion set connected to the saline container and the packed red cell bag. Invert the bag, and open the roller clamps from the saline to the packed red cells.

ADMINISTRATION

Direct injection: Appropriate only for neonatal transfusion. Draw pre-filtered red cells into a 50-ml syringe and inject slowly through a 19G to 21G needle or catheter.

Intermittent infusion: not used.

Continuous infusion: Infuse through a Y-type set with at least a 170-micron filter at a rate of 1 unit over 2 to 3 hours for adults and 2 to 5 ml/kg hourly for children. (The blood bank can divide units into several bags with small volumes if infusion will exceed 4 hours.) For optimal flow rate, use at least a 19G needle. In children and adults with small veins, use a 21G or 23G needle, if necessary.

Use automatic infusion devices, such as IMED and IVAC, only if they've been tested and approved for .transfusion by the manufacturer. Don't inflate manual pressure cuffs above 300 mm Hg.

Begin the infusion slowly, and remain at the bedside. Take vital signs. If patient shows no signs of transfusion reaction, adjust flow to the prescribed rate. During rapid, massive infusion, use a microaggregate filter (20- to 40-micron pore size). Used with or as replacement for standard blood filters, these filters remove small WBC particulates that aggregate during storage. Aggregates may migrate to the lungs and cause dyspnea.

INCOMPATIBILITY

Incompatible with all drugs and solutions except 0.9% sodium chloride.

ADVERSE REACTIONS

Life-threatening: acute hemolytic reaction, graft-versus-host disease (rare, occurring in immunocom-promised patients receiving red cells with viable lymphocytes), hemosiderosis, viral infection (acquired immune deficiency syndrome, hepatitis), volume overload (cough, crackles at lung bases, distended neck veins, dyspnea).

Other: anxiety, fever above 100.4° F. (38° C.) or an increase of more than about 2° F. (1° C.), flushing, headache, myalgia, pruritus, sudden chills, urticaria.

INTERACTIONS

None reported.

EFFECTS ON DIAGNOSTIC TESTS

Direct Coombs' test: possible detection of antibody attached to RBCs after transfusion of incompatible plasma or in delayed hemolytic reaction.

Hematocrit: increased over pretransfusion level (expected increase, 3%/unit).

Hemoglobin: increased over pretransfusion level (expected increase, 1 g/dl/unit).

Indirect Coombs' test: possible detection of antibody formed after exposure to minor red cell antigens.

SPECIAL CONSIDERATIONS

• Allow at least 1 hour for a routine crossmatch. In an emergency, O-negative red cells may be safely transfused.

• Take vital signs, record results, and establish a patent venous catheter before requesting release of red cells from the blood bank.

• Confirm recipient's identity by comparing name and ID number on blood bag tag with patient ID bracelet. Verify blood compatibility by matching blood group and type on bag to chart or other blood bank record. Have another qualified staff member perform this check, too.

• Red cells needn't always match the patient's group and type, but they must always be compatible. Type O is compatible with red cell type O; type A, with A or O; type B, with B or O; and type AB, with AB, O, A, or B. If the recipient's blood is Rh-positive, it's compatible with Rh-positive and Rh-negative red cells; if it's Rh-negative, it's compatible with Rh-negative red cells.

• Don't administer any drug through a line used for blood product transfusion.

• Monitor vital signs every 15 minutes until 1 hour after transfusion. Record vital signs, product number, starting and ending times, volume, and response to transfusion.

• Monitor for chills, disseminated intravascular coagulation, fever, hemoglobinemia, hemoglobinuria, hypotension, low back pain, acute renal failure, tachycardia, tachypnea, and vascular collapse. These may signal an acute hemolytic reaction, especially if they occur during administration of the first 50 ml of red cells.

• If acute hemolytic reaction occurs, stop the transfusion at the needle hub and rapidly infuse 0.9% sodium chloride. Contact the doctor and the blood bank, and treat symptomatically to maintain renal blood flow. Also arrange serologic evaluation of urine and blood.

• Monitor for hemosiderosis if patient has received multiple, long-term transfusions (exceeding 100 units).

• For patients having repeat febrile reactions, provide leukocyte-poor blood, as ordered. Use a leukocyte-depleting filter with the standard blood filter or as a replacement for it.

• Blood warmers may be used during transfusion to prevent dysrhyth-

mias associated with rapid infusion of cold blood. Prewarmed blood should also be used in transfusions to patients with cold agglutinin disease. Use coil-tubing or heated-plate warmers designed to allow close temperature monitoring; red cell hemolysis can occur if temperature exceeds 104° F. (40° C.).

• Alloimmunization, the development of antibodies to foreign antigens, occurs in 1% to 2% of previously transfused or pregnant patients and may be responsible for delayed hemolytic reactions. Subsequent crossmatching is more difficult in these patients.

---

red blood cells, washed (leukocyte-poor red cells, washed packed cells)

Pregnancy Risk Category: Not applicable

COMPOSITION
Washed red blood cells are derived from whole blood. About 200 to 250 ml of plasma are first removed from a collected pint of blood (about 500 ml). Then the red cell buffy coat, consisting of WBCs and platelets, is removed by saline washing, inverted centrifugation, or microaggregate blood filters. The American Association of Blood Banks standards specify elimination of 70% of WBCs with less than 30% loss of red cells. After washing, the concentration of red cells is approximately 70% to 90%. The volume of each unit of washed red cells is 250 to 300 ml.

INDICATIONS & DOSAGE
• Restoration or maintenance of adequate oxygenation with minimal expansion of blood volume in severe or recurrent febrile nonhemolytic trans-

fusion reactions or urticarial allergic reactions. *Adults:* number of units determined by clinical status.

CONTRAINDICATIONS & CAUTIONS
• Contraindicated in patients with only one previous transfusion reaction.
• Use cautiously if infusing large amounts of washed red cells because of the risk of hypervolemia.

PREPARATION & STORAGE
Storage of frozen, thawed red blood cells is limited to 24 hours at 34° to 43° F. (1° to 6° C.) because deglycerolization and resuspension occur in transfer from the original bag for washing.

ADMINISTRATION
Direct injection: not used.
Intermittent infusion: not used.
Continuous infusion: Infuse through a Y-type set with at least a 170-micron filter. Give at a rate of 1 unit over 2 to 3 hours for adults and 2 to 5 ml/kg hourly for children. (The blood bank can divide units into several bags containing small volumes if infusion will exceed 4 hours.) For optimal rate, use at least a 19G needle or, in children and adults with smaller veins, a 21G or 23G winged infusion set.

Begin the infusion slowly. Take vital signs. If patient shows no evidence of transfusion reaction, adjust flow to the prescribed rate.

Infusion devices are useful for exceedingly slow rates, especially in children and neonates, but packed or washed cells are likely to undergo hemolysis when given through a pressurized infusion pump. Consult pump manufacturer before use.

INCOMPATIBILITY
Incompatible with all drugs and solutions except 0.9% sodium chloride.

ADVERSE REACTIONS
Life-threatening: acute hemolytic reaction, hypervolemia (cough; dyspnea; EKG abnormalities, usually premature ventricular contractions; hypertension), viral infection ((acquired immune deficiency syndrome, hepatitis).
Other: fever, jaundice, malaise.

INTERACTIONS
None reported.

EFFECTS ON DIAGNOSTIC TESTS
Hematocrit: increased over pretransfusion level (expected increase, 3%/unit).
Hemoglobin: increased over pretransfusion level (expected increase, 1 g/dl/unit).

SPECIAL CONSIDERATIONS
• Allow at least 1 hour for a routine blood crossmatch. In an emergency, O-negative red cells may be safely transfused to all patients.
• Take vital signs, record results, and establish a patent venous catheter before requesting release of red cells from the blood bank.
• Confirm the recipient's identity by comparing name and ID number on blood bag tag with patient ID bracelet. Verify blood compatibility by matching blood group and type on bag with chart or other blood bank record. Have another qualified staff member perform this check, too.
• Red cells needn't always match the patient's blood group and type, but they must always be compatible. Type O is compatible with red cell type O; type A, with A or O; type B, with B or O; and type AB, with

AB, O, A, or B. If the recipient's blood is Rh-positive, it's compatible with Rh-positive and Rh-negative red cells; if it's Rh-negative, it's compatible with Rh-negative cells.
• Don't administer any drug through a line used for transfusion.
• Monitor vital signs every 15 minutes until 1 hour after transfusion. Record vital signs, product number, starting and ending times, volume, and response to transfusion.
• Monitor for hemosiderosis if patient has received multiple, long-term transfusions (exceeding 100 units).
• Observe the patient for delayed hemolytic reaction characterized by fever, falling hematocrit, jaundice, and malaise.
• If patient has had one febrile or allergic transfusion reaction, he usually doesn't have a second. Repeat reactions are more common in women who have had multiple pregnancies and in patients who receive frequent transfusions. Repeated transfusion reactions are required before receiving washed red blood cells.
• Blood warmers may be used during transfusion to prevent dysrhythmias associated with rapid infusion of cold blood. Prewarmed blood should also be used in transfusions to patients with cold agglutinin disease. Use coil-tubing or heated-plate warmers designed to allow close monitoring of temperature; red cell hemolysis can occur if temperature exceeds 104° F. (40° C.). However, routine bloodwarming is unnecessary and usually slows infusion rate.
• Alloimmunization occurs in 1% to 2% of previously transfused or pregnant patients and may be responsible for delayed hemolytic transfusion reactions. Subsequent blood cross-matching is more difficult in these patients.

• If a patient continues to have reactions even after administration of washed cells, the use of frozen-thawed-deglycerolized red blood cells may be effective.
• Washing red blood cells removes plasma and WBCs, further reducing the risk of allergic reaction to donor plasma.
• Washing red blood cells may result in loss of some red blood cells. Frequent transfusions may be needed.
• Urticarial reactions are nearly eliminated by using washed red blood cells.

Ringer's Injection

Pregnancy Risk Category: C

COMPOSITION
An isotonic multiple electrolyte solution, Ringer's injection contains the principal ionic constituents of normal plasma. Each 100 ml contains 860 mg of sodium chloride, 30 mg of potassium chloride, and 33 mg of calcium chloride dehydrate. A liter of Ringer's injection provides 147 mEq of sodium, 4 mEq of potassium, 4 mEq of calcium, and 155 mEq of chloride. The solution's pH is approximately 6.0.

INDICATIONS & DOSAGE
• Replacement of extracellular fluid and electrolyte losses. *Adults and children:* dose highly individualized but usually 1.5 to 3 liters (2% to 6% of body weight) daily.

CONTRAINDICATIONS & CAUTIONS
• Contraindicated in renal failure, except as an emergency volume expander.

• Avoid use as a blood replacement or a substitute for plasma volume expanders, except in emergencies.
• Use cautiously in congestive heart failure, hyperkalemia, hypoproteinemia, severe renal failure, and sodium retention because Ringer's injection may worsen these conditions.

PREPARATION & STORAGE

Available in 500 and 1,000 ml containers. Store at room temperature. Avoid excessive heat; however, brief exposure to higher temperatures (up to 104° F. [40° C.]) doesn't adversely affect solution. Protect from freezing.

Before administration, inspect for particulate matter and discoloration. Don't use unless solution is clear and container undamaged.

ADMINISTRATION

Direct injection: not used.
Intermittent infusion: not used.
Continuous infusion: Infuse through central or peripheral I.V. line over ordered duration.

INCOMPATIBILITY

Incompatible with ampicillin sodium, cefamandole, cephradine, chlordiazepoxide, diazepam, erythromycin lactobionate, methicillin, potassium phosphate, sodium bicarbonate, and thiopental.

ADVERSE REACTIONS

Life-threatening: none reported.
Other: electrolyte imbalance, fever, fluid overload, infection at injection site, phlebitis or venous thrombosis, pulmonary edema.

INTERACTIONS

Corticosteroids, corticotropin: increased risk of hypernatremia.
Potassium-sparing diuretics, potassium supplements: enhanced risk of hyperkalemia.

EFFECTS ON DIAGNOSTIC TESTS

None significant.

SPECIAL CONSIDERATIONS

• Solution may be given with dextrose, other carbohydrates, or sodium lactate.
• I.V. administration of Ringer's injection can cause fluid or solute overload, resulting in dilution of serum electrolyte concentrations, overhydration, or pulmonary edema.
• If an adverse reaction occurs, discontinue infusion, institute symptomatic treatment, and save the remainder of the solution for examination, if necessary.
• Monitor changes in fluid and electrolyte balance during prolonged therapy.
• Administer to pregnant women only if clearly indicated. Not known if Ringer's injection can cause fetal harm.
• Electrolyte content is insufficient for treating severe electrolyte deficiencies.

Ringer's injection, lactated (Hartmann's solution, Ringer's lactate solution)

Pregnancy Risk Category: C

COMPOSITION

Lactated Ringer's injection consists of multiple electrolytes—130 mEq of sodium, 4 mEq of potassium, 3 mEq of calcium, 109 mEq of chloride, and 28 mEq of lactate per liter. A liter of this isotonic solution contains 9 calories (from lactate). Solutions containing dextrose 5% or 10% provide additional calories.

INDICATIONS & DOSAGE

• Replacement of extracellular fluid and electrolyte losses. *Adults and children:* dose highly individualized, but usually 1.5 to 3 liters (2% to 6% of body weight) daily.

CONTRAINDICATIONS & CAUTIONS

• Contraindicated in hyperkalemia, severe renal failure, and potassium retention because of possible worsening of these conditions.
• Avoid use in lactic acidosis.
• Give carefully in congestive heart failure, edema, severe renal insufficiency, sodium retention, and metabolic or respiratory alkalosis because lactated Ringer's injection may exacerbate these conditions.
• Use cautiously in patients with hepatic insufficiency because of increased level or impaired use of lactate ions.
• Use cautiously because excess lactate levels may cause metabolic acidosis.

PREPARATION & STORAGE

Available in 250-, 500-, and 1,000-ml containers. Store at room temperature. Avoid excessive heat; however, brief exposure to temperatures up to 104° F. (40° C.) doesn't affect solution adversely.

ADMINISTRATION

Direct injection: not used.
Intermittent infusion: not used.
Continuous infusion: Infuse ordered amount through peripheral or central I.V. line over 18 to 24 hours.

INCOMPATIBILITY

Incompatible with amphotericin B, ampicillin sodium, cefamandole, cephradine, chlordiazepoxide, diazepam, erythromycin lactobionate, methicillin, methylprednisolone sodium succinate, oxytetracycline, phenytoin sodium, potassium phosphate, sodium bicarbonate, thiopental, warfarin, and whole blood.

ADVERSE REACTIONS

Life-threatening: none reported.
Other: electrolyte imbalance, extravasation, fever, hypervolemia, infection at injection site.

INTERACTIONS

Corticosteroids, corticotropin: increased risk of hypernatremia.
Potassium-sparing diuretics, potassium supplements: enhanced risk of hyperkalemia.

EFFECTS ON DIAGNOSTIC TESTS

None significant.

SPECIAL CONSIDERATIONS

• During long-term therapy, monitor fluid and electrolyte balance.

---

ritodrine hydrochloride
Yutopar♦

Pregnancy Risk Category: B

PHARMACOKINETICS

Distribution: 32% bound to plasma proteins, almost exclusively to albumin. Drug crosses the placenta and probably the blood-brain barrier.
Metabolism: in the liver, primarily to inactive metabolites.
Excretion: in urine, with 70% to 90% excreted in 10 to 12 hours as unchanged drug and inactive metabolites. Half-life is triphasic: 6 to 9 minutes in first (distribution) phase; about 1½ to 3 hours in second phase; and more than 10 hours in third (elimination) phase. Not known if drug appears in breast milk.
Action: peak serum level, 60 minutes.

MECHANISM OF ACTION
This beta-receptor agonist inhibits uterine contractions by relaxing uterine smooth muscles. Stimulation of $beta_2$-adrenergic receptors results in increased uptake of intracellular calcium, preventing activation of contractile proteins in smooth muscle. Ritodrine also acts on $beta_2$-receptors in bronchial and vascular smooth muscle and has some effect on $beta_1$-receptors in the heart.

INDICATIONS & DOSAGE
• Management of uncomplicated preterm labor after gestation of 20 or more weeks, but less than 36 weeks. *Adults:* initially 50 to 100 mcg/minute, increasing q 10 minutes in 50-mcg increments until contractions cease. (Usual effective dosage, 150 to 350 mcg/minute.) Maintenance dosage, 150 to 350 mcg/minute for 12 to 24 hours after contractions stop. Maximum dosage, 350 mcg/minute.

CONTRAINDICATIONS & CAUTIONS
• Contraindicated before the 20th week of pregnancy because of inadequate research; in antepartum hemorrhage, chorioamnionitis, pregnancy-induced hypertension, or pulmonary hypertension because continuation of pregnancy would be hazardous to patient or fetus; and in intrauterine fetal death or any known abnormality that requires immediate delivery.
• Also contraindicated in hypersensitivity to sulfites, ritodrine, and other $beta_2$-adrenergic receptor agonists.
• Avoid use in hyperthyroidism or cardiac disorders, especially those associated with dysrhythmias, because drug may precipitate dysrhythmias or heart failure.

• Give cautiously in diabetes mellitus because drug may aggravate the disorder.
• In mild to moderate hypertension, also give drug cautiously because of the risk of blood pressure changes secondary to vascular smooth muscle relaxation.
• Ritodrine's effectiveness in advanced labor (cervical dilation of more than 4 cm or effacement of more than 80%) hasn't been established.

PREPARATION & STORAGE
Available in concentrations of 10 and 15 mg/ml in 5 and 10 ml ampules, vials, and syringes. Store at room temperature.

For infusion, add 150 mg of ritodrine to 500 ml of dextrose 5% in water to yield 300 mcg/ml. In patients with fluid restrictions, prepare a more concentrated solution, as ordered. Drug may also be diluted with 10% Dextran 40 in sodium chloride or 10% invert sugar solution. Avoid diluting with Ringer's injection, 0.9% sodium chloride, or Ringer's lactate. Also avoid diluting in sodium chloride solutions except in maternal diabetes because of the increased risk of pulmonary edema. Use solution within 48 hours. Discard if discoloration or precipitation is present.

ADMINISTRATION
Ritodrine should be used only by skilled personnel equipped to manage its complications.
Direct injection: not used.
Intermittent infusion: not used.
Continuous infusion: Using a pump to control rate, infuse by I.V. piggyback into a patent primary line at the port closest to the infusion needle. Adjust delivery to 50 to 100 mcg/ml (10 to 20 drops/minute, using microdrip chamber). Increase by

50 mcg/minute every 10 minutes until contractions or dilation stops, adverse maternal or fetal effects occur, or maximum dosage of 350 mcg/minute (70 drops/minute) is reached. At the recommended dilution, maximum fluid volume after 12 hours is 850 ml.

INCOMPATIBILITY
No incompatibilities reported.

ADVERSE REACTIONS
Most common adverse effects are dose-related.
Life-threatening: anaphylaxis, ketoacidosis, pulmonary edema.
Other: anxiety, blood pressure changes (increased systolic and decreased diastolic), chest pain or tightness, chills, drowsiness, dyspnea, emotional upset, fetal hyperglycemia and tachycardia, glycosuria, headache, hemolytic icterus, nausea, rapid or irregular heartbeat, rash, reddened skin, restlessness, sweating, trembling, vomiting, weakness.
In neonates: hyperglycemia, hypoglycemia, ileus, tachycardia.

INTERACTIONS
Beta-adrenergic blockers: reduced effectiveness of ritodrine.
Corticosteroids: increased incidence of pulmonary edema; increased insulin requirements in diabetics.
General anesthetics, parenteral diazoxide: potentiated cardiovascular effects of ritodrine.
Magnesium sulfate: cardiac disturbances.
Other sympathomimetic drugs: enhanced effects of both drugs and potential for adverse effects.

EFFECTS ON DIAGNOSTIC TESTS
Serum free fatty acids, glucose, insulin: possible transient increases, usually returning to pretherapy levels within 72 hours during continuous infusion.
Serum cAMP, iron, lactic acids: possible elevated levels.
Serum potassium: possible decreased levels, reaching nadir within 2 hours after start of infusion. Effect continues for 30 minutes to 24 hours after stopping therapy.

SPECIAL CONSIDERATIONS
• *Treatment of overdose:* Discontinue infusion and administer a beta-adrenergic blocker, if necessary.
• Before therapy, obtain baseline glucose and potassium levels and EKG to rule out latent cardiac disease.
• Sinus bradycardia may follow drug withdrawal.
• For most effective results, start therapy as soon as preterm labor diagnosis is confirmed.
• Place patient in left lateral position to minimize hypotension.
• Closely monitor intake and output. Also check fetal and maternal heart rates as well as maternal blood pressure, breath sounds, respirations, and uterine activity. Carefully adjust dosage and duration of infusion, as ordered.
• Maternal tachycardia or decreased diastolic blood pressure usually resolves when dosage is reduced.
• As ordered, stop ritodrine therapy if labor persists after maximum dose.
• During prolonged therapy, monitor serum glucose and electrolytes carefully, especially if patient has diabetes or is taking corticosteroids, potassium-depleting diuretics, or cardiac glycosides.
• Oral therapy usually follows I.V. therapy.
• If preterm labor recurs, I.V. infusion may be repeated. If contractions don't recur after 36 to 48

hours, patient may gradually resume ambulation.

scopolamine hydrobromide (hyoscine hydrobromide)

Pregnancy Risk Category: C

PHARMACOKINETICS
Distribution: not fully character-ized. Drug binds minimally to plasma proteins and crosses the placenta and blood-brain barrier.
Metabolism: in the liver by enzymatic hydrolysis.
Excretion: in urine, as unchanged drug and metabolites. Half-life is 8 hours. Not known if drug appears in breast milk.
Action: onset, 10 minutes; duration 2 hours.

MECHANISM OF ACTION
Acts on the iris and ciliary body of the eye and on salivary, bronchial, and sweat glands. Unlike other anti-muscarinics, scopolamine also produces CNS depression. As an antiemetic, the drug reduces excitability of the labyrinthine receptors and depresses conduction in the vestibular cerebellar pathway. It also has antivertigo effects, probably resulting from action on the cerebral cortex or the membranous labyrinth of the vestibular system.

INDICATIONS & DOSAGE
• Premedication to reduce secretions; treatment or prophylaxis for nausea. *Adults:* 300 to 600 mcg (0.3 to 0.6 mg) as single dose. *Children:* 6 mcg (0.006 mg)/kg or 200 mcg (0.2 mg)/m² as single dose.
• Premedication as anesthesia adjunct for amnesia. *Adults:* 320 to 650 mcg (0.32 to 0.65 mg) in single dose.
• Premedication as anesthesia adjunct for sedation. *Adults:* 600 mcg (0.6 mg) given 30 minutes before procedure. May be repeated three or four times.

CONTRAINDICATIONS & CAUTIONS
• Contraindicated in scopolamine hypersensitivity.
• Also contraindicated in paralytic ileus because drug further slows gastric emptying and heightens the risk of obstruction; in bladder neck obstruction caused by prostatic hypertrophy because drug may worsen urine retention; in pyloric obstruction because drug may aggravate disorder; and in angle-closure glaucoma because antimuscarinic action may raise intraocular pressure.
• Avoid use in tachycardia stemming from cardiac insufficiency or thyrotoxicosis because of possible exacerbation.
• Use cautiously in children with brain damage because drug may exacerbate CNS effect, and in children with spastic paralysis because of possible enhanced response.
• In Down's syndrome, administer carefully because of the risk of abnormally increased pupillary dilation and tachycardia.
• Use with caution in reflux esophagitis or hiatal hernia because drug promotes gastric retention and aggravates reflux; in obstructive GI diseases, such as achalasia and pyloroduodenal stenosis, because drug may decrease GI motility and tone, resulting in obstruction and gastric retention; in elderly or debilitated patients with intestinal atony because of possible obstruction; and in ulcerative colitis because large doses may suppress GI motility and cause paralytic ileus. Drug may also cause or aggravate megacolon.

- Give cautiously in fever, which may rise because of suppressed sweat gland activity.
- Also give cautiously in cardiac disease, especially dysrhythmias, congestive heart failure, coronary heart disease, and mitral stenosis because increased heart rate may be hazardous; in acute hemorrhage related to unstable cardiovascular status because heart rate may rise; in hypertension because drug may aggravate disorder; in toxemia of pregnancy because hypertension may worsen; and in hepatic or renal impairment because of the heightened risk of adverse reactions.
- In chronic lung disease, especially in infants, young children, and debilitated patients, use cautiously because drug may promote bronchial mucus plug formation.
- Also use cautiously in myasthenia gravis, which may be aggravated.
- Administer scopolamine carefully in nonobstructive prostatic hypertrophy, urine retention, or obstructive uropathy because drug may aggravate or precipitate urine retention; and in autonomic neuropathy because drug may worsen urine retention and cycloplegia.
- In xerostomia, prolonged use may further curtail salivary flow. Use cautiously.
- Use cautiously in breastfeeding women.

PREPARATION & STORAGE
Available in 1 ml vials containing 300 mcg/ml and in 1 ml ampules and vials containing 400 mcg/ml, 500 mcg/ml, or 1 mg/ml. Store at room temperature. Protect from light and freezing. For direct injection, dilute with sterile water for injection according to manufacturer's instructions.

ADMINISTRATION
Direct injection: Inject diluted drug at ordered rate through patent I.V. line.
Intermittent infusion: not recommended.
Continuous infusion: not recommended.

INCOMPATIBILITY
Incompatible with alkalies and methohexital sodium.

ADVERSE REACTIONS
Life-threatening: anaphylaxis, respiratory depression.
Other: anhidrosis; bloated sensation; blurred vision; clumsiness; confusion; constipation; decreased lactation; dizziness; drowsiness (especially with large doses); dry mouth, nose, or throat; dysphagia; excitement; eye pain; false sense of well-being; fatigue; fever; hallucinations; headache; insomnia; irritability; memory loss (especially with large doses); mydriasis; nervousness; photophobia; rash; restlessness; seizures; slurred speech; tachycardia; warm, dry, and flushed skin; urinary hesitancy or retention; weakness.

INTERACTIONS
Amantadine, antihistamines, antimuscarinics, buclizine, cyclizine, cyclobenzaprine, disopyramide: enhanced antimuscarinic effects.
Antimyasthenics: further reduced GI motility.
Apomorphine: decreased emetic effect in treatment of poisoning; deepened CNS depression.
Corticosteroids, corticotropin: increased intraocular pressure.
Digoxin: elevated serum levels.
Guanadrel, guanethidine, reserpine: antagonized inhibition of scopolamine on gastric acid secretion.
Haloperidol: decreased antipsychotic effects in schizophrenic patients.

Ipratropium, loxapine, maprotiline, meclizine, methylphenidate, molindone, orphenadrine: heightened antimuscarinic effects.

Lorazepam (parenteral): increased sedation, hallucinations, and irrational behavior. (Concurrent use has no benefit.)

MAO inhibitors: intensified antimuscarinic effects; possible blocked detoxification of scopolamine.

Opioid analgesics: heightened risk of severe constipation, which may cause urine retention and paralytic ileus.

Other CNS depressants: increased sedation.

Phenothiazines, pimozide, procainamide, thioxanthenes, tricyclic antidepressants: intensified antimuscarinic effects.

Potassium chloride (especially wax-matrix preparations): magnified risk of GI lesions.

Urine alkalinizers (calcium- or magnesium-containing antacids, carbonic anhydrase inhibitors): delayed scopolamine excretion.

EFFECTS ON DIAGNOSTIC TESTS

Gastric acid secretion test: possible antagonized effects of pentagastrin.

SPECIAL CONSIDERATIONS

• ***Treatment of overdose:*** Give physostigmine I.V. slowly (less than 1 mg/minute) to reverse severe antimuscarinic symptoms. As needed, repeat doses of 0.5 to 2 mg (up to total dose of 5 mg) in adults or 0.5 to 1 mg (up to total dose of 2 mg) in children. Or in adults, give 0.5 to 1 mg neostigmine methylsulfate I.M., repeated every 2 to 3 hours, or 0.5 to 2 mg I.V., repeated as necessary.

To control excitement or delirium, give small doses of a short-acting barbiturate (100 mg of thiopental sodium) or a benzodiazepine, or rectally infuse 2% solution of chloral hydrate. Respiratory depression may require mechanical ventilation. Maintain adequate hydration and provide symptomatic treatment.

• Expect adverse reactions.

• Raise the bed's side rails and take other safety precautions for elderly patients. Confusion, agitation, excitement, and drowsiness may occur even with usual doses. Reorient patients as necessary. Lower doses may be necessary.

• Elderly patients and children are especially susceptible to adverse antimuscarinic effects.

• Encourage good oral hygiene, and monitor bowel sounds and intake and output.

• When given for pain without concurrent use of morphine or meperidine, scopolamine can act as a stimulant, producing delirium.

• Parenteral use in pregnant women before onset of labor may cause neonatal CNS depression and hemorrhage.

• With prolonged use, patients may develop tolerance to some adverse effects and scopolamine's effectiveness may be reduced.

• After drug discontinuation, be alert for rebound reduction in duration of rapid-eye-movement sleep. Symptoms include anxiety, irritability, nightmares, and insomnia. Treatment may be necessary.

• Avoid giving drug for 24 hours before gastric acid secretion test.

secobarbital
Seconal♦

Controlled Substance Schedule II
Pregnancy Risk Category: D

PHARMACOKINETICS
Distribution: rapidly distributed to all tissues and fluids, with high concentrations in the brain, liver, and kidneys. About 30% to 45% is bound to plasma proteins. Drug rapidly crosses the blood-brain barrier and placenta. Fetal blood levels approach maternal levels within a few minutes after administration.
Metabolism: in the liver, to inactive metabolites.
Excretion: in urine as inactive metabolites or glucuronide conjugates. Trace amounts are eliminated in feces and sweat. Half-life is about 30 hours. Drug appears in breast milk.
Action: onset, 1 to 3 minutes; duration, 15 minutes after 100 to 150 mg dose.

MECHANISM OF ACTION
Not fully understood. As a sedative-hypnotic, this barbiturate depresses the sensory cortex, decreasing motor activity, altering cerebral function, and promoting drowsiness, sedation, and hypnosis. As an anticonvulsant, it depresses monosynaptic and polysynaptic transmission in the CNS. The drug also increases the threshold for electrical stimulation of the motor cortex.

INDICATIONS & DOSAGE
● Acute agitation in psychosis.
Adults: initially, no more than 250 mg; additional doses given cautiously after 5 minutes if initial dose doesn't produce desired response. Usually a dose of 1.1 to 1.7 mg/kg produces moderate to heavy sedation, 2.2 mg/kg produces hypnosis, and 3.3 to 4.4 mg/kg calms extremely agitated patients. Maximum dose, 500 mg.
● Status epilepticus. *Adults:* 250 to 350 mg.
● Tetanic seizures. *Adults:* 5.5 mg/kg, repeated q 3 to 4 hours, p.r.n. *Children:* 3 to 5 mg/kg or 12.5 mg/m².
● Preoperative anesthesia. *Adults:* 50 to 250 mg in divided doses.
● Insomnia. *Adults:* 100 to 150 mg.

CONTRAINDICATIONS & CAUTIONS
● Contraindicated in hypersensitivity to barbiturates and in acute intermittent porphyria or variegate porphyria because drug may aggravate symptoms.
● Also contraindicated in bronchial pneumonia or other severe pulmonary insufficiency because drug causes respiratory depression.
● Use cautiously in debilitated or elderly patients because usual doses may cause marked excitement, depression, and confusion.
● During pregnancy or labor and delivery, give carefully because of adverse fetal effects or neonatal respiratory depression. Contraindicated in breastfeeding women.
● Also give carefully in severe anemia, hyperkinesis, and hyperthyroidism because the drug may aggravate these conditions, and in asthma because of the increased risk of hypersensitivity reactions.
● Take special care in giving this drug to patients with a history of drug abuse or dependence; these patients are at increased risk for habituation. Also give carefully to depressed patients because drug may worsen depression or suicidal tendencies.

• Use cautiously in patients with borderline hypoadrenalism because drug may decrease systemic effects of exogenous hydrocortisone and endogenous cortisol; to patients with acute or chronic pain because it may mask symptoms or induce paradoxical excitement; to patients with hepatic impairment or in hepatic coma because of decreased drug metabolism; and to those with renal impairment because of reduced drug excretion.

• Also use cautiously in cardiac disease because of the risk of adverse reactions (especially with rapid administration) and in hypertension because of the enhanced risk of hypotension.

PREPARATION & STORAGE
Available in concentration of 50 mg/ml in 1 and 2 ml prefilled syringe cartridges and 20 ml vials. Store in refrigerator at 36° to 46° F. (2° to 8° C.). Protect from light. Don't use if solution is discolored or contains a precipitate. Drug may be administered as supplied or diluted with sterile water for injection, 0.9% sodium chloride injection, or Ringer's injection.

ADMINISTRATION
Direct injection: Inject drug slowly (not exceeding 50 mg/15 seconds) through a primary I.V. line containing a free-flowing compatible solution. Slow administration usually prevents hypotension in hypertensive patients.

Avoid extravasation. Use large veins to minimize irritation and risk of thrombosis. Parenteral solutions of barbiturate salts are highly alkaline and may cause local tissue damage and necrosis. Also avoid inadvertent intraarterial injection, which may cause spasm, severe pain, and gangrene.

Intermittent infusion: not recommended.
Continuous infusion: not recommended.

INCOMPATIBILITY
Incompatible with alkali-labile drugs (such as penicillin), atracurium, benzquinamide, chlorpromazine, cimetidine, clindamycin phosphate, codeine phosphate, diphenhydramine, droperidol, ephedrine, erythromycin glucepate, glycopyrrolate, hydrocortisone sodium succinate, isoproterenol hydrochloride, lactated Ringer's injection, levorphanol, metaraminol, methadone hydrochloride, methyldopate hydrochloride, norepinephrine, oxytetracycline, pancuronium, pentazocine lactate, phenytoin sodium, procaine, propiomazine hydrochloride, regular insulin, sodium bicarbonate, streptomycin, succinylcholine, tetracycline hydrochloride, and vancomycin.

ADVERSE REACTIONS
Life-threatening: bronchospasm, congestive heart failure, exfoliative dermatitis, hypertension, laryngospasm, pulmonary edema, renal failure, respiratory depression, Stevens-Johnson syndrome.
Other: anxiety; bleeding sores on lips; bradycardia; chest pain; clumsiness or unsteadiness; confusion; constipation; depression; drowsiness (severe); dyspnea; excitement (paradoxical reaction); faintness; fatigue; fever; hallucinations; hangover; headache; insomnia; lightheadedness; muscle or joint pain; nausea; nightmares; rash; red, thickened, or scaly skin; slurred speech; soreness, redness, swelling, or pain at injection site; sore throat; swelling of eyelids, face, or lips; trembling; unusual bleeding or bruising; unusual eye movements; urticaria; vomiting; weakness.

Unmarked trade names available in the United States only.
♦ Also available in Canada.   ♦♦ Available in Canada only.

INTERACTIONS

Alcohol, CNS depressant drugs: deepened CNS depression.
Ascorbic acid: increased excretion.
Calcium channel blockers: excessive hypotension.
Carbamazepine: increased metabolism and decreased serum levels of either interacting drug.
Carbonic anhydrase inhibitors: enhanced risk of osteopenia.
Contraceptives (oral): reduced reliability.
Cardiac glycosides, corticosteroids, cyclosporine, dacarbazine, levothyroxine, quinidine: diminished effects.
Cyclophosphamide: intensified leukopenia.
Disopyramide: reduced serum levels (to ineffective levels).
Divalproex sodium, valproic acid: deepened CNS depression and neurotoxicity.
Doxycycline: shortened half-life.
Estramustine, systemic estrogens, vitamin D: reduced effects.
Griseofulvin: lessened absorption.
Guanadrel, guanethidine, loop diuretics: increased orthostatic hypotension.
Haloperidol: altered pattern or frequency of seizures.
Hydantoin anticonvulsants: unpredictable metabolism.
Hypothermia-producing medications: enhanced risk of hypothermia.
Ketamine: heightened potential for hypotension and respiratory depression.
Loxapine, phenothiazines, thioxantheines: lowered seizure threshold.
MAO inhibitors: prolonged CNS depression and possible altered seizure pattern.
Maprotiline: enhanced CNS depression, lowered seizure threshold, and decreased secobarbital effects.

Methylphenidate: elevated secobarbital levels, risking toxicity.
Mexiletine: decreased levels.
Other dermatitis-causing drugs: heightened risk of dermatologic reactions.
Posterior pituitary hormone: enhanced risk of dysrhythmias and coronary insufficiency.
Primidone: altered seizure pattern.
Tricyclic antidepressants: decreased effects, deepened CNS depression, and lowered seizure threshold.
Warfarin sodium, indanedione-derived anticoagulants: decreased effects.
Xanthines: subtherapeutic serum levels, stemming from increased theophylline clearance.

EFFECTS ON DIAGNOSTIC TESTS

Cyanocobalamin (Co 57): impaired absorption.
Phentolamine test: possible false-positive results.
Serum bilirubin: decreased levels in neonates and patients with seizures or congenital nonhemolytic unconjugated hyperbilirubinemia.

SPECIAL CONSIDERATIONS

• Always keep resuscitation and mechanical ventilation equipment available.
• Monitor vital signs.
• Maintain airway with ventilation and oxygen administration as needed. Administer chest physiotherapy. Respiratory difficulty can occur 2 to 10 minutes after I.V. dose. Such reactions are cumulative and potentiated with repeated administration.
• Administer a vasopressor, as ordered, for hypotension.
• Discontinue drug if skin eruptions occur; these may precede potentially fatal reactions.

• Monitor fluid balance. Avoid sodium or fluid overload, especially in cardiac disorders.

• Degree of CNS depression (from mild sedation to hypnosis to deep coma or even death) with I.V. barbiturates depends on dosage, drug's pharmacokinetics, patient's age and physical and emotional state, and concurrent use of other drugs.

• Forced diuresis may help to eliminate the drug in normal renal function.

• Although not recommended, hemodialysis or hemoperfusion may be used in patients with severe barbiturate poisoning, anuria, or shock.

• After drug discontinuation, be alert for withdrawal symptoms. Those that require medical attention include anxiety or unusual restlessness, dizziness, hallucinations, lightheadedness, muscle twitching, nausea and vomiting, seizures, insomnia, trembling hands, vision problems, and unusual weakness.

• In suspected pneumonia, take appropriate specimens for cultures and administer antibiotics, as ordered.

• Full anesthetic dose decreases the force and frequency of uterine contractions.

• Drug has little analgesic action at subanesthetic doses and may increase reaction to painful stimuli.

• Patients receiving dialysis may require increased dosage.

• The risk of barbiturate-induced hypothermia may increase in elderly patients, especially with high doses or acute overdose.

• Secobarbital should be administered I.V. only when oral or I.M. administration isn't feasible.

• Withhold drug for at least 24 hours, preferably for 48 to 72 hours, before the phentolamine test.

sodium bicarbonate
Sodium Bicarbonate

Pregnancy Risk Category: C

PHARMACOKINETICS
Distribution: throughout extracellular fluid. Drug probably crosses the placenta.
Metabolism: dissociated in water to sodium and bicarbonate ions. Bicarbonate anion is converted to carbonic acid, then to its volatile form, carbon dioxide.
Excretion: in urine, by glomerular filtration as bicarbonate. Usually less than 1% is excreted. Carbon dioxide is excreted by the lungs. Drug probably appears in breast milk.
Action: onset, immediate; duration, unknown.

MECHANISM OF ACTION
As a systemic alkalinizing agent, sodium bicarbonate increases plasma bicarbonate and buffers excess hydrogen ion concentration.

INDICATIONS AND DOSAGE
Dosage reflects severity of acidosis, test results, and the patient's age, weight, and condition.
• Cardiac arrest. *Adults and children age 2 and older:* 1 mEq/kg initially, then 0.5 mEq/kg q 10 minutes, depending on arterial blood gas (ABG) measurements, if available. *Children under age 2:* 1 mEq/kg initially. If ABGs and pH levels are available, further doses are given q 10 minutes and calculated in milliequivalents of NaHCO$_3$. Multiply 0.3 by body weight (kg). Then multiply this figure by base deficit (mEq/liter). If ABGs and pH levels are unavailable, further doses of 1 mEq/kg are given q 10 minutes dur-

ing arrest. Maximum dosage, 8 mEq/kg daily.

• *Metabolic acidosis associated with chronic renal failure.* *Adults and older children:* initially, 2 to 5 mEq/kg; subsequent doses are determined by response to drug and test results (total CO_2, blood pH).

• *Urinary alkalinization.* *Adults and children:* 2 to 5 mEq/kg.

CONTRAINDICATIONS & CAUTIONS

• Contraindicated in metabolic or respiratory alkalosis because sodium bicarbonate may exacerbate them.

• Also contraindicated in chloride loss from vomiting or continuous GI suctioning because of the increased risk of severe alkalosis; in hypocalcemia because of the heightened risk of alkalosis resulting in tetany; and in patients at risk for developing diuretic-induced hypochloremic alkalosis.

• Because sodium content may cause exacerbation, give cautiously in renal insufficiency; in edematous sodium-retaining conditions, such as cirrhosis of the liver, congestive heart failure, or toxemia of pregnancy; and in hypertension.

• During pregnancy, this drug should be given only when clearly needed. Potential for fetal harm is unknown.

PREPARATION & STORAGE

Available in 5 ml (2.4 mEq) flip-top and pin-top vials containing 4% solution (6.48 mEq/ml); 10 ml (5 mEq) disposable syringes containing 4.2% solution (0.5 mEq/ml); 500 ml (297.5 mEq) containers of 5% solution (0.595 mEq/ml); 10 ml (8.9 mEq) ampules and 50 ml (44.6 mEq) ampules and disposable syringes containing 7.5% solution (0.892 mEq/ml); and 10 ml (10 mEq) disposable syringes and 50 ml

(50 mEq) vials and disposable syringes containing 8.4% solution (1 mEq/ml).

Store at room temperature, always below 104° F. (40° C.), and protect from freezing and heat. Stability may be increased by refrigerating sodium bicarbonate injection and syringes before preparation, rinsing syringes twice with refrigerated sterile water for injection, and minimizing contact with air. To do this, expel air from syringes and tape the plungers in place to reduce movement caused by escaping CO_2. The 7.5% solution in polypropylene syringes is stable up to 100 days if refrigerated or up to 45 days at room temperature. Don't use solution if it is cloudy or contains a precipitate.

To dilute for infusion, follow manufacturer's instructions, using sterile water for injection or other standard electrolyte solutions. In neonates and children under age 2, use 4.2% sodium bicarbonate solution or dilute 7.5% or 8.4% sodium bicarbonate solution 1:1 with dextrose 5% in water.

ADMINISTRATION

Direct injection: For cardiac arrest, flush I.V. line before and after use. In adults, inject rapidly into patent primary I.V. line. In neonates and children under age 2, inject ordered dose into patent primary I.V. line over 1 to 2 minutes. Overly rapid injection (10 ml/minute) can cause hypernatremia, decreased cerebrospinal fluid pressure, intracranial hemorrhage, and severe alkalosis, accompanied by hyperirritability or tetany.
Intermittent infusion: not recommended.
Continuous infusion: Flush I.V. line before and after use. Infuse ordered amount of diluted drug into patent I.V. line over 4 to 8 hours, as ordered, for metabolic acidosis.

INCOMPATIBILITY

Incompatible with ACTH, alcohol 5% in dextrose 5%, amino acids, ascorbic acid injection, calcium salts, carmustine, cisplatin, codeine phosphate, corticotropin, dextrose 5% in lactated Ringer's injection, dobutamine, dopamine, epinephrine hydrochloride, fat emulsion 10%, glycopyrrolate, hydromorphone, insulin (regular), Ionosol B, D, or G with invert sugar 10%, isoproterenol hydrochloride, labetalol hydrochloride, levorphanol, magnesium sulfate, meperidine, methadone hydrochloride, methicillin sodium, methylprednisolone sodium succinate, metoclopramide, morphine sulfate, norepinephrine bitartrate, oxytetracycline hydrochloride, penicillin G potassium, pentazocine lactate, pentobarbital sodium, phenobarbital sodium, procaine hydrochloride, promazine hydrochloride, Ringer's injection and lactated Ringer's injection, secobarbital sodium, sodium lactate (⅙ M), streptomycin sulfate, succinylcholine chloride, tetracycline hydrochloride, thiopental sodium, vancomycin hydrochloride, and vitamin B complex with vitamin C.

ADVERSE REACTIONS

Life-threatening: intracranial hemorrhage in children under age 2 (with rapid administration), metabolic alkalosis.
Other: bradypnea; fatigue; increased thirst; irregular heartbeat; mental changes; muscle cramps, pain, or twitching; necrosis, sloughing, or ulceration with extravasation; nervousness; restlessness; swollen feet or lower legs; unpleasant taste; weakness.

INTERACTIONS

Amphetamines, quinidine: possible toxicity, resulting from inhibited urinary excretion.
Anabolic steroids, androgens: heightened risk of edema.
Antidyskinetics: reduced therapeutic effects.
Antimuscarinics, especially atropine-related compounds: reduced effectiveness, delayed excretion, and increased adverse effects.
Corticosteroids: increased risk of hypernatremia with frequent or high-dose administration of sodium bicarbonate.
Ephedrine: lengthened half-life and prolonged action, especially if alkaline urine persists for several days.
Lithium: enhanced excretion and possible decreased effectiveness.
Mecamylamine: delayed excretion and prolonged effects.
Methenamine: reduced effectiveness.
Mexiletine: delayed excretion.
Potassium-wasting diuretics: enhanced risk of hypochloremic alkalosis.
Potassium-sparing diuretics, potassium supplements: altered serum potassium levels.
Salicylates: increased excretion.
Warfarin, indanedione-derived anticoagulants: reduced effectiveness, resulting from decreased absorption.

EFFECTS ON DIAGNOSTIC TESTS

Blood and urine pH: possible rise.
Gastric acid secretion: antagonized response to pentagastrin. Don't give sodium bicarbonate on the morning of test.
Serum potassium: possible elevated levels.

SPECIAL CONSIDERATIONS

• *Treatment of overdose:* For alkalosis, have patient rebreathe expired air from a mask or paper bag. If alkalosis is severe, administer calcium gluconate I.V., as ordered.
• Correct electrolyte imbalances, especially hypokalemia and hypocalcemia, before or during therapy.

• Throughout therapy, monitor ABGs and pH, serum bicarbonate, renal function (especially in long-term therapy), and urine pH (especially when drug is used for alkalinization).

• Administer repeated small doses to avoid overdose and resultant metabolic alkalosis. Excessive doses may induce hypokalemia and predispose the patient to dysrhythmias.

• Use of this drug in cardiac arrest should be preceded by manual or mechanical hyperventilation to lower PCO_2 levels.

• Don't attempt full correction of bicarbonate deficit during the first 24 hours of therapy; this may produce metabolic alkalosis from delayed compensatory mechanisms.

• Sodium bicarbonate is frequently overused during cardiac arrest. American Heart Association no longer recommends its routine use in the initial stages of advanced life support. Instead, initial treatment should include basic life support and defibrillation, hyperventilation, or pharmacologic therapy.

---

sodium chloride
0.45% Sodium Chloride Injection,
0.9% Sodium Chloride Injection,
3% Sodium Chloride Injection,
5% Sodium Chloride Injection

Pregnancy Risk Category: C

COMPOSITION
These solutions consist of sodium chloride and sterile water with no bacteriostatic or antimicrobial agents or added buffers. They have a pH of 4.5 to 7.

The 0.45% concentration is hypotonic with 77 mEq/liter of sodium and of chloride and an osmolarity of 154 to 155 mOsm/liter. The 0.9% concentration is isotonic, contains 154 mEq/liter of sodium and of chloride, and has an osmolarity of 308 to 310 mOsm/liter. The 3% concentration is hypertonic and contains 513 mEq/liter of sodium and of chloride with an osmolarity of 1,026 to 1,030 mOsm/liter. Also hypertonic, 5% sodium chloride contains 855 mEq/liter of sodium and of chloride. Its osmolarity is 1,710 to 1,711 mOsm/liter.

Concentrations of 0.225% and 0.3% sodium chloride are not commercially available. These hypotonic solutions contain 38.5 mEq/liter of sodium and of chloride for the 0.225% concentration and 51 mEq/liter for the 0.3% concentration.

INDICATIONS & DOSAGE
Dosage depends on the disorder and the patient's age, weight, and fluid, electrolyte, and acid-base balance. For children, concentration and dosage are based on weight or body surface area.

• Fluid and electrolyte replacement. *Adults:* usually 1 liter daily of 0.9% sodium chloride or 1 to 2 liters daily of 0.45% sodium chloride.

• Fluid and electrolyte replacement in ketoacidosis. *Children:* 0.225% or 0.3% sodium chloride.

• Severe sodium chloride depletion requiring rapid replacement. *Adults:* 100 ml of 3% or 5% sodium chloride over 1 hour, then additional doses determined by serum electrolyte measurement.

• Adjunct to blood transfusions and hemodialysis. *Adults:* 0.9% sodium chloride.

• Hyperosmolar diabetes. *Adults:* 0.45% sodium chloride.

CONTRAINDICATIONS & CAUTIONS

• Contraindicated in conditions in which sodium and chloride administration is hazardous.
• Use hypertonic solutions only in patients with severe sodium and chloride deficits.
• Use with extreme caution in patients with CHF, other sodium-retaining conditions, and severe renal disease or insufficiency because of the increased risk of fluid retention.
• Give carefully in elderly or postoperative patients because fluid retention may worsen.

PREPARATION & STORAGE

Available in glass or flexible PVC containers. Solutions of 0.45% NaCl come in 500 and 1,000 ml containers; 0.9% NaCl in 50, 100, 150, 250, 500, and 1,000 ml containers; and 3% and 5% NaCl in 500 ml containers. Solutions of 0.9% NaCl are also supplied in 25, 50, and 100 ml containers as diluents for drug delivery. Store solutions at room temperature.

ADMINISTRATION

Direct injection: used only as drug diluent.
Intermittent infusion: used only as drug diluent.
Continuous infusion: Infuse through a peripheral or central vein at ordered rate. Infuse 3% or 5% solutions through a large vein, at a rate not exceeding 100 ml/hr. Avoid extravasation. Observe infusion site carefully for signs of phlebitis.

INCOMPATIBILITY

Incompatible with amphotericin B, benzquinamide, chlordiazepoxide, diazepam, fat emulsion, methylprednisolone sodium succinate, and phenytoin sodium.

ADVERSE REACTIONS

Life-threatening: acidosis, congestive heart failure, pulmonary edema.
Other: extravasation, fever, fluid and electrolyte overload, hypernatremia, hypokalemia, infection at injection site, phlebitis, venous thrombosis.

INTERACTIONS

Corticosteroids: increased risk of hypernatremia.

EFFECTS ON DIAGNOSTIC TESTS

None reported.

SPECIAL CONSIDERATIONS

• If fluid overload occurs, discontinue the infusion and initiate corrective measures.
• Monitor serum electrolytes, especially sodium and potassium. Also check chloride and bicarbonate levels.

---

sodium lactate
(⅙ M sodium lactate)

Pregnancy Risk Category: C

PHARMACOKINETICS

Distribution: not well characterized.
Metabolism: in the liver by oxidation to bicarbonate and glycogen. Conversion usually requires 1 to 2 hours.
Excretion: not well characterized.
Action: unknown.

MECHANISM OF ACTION

This alkalinizing agent's action depends on conversion to bicarbonate, the principal extracellular buffer, which acts to maintain acid-base balance.

INDICATIONS & DOSAGE
• Mild to moderate metabolic acidosis. *Adults:* To calculate suggested dosage in ml, multiply 0.8 by body weight (lb). Then multiply this figure by 60 and subtract from plasma CO_2 level. Actual dosage depends on severity of acidosis, test results (plasma glucose, serum electrolyte levels), and patient's age, weight, and underlying disorder.

CONTRAINDICATIONS & CAUTIONS
• Contraindicated in lactic acidosis because lactate metabolism is impaired and bicarbonate doesn't form.
• Also contraindicated in hypernatremia and other conditions in which sodium administration is harmful.
• Use cautiously in patients with edema or sodium-retaining conditions, such as congestive heart failure, oliguria, or anuria.
• Sodium lactate can exacerbate metabolic or respiratory alkalosis because it's an alkalinizing agent. Use cautiously.
• Administer cautiously in conditions that increase lactate use, such as severe hepatic insufficiency, shock, hypoxia, or beriberi. Additional lactate may worsen these conditions.
• Also administer cautiously in metabolic acidosis associated with circulatory insufficiency, extracorporeal circulation, hypothermia, glycogen storage disease, liver dysfunction, respiratory alkalosis, shock, cardiac decompensation, or other conditions involving reduced tissue perfusion. Tissue anoxia and impaired lactate metabolism reduce lactate conversion to bicarbonate.

PREPARATION & STORAGE
Available in 150, 250, 500, and 1,000 ml containers of solution having sodium and lactate ions, each in concentrations of 167 mEq/liter. Also available in 10 ml flip-top vials containing 5 mEq/ml. Store at 104° F. (40° C.) or below. Protect from freezing and extreme heat. Discard any unused portions.

For infusion, dilute sodium lactate in ordered volume of solution if desired concentration isn't commercially available.

ADMINISTRATION
Direct injection: not recommended.
Intermittent infusion: not recommended.
Continuous infusion: Infuse diluted solution through primary I.V. line or piggyback at ordered rate. Don't exceed 300 ml/hour in adults.

INCOMPATIBILITY
Incompatible with oxytetracycline and sodium bicarbonate.

ADVERSE REACTIONS
Life-threatening: hypokalemia, metabolic alkalosis (overdose), pulmonary edema.
Other: hypernatremia (with or without edema), hypovolemia.

INTERACTIONS
None significant.

EFFECTS ON DIAGNOSTIC TESTS
Arterial blood gas levels: findings indicative of improved metabolic acidosis.

SPECIAL CONSIDERATIONS
• Throughout therapy, carefully monitor plasma glucose, fluid and electrolyte balance, and acid-base balance.
• When administering sodium lactate, determine needed volume of I.V. fluid by calculating the patient's maintenance or replacement requirements.

• Discontinue infusion if an adverse reaction occurs. Evaluate the patient, begin symptomatic treatment, and save remaining solution for examination, if necessary.
• One gram of sodium lactate provides 8.9 mEq of sodium and 8.9 mEq of lactate.

sodium salicylate
Uracel

Pregnancy Risk Category: C

PHARMACOKINETICS
Distribution: widespread. Drug is highly bound to plasma proteins, primarily to albumin; however, binding diminishes with increased plasma salicylate levels, reduced plasma albumin levels, renal dysfunction, and pregnancy. Drug readily crosses the placenta.
Metabolism: in the liver and blood by hydrolysis to salicylate, then further metabolized in liver.
Excretion: in urine, primarily as free salicylic acid and conjugated metabolites. Half-life depends on dose and urine pH, and ranges from 2 to 20 hours. Drug appears in breast milk.
Action: unknown.

MECHANISM OF ACTION
Unknown, but drug's anti-inflammatory effect may peripherally inhibit synthesis of prostaglandin and synthesis and action of other substances that sensitize pain receptors to mechanical or chemical stimulation. Drug produces analgesia by acting on the hypothalamus and peripherally blocking pain impulses. As an antipyretic, it acts on the hypothalamic heat-regulating center to produce peripheral vasodilation.

INDICATIONS & DOSAGE
• Pain. *Adults:* 500 mg in a single dose. Maximum dosage, 1 g daily. Always use lowest effective dose. Elderly patients may need dosage adjustment.
• Rheumatic fever. *Adults:* not typically used because of drug's high sodium content, but single daily I.V. infusions up to 10 g have been given.

CONTRAINDICATIONS & CAUTIONS
• Contraindicated in hypersensitivity to this drug or other salicylates, and in breastfeeding women.
• Also contraindicated in bleeding ulcers or hemorrhage because drug may worsen these conditions, and in hemophilia because of an increased risk of hemorrhage.
• Use cautiously in anemia because vasodilation may cause pseudoanemia; in gout because salicylates' variable dose-dependent effects on serum uric acid levels may interfere with effectiveness of antigout drug; and in thyrotoxicosis because high doses may exacerbate the disorder.
• Use cautiously in patients with conditions that predispose them to fluid retention, such as compromised cardiac function or hypertension, because sodium may be detrimental. High doses may cause edema in compromised cardiac function. In patients with congestive heart failure, the drug may increase the risk of adverse renal effects.
• Use cautiously in hepatic and renal impairment because of increased risk of adverse effects and in hypoprothrombinemia or vitamin K deficiency because of enhanced potential for bleeding.

PREPARATION & STORAGE
Available in 10 ml ampules containing 1 g/10 ml. Protect from light.

For infusion, dilute in 1 liter of 0.9% sodium chloride injection or lactated Ringer's injection.

ADMINISTRATION
Direct injection: not used.
Intermittent infusion: not recommended.
Continuous infusion: Infuse diluted drug slowly through patent I.V. line, usually the primary line, over ordered time (usually 4 to 8 hours). Always infuse slowly; rapid infusion may cause thrombophlebitis and extravasation.

INCOMPATIBILITY
No incompatibilities reported.

ADVERSE REACTIONS
Life-threatening: anaphylaxis.
Other: acid-base imbalance, chest tightness, confusion, deep breathing, diaphoresis, diarrhea, (severe or continuing), dizziness, dyspnea, excitement, extreme drowsiness, fatigue, fever, hallucinations, headache (severe or continuing), hearing loss, hematuria, hyperglycemia, hypoglycemia, hypokalemia, hyponatremia, ketonuria, light-headedness, nervousness, proteinuria, pruritus, rash, seizures, tachypnea, thirst, tinnitus, uncontrollable hand flapping (especially in the elderly), urticaria, vision problems, weakness, wheezing.

INTERACTIONS
ACTH, androgens, glucocorticoids, mineralocorticoids (especially anabolic steroids, fludrocortisone): magnified risk of hypernatremia, edema, and hypertension, especially with chronic use.
Aminoglycosides, bumetanide, capreomycin, cisplatin, ethacrynic acid, high-dose erythromycin (in renal impairment), vancomycin: enhanced risk of ototoxicity.

Anticoagulants, streptokinase, urokinase: heightened risk of bleeding.
Antiemetics: masked symptoms of salicylate toxicity (dizziness, tinnitus, vertigo).
Carbonic anhydrase inhibitors: possible metabolic acidosis and reduced salicylate levels, resulting from increased salicylate excretion.
Furosemide: increased risk of ototoxicity; salicylate toxicity with high-dose salicylate therapy.
High-dose antacids (especially chronic use of calcium- or magnesium-containing antacids), urine alkalinizers (such as citrates and sodium bicarbonate): reduced salicylate levels, resulting from increased salicylate excretion.
Insulin or oral antidiabetic drugs: enhanced hypoglycemic effects with high salicylate doses.
Methotrexate: toxic plasma levels.
Nifedipine, verapamil: amplified risk of toxicity for these calcium channel blockers and sodium salicylate.
Probenecid: diminished effects of probenecid; possible salicylate toxicity, resulting from reduced renal clearance and elevated plasma levels.
Salicylic acid (topical): enhanced potential for salicylate toxicity if significant quantities absorbed.
Sulfinpyrazone: decreased sulfinpyrazone effects; diminished salicylate excretion.
Urine acidifiers (such as ammonium chloride, ascorbic acid, potassium phosphate, sodium phosphate): elevated salicylate levels, stemming from suppressed salicylate excretion.

EFFECTS ON DIAGNOSTIC TESTS
Gerhardt's test for urine acetoacetic acid: interference with results because of reaction with ferric chloride.

Prothrombin time: increased with large salicylate doses, especially if plasma levels exceed 300 mcg/ml.
Serum alkaline phosphatase, SGOT, SGPT: abnormal results.
Serum potassium: possible decreased levels.
Serum uric acid: increased levels in plasma salicylate levels below 150 mcg/ml; reduced levels in salicylate levels above 150 mcg/ml; falsely elevated results of colorimetric assay when salicylate levels exceed 130 mcg/ml.
Thyroid function: with high doses of salicylates, reduced levels of serum thyroxine (T_4) and serum triiodothyronine (T_3), and possible enhanced T_3 resin uptake.
Urine phenolsulfonphthalein: possible diminished levels.
Urine vanillylmandelic acid: falsely increased or decreased levels, depending on method used.

SPECIAL CONSIDERATIONS

• *Treatment of overdose:* Discontinue drug, and monitor and support vital functions. Then correct hyperthermia; fluid, electrolyte, and acid-base imbalances; and plasma glucose level, as needed. Monitor serum salicylate levels until they're nontoxic. Also induce alkaline diuresis to increase salicylate excretion. As needed to correct severe overdose, begin exchange transfusion, hemodialysis, peritoneal dialysis, or hemoperfusion. Monitor for pulmonary edema and begin appropriate therapy as necessary. Administer blood or vitamin K, if necessary, to treat hemorrhage.
• Children, especially those with fever and dehydration, may be at increased risk for salicylate toxicity.
• Children and teenagers shouldn't be given salicylates for chicken pox or influenza symptoms because Reye's syndrome may occur.

streptokinase
Kabikinase, Streptase♦

Pregnancy Risk Category: C

PHARMACOKINETICS
Distribution: in plasma. Drug crosses the placenta minimally.
Metabolism: not metabolized.
Excretion: rapidly cleared from the circulation by antibodies and the reticuloendothelial system. Initial half-life is about 18 minutes (from antibody action against streptokinase); subsequent half-life, about 83 minutes (in absence of antibodies). Not known if drug appears in breast milk.
Action: onset, rapid; duration, a few hours after therapy is discontinued.

MECHANISM OF ACTION
Streptokinase promotes thrombolysis by converting residual plasminogen to plasmin (fibrinolysin), which degrades fibrin clots, fibrinogen, and precoagulant factors V and VII. Drug also decreases blood and plasma viscosity and reduces erythrocytes' tendency to form aggregates, thereby increasing perfusion of collateral blood vessels. Streptokinase is strongly antigenic. It promotes antibody formation, which diminishes its effects and may cause allergic reactions.

INDICATIONS & DOSAGE
• Pulmonary embolism, deep vein thrombosis, arterial embolism or thrombosis. *Adults:* loading dose 250,000 IU; maintenance dose 100,000 IU/hour.

- Acute, obstructing coronary artery thrombi associated with evolving acute MI. *Adults:* 1.5 million IU over 30 to 60 minutes.
- Arteriovenous cannula occlusion. *Adults:* 100,000 to 250,000 IU in 2 ml of I.V. solution.

CONTRAINDICATIONS & CAUTIONS

- Contraindicated in active internal bleeding, intracranial neoplasm, severe uncontrolled hypertension, or recent (within 2 months) cerebrovascular accident or intracranial or intraspinal surgery because thrombolytic therapy increases the risk of bleeding.
- Also contraindicated in previous severe allergic reaction to the drug.
- Use with extreme caution in conditions with associated risk of bleeding, such as dissecting aneurysm, cerebrovascular accident or disease (within 2 months), childbirth, invasive procedures or surgery within the past 10 days, uncontrolled coagulation defects or other hemostatic defects (including those secondary to severe hepatic or renal disease), subacute bacterial endocarditis, diabetic hemorrhagic retinopathy, severe GI bleeding within the past 10 days, GI lesion or ulcer, moderate hypertension, recent trauma (minor or severe, including possible internal injury caused by cardiopulmonary resuscitation), and active tuberculosis with cavitation of recent onset.
- Use cautiously in mitral stenosis with atrial fibrillation or other indications of probable left heart thrombus and in conditions with risk of cerebral embolism.
- Give cautiously in sepsis at or near thrombus site, obstructed intravenous catheter, or occluded arteriovenous cannula because of enhanced risk of systemic infection.

- Administer carefully in patients with recent streptococcal infection (and in any patient receiving drug) because elevated streptokinase antibody levels may cause resistance to therapy.

PREPARATION & STORAGE

Available in powder form in 5 ml vials containing 250,000, 600,000, or 750,000 IU; in 6.5 ml vials containing 250,000, 750,000, or 1.5 million IU; and in 50 ml infusion bottle of 1.5 million IU. Store unopened vials at room temperature.

For arteriovenous cannula clearance, reconstitute using 2 ml of 0.9% sodium chloride injection or dextrose 5% injection for each 250,000 IU of streptokinase. Add diluent slowly, directed at the side of the vial (rather than onto the powder). Roll and tilt the vial gently; avoid shaking, which may cause foaming and an increase in flocculation. Slight flocculation doesn't interfere with safe use; however, solutions containing many particles should be discarded.

For infusion, reconstitute with 0.9% sodium chloride injection or dextrose 5% injection. Further dilute, generally to a volume of 45 ml (loading dose infusion) or to a multiple of 45 ml to a maximum of 500 ml (continuous maintenance infusion), with the same solution used for reconstitution. Infusions should be administered through a .22- or .45-micron filter. Use volumetric or syringe pumps because reconstituted streptokinase solution may alter drop size, influencing the accuracy of drop-counting infusion devices.

Store reconstituted solutions at 36° to 39° F. (2° to 4° C.); discard after 24 hours. Don't add any other drugs to the solution.

ADMINISTRATION

Streptokinase should be administered only by staff trained in managing thrombotic disease and working in hospitals equipped to monitor thrombin time and perform other necessary laboratory tests.

Direct injection: To clear arteriovenous cannula obstruction, use an infusion pump to slowly deliver 250,000 IU of reconstituted drug into each occluded cannula over 25 to 35 minutes. Then clamp off the cannula(s) for 2 hours. Closely observe patient for possible adverse reactions. After 2 hours, aspirate contents of the cannula(s) and flush with 0.9% sodium chloride. Reconnect cannula.

Intermittent infusion: not recommended.

Continuous infusion: For loading dose in pulmonary embolism, deep vein thrombosis, or arterial embolism or thrombosis, give diluted drug through a peripheral I.V. line, using an infusion pump to deliver 250,000 IU over 30 minutes. Set rate at 30 ml/hour (for 750,000 IU vial) or 90 ml/hour (for 250,000 IU vial) with dilution equaling 45 ml.

For maintenance dose, set infusion pump to deliver 100,000 IU/hour. Continue infusion for 24 hours for pulmonary embolism, for 24 to 72 hours for arterial embolism or thrombosis, and for 72 hours for deep vein thrombosis.

For coronary artery thrombi, give diluted drug through a peripheral I.V. line, using an infusion pump with rate set at 1.5 million IU/hour for 1 hour. No maintenance dose required.

INCOMPATIBILITY

Incompatible with dextrans.

ADVERSE REACTIONS

Life-threatening: anaphylaxis, severe hemorrhage.

Other: abdominal pain or swelling; backache; bleeding or oozing from cuts or wounds; bloody or black, tarry stools; constipation (paralytic ileus or intestinal obstruction caused by hemorrhage); dizziness; dyspnea; epistaxis; fast, slow, or irregular heartbeat; fever; headache (mild or severe); hematemesis; hematuria; hemoptysis; hypotension (sudden or severe); muscle pain or stiffness; nausea; phlebitis at infusion site; pruritus; rash; swelling of eyes, face, lips, or tongue; unexpected or unusually heavy vaginal bleeding; urticaria; wheezing.

INTERACTIONS

ACTH (long-term), corticosteroids (glucocorticoids), ethacrynic acid, nonacetylated salicylates: heightened risk of severe hemorrhage because GI ulceration or hemorrhage may occur with these drugs.

Antifibrinolytic drugs (aminocaproic acid): reversal of streptokinase effects.

Aspirin, azlocillin, carbenicillin (parenteral), indomethacin, mezlocillin, piperacillin, ticarcillin: heightened risk of bleeding because of altered platelet function.

Cefamandole, cefoperazone, moxalactam, plicamycin: enhanced risk of severe hemorrhage.

Dextran, dipyridamole, divalproex, phenylbutazone, sulfinpyrazone, valproic acid: increased risk of bleeding because of altered platelet function.

Heparin, oral anticoagulants: magnified risk of hemorrhage.

EFFECTS ON DIAGNOSTIC TESTS

Erythrocyte sedimentation rate: possible increase or temporary decrease.

Fibrin split products: elevated levels.

Fibrinogen and other plasma proteins: reduced levels.

Hematocrit, hemoglobin: possible diminished levels.

SGOT, SGPT: transient elevations during or shortly after streptokinase infusion.

Thrombin time: prolonged; 2 to 5 times greater than the normal control value. Effects may persist up to 24 hours after drug discontinuation.

SPECIAL CONSIDERATIONS

• *Treatment of overdose:* In hemorrhage, discontinue drug immediately. If necessary, administer whole blood (fresh blood preferred), packed red blood cells, and cryoprecipitate or fresh frozen plasma. Don't use dextrans. Aminocaproic acid may be administered in an emergency, although its use as an antidote hasn't been established.

• Before initiating therapy, obtain a blood sample to determine thrombin time, activated partial thromboplastin time, prothrombin time, hematocrit, and platelet count. This is especially important in pretreatment with heparin.

• Monitor vital signs and clotting status.

• Avoid invasive arterial procedures before and during therapy. If necessary, use an upper extremity.

• Perform venipunctures carefully and infrequently if possible.

• Avoid I.M. injections and unnecessary handling of the patient.

• To avoid dislodging deep venous thrombi, don't take blood pressure in the patient's lower extremities.

• Assess percutaneous puncture sites and cuts for oozing because streptokinase may lyse fibrin deposits at these sites.

• Because exposure to streptococci (source of streptokinase) is common, a loading dose is used to neutralize the antibodies present in many patients. To help establish dose, determine patient resistance to streptokinase. Don't give loading dose greater than 1 million IU.

• Although heparin isn't recommended during streptokinase therapy, it may be used soon afterward to minimize the risk of recurrent thrombosis and pulmonary emboli.

---

streptozocin
Zanosar♦

Pregnancy Risk Category: C

PHARMACOKINETICS
Distribution: not fully characterized. Only small amounts of drug cross the blood-brain barrier, but metabolites readily enter cerebrospinal fluid. Streptozocin crosses the placenta.

Metabolism: probably altered in the liver and kidneys, with extensive conversion to metabolites.

Excretion: principally removed as metabolites in urine. Significant amounts are eliminated in respiration. Less than 1% is excreted in feces. Plasma half-life is biphasic for unchanged drug and triphasic for metabolites. Initial half-life is 5 to 15 minutes for unchanged drug and 6 minutes for metabolites. Intermediate phase half-life of metabolites is 3.5 hours. Terminal phase half-life is 35 minutes for unchanged drug and 40 hours for metabolites. Not known if drug appears in breast milk.

Action: unknown.

MECHANISM OF ACTION

The cytotoxic action of streptozocin, an antineoplastic antibiotic, probably stems from cross-linking of DNA strands, impairing DNA synthesis. Its action is cell cycle–nonspecific, although it inhibits progression of the G_2 phase of cell division.

The drug has diabetogenic or hyperglycemic effects with selective uptake by pancreatic islet beta cells. Irreversible cell damage results in degranulation and stops insulin secretion.

INDICATIONS & DOSAGE

Dosage depends on renal, hematologic, and hepatic response and tolerance to the drug.
• *Metastatic islet cell carcinoma of pancreas. Adults:* 500 mg/m² daily for 5 consecutive days q 4 to 6 weeks. Alternatively, 1 g/m² in a single dose weekly for 2 weeks; after that, if necessary, up to 1.5 g/m² weekly. A single course usually consists of 4 to 6 weekly doses, but therapy may be extended.

CONTRAINDICATIONS & CAUTIONS

• Contraindicated in current or recent chickenpox or herpes zoster because of the risk of severe generalized disease.
• Use cautiously in bone marrow depression or infection because of possible hematologic toxicity; in diabetes mellitus because the drug aggravates the disorder; in renal and hepatic impairment because of the increased risk of toxicity; and in previous cytotoxic or radiation therapy because drug causes further bone marrow depression.

PREPARATION & STORAGE

To avoid mutagenic, teratogenic, and carcinogenic risks, use a biological containment cabinet, wear gloves and mask, and use syringes with Luer-Lok fittings to prevent leakage of drug solution. Also correctly dispose of needles, vials, and unused drug, and avoid contaminating work surfaces. If skin or mucous membrane contact occurs, wash area with copious amounts of soap and water.

Supplied in powder form in 1 g vials. Store vials at 36° to 46° F. (2° to 8° C.) and protect from light. Reconstitute with 9.5 ml of dextrose 5% injection or 0.9% sodium chloride injection to yield 100 mg/ml.

Dilute reconstituted drug with dextrose 5% injection, 0.9% sodium chloride, or dextrose 5% in 0.9% sodium chloride injection. Usual dilution for intermittent infusion is 100 mg/ml of streptozocin solution added to 10 to 200 ml of dextrose 5% injection.

If kept at room temperature, reconstituted drug should be used within 12 hours. Discard if color changes from pale gold to dark brown, indicating decomposition.

ADMINISTRATION

Direct injection: Rapidly inject reconstituted drug through port of primary I.V. line containing a free-flowing compatible solution.
Intermittent infusion: Infuse diluted drug over ordered duration (usually 15 minutes to 6 hours) via I.V. line containing a free-flowing compatible solution.
Continuous infusion: Infuse diluted drug over ordered duration. Continuous 5-day I.V. infusions have been given, but prolonged continuous administration may cause CNS toxicity.

INCOMPATIBILITY

No incompatibilities reported.

ADVERSE REACTIONS

Life-threatening: hematologic toxicity (rare), renal toxicity (azotemia,

glycosuria, hypophosphatemia, proteinuria, renal tubular acidosis).
Other: anemia; anxiety; chills; cold sweats; cool, pale skin; drowsiness; fatigue; fever; headache; hypoglycemia; jaundice; leukopenia; nausea and vomiting (common, progressively worsens during therapy); oliguria; rapid pulse; shakiness; sore throat; swelling of feet or lower legs; thrombocytopenia; unusual bleeding or bruising; weakness.

INTERACTIONS
ACTH, corticosteroids: heightened hyperglycemic effect of streptozocin.
Bone marrow depressants, radiation therapy: enhanced bone marrow depression.
Doxorubicin: prolonged half-life.
Live-virus vaccines: increased viral replication, increased adverse effects of vaccines, decreased antibody response to vaccines.
Nephrotoxic drugs: cumulative nephrotoxicity.
Nicotinamide: reduced diabetogenic effect of streptozocin.
Phenytoin: diminished therapeutic effects of streptozocin.

EFFECTS ON DIAGNOSTIC TESTS
BUN, serum creatinine, urine protein: possible increased levels because of drug's nephrotoxicity.
Plasma glucose: initially reduced, from sudden insulin release.
Serum albumin: decreased levels stemming from drug's hepatotoxicity.
Serum bilirubin, LDH, SGPT: possible elevated levels resulting from drug's hepatotoxicity.
Serum phosphate: possible depressed levels because of drug's nephrotoxicity.

SPECIAL CONSIDERATIONS
• Keep I.V. dextrose available, especially with first dose of streptozocin, because of the risk of hypoglycemia.

• If extravasation occurs, stop infusion. Apply cold compresses and elevate the arm. Complete administration in another vein.
• To detect nephrotoxicity, monitor BUN, serum creatinine, serum electrolyte, and urine creatinine levels and urinalysis before and at least weekly during therapy. After each course, monitor weekly for 4 to 6 weeks. Also watch for proteinuria, often the first sign of dose-related, cumulative nephrotoxicity.
• Encourage fluids to aid clearance of active metabolites.
• Warn patient to watch for signs of infection (chills, fever, sore throat) and to report these immediately.
• Monitor CBC and liver function studies weekly during and after therapy.
• Streptozocin has a low therapeutic index; toxicity usually accompanies therapeutic effects.

succinylcholine chloride
Anectine♦, Flo-Pack, Quelicin, Succinylcholine Chloride Min-I-Mix, Sucostrin

Pregnancy Risk Category: C

PHARMACOKINETICS
Distribution: widely dispersed by plasma. Drug doesn't cross the blood-brain barrier but does cross the placenta in small amounts.
Metabolism: rapidly hydrolyzed by plasma pseudocholinesterase to the active metabolite succinylmonocholine, and choline. Succinylmonocholine is further metabolized, principally by alkaline hydrolysis, to inactive succinate acid and choline.
Excretion: in urine as active and inactive metabolites and small

amounts (about 10%) of unchanged drug. Not known if drug appears in breast milk.

Action: onset, 30 to 60 seconds; duration, usually 4 to 10 minutes after a single injection (longer with continuous I.V. infusion).

MECHANISM OF ACTION

A depolarizing neuromuscular blocker, succinylcholine paralyzes skeletal muscle by blocking impulse transmission at the neuromuscular junction. Drug competes with acetylcholine for cholinergic receptors of the motor end-plate. Like acetylcholine, succinylcholine binds with these receptors and produces depolarization; however, depolarization is more prolonged.

INDICATIONS & DOSAGE

Dosages below are guidelines.

• Skeletal muscle relaxant for short procedures, such as endotracheal intubation, endoscopy, and orthopedic manipulations. *Adults:* initially, 0.6 mg/kg (range 0.3 to 1.1 mg/kg). Subsequent doses based on response to drug. *Children:* initially, 1 to 2 mg/kg. Subsequent doses based on first dose.

• Skeletal muscle relaxant for prolonged surgical procedures. *Adults:* 2.5 mg/minute (0.5 to 10 mg/minute) by continuous infusion (preferred method). Or initially, 0.3 to 1.1 mg/kg by intermittent infusion; subsequent doses 0.04 to 0.07 mg/kg p.r.n. to maintain relaxation.

• Electroshock therapy. *Adults:* 10 to 100 mg given about 1 minute before shock is administered.

CONTRAINDICATIONS & CAUTIONS

• Contraindicated in patients with low pseudocholinesterase levels because of the risk of apnea or prolonged muscle paralysis, and in myopathies associated with elevated serum creatine kinase levels because drug may worsen the disorder.

• Also contraindicated in patients with a personal or family history of malignant hyperthermia because drug may induce the disorder, and in angle-closure glaucoma and penetrating eye injuries because drug may increase intraocular pressure.

• Use cautiously in recent digitalis therapy or digitalis toxicity, severe burns, degenerative or dystrophic neuromuscular disease, paraplegia, spinal cord injury, or severe trauma because of enhanced risk of dysrhythmias or cardiac arrest.

• Give carefully in bronchogenic carcinoma because the drug may enhance neuromuscular blocking action; in dehydration or electrolyte or acid-base imbalance because drug action may be altered; in conditions in which histamine release would be hazardous because drug may cause histamine release; and in hyperkalemia because drug may worsen the disorder.

• Also give carefully in anemia, dehydration, exposure to neurotoxic insecticides, severe hepatic disease or cirrhosis, malnutrition, pregnancy, or recessive hereditary trait (plasma pseudocholinesterase) because of potential for prolonged respiratory depression or apnea, and in pulmonary impairment or respiratory depression because of risk of further respiratory depression.

• In severe obesity or neuromuscular disease, also use cautiously because of possible airway or ventilation problems.

• In open eye injury or chronic open-angle glaucoma or during ocular surgery, use drug cautiously because of risk of increased intraocular pressure.

• Also use cautiously in fractures or muscle spasm because initial muscle fasciculations may result in additional trauma.

• Administer carefully in hepatic impairment because decreased pseudocholinesterase activity may result in apnea or respiratory depression and in renal impairment because of possible slowed drug clearance and prolonged effect.

• In hyperthermia, drug intensity and duration may decrease; in hypothermia, they may increase. Use succinylcholine cautiously.

• Use cautiously in severe obesity or neuromuscular disease because of possible airway or ventilation problems.

• Continuous I.V. infusion is considered unsafe in infants and children because of risk of malignant hypertension.

PREPARATION & STORAGE

Available in 10 ml vials containing 20 or 100 mg/ml and in 10 and 20 ml ampules containing 50 mg/ml. Also available in powder form in strengths of 100 mg, 500 mg, and 1 g in 5 ml unit dose vials (with diluent and Min-I-Mix injector).

Reconstitute powder with compatible diluent, such as dextrose 5% injection or 0.9% sodium chloride, according to manufacturer's instructions. Store solutions at 36° to 46° F. (2° to 8° C.). Multidose vials are stable for 14 days at room temperature. Powders don't require refrigeration.

For continuous infusion, dilute to a concentration of 1 to 2 mg/ml. Add 1 g of powder, 10 ml of solution (100 mg/ml), or 20 ml of solution (500 mg/ml) to 1 liter or 500 ml of compatible diluent, such as dextrose 5% injection, dextrose 5% in 0.9% sodium chloride, 0.9% sodium chloride, or 1/6 M sodium lactate. Alternatively, add 500 mg of powder, 5 ml of solution (100 mg/ml), or 10 ml of solution (50 mg/ml) to 500 or 250 ml of diluent to yield 1 or 2 mg/ml succinylcholine, respectively.

For direct injection, use prepared solution if possible, or dilute with compatible solution to yield concentration, volume, and dosage ordered.

Discard unused solutions within 24 hours.

ADMINISTRATION

Succinylcholine should be administered only by staff trained to administer anesthetics and manage their adverse reactions.

Direct injection: Inject ordered amount of commercially prepared or diluted drug over 10 to 30 seconds into a primary I.V. line containing a free-flowing compatible solution.

Intermittent infusion: not recommended. Administration of repeated intermittent doses may produce tachyphylaxis and prolonged apnea.

Continuous infusion: Infuse diluted drug through an I.V. line containing a free-flowing compatible solution at 2.5 mg/minute initially; then adjust to 0.5 to 10 mg/minute, depending on patient response.

To avoid overdose and detect development of nondepolarizing neuromuscular blockade, monitor neuromuscular function with a peripheral nerve stimulator when giving drug by infusion.

INCOMPATIBILITY

Decomposes in any solution having a pH greater than 4.5. Incompatible with barbiturates, nafcillin, and sodium bicarbonate.

ADVERSE REACTIONS

Life-threatening: anaphylaxis, apnea, asystole or severe bradycardia (especially after second bolus), cardiac arrest (especially in infants and children), malignant hyperthermia. *Other:* blood pressure changes (increased or decreased), bradycardia, dyspnea, high fever, increased intraocular pressure, irregular heartbeat, muscle pain and stiffness (postoperative), myoglobinuria or myoglobinemia (especially in children), rash, unusual watering of mouth, wheezing.

INTERACTIONS

Aminoglycosides (including oral neomycin), anesthetics (parenteral or local), capreomycin, citrate-anti-coagulated blood (massive transfusions): increased neuromuscular blockade.

Antimyasthenics, edrophonium: prolonged neuromuscular blockade; antagonized antimyasthenic effects on skeletal muscle.

Cardiac glycosides: possible increased cardiac effects.

Cholinesterase inhibitors (especially demecarium, echothiophate, and isoflurophate), cyclophosphamide: heightened neuromuscular blockade.

Clindamycin, lidocaine (in I.V. doses greater than 5 mg/kg), lincomycin, polymyxins, procaine (I.V.), trimethaphan (high doses): additive neuromuscular blockade.

Doxapram: possible masking of succinylcholine's residual effects.

Fentanyl, sufentanil: additive respiratory depression and reversal of fentanyl- or sufentanil-induced muscle rigidity.

Halogenated hydrocarbon anesthetics: potentiated neuromuscular blockade.

Hexafluorenium: prolonged neuromuscular blockade and diminished or absent succinylcholine-induced fasciculations or pain.

Inhalation anesthetics: increased risk of malignant hyperthermia; also with repeated, concurrent use, possible enhanced initial transient bradycardia produced by succinylcholine.

Lithium: prolonged neuromuscular blockade.

Magnesium salts (parenteral), procainamide, quinidine: heightened neuromuscular blockade.

Neurotoxic insecticides (including large quantities of topical malathion, phenelzine, or thiotepa): enhanced neuromuscular blockade.

Nondepolarizing neuromuscular blocking agents: if administered long-term, increased blockade.

Opioid analgesics: additive respiratory depression.

Physostigmine: at high doses, additive muscle fasciculation and depolarization block.

EFFECTS ON DIAGNOSTIC TESTS

Serum potassium: possible increased levels.

SPECIAL CONSIDERATIONS

• *Treatment of overdose:* Use a peripheral nerve stimulator to determine nature and degree of neuromuscular blockade. Overdose may result in prolonged respiratory depression or apnea and cardiovascular collapse. If apnea or prolonged paralysis occurs, maintain airway and administer manual or mechanical ventilation until independent respiration resumes. Administer fluids and vasopressors as needed to treat shock or severe hypotension.

In prolonged administration, if the depolarizing neuromuscular blockade changes to nondepolarizing blockade (determined by nerve stimulator), give small doses of an anticholinesterase drug (antagonist), as ordered. Administer atropine with an anticholinesterase agent to counteract muscarinic side effects. Observe the patient for at least 1 hour after reversal of nondepolarizing blockade

for possible return of muscle relaxation.
• When administering succinylcholine, keep emergency resuscitation equipment available.
• As ordered, administer test dose of 10 mg I.V. to determine patient's sensitivity and recovery time.
• Premedicate with atropine or scopolamine to prevent excessive salivation. Also premedicate with atropine or thiopental sodium to inhibit transient bradycardia accompanied by hypotension, dysrhythmias, and temporary sinus arrest resulting from vagal stimulation.
• Succinylcholine fasciculations can cause postoperative myalgia, which may be quite intense. Reassure patient that this will pass in 24 to 48 hours. Some doctors advocate giving a small dose of succinylcholine to reduce severity of fasciculations.
• Administration of small doses of tubocurarine before succinylcholine may decrease the incidence of myoglobinuria in children.
• Neuromuscular blockers have no known effect on consciousness or pain threshold. To avoid upsetting patient, give drug after unconsciousness has been induced.

sufentanil citrate
Sufenta

Controlled Substance Schedule II
Pregnancy Risk Category: C

PHARMACOKINETICS
Distribution: rapidly and extensively dispersed throughout body tissues. Not known if drug crosses the placenta.
Metabolism: primarily metabolized in the liver and small intestine.
Excretion: mainly eliminated in urine, but also in feces. Half-life is about 2.5 hours. Not known if drug appears in breast milk.
Action: onset, about 1 to 3 minutes; duration, dose-dependent, ranging from 5 minutes with analgesic doses (less than 8 mcg/kg) to about 3 hours with anesthetic doses (more than 8 mcg/kg).

MECHANISM OF ACTION
Sufentanil acts as an agonist at stereospecific opioid receptor sites in the CNS. The drug alters both the perception of pain and the emotional response to it.

INDICATIONS & DOSAGE
Dosage depends on concurrent drug administration (especially anesthetics), type and expected length of surgery, and the patient's age, ideal weight, size, physical condition, underlying disorder, and response to the drug.
• **Adjunct in anesthesia.** *Adults:* low initial dose, 0.5 to 1 mcg/kg, with supplemental doses of 10 to 25 mcg p.r.n. to maintain analgesia or anesthesia; moderate initial dose, 2 to 8 mcg/kg, with supplemental doses of 10 to 50 mcg p.r.n.

If used with nitrous oxide and oxygen for procedures lasting 8 hours or longer, total dosage is 1 mcg/kg/hour or less.
• **Primary anesthesia.** *Adults:* initially, 8 to 30 mcg/kg with 100% oxygen, with supplemental doses of 25 to 50 mcg p.r.n. to maintain anesthesia. Loading dose followed by continuous infusion is recommended for prolonged procedures. *Children:* initially, 10 to 25 mcg/kg with 100% oxygen, with supplemental doses of 25 to 50 mcg p.r.n. (maximum total, 1 to 2 mcg/kg) to maintain anesthesia.

CONTRAINDICATIONS & CAUTIONS

• Contraindicated in sensitivity to sufentanil or other fentanyl derivatives.
• Use with extreme caution in patients receiving MAO inhibitors within the previous 14 days (sufentanil test dose recommended).
• Also use with extreme caution in altered respiratory function because of the risk of further respiratory depression and increased airway resistance.
• Use cautiously in patients with head injury and increased intracranial pressure. Sufentanil can obscure changes in level of consciousness and raise intracranial pressure, resulting from hypercarbia associated with respiratory depression.
• Give lowered doses in hepatic or renal impairment because of the increased risk of toxicity, and in hypothyroidism because of the risk of respiratory depression and prolonged CNS depression.
• In elderly and debilitated patients and in neonates, give cautiously because of increased sensitivity to sufentanil, especially respiratory depression. Lower doses may be necessary.
• Administer carefully in patients with bradydysrhythmias because drug may worsen the condition, and in patients with poor cardiac reserve because of enhanced risk of severe bradycardia or large decrease in blood pressure.

PREPARATION & STORAGE

Available in preservative-free 1, 2, and 5 ml ampules containing 50 mcg/ml. Store at room temperature, always below 104° F. (40° C.). Protect from light and freezing. For continuous infusion, dilute with a compatible solution.

ADMINISTRATION

Sufentanil should be given only by staff trained in administering I.V. anesthetics and managing their adverse reactions.
Direct injection: Inject slowly, especially with large doses, over 1 to 2 minutes. Use a 1 ml syringe for small doses.
Intermittent infusion: not recommended.
Continuous infusion: After loading dose, infuse 1 mcg/kg or less over 1 hour.

INCOMPATIBILITY

No incompatibilities reported.

ADVERSE REACTIONS

Life-threatening: bronchospasm or laryngospasm, hypotension, peripheral vascular collapse or cardiac arrest (with rapid injection), respiratory depression.
Other: changes in blood pressure (increased or decreased), chest wall rigidity, chills, confusion, decreased systemic vascular resistance, delirium, depression, drowsiness, dysrhythmias, excitement, nausea, pruritus, seizures, unusual muscle movements (intraoperative), vomiting.

INTERACTIONS

Anesthetics (spinal or peridural): additive respiratory depression, bradycardia, or hypotension.
Benzodiazepines: quickened loss of consciousness. Lower dose of sufentanil may be necessary.
Beta-adrenergic blockers: reduced severity or frequency of hypertensive response; enhanced risk of bradycardia.
CNS depressants: heightened risk of CNS and respiratory depression and hypotension.
Diuretics: increased hypotensive effects.

Droperidol: augmented risk of CNS and respiratory depression and elevated blood pressure.

MAO inhibitors: increased risk of severe hypertension, hypotension, and tachycardia if drugs are taken within 14 days of each other.

Nalbuphine, pentazocine: partial antagonism of sufentanil's anesthetic and CNS and respiratory depressant effects.

Naloxone, naltrexone: antagonized sufentanil effects.

Neuromuscular blockers: additive respiratory depression. High doses of sufentanil may allow lower doses of blocking agents.

Nitrous oxide: deepened CNS and respiratory depression and increased hypotension; reduced blood pressure, heart rate, and cardiac output.

Opiate narcotics: additive CNS and respiratory depression.

EFFECTS ON DIAGNOSTIC TESTS

Cerebrospinal fluid (CSF) analysis: possible increased CSF pressure.

SPECIAL CONSIDERATIONS

• *Treatment of overdose:* Maintain airway patency and provide respiratory support. Give naloxone as needed to reverse respiratory depression. Also administer I.V. fluids and vasopressors, as ordered, to maintain blood pressure and neuromuscular blockers to relieve muscle rigidity.

• During therapy with sufentanil, keep resuscitation equipment available.

• Monitor patient's breathing for at least 1 hour after dose. If rate drops below 8 breaths/minute, arouse patient to stimulate breathing and notify doctor.

• Administer drug with patient lying down to minimize hypotensive effects. Tell him to get up slowly to reduce dizziness and faintness.

• Sufentanil is used to supplement general, regional, or local anesthetics and as a primary agent to maintain anesthesia in certain types of major surgery.

• Sufentanil is five to seven times more potent than fentanyl.

• Patients who are tolerant of other opioids may be tolerant of sufentanil.

• High doses may produce muscle rigidity, which can be reversed by administering neuromuscular blocking agents.

• Concomitant use of a benzodiazepine or other amnestic agent is recommended during surgical anesthesia with sufentanil.

• Closely monitor for signs of withdrawal when discontinuing sufentanil after prolonged use. Physical dependence is possible.

teniposide (VM-26)
Vumon♦♦

Investigational Drug
Pregnancy Risk Category: D

PHARMACOKINETICS

Distribution: accumulates in the kidneys, small intestine, liver, and adrenals. Minimal amounts cross the blood-brain barrier into the CNS. Drug may cross the placenta.

Metabolism: in liver. Drug is extensively bound to plasma proteins.

Excretion: primarily removed in feces. Significant amounts also excreted in urine. Drug probably appears in breast milk.

Action: peak serum level, immediately after infusion.

MECHANISM OF ACTION

A podophyllotoxin derivative, teniposide arrests cell mitosis in metaphase, causing a marked decrease in the mitotic index.

INDICATIONS & DOSAGE

• Hodgkin's lymphomas. *Adults:* 30 mg/m² daily for 5 days, 30 mg/m² daily for 10 days, 50 to 100 mg/m² weekly, 60 to 70 mg/m² weekly in combination therapy.
• Neuroblastomas. *Adults:* 130 to 180 mg/m² as a single dose, or 100 mg/m² daily for 21 days in combination therapy.
• Acute lymphocytic leukemia. *Adults:* 165 mg/m² twice weekly in combination therapy.

CONTRAINDICATIONS & CAUTIONS

None reported.

PREPARATION & STORAGE

Use extreme caution when preparing and administering teniposide to avoid mutagenic, teratogenic, and carcinogenic risks. Use a biological containment cabinet, wear gloves and mask, and use syringes with Luer-Lok fittings to prevent drug leakage. Avoid contaminating work surfaces, and dispose of needles, syringes, ampules, and unused drug correctly. Avoid inhaling teniposide particles or solutions or allowing contact with skin or mucosa. If contact occurs, wash the area immediately with soap and water.

Teniposide is supplied in ampules of 50 mg/5 ml that must be protected from light. Dilute for infusion with at least 5 to 20 equal volumes of dextrose 5% in water or 0.9% sodium chloride. In glass containers, solutions of 100 to 200 mcg/ml are stable for 24 hours using dextrose 5% in water or sterile water; 100 to 400 mcg/ml solutions are stable for 24 hours using 0.9% sodium chloride. In plastic containers, 100 mcg/ml solutions are stable for 8 hours using 0.9% sodium chloride or sterile water. However, drug is unstable in plastic containers at concentrations greater than 100 mcg/ml. Solution may appear slightly opalescent from surfactants in the formulation.

ADMINISTRATION

Direct injection: not recommended.
Intermittent infusion: not recommended.
Continuous infusion: Using a 23G or 25G winged-tip needle, administer over at least 45 minutes to avoid hypotension. Use distal rather than major veins. Choose a new site for each infusion.

If extravasation occurs, apply ice to the area. Injection of a corticosteroid and irrigation with copious amounts of 0.9% sodium chloride may decrease swelling.

INCOMPATIBILITY

No incompatibilities reported.

ADVERSE REACTIONS

Life-threatening: anaphylaxis.
Other: alopecia, diarrhea, headache, hepatotoxicity, hypotension, myelosuppression, nausea, phlebitis at infusion site, renal toxicity, stomatitis, vomiting.

INTERACTIONS

Cyclophosphamide: increased effect.
Dactinomycin: decreased activity.
Fluorouracil, methotrexate, mitomycin: enhanced cytotoxic effects.

EFFECTS ON DIAGNOSTIC TESTS

None reported.

SPECIAL CONSIDERATIONS

• Keep diphenhydramine, epinephrine, hydrocortisone, and an airway available in case of anaphylaxis.

- Monitor blood pressure before, during, and after infusion. Stop infusion and notify doctor if systolic pressure falls below 90 mm Hg.
- Monitor CBC during and after treatment (leukopenia nadir occurs in 3 to 14 days). Instruct patient to report signs of bleeding or infection.
- Monitor for phlebitis at injection site.
- Encourage adequate fluid intake to increase urine output and facilitate uric acid excretion.
- Monitor liver function studies.
- Advise patient that alopecia is temporary.
- Advise home care patients to avoid exposure to persons with infections.

---

terbutaline sulfate
Brethine, Bricanyl

Pregnancy Risk Category: B

PHARMACOKINETICS
Distribution: widespread. Drug crosses the placenta and the blood-brain barrier.
Metabolism: partly altered in the liver, mainly to inactive metabolites.
Excretion: about 60% removed unchanged in urine. Drug appears in breast milk at concentrations 1% less than maternal levels.
Action: onset, within 15 minutes; duration, 1.5 to 4 hours.

MECHANISM OF ACTION
This drug stimulates beta$_2$-adrenergic receptors and causes uterine relaxation, along with other sympathetic effects.

INDICATIONS & DOSAGE
- Treatment of premature labor (after 20 weeks' gestation). *Adults:* initially, 10 mcg/minute, increased by 10 mcg/minute q 20 minutes until

contractions stop or until reaching maximum rate of 80 mcg/minute. Once contractions have ceased for 30 to 60 minutes, reduce dose by 5 mcg/minute and maintain at minimum effective rate for 4 hours. Then switch to oral form.

CONTRAINDICATIONS & CAUTIONS
- Contraindicated in hypersensitivity to sympathomimetics.
- Also contraindicated in dysrhythmias caused by digitalis intoxication because of the enhanced risk of drug-induced tachycardia.
- Use cautiously in patients with diabetes mellitus, glaucoma, pheochromocytoma, hypertension, vasomotor instability, or a history of seizures because terbutaline may exacerbate these conditions.
- In hyperthyroidism, give cautiously because of enhanced risk of adverse reactions.

PREPARATION & STORAGE
Available in 2 ml ampules containing 1 mg/ml. Solution is clear and colorless; don't use if discolored. Store ampules at room temperature and protect from light. For infusion, add 10 mg of drug to 250 ml of dextrose 5% in water, 0.9% sodium chloride, or 0.45% sodium chloride to yield 40 mcg/ml.

ADMINISTRATION
Direct injection: not recommended.
Intermittent infusion: not recommended.
Continuous infusion: Before administration, start a primary I.V. Hang terbutaline solution as a secondary I.V. to allow immediate discontinuation if adverse effects occur. Use an infusion pump and continuously monitor cardiac status.

INCOMPATIBILITY
Incompatible with bleomycin sulfate.

ADVERSE REACTIONS
Life-threatening: anaphylaxis, dysrhythmias, pulmonary edema.
Other: angina, anxiety, bradycardia, chest pain, chills, dizziness, drowsiness, dry mouth, dyspnea, fever, flushing, hallucinations, headache, hypertension, insomnia, mood changes, nausea, palpitations, restlessness, sweating, tachycardia, tinnitus, tremor, vertigo, vomiting.

INTERACTIONS
Anesthetics: increased risk of severe ventricular dysrhythmias.
CNS stimulants, other sympathomimetics, xanthines: possible additive CNS stimulation.
Digitalis, levodopa, MAO inhibitors, tricyclic antidepressants: enhanced cardiovascular effects.
Diuretics: possible reduced antihypertensive effects.
Glucocorticoids (inhalation forms): possible increased risk of fluorocarbon toxicity.
Nitrates: possible decreased antianginal effects.
Thyroid hormones: possible heightened effects of both interacting drugs.

EFFECTS ON DIAGNOSTIC TESTS
Allergy tests: inhibited responses.
Serum glucose: elevated levels.
Serum potassium: decreased levels.
Serum thyroid hormones: interference with results.

SPECIAL CONSIDERATIONS
• Monitor serum potassium and glucose levels closely during infusion.
• Record intake and output and assess for signs of pulmonary edema. Limit I.V. fluids to 50 ml/hour.

• Monitor the fetus continuously for cardiovascular effects.
• After delivery, observe the neonate for hypoglycemia.
• To reduce the risk of pulmonary edema, avoid using sodium chloride as a diluent when possible.
• Although drug isn't recommended by manufacturers for treating premature labor nor approved for this use by the FDA, it's used effectively in some hospitals. However, studies demonstrate that S.C. administration followed by maintenance oral administration is equally effective and poses less risk to the patient.

teriparatide acetate
Parathar

Pregnancy Risk Category: C

PHARMACOKINETICS
Distribution: obscure, but drug disappears rapidly from plasma.
Metabolism: not well characterized.
Excretion: unknown. Half-life is less than 15 minutes.
Action: onset, less than 30 minutes; duration, less than 1 hour.

MECHANISM OF ACTION
A synthetic polypeptide hormone, teriparatide stimulates adenylate cyclase in bone and kidneys, promoting increased calcium release from bone to blood. It also reduces renal calcium excretion.

INDICATIONS & DOSAGE
As a diagnostic agent to help determine cause of hypocalcemia (hypoparathyroidism or pseudohypoparathyroidism). *Adults:* 200 units. *Children 3 years and over:* 3 units/kg. Maximum 200 units.

CONTRAINDICATIONS & CAUTIONS
• Contraindicated in hypersensitivity to teriparatide or to any of its components.

PREPARATION & STORAGE
Available in 10-ml vials containing 200 units of teriparatide. Reconstitute for infusion by adding 10 ml of the diluent provided by the manufacturer to the 10-ml vial. Store at room temperature; use reconstituted solution within 4 hours.

ADMINISTRATION
Direct injection: not recommended.
Intermittent infusion: not recommended.
Continuous infusion: Infuse reconstituted solution over 10 minutes.

INCOMPATIBILITY
None reported.

ADVERSE REACTIONS
Life-threatening: anaphylaxis, hypertensive crisis, hypocalcemic seizures.
Other: abdominal cramps, diarrhea, metallic taste, nausea, pain at infusion site, tingling of extremities, urge to defecate.

INTERACTIONS
None reported.

EFFECTS ON DIAGNOSTIC TESTS
None reported.

SPECIAL CONSIDERATIONS
• *Treatment of overdose:* In hypercalcemia (possible with doses of 500 units or more), discontinue drug and provide adequate hydration.
• To distinguish between hypoparathyroidism and pseudohypoparathyroidism as a cause of hypocalcemia in the modified Ellsworth Howard test, have patient fast before test and maintain urine output by ingesting 200 ml of water/hour for 2 hours before and during the test. Obtain a baseline urine sample in the 60-minute period before teriparatide infusion. After infusion (time 0), collect separate urine samples for the 0-to-30 minute, 30-to-60 minute, and 60-to-120 minute periods. The change in urinary cAMP excretion in the 0-to-30 minute urine sample is the most sensitive discriminator of the cause of hypocalcemia.

---

tetracycline hydrochloride
Achromycin Intravenous

Pregnancy Risk Category: D

PHARMACOKINETICS
Distribution: readily dispersed throughout body fluids, including synovial, pleural, ascitic, and gingival crevicular fluids; sinus secretions; and bile. Drug binds variably to plasma proteins and localizes in bone, liver, spleen, tumors, and teeth. It crosses the placenta and also appears in CSF in varying concentrations.
Metabolism: not metabolized.
Excretion: excreted unchanged in urine by glomerular filtration, with 48% to 60% removed within 72 hours. Half-life is 6 to 11 hours, 57 to 120 hours in anuria. Drug is also excreted in feces in high concentrations and appears in breast milk.
Action: onset, immediately after administration; peak serum level, 30 minutes.

MECHANISM OF ACTION
This broad-spectrum antibiotic, bacteriostatic, and antiprotozoal agent inhibits protein synthesis by binding

---

to the 30S ribosomal subunit of microorganisms.

Susceptible gram-negative bacteria include *Bartonella bacilliformis, Bordetella pertussis, Brucella, Calymmatobacterium granulomatis, Campylobacter fetus, Francisella tularensis, Haemophilus ducreyi, H. influenzae, Legionella pneumophilia, Leptotrichia buccalis, Neisseria gonorrhoeae, N. meningitidis, Pasteurella multocida, Pseudomonas pseudomallei, Ps. mallei, Shigella, Spirillum minor, Streptobacillus moniliformis, Vibrio cholerae, V. parahemolyticus, Yersinia enterocolitica, Y. pestis,* and some strains of *Acinetobacter, Bacteroides, Enterobacter aerogenes, Escherichia coli,* and *Klebsiella.*

Susceptible gram-positive bacteria include *Actinomyces israelii, Arachnia propionica, Bacillus anthracis, Clostridium perfringens, C. tetani, Listeria monocytogenes, Nocardia,* and *Propionibacterium acnes.*

The drug also proves effective against *Balantidium coli, Borrelia recurrentis, B. burgdorferi, Chlamydia trachomatis, C. psittaci, Coxiella burnetti, Leptospira, Mycobacterium mannum, Mycoplasma hominus, M. pneumoniae, Rickettsia akari, R. prowazeki, R. rickettsii, R. tsutsugamushi, R. typhi, Trepanoma pallidum,* and *T. pertenue.*

INDICATIONS & DOSAGE

● Infections caused by susceptible organisms. *Adults:* 250 to 500 mg q 8 to 12 hours for 7 days. Maximum 2 g daily. *Children 8 years and over:* 6 mg/kg q 12 hours for at least 5 days. Maximum 10 to 20 mg daily, depending on severity of infection.
● Pelvic inflammatory disease. *Children over 7 years:* 10 mg/kg q 8 hours (in combination with cephalosporin antibiotics) for at least 6 days (including at least 2 days after im-

provement). Then, switch to oral form.

Note: Adjust dosage for renal impairment. For adults, if creatinine clearance is 10 to 50 ml/minute, increase dosing interval to 12 to 24 hours.

CONTRAINDICATIONS & CAUTIONS

● Because of possible tooth discoloration, enamel hypoplasia, and bone growth retardation in children, drug is contraindicated during the last half of pregnancy, during breast-feeding, and in children under 8 years. Also contraindicated in tetracycline hypersensitivity.
● Use cautiously in renal or hepatic impairment because of the enhanced risk of toxicity. Also use cautiously in systemic lupus erythematosus.

PREPARATION & STORAGE

Available as a yellow crystalline powder in 250 and 500 mg vials. Reconstitute with sterile water for injection, dextrose 5% in water, or 0.9% sodium chloride injection. Add 5 ml to a 250 mg vial or 10 ml to a 500 mg vial. For direct injection, dilute further to 10 mg/ml. For intermittent infusion, dilute to 1 mg/ml in 100 to 1,000 ml of Ringer's injection, Ringer's lactate, dextrose 5% in water, 0.9% sodium chloride, or combinations of dextrose and sodium chloride. Give immediately.

Use Ringer's injection and Ringer's lactate injection cautiously for dilution because these contain calcium. However, the calcium in these diluents usually doesn't precipitate tetracycline in an acid medium. Discoloration with no significant loss of potency may occur with dilution in multielectrolyte solutions.

Before reconstitution, store vials at room temperature and protect from light. Reconstituted solutions are stable at room temperature for 12 hours or at 41° F. (5° C.) for 24 hours. Nephrotoxicity has been associated with use of outdated or improperly stored drug.

ADMINISTRATION

Avoid rapid administration and extravasation. Thrombophlebitis is more likely with high concentrations. If patient complains of vein irritation, reduce infusion rate.

Direct injection: Using diluted dose, inject each 100 mg over 5 minutes.

Intermittent infusion: Infuse prescribed diluted dose at a rate of 2 mg/minute.

Continuous infusion: Infuse diluted drug over 8 to 12 hours, depending on ordered fluid volume.

INCOMPATIBILITY

Incompatible with amikacin, aminophylline, amobarbital sodium, amphotericin B, ampicillin sodium, calcium, carbenicillin disodium, cefazolin, cephalothin, cephapirin, chloramphenicol sodium succinate, chlorothiazide sodium, dimenhydrinate, erythromycin glucepate, erythromycin lactobionate, 10% fat emulsions, heparin sodium, hydrocortisone sodium succinate, Ionosol MB with dextrose 5%, Ionosol T with dextrose 5%, magnesium, methicillin, methohexital, methyldopate, methylprednisolone sodium succinate, metoclopramide, oxacillin, penicillin G potassium, pentobarbital sodium, phenobarbital sodium, phenytoin sodium, polymyxin B, secobarbital sodium, sodium bicarbonate, thiopental, and warfarin.

ADVERSE REACTIONS

Life-threatening: anaphylaxis, exfoliative dermatitis, liver failure (with renal dysfunction in pregnancy and with doses exceeding 2 g).

Other: angioneurotic edema, anorexia, bacterial and fungal superinfection, bulging fontanels with increased intracranial pressure in infants (reversible), diarrhea, dizziness, dysphagia, enamel hypoplasia, eosinophilia, glossitis, headache, hemolytic anemia, hepatotoxicity (with large doses), increased pigmentation, inflammatory anogenital lesions, meningeal irritation, nausea, neutropenia, paresthesias, pericarditis, photosensitivity, pseudomembranous colitis, rash, thrombocytopenia, thrombophlebitis, tooth discoloration, urticaria, vomiting.

INTERACTIONS

Anticoagulants: decreased prothrombin activity and impaired thromboplastin regeneration, possibly requiring lower dosage.

Corticosteroids: emergence of tetracycline-resistant organisms; diminished resistance to infection.

Diuretics: increased BUN.

Hepatotoxic drugs: enhanced toxicity.

Lithium carbonate: toxicity.

Methoxyflurane: nephrotoxicity.

Oral contraceptives: ineffectiveness and breakthrough bleeding.

Penicillin: interference with bactericidal action.

EFFECTS ON DIAGNOSTIC TESTS

BUN: elevated levels.

CBC: anemia, eosinophilia, neutropenia, thrombocytopenia.

Prothrombin time: increased.

Serum alkaline phosphatase, amylase, bilirubin; SGOT, SGPT: elevated levels.

Urine catecholamines: falsely elevated results when using Hingerty method.

Urine glucose: false-positive results when tested with cupric sulfate (Benedict's solution, Clinitest); false-negative results when tested with glucose oxidase (Clinistix, Tes-Tape).

SPECIAL CONSIDERATIONS

• Use I.V. route only when oral therapy is inadequate or not tolerated. Change to oral therapy as soon as possible.

• Obtain specimens for culture and sensitivity tests before therapy. Therapy may begin ahead of results.

• Change I.V. site every 48 to 72 hours. Also reduce infusion rate and apply ice to I.V. site to reduce discomfort from vein irritation.

• Advise patient to avoid exposure to sun because of possible photosensitivity reaction.

• Observe for signs of overgrowth of nonsusceptible organisms, including fungi. If this occurs, discontinue drug and start appropriate therapy.

• If diarrhea persists during therapy, obtain specimens for stool culture to rule out pseudomembranous colitis.

• Treat Group A beta-hemolytic streptococcal infections for at least 10 days. Discontinue drug if erythema occurs.

• With long-term therapy, monitor hematopoietic, renal, and hepatic studies.

• Obtain serum drug levels if therapy is prolonged. High levels may cause azotemia, hyperphosphatemia, and acidosis in significant renal dysfunction.

• In patients with diabetes mellitus, monitor blood glucose levels.

• In pregnant or postpartum patients with pyelonephritis, make sure serum drug levels don't exceed 15 mcg/ml. Monitor liver function tests.

• If the patient has a sexually transmitted disease with suspected coexistent syphilis, arrange for a darkfield microscopic examination before starting treatment and perform blood serology monthly for at least 4 months.

• Dialysis removes significant amounts of tetracycline.

theophylline ethylenediamine (aminophylline)
Aminophyllin Injection

Pregnancy Risk Category: C

PHARMACOKINETICS

Distribution: rapidly dispersed throughout extracellular fluids and body tissues. Drug crosses the placenta and partially penetrates RBCs.

Metabolism: in liver.

Excretion: mainly excreted in urine with small amounts removed unchanged in feces. Drug also appears in breast milk in concentrations about 70% of serum levels. Serum half-life is 3 to 12 hours in nonsmoking asthmatic adults; 1½ to 9½ hours in children.

Action: onset, upon completion of infusion; duration, varies with age, sex, and activities.

MECHANISM OF ACTION

Not fully understood, but this xanthine derivative either acts as an adenosine receptor antagonist or inhibits phosphodiesterase (the enzyme that degrades cyclic AMP). This action alters intracellular calcium levels, relaxing bronchial smooth muscles and pulmonary vessels. Theophylline also causes coronary vasodilation, diuresis, and cardiac, cerebral, and skeletal muscle stimulation; it also increases medullary sensitivity to carbon dioxide.

INDICATIONS & DOSAGE

• Acute bronchial asthma and reversible bronchospasm associated with chronic bronchitis and emphysema. *Adults not currently receiving theophylline:* initially, 4.7 mg/kg, followed by maintenance doses—for nonsmoking adults, 0.55 mg/kg/hour for the first 12 hours, then 0.39 mg/

kg/hour for the next 12 hours; for elderly patients and those with cor pulmonale, 0.47 mg/kg/hour for the first 12 hours, then 0.24 mg/kg/hour for the next 12 hours; for patients with congestive heart failure (CHF) or liver failure, 0.39 mg/kg/hour for the first 12 hours, then 0.08 to 0.16 mg/kg/hour for the next 12 hours. *Children not currently receiving theophylline:* initially, 4 to 7 mg/kg, followed by maintenance doses—for children 6 months to 9 years, 0.95 mg/kg/hour for the first 12 hours, then 0.79 mg/kg/hour for the next 12 hours; for children 9 to 16 years, 0.79 mg/kg/hour for the first 12 hours, then 0.63 mg/kg/hour for the next 12 hours. *Adults and children currently receiving theophylline:* dosage form, amount, time, and administration rate of last theophylline dose determine initial dose. Ideally, initial dose deferred until serum theophylline level can be obtained.

CONTRAINDICATIONS & CAUTIONS

• Contraindicated in hypersensitivity to theophylline, caffeine, theobromine, and other xanthine compounds.
• Use cautiously in severe cardiac disease, severe hypoxemia, hypertension, hyperthyroidism, peptic ulcer, diabetes mellitus, acute MI, and CHF because drug may exacerbate symptoms.
• Also use cautiously in neonates, elderly patients, and those with liver disease because of the increased risk of toxicity.
• In prostatic enlargement, give cautiously because of the increased risk of urinary retention.
• Also give cautiously in cor pulmonale, prolonged fever, and febrile viral respiratory infections because of prolonged theophylline half-life.

PREPARATION & STORAGE

Available as a 25 mg/ml solution in 10 ml (250 mg) and 20 ml (500 mg) ampules. Also available in 500 and 1,000 ml containers with 1 or 2 mg/ml in 0.45% sodium chloride, and in 500 and 1,000 ml containers with 0.4, 0.8, 1.6, 2, 3.2, or 4 mg/ml in dextrose 5%. Drug may be administered undiluted or may be diluted with 0.9% sodium chloride or dextrose 5% in water.

Store containers at room temperature and protect from freezing and light. Inspect for particulate matter and discoloration before use.

ADMINISTRATION

Direct injection: Give undiluted loading dose (25 mg/ml) slowly, not exceeding 25 mg/minute. Don't give through a central venous catheter. Rapid injection can be fatal.
Intermittent infusion: not recommended.
Continuous infusion: For maintenance therapy, administer desired dose in a large volume (500 to 1,000 ml) of compatible solution. Adjust infusion rate to deliver prescribed amount each hour.

INCOMPATIBILITY

Incompatible with ascorbic acid, cephalothin, cephapirin, chlorpromazine, clindamycin, codeine phosphate, corticotropin, dimenhydrinate, dobutamine, doxorubicin, epinephrine hydrochloride, erythromycin gluceptate, 10% fat emulsion, fructose 10% in 0.9% sodium chloride, hydrazaline, hydroxyzine hydrochloride, insulin, invert sugar 10% in 0.9% sodium chloride, levorphanol bitartrate, meperidine, methadone hydrochloride, methylprednisolone, morphine sulfate, norepinephrine sulfate, oxytetracycline, penicillin G potassium, pentazocine lactate, phenobarbital sodium, phenytoin sodium, prochlorperazine edisylate, promazine hydrochloride, promethazine hydrochloride, tetracycline, vancomycin, and vitamin B complex with C.

ADVERSE-REACTIONS

Life-threatening: bradycardia, cardiac arrest, circulatory collapse, generalized tonic-clonic seizures, hypotension, ventricular fibrillation.
Other: albuminuria, diarrhea, dizziness, dysrhythmias, epigastric pain, flushing, headache, hematemesis, hyperglycemia, syndrome of inappropriate ADH secretion, insomnia, irritability, light-headedness, muscle twitching, nausea, palpitations, precordial pain, reflex hyperexcitability, restlessness, severe dehydration, syncope, tachycardia, tinnitus, vomiting.

INTERACTIONS

Allopurinol (high-dose), cimetidine, erythromycin, propranolol, troleandomycin: possible increased serum theophylline levels.
Barbiturates, carbamazepine, phenytoin, rifampin: enhanced metabolism and decreased theophylline levels.
Beta-adrenergic agonists: possible heightened risk of dysrhythmias.
Beta-adrenergic blockers, levobunolol, timolol: antagonism with possible mutual inhibition of therapeutic effects and reduced theophylline clearance; propranolol and nadalol, especially, may also cause bronchospasm.
Caffeine, other xanthines: heightened potential for toxic effects.
CNS stimulants: additive CNS stimulation.
Ephedrine: possible toxic synergism.
Estrogen-containing contraceptives: altered effectiveness.
Hydrocarbon inhalation anesthetics: enhanced risk of dysrhythmias.
Influenza vaccine: possible reduced serum theophylline levels.

Lithium carbonate: increased excretion.
Nicotine chewing gum, other smoking cessation products: augmented theophylline effects.
Oral anticoagulants: enhanced effects, with increased plasma prothrombin and Factor V.

EFFECTS ON DIAGNOSTIC TESTS

Serum uric acid: falsely elevated levels with Bittner or colorimetric method.

SPECIAL CONSIDERATIONS

• *Treatment of overdose:* Discontinue drug immediately and provide supportive and symptomatic treatment. Avoid giving sympathomimetic drugs.
• Base dosage on lean body weight and serum theophylline level. Monitor serum trough level to manage regimen; monitor serum peak levels to assess for toxicity. Optimum therapeutic levels: 10 to 20 mcg/ml.
• I.V. administration can cause vein irritation and burning. Dilute drug with compatible solution if necessary.
• Expect to reduce dosage in neonates; elderly patients; and in patients with COPD, active influenza, and cardiac, renal, or hepatic dysfunction because of decreased theophylline clearance.
• Exercise care when interpreting orders—don't confuse aminophylline with theophylline. Aminophylline is approximately 79% theophylline.
• When changing from continuous infusion to the oral preparation, first give extended-release form when discontinuing I.V. form; then give intermediate-release form 4 to 6 hours later.
• I.V. theophylline has also been used to treat cystic fibrosis in infants and to promote diuresis and

treat Cheyne-Stokes respirations and paroxysmal nocturnal dyspnea in adults.

thiamine hydrochloride (vitamin B₁)
Betalin S, Betaxin♦♦, Biamine, Thiamine

Pregnancy Risk Category: A
(C if greater than RDA)

PHARMACOKINETICS
Distribution: throughout tissues. Drug probably crosses the placenta.
Metabolism: in liver.
Excretion: in urine as metabolites after therapeutic dose and as unchanged thiamine and metabolites after higher doses, resulting from tissue saturation. Drug probably appears in breast milk.
Action: onset, immediately after administration; duration, unknown.

MECHANISM OF ACTION
This water-soluble vitamin, isolated from rice bran, combines with ATP to form a coenzyme needed for carbohydrate metabolism.

INDICATIONS & DOSAGE
• Severe thiamine deficiency (beriberi). *Adults:* 5 to 100 mg t.i.d.
Children: 10 to 25 mg daily.
• Wernicke's encephalopathy.
Adults: 500 to 1,000 mg daily.
• During TPN therapy. *Adults:* 3 to 21 mg daily.

CONTRAINDICATIONS & CAUTIONS
• Contraindicated in thiamine hypersensitivity.

PREPARATION & STORAGE
Supplied in 1 ml ampules, prefilled syringes, and cartridges, as well as 10 and 30 ml vials, each containing 100 or 200 mg/ml. Dilute if necessary in 0.9% sodium chloride, dextrose 5% in water, or a combination of these solutions. Refrigerate drug (don't freeze) and protect from light.

ADMINISTRATION
Direct injection: not recommended.
Intermittent infusion: Administer ordered amount at a rate not to exceed 20 mg/minute. Use an infusion pump for high doses.
Continuous infusion: Add ordered dose to maintenance fluids and infuse at a rate not to exceed 20 mg/minute.

INCOMPATIBILITY
Incompatible with acetates, alkali carbonates, amobarbital, barbiturates, citrates, erythromycin estolate, kanamycin sulfate, phenobarbital, streptomycin sulfate, and sulfites.

ADVERSE REACTIONS
Life-threatening: anaphylaxis, respiratory distress, severe pulmonary edema, vascular collapse.
Other: angioedema, cyanosis, diarrhea, GI bleeding, hemorrhage, hypotension, nausea, pain, paresthesias, pruritus, restlessness, sweating, throat tightness, transient vasodilation, urticaria, warmth, weakness, wheezing.

INTERACTIONS
Neuromuscular blockers: possible enhanced effects.

EFFECTS ON DIAGNOSTIC TESTS
Serum theophylline: with high doses, altered levels using Schack and Waxler spectrophotometric method.
Serum uric acid: with high doses, possible false-positive results using phototungstate method.

Urine urobilinogen: possible false-positive results using Ehrlich's reagents.

SPECIAL CONSIDERATIONS
• Never give thiamine by direct injection because of the risk of anaphylaxis. Perform a skin test before administration, and keep epinephrine available.
• Use I.V. route only if oral or I.M. administration isn't feasible.
• Signs and symptoms of mild thiamine deficiency include paresthesia, hyperesthesia, anesthesia and weakness, and possible foot and wrist drop. Severe thiamine deficiency may be marked by cardiomegaly, tachycardia, and dependent edema.
• Acute pernicious beriberi may occur if patient becomes thiamine deficient during TPN. Disorder has mortality rate approaching 50%.

thiopental sodium
Pentothal♦

Controlled Substance Schedule III
Pregnancy Risk Category: C

PHARMACOKINETICS
Distribution: rapidly dispersed to CNS, then redistributed first to highly perfused tissues and eventually to fatty tissue. Drug crosses the placenta and is 80% bound to plasma proteins.
Metabolism: in liver and and kidneys.
Excretion: minimally, in urine. In large doses, drug appears in small amounts in breast milk.
Action: onset, 30 to 60 seconds; duration, 10 to 30 minutes.

MECHANISM OF ACTION
Anesthetic actions aren't fully understood, but the drug may facilitate synaptic actions of inhibitory neurotransmitters and block synaptic actions of excitatory neurotransmitters.

INDICATIONS & DOSAGE
Dosage individualized, based on desired depth of anesthesia, concurrent use of other drugs, and patient's age, weight, sex, and condition.
• Sole anesthesia for brief (15-minute) procedures. *Adults:* initially, 50 to 75 mg q 20 to 40 seconds until anesthesia is established, then 25 to 50 mg p.r.n. *Children 15 years and under:* initially, 3 to 5 mg/kg, then 1 mg/kg p.r.n.
• Induction of general anesthesia before administration of other agents. *Adults:* 3 to 4 mg/kg.
• Supplement to regional anesthesia. *Adults:* 25 to 50 mg p.r.n.
• Hypnosis during balanced anesthesia with other agents for analgesia or muscle relaxation. *Adults:* 50 to 100 mg p.r.n.
• Seizure control during or after inhalation or local anesthesia. *Adults:* 75 to 125 mg as soon as possible after start of seizure.
• Increased intracranial pressure in neurosurgery (with adequate ventilation). *Adults:* 1.5 to 3.5 mg/kg, repeated p.r.n.
• Narcoanalysis and narcosynthesis in psychiatric patients. *Adults:* 100 mg/minute (2.5% solution) until patient is semidrowsy but can speak and respond.

CONTRAINDICATIONS & CAUTIONS
• Contraindicated in barbiturate hypersensitivity.
• Contraindicated in status asthmaticus because drug provokes histamine release, which could precipitate an asthma attack. Also contraindicated in porphyria because of possible aggravated symptoms.

• Use cautiously in severe cardiovascular disease, hypotension, and shock because of worsened cardiovascular depression.

• In severe obesity or neuromuscular disease, also use cautiously because of possible airway or ventilation problems.

• Use cautiously in conditions that may prolong hypnotic effect.

PREPARATION & STORAGE

Available in 250, 400, and 500 mg syringes; in 500 and 1,000 mg vials; and in 1, 2.5, and 5 g containers in kits. Reconstitute with 20 to 500 ml of sterile water for injection, 0.9% sodium chloride, or dextrose 5% in water to yield 0.2% to 5% concentration (usually 2.5%). Compatible solutions include dextrose 2.5% in water, dextrose 5% in water, Ionosol PSL, 0.45% sodium chloride, Dextran 6% in dextrose 5% in water or 0.9% sodium chloride, and ⅙ M sodium lactate. Store thiopental at room temperature before reconstituting. Refrigerate reconstituted solutions and discard after 24 hours. Drug contains no bacteriostatic agents.

ADMINISTRATION

Drug should be administered only by staff specially trained to give anesthetics and to manage their adverse effects.

Direct injection: Inject ordered dose through I.V. tubing containing a free-flowing compatible solution. Repeat as needed to maintain anesthesia.

Intermittent infusion: not recommended.

Continuous infusion: Infuse a concentration of 0.2% to 0.4% (200 to 400 mg/100 ml) at a rate not exceeding 50 ml/hour. Monitor serum drug levels. Prolonged continuous infusion may cause respiratory and circulatory depression.

INCOMPATIBILITY

Incompatible with amikacin, benzquinamide, cephapirin, chlorpromazine, codeine phosphate, dextrose 10% in water or 0.9% sodium chloride, dimenhydrinate, diphenhydramine, ephedrine, fructose 10%, glycopyrrolate, human fibrinolysin, hydromorphone, insulin (regular), invert sugar 5% and 10% in 0.9% sodium chloride, levorphanol bitartrate, meperidine, metaraminol, methadone, morphine, norepinephrine bitartrate, Normosol solutions (except Normosol R), penicillin G potassium, prochlorperazine edisylate, promazine, promethazine hydrochloride, Ringer's injection, Ringer's lactate, sodium bicarbonate, succinylcholine chloride, and tetracycline hydrochloride.

ADVERSE REACTIONS

Life-threatening: anaphylaxis, bronchospasm, dysrhythmias, hypotension, laryngospasm, myocardial depression, respiratory depression.

Other: coughing, headache, nausea, prolonged drowsiness and recovery, rash, shivering, sneezing, thrombophlebitis, vomiting.

INTERACTIONS

Antihypertensives, barbiturates, ethacrynic acid, furosemide, other diuretics: possible orthostatic hypotension.

CNS depressants (including alcohol): possible deepened CNS depression.

Hypothermia-producing drugs: increased risk of hypothermia.

[131]I: reduced thyroid uptake of thiopental.

Ketamine: increased risk of hypotension and respiratory depression.

Magnesium sulfate (parenteral): deepened CNS depression.

Phenothiazines: deepened CNS depression and potentiated hypotensive and CNS excitatory effects.

EFFECTS ON DIAGNOSTIC TESTS
EEG: slowed.
Radioactive iodine tests: possible decreased uptake of ^{123}I and ^{131}I.

SPECIAL CONSIDERATIONS
• Patients tolerant to other barbiturates or alcohol may require higher doses.
• Avoid administering drug subcutaneously or intra-arterially; drug may cause sloughing and necrosis. If inadvertent intra-arterial injection occurs, dilute injected thiopental by removing the tourniquet. Leave the needle or I.V. catheter in place and inject the artery with 40 to 80 mg of papaverin or 1% procaine.
• Use warming blankets, chlorpromazine, or methylphenidate, as ordered, to treat shivering.
• After administration, warn the patient to avoid alcohol or other CNS depressants and that psychomotor skills may be impaired for 24 hours.

---

thiotepa
(TSPA, TESPA)

Pregnancy Risk Category: D

PHARMACOKINETICS
Distribution: rapidly cleared from plasma and found primarily within cells. Drug crosses the placenta.
Metabolism: partially metabolized to triethylene phosphoramide (TEPA).
Excretion: in urine with 60% to 85% excreted within 24 to 72 hours. Not known if drug or its metabolites appear in breast milk.
Action: onset, unknown; duration, unknown.

MECHANISM OF ACTION
An alkylating agent, thiotepa interferes with DNA replication and RNA transcription, ultimately disrupting nucleic acid function. Drug also has some immunosuppressive activity.

INDICATIONS & DOSAGE
Dosage reflects response to the drug and appearance or degree of toxicity. Maintenance doses are based on hematologic studies.
• Adenocarcinomas of breast and ovary, lymphomas, bronchogenic carcinoma (palliative treatment).
Adults and children 12 years and over: 0.3 to 0.4 mg/kg q 1 to 4 weeks. Or 0.2 mg/kg (or 6 mg/m²) daily for 4 or 5 days q 2 to 4 weeks.
Children under 12 years: dosage not established.

CONTRAINDICATIONS & CAUTIONS
• Contraindicated in thiotepa hypersensitivity.
• Also contraindicated in existing or recent exposure to chicken pox or herpes zoster because of the risk of severe generalized disease.
• Use cautiously in bone marrow depression, gout, or history of urate renal calculi because of the risk of hyperuricemia.
• In infection, use cautiously because myelosuppression complicates treatment.
• Also use cautiously in tumor cell infiltration of bone marrow, previous cytotoxic drug therapy, or radiation therapy because of possible further myelosuppression.
• Give cautiously in renal or hepatic impairment because of the increased risk of toxicity.

PREPARATION & STORAGE

Take extreme caution in preparing and administering thiotepa to avoid mutagenic, teratogenic, and carcinogenic risks. Use a biologic containment cabinet, wear gloves and mask, and use syringes with Luer-Lok fittings to prevent drug leakage. Also dispose of needles, vials, and unused drug correctly, and avoid contaminating work surfaces.

Thiotepa is available as a powder in 15-mg vials. Reconstitute with 1.5 ml of sterile water for injection to yield a concentration of 10 mg/ml. For infusion, further dilute drug in sodium chloride injection, dextrose injection, dextrose and sodium chloride injection, Ringer's injection, or lactated Ringer's injection.

Refrigerate powder and reconstituted solution at 36° to 46° F. (2° to 8° C.), and protect from light. Reconstituted solution is stable for 5 days if refrigerated (0.5 mg/ml solution in Ringer's injection is stable for 15 days refrigerated or at room temperature). Don't use if solution is grossly opaque or contains precipitates—microbiologic contamination is possible.

ADMINISTRATION

Direct injection: Using a 21G or 23G needle, inject rapidly.
Intermittent infusion: Give diluted drug over ordered duration. Start a primary I.V. line or use the infusion port of an existing primary line.
Continuous infusion: not recommended.

INCOMPATIBILITY

No incompatibilities reported.

ADVERSE REACTIONS

Life-threatening: anaphylaxis, leukopenia, pancytopenia, thrombocytopenia.

Other: alopecia, amenorrhea, anorexia, chills, delayed menses, dizziness, exudates from S.C. lesions (from tumor breakdown), fever, headache, hyperuricemia, nausea, pain at injection site, pruritus, rash, sore throat, stomatitis, throat tightness, ulceration of intestinal mucosa, unusual bleeding or bruising, urticaria, vomiting, wheezing.

INTERACTIONS

Allopurinol, colchicine, probenecid, sulfinpyrazone: possible increased doses required because thiotepa causes hyperuricemia.
Anticoagulants, aspirin: increased risk of bleeding.
Live virus vaccines: potentiated vaccine virus replication, increased adverse reactions, decreased antibody response.
Myelosuppressive drugs, radiation therapy: additional myelosuppression.
Succinylcholine: possible enhanced neuromuscular blockade.

EFFECTS ON DIAGNOSTIC TESTS

Serum cholinesterase: possible reduced levels.
Serum uric acid: possible increased levels.
WBC and platelet counts: decreased.

SPECIAL CONSIDERATIONS

• *Treatment of overdose:* As ordered, give transfusions of whole blood, platelets, or WBCs, which may relieve hematopoietic toxicity.
• Drug is highly toxic with a low therapeutic index; many adverse effects are unavoidable. Some effects, such as leukopenia, are used to indicate the drug's effectiveness to aid dosage titration.
• Expect to administer lower doses in renal, hepatic, or hematopoietic impairment. Monitor carefully.

Unmarked trade names available in the United States only.
♦ Also available in Canada.   ♦♦ Available in Canada only.

• In recent cytotoxic drug or radiation therapy, therapy isn't recommended until depressed WBC and platelet counts start to recover (WBC counts above 2,000/mm³; platelet counts above 50,000/mm³).

• Before and during therapy, monitor WBC and platelet counts and BUN, hematocrit, SGOT, SGPT, bilirubin, creatinine, LDH, and uric acid levels.

• At the first sign of a sudden large drop in WBC (particularly granulocyte) or platelet counts, discontinue drug or reduce dosage, as ordered, to prevent irreversible myelosuppression. WBC nadir may occur at 10 to 14 days when given weekly. Resume therapy when counts return to acceptable levels.

• Watch carefully for signs of infection in patients with leukopenia. If infection develops, give antibiotics, as ordered.

• Provide adequate oral hydration, which may prevent or delay uric acid nephropathy. Allopurinol administration may also be helpful.

• Inform the patient of the drug's adverse effects, and stress the importance of adequate fluid intake.

• Advise home care patients to avoid contact with people with infections, and to avoid taking nonprescription products containing aspirin.

ticarcillin disodium
Ticar♦

Pregnancy Risk Category: B

PHARMACOKINETICS
Distribution: readily dispersed to pleural and interstitial fluid, skin, kidneys, bone, bile, and sputum. Usually low CSF concentration increases with meningeal irritation. Drug is 45% to 65% bound to plasma proteins and probably crosses the placenta.

Metabolism: in liver where 10% to 15% is metabolized to inactive penicilloic acids.

Excretion: principally excreted in urine, by renal tubular secretion and glomerular filtration. Drug is partially excreted in feces. Usual half-life is about 1 hour, with 80% to 93% excreted within 24 hours (most within the first 2 to 6 hours). Half-life is prolonged in renal or hepatic impairment. Drug appears in breast milk in small quantities.

Action: peak serum level, immediately after administration.

MECHANISM OF ACTION
An extended-spectrum penicillin, ticarcillin inhibits bacterial septum and cell-wall synthesis by preventing cross-linkage of peptidoglycan chains. It also inhibits cell division and growth. Rapidly dividing bacteria are most susceptible.

Susceptible gram-positive bacteria include *Staphylococcus aureus; S. epidermis;* groups A, B, C, and G streptococci; *Streptococcus pneumoniae; S. viridans;* and some strains of enterococci. Susceptible gram-negative bacteria include *Acinetobacter, Eikenella corrodens, Escherichia coli, Haemophilus influenzae, Morganella morganii, Moroxella, Neisseria gonorrhoeae, N. menigitidis, Pasteurella multocida, Proteus mirabilis, P. vulgaris, Providencia rettgeri, Pseudomonas, Salmonella,* and *Shigella.*

Drug may also be used against the anaerobic bacteria *Actinomyces, Bacteroides, Bifidobacterium, Clostridium, Eubacterium, Fusobacterium, Lactobacillus, Peptococcus, Proprionibacterium,* and *Veillonella.*

INDICATIONS & DOSAGE

• Septicemia; respiratory tract, skin, soft tissue, intra-abdominal, female pelvic, and genital tract infections. *Adults and children weighing over 40 kg:* 200 to 300 mg/kg per day in divided doses given q 3, 4, or 6 hours. *Children weighing up to 40 kg:* 200 to 300 mg/kg per day, q 4 to 6 hours. *Neonates weighing 2 kg and over:* 75 mg/kg q 8 hours for first week of life; then 100 mg/kg q 8 hours.

• Urinary tract infections (complicated). *Adults and children weighing over 40 kg:* 150 to 200 mg/kg per day in divided doses given q 4 to 6 hours. *Children weighing up to 40 kg:* 25 to 33.3 mg/kg q 4 hours; or 37.5 to 50 mg/kg q 6 hours.

• Urinary tract infections (uncomplicated). *Adults and children weighing over 40 kg:* 1 g q 4 to 6 hours. *Children weighing up to 40 kg:* 12.5 to 25 mg/kg q 6 hours; or 16.7 to 33.3 mg/kg q 8 hours.

Note: Dosage in renal failure reflects creatinine clearance. Recommended adult dosage: 3 g every 4 hours for creatinine clearance of 60 ml/minute; 2 g every 4 hours for clearance of 30 to 60 ml/minute; 2 g every 8 hours for clearance of 10 to 30 ml/minute; 2 g every 12 hours for clearance of 10 ml/minute; and 2 g every 24 hours for clearance of 10 ml/minute with hepatic impairment.

CONTRAINDICATIONS & CAUTIONS

• Contraindicated in hypersensitivity to penicillin and other beta-lactam antibiotics.

• Use cautiously in renal impairment because of increased risk of toxicity and in sodium restriction; sodium content is 6.5 mEq/g of drug.

• In hypokalemia, use cautiously because condition may be aggravated. Check serum potassium frequently.

• Give cautiously in patients with a history of allergic disorders because of the increased risk of hypersensitivity.

• In bleeding disorders, also give cautiously because drug may cause platelet dysfunction, increasing the risk of hemorrhage.

• Use cautiously in patients with a history of ulcerative colitis, regional enteritis, or antibiotic-associated colitis because of the enhanced risk of pseudomembranous colitis.

PREPARATION & STORAGE

Supplied as a white to pale yellow powder or lyophilized cake in 1, 3, and 6 g vials and 3 g piggyback vials. Reconstitute by adding 4 ml of 0.9% sodium chloride, dextrose 5% in water, or Ringer's lactate for each gram of ticarcillin. For continuous infusion, dilute further with 10 to 100 ml of a compatible I.V. solution. Reconstituted solution is clear and colorless or pale yellow.

Store powder at room temperature. Refrigerate reconstituted solution or use within 30 minutes. Diluted solutions are stable for 72 hours at room temperature with sterile water for injection, dextrose 5% in water, and 0.9% sodium chloride; and for 48 hours at room temperature with Ringer's injection or Ringer's lactate (10 to 100 mg/ml). Solutions with dextrose 5% in 0.225% or 0.45% sodium chloride or with 5% alcohol are stable at room temperature for 72 hours (10 to 50 mg/ml). All solutions are stable for 14 days when refrigerated at 39° F. (4° C.) but shouldn't be used for multiple doses if stored longer than 72 hours. Reconstituted solutions may also be frozen at 0° F. (−18° C.) and are stable for up to 30 days. Use thawed solution within 24 hours.

ADMINISTRATION

Direct injection: not recommended.
Intermittent infusion: Infuse diluted solution directly into vein via an established I.V. line. To minimize vein irritation, use solutions containing 50 mg/ml or less and infuse slowly—over 30 minutes to 2 hours in adults or 10 to 20 minutes in neonates.
Continuous infusion: Add the total daily dosage of reconstituted drug to ordered volume of compatible solution. Adjust rate to deliver required 24-hour volume.

INCOMPATIBILITY

Incompatible with aminoglycosides.

ADVERSE REACTIONS

Life-threatening: anaphylaxis.
Other: anemia, bacterial and fungal superinfection, bleeding, diarrhea, dizziness, eosinophilia, fever, leukopenia, muscle weakness, nausea, neuromuscular irritability or seizures, neutropenia, pain at injection site, phlebitis, platelet dysfunction, pruritus, pseudomembranous colitis, rash, thrombocytopenia, unusual bleeding, urticaria, vein irritation, vomiting.

INTERACTIONS

Anticoagulants, thrombolytic agents: possible increased risk of hemorrhage.
Antidiarrheals, antiperistaltics: heightened risk of pseudomembranous colitis.
Chloramphenicol, erythromycin, sulfonamides, tetracyclines: possible interference with ticarcillin's bactericidal effect.
NSAIDs, platelet aggregation inhibitors, salicylates, sulfinpyrazone: further inhibition of platelet function and enhanced risk of hemorrhage.
Probenecid: increased risk of toxicity, stemming from decreased ticarcillin elimination.

EFFECTS ON DIAGNOSTIC TESTS

Bleeding time: increased.
BUN, serum creatinine, sodium: possible elevated levels.
Coombs' test: possible false-positive results.
Hematocrit: hemoglobin, possible reduced levels.
Partial thromboplastin time: prothrombin time, prolonged (especially in renal impairment).
Serum alkaline phosphatase, bilirubin, LDH, uric acid; SGOT, SGPT: possible elevated levels.
Serum potassium: possible depressed levels.
Urine protein: possible false-positive reactions with sulfosalicylic acid and boiling test, acetic acid test, or biuret reaction and nitric acid test.

SPECIAL CONSIDERATIONS

● *Treatment of overdose:* Treat symptomatically and supportively. Hemodialysis may be used if needed.
● Before giving ticarcillin, ask patient if he's had any allergic reactions to penicillin or other beta-lactam drugs. However, a negative history doesn't rule out a future allergic reaction.
● Obtain specimens for culture and sensitivity tests before giving first dose. Therapy may begin before results are complete. Give drug at least 1 hour before bacteriostatic antibiotics.
● Monitor electrolyte levels (especially potassium) and cardiac status frequently because drug's high sodium content may cause electrolyte imbalance and dysrhythmias.
● Observe patient for fungal and bacterial superinfection with prolonged use.
● With prolonged treatment, monitor for renal, hepatic, and hematopoietic dysfunction. Monitor bleeding times closely.

• Monitor neurologic status. High concentrations may cause seizures.

ticarcillin disodium/clavulanate potassium
Timentin

Pregnancy Risk Category: B

PHARMACOKINETICS
Distribution: readily dispersed into pleural and interstitial fluid, blister fluid, skin, kidneys, bone, lymph tissue, urine, and gallbladder. Clavulanic acid is distributed poorly into respiratory tract. Usually low CSF concentration rises with meningeal irritation. Drug is 45% to 65% bound to plasma proteins. Clavulanic acid and probably ticarcillin cross the placenta.
Metabolism: in liver—extensively for clavulanic acid, minimally for ticarcillin.
Excretion: in urine, with 60% to 70% of ticarcillin and 35% to 45% of clavulanic acid excreted unchanged within 6 to 12 hours. Halflife of ticarcillin is about 1 hour; of clavulanic acid, about 1 to 1½ hours. Half-lives lengthen renal dysfunction. Both drugs appear in breast milk in small amounts.
Action: peak serum levels, immediately after infusion.

MECHANISM OF ACTION
Ticarcillin, a bactericidal agent, inhibits bacterial cell-wall synthesis. Clavulanic acid, a beta-lactamase inhibitor, provides a synergistic bactericidal effect. It binds to certain beta-lactamases that usually inhibit ticarcillin. This results in a broadened spectrum of activity.

Susceptible gram-positive bacteria include *Staphylococcus aureus, S. epidermis, S. saprophyticus,* group A beta-hemolytic streptococci, group B streptococci, *Streptococcus pneumoniae, S. faecalis, S. bovis,* and *S. viridans.*

Susceptible gram-negative bacteria include some strains of *Acinetobacter, Branhamella catarrhalis, Citrobacter amalonaticus, C. diversus, C. freundii, Enterobacter agglomerans, Escherichia coli, Haemophilus influenzae, Klebsiella, Morganella morganii, Neisseria meningitidis, N. gonorrhoeae, Proteus mirabilis, P. vulgaris, Providencia rettgeri, Pseudomonas acidovorans, P. moltaphilia, P. aeruginosa, Salmonella,* and *Shigella.*

The drugs are also active against susceptible anaerobic bacteria, such as *Bacteroides, Clostridium, Eubacterium, Fusobacterium, Peptococcus, Peptostreptococcus,* and *Veillonella.*

INDICATIONS & DOSAGE
• Systemic infections and urinary tract infections, particularly those caused by beta-lactamase producing organisms. *Adults weighing over 60 kg:* 3.1 g ticarcillin (as 3 g ticarcillin and 100 mg clavulanic acid) q 4 to 6 hours. *Adults weighing under 60 kg and children 12 years and over:* 33.3 to 50 mg ticarcillin/kg q 4 hours; or 50 to 75 mg ticarcillin/kg q 6 hours.
Note: Dosage in renal failure reflects creatinine clearance. Loading dose for adults is 3.1 g (3 g ticarcillin with 100 mg clavulanate). If clearance is less than 10 ml/min (with liver failure), dosage is 2 g q 24 hours; if clearance is less than 10 ml/min (absence of liver failure), dosage is 2 g q 12 hours; if clearance is 10 to 30 ml/min, dosage is 2 g q 8 hours; if clearance is 30 to 60 ml/min, dosage is 2 g q 4 hours; if clearance is more than 60 ml/min, dosage is 3.1 g q 4 hours. In patients on hemodialysis, dosage is 2 g

q 12 hours, then 3.1 g after treatment; in patients on peritoneal dialysis, dosage is 3.1 g q 12 hours.

CONTRAINDICATIONS & CAUTIONS
• Contraindicated in hypersensitivity to penicillin and other beta-lactam antibiotics.
• Use cautiously in renal impairment because of increased risk of toxicity; in sodium restriction because of ticarcillin's high sodium content (about 4.75 mEq/g of ticarcillin); and in electrolyte imbalance because of risk of dysrhythmias.
• Give cautiously in patients with a history of allergic disorders because of the increased risk of hypersensitivity.
• Also give cautiously in ulcerative colitis, regional enteritis, or antibiotic-associated colitis because of the enhanced risk of pseudomembranous colitis.

PREPARATION & STORAGE
Supplied as a white to pale yellow powder in vials containing 3.1 g (3 g ticarcillin and 100 mg clavulanic acid). Reconstitute by adding 13 ml of sterile water or 0.9% sodium chloride for a ticarcillin concentration of 200 mg/ml and a clavulanate concentration of 6.7 mg/ml. Before infusion, dilute solution in 50 to 100 ml of 0.9% sodium chloride, dextrose 5% in water, or Ringer's lactate. Drug is also available in pharmacy-mixed reconstituted piggyback infusion bottles.

Store powder at 70° to 75° F. (21° to 24° C.). After reconstitution, solutions of 200 mg ticarcillin/ml are potent for 6 hours at room temperature and for up to 72 hours if refrigerated. Ringer's lactate and 0.9% sodium chloride solutions of 10 to 100 mg ticarcillin/ml remain potent for 24 hours at room temperature and for 7 days if refrigerated; dextrose 5% in water solutions remain potent for 12 hours at room temperature and for 3 days if refrigerated. Solutions of 100 mg ticarcillin/ml or less in 0.9% sodium chloride or Ringer's lactate may be frozen and stored up to 30 days; 7 days for solutions in dextrose 5% in water. Use thawed solutions within 8 hours.

ADMINISTRATION
Direct injection: not recommended.
Intermittent infusion: Give diluted dose over 30 minutes by infusion through a Y tubing, or use the piggyback method. Temporarily discontinue administration of primary solutions during administration.
Continuous infusion: not recommended.

INCOMPATIBILITY
Incompatible with aminoglycosides and sodium bicarbonate. Not recommended for use with other anti-infective agents.

ADVERSE REACTIONS
Life-threatening: anaphylaxis, bronchospasm.
Other: arthralgia, bacterial and fungal superinfection, chest discomfort, chills, diarrhea, eosinophilia, epigastric pain, fever, flatulence, giddiness, headache, impaired taste and smell, leukopenia, myalgia, nausea, neuromuscular irritability, neutropenia, pruritus, pseudomembranous colitis, rash, seizures, stomatitis, thrombocytopenia, thrombophlebitis, urticaria, vomiting, wheezing.

INTERACTIONS
Anticoagulants, thrombolytic agents: increased risk of hemorrhage.
Antidiarrheals, antiperistaltics: heightened risk of pseudomembranous colitis.

Chloramphenicol, erythromycin, sulfonamides, tetracyclines: may reduce ticarcillin's effects.

Diflunisal, NSAIDs, platelet aggregation inhibitors, salicylates, sulfinpyrazone: impaired platelet function, enhanced risk of hemorrhage.

Probenecid: increased and prolonged ticarcillin serum concentrations.

EFFECTS ON DIAGNOSTIC TESTS

Bleeding time, partial thromboplastin time, prothrombin time: prolonged.

BUN, serum creatinine: possible increased levels.

Coombs' test: possible false-positive results.

Hematocrit, hemoglobin: reduced levels.

Serum alkaline phosphatase, bilirubin, LDH; SGOT, SGPT: possible increased levels.

Serum potassium: possible elevated or reduced levels.

Serum sodium, uric acid: possible decreased levels.

Urine protein: possible false-positive results with turbidometric methods using sulfosalicylic acid, trichloroacetic acid, acetic acid, or nitric acid.

SPECIAL CONSIDERATIONS

• *Treatment of overdose:* Both ticarcillin and clavulanic acid may be removed by hemodialysis.

• Obtain specimens for culture and sensitivity tests before first dose. Therapy may begin before results are complete.

• Before giving drug, ask patient about allergic reactions to penicillin. A negative allergy history doesn't rule out a future reaction.

• Drug is particularly useful in infections caused by ticarcillin-resistant organisms (for example, peritonitis) and in nosocomial urinary or respiratory tract infections.

• Monitor serum sodium and potassium levels closely. Ticarcillin has a high sodium content, and clavulanic acid contributes about 0.15 mEq (6 mg) of potassium per 100 mg.

• Monitor CBC, prothrombin time, and bleeding times. Watch for bleeding tendencies and discontinue drug if bleeding occurs.

• If diarrhea persists during therapy, obtain stool culture to rule out pseudomembranous colitis.

• If patient is receiving dialysis, administer drug after session is complete.

• Observe patient for fungal and bacterial superinfection with prolonged use.

---

tobramycin sulfate
Nebcin♦

Pregnancy Risk Category: D

PHARMACOKINETICS

Distribution: widely distributed to tissues and fluids, including sputum and peritoneal, synovial, ascitic, and abscess fluid. Drug readily crosses the placenta. CSF penetration varies.

Metabolism: not metabolized.

Excretion: in urine by glomerular filtration, with 84% excreted within 8 hours and nearly all removed within 24 hours. Small amounts appear in breast milk.

Action: peak serum level, on completion of the infusion.

MECHANISM OF ACTION

This drug inhibits protein synthesis by binding to the 30S subunit, which results in production of a nonfunctional protein.

Susceptible gram-negative bacteria include *Acinetobacter, Citrobacter, Enterobacter, Escherichia coli, Klebsiella, Proteus, Providencia, Pseudomonas, Salmonella,* and *Serratia.*

Susceptible gram-positive bacteria include most strains of *Staphylococcus aureus* and *S. epidermis.*

INDICATIONS & DOSAGE
• Serious bacterial infections, including septicemia, lower respiratory tract infections, meningitis, intra-abdominal infections, complicated or recurrent urinary tract infections, and infections of skin, bone, and skin structures. Dosages are based on ideal body weight. *Adults:* 3 mg/kg daily in equal doses q 8 hours. May be increased to 5 mg/kg daily in three or four equal doses for life-threatening infections. *Children:* 6 to 7.5 mg/kg daily in three or four equal doses. *Neonates under 1 week:* 4 mg/kg daily or less in equal doses q 12 hours.
• Endocarditis prophylaxis before dental or other minor surgery. *Adults and children weighing 27 kg or more:* 1.5 mg/kg in combination with ampicillin given 30 minutes before procedure. *Children weighing less than 27 kg:* 2 mg/kg in combination with ampicillin given 30 minutes before procedure.
• Acute pelvic inflammatory disease. *Adults:* initially, 2 mg/kg, then 1.5 mg/kg q 8 hours.
Note: Adjust dosage in renal impairment. For adults, initial dosage is same as for patients with normal renal function. Subsequent doses and frequency determined by renal function study results and blood levels; keep peak serum concentrations between 4 and 10 mcg/ml, and trough serum concentrations between 1 and 2 mcg/ml.

CONTRAINDICATIONS & CAUTIONS
• Contraindicated in hypersensitivity to tobramycin or any other aminoglycoside.

• Use cautiously in elderly patients, neonates, premature infants, and patients with renal impairment or dehydration because of the increased risk of nephrotoxicity.
• Also use cautiously in cranial nerve VIII damage because of the heightened risk of ototoxicity.
• In infant botulism, myasthenia gravis, and Parkinson's disease, give cautiously because of the risk of neuromuscular blockade and increased skeletal muscle weakness.

PREPARATION & STORAGE
Available as a clear, colorless solution in rubber-stopped vials containing 80 mg/2 ml or 20 mg/2 ml and as pediatric injection in 2 ml vials containing 10 mg/ml. Also available as a dry powder (1.2 g), which should be reconstituted with 30 ml of sterile water for injection to a 40 mg/ml concentration. For adults, further dilute the calculated dose in 50 to 100 ml of 0.9% sodium chloride or dextrose 5% injection. For children, dilution depends on patient needs.

Diluted tobramycin is stable for 24 hours at room temperature.

ADMINISTRATION
Direct injection: not recommended.
Intermittent infusion: Infuse diluted solution over 20 to 60 minutes.
Continuous infusion: not recommended.

INCOMPATIBILITY
Incompatible with beta-lactam antibiotics; cefamandole nafate; cefoperazone; cefotaxime sodium; dextrose 5% in Polysal, Polysal M, or Isolyte E, M, or P; heparin sodium; and I.V. solutions containing alcohol. Because of other potential incompatibilities, manufacturer recommends mixing no other drugs with tobramycin.

ADVERSE REACTIONS
Life-threatening: anaphylaxis.
Other: anemia, arthralgia, disorientation, encephalopathy, fever, granulocytopenia, headache, hypocalcemia, hypokalemia, hypomagnesemia, hypotension, lethargy, leukopenia, local irritation, nausea, nephrotoxicity (cylinduria; increased proteinuria; oliguria; rising BUN, nonprotein nitrogen, and serum creatinine), ototoxicity, paresthesias, peripheral neuritis, rash, splenomegaly, tachycardia, thrombocytopenia, thrombophlebitis, transient hepatomegaly, tremor, tubular necrosis, urticaria, vomiting.

INTERACTIONS
Antihistamines, loxapine, phenothiazines, thioxanthenes: possible masked signs of ototoxicity.
Antimyasthenics: possible antagonized effects.
Diuretics: possible altered serum and tissue tobramycin levels, possible increased toxicity.
Hydrocarbon inhalation anesthetics, massive transfusions of citrated blood, neuromuscular blockers: possible heightened neuromuscular blockade, resulting in respiratory depression.
Indomethacin (I.V.): augmented risk of toxicity in neonates.
Nephrotoxic or neurotoxic antibiotics: enhanced risk of toxicity.
Opioid analgesics: deepened respiratory depression.

EFFECTS ON DIAGNOSTIC TESTS
BUN, serum creatinine: elevated levels.
Serum bilirubin, LDH; SGOT, SGPT: increased levels.
CBC: eosinophilia, leukocytosis, leukopenia.
Serum calcium, magnesium, potassium, sodium: reduced levels.

SPECIAL CONSIDERATIONS
• *Treatment of overdose:* Hemodialysis effectively reduces serum drug levels.
• Obtain specimens for culture and sensitivity tests before giving first dose. Therapy may begin before results are complete.
• Monitor serum drug levels, especially in neonates, elderly patients, and those with renal impairment. Therapeutic concentration is 4 to 10 mcg/ml. Peak serum levels should be no greater than 10 mcg/ml; trough levels, no greater than 2 mcg/ml. Coordinate blood sampling and drug administration with the laboratory. Draw trough levels before next dose; peak levels ½ hour after infusion.
• Obtain periodic BUN and serum creatinine levels to help assess renal function.
• Question patients about tinnitus or hearing loss. If possible, obtain serial audiograms for patients at high risk for ototoxicity.
• Observe patient for fungal and bacterial superinfection with prolonged use.
• May contain sulfites.

trace elements (chromium, copper, manganese, selenium, zinc)
Multitrace

Pregnancy Risk Category: C

PHARMACOKINETICS
Distribution: varies. *Chromium* tends to accumulate in skin, muscle, fat, and hair. *Copper,* found in all tissues, reaches its highest concentrations in the brain and liver. *Manganese* appears in small amounts in bone, the pituitary, pancreas, intestinal mucosa, liver, and

other tissues. It also crosses the placenta. Only small amounts (12 to 20 mg) are stored in the body. *Selenium* appears in all tissues except fat, with highest concentrations in the kidneys, heart, spleen, and liver. *Zinc* is distributed to all tissues, with about 70% concentrated in the skeleton and high amounts in the skin, hair, and testes. Most zinc is protein-bound.

Metabolism: not metabolized.

Excretion: varies. *Chromium* is primarily excreted in urine, with small amounts in feces. *Copper* and *manganese* are eliminated primarily in bile. A small amount of manganese is excreted in urine. *Selenium's* excretion isn't well-defined. *Zinc* is eliminated primarily in feces, with small amounts in urine.

Action: onset, unknown; duration, unknown.

MECHANISM OF ACTION

Exogenous trace elements help maintain serum trace element levels and prevent excretion of endogenous stores and resultant deficiency. Their mechanism of action isn't well understood. *Chromium* maintains normal glucose metabolism and peripheral nerve function and also activates insulin-mediated reactions. Essential in many enzymes, *copper* maintains normal rates of RBC and WBC formation and is a cofactor for serum ceruloplasmin. *Manganese* aids in developing normal skeletal and connective tissue and activates enzymes involved in the synthesis of fatty acids, cholesterol, and mucopolysaccharides; the formation of urea; and the structure and function of mitochondria. An essential component of the enzyme glutathione peroxidase, *selenium* aids in cell growth, release of energy to cells, development of sperm cells, and liver function. *Zinc* facilitates wound healing, promotes growth, and plays a role in skin hydration and the senses of taste and smell. It acts as cofactor for numerous enzymes.

INDICATIONS & DOSAGE

Prevention of trace element deficiencies in long-term total parenteral nutrition (TPN). *As a combination product: Adults:* 5 ml/day. *As a single element product:*

• Chromium. *Adults:* 10 to 15 mcg daily (20 mcg daily with intestinal fluid loss). *Children:* 0.14 to 0.2 mcg/kg daily.

• Copper. *Adults:* 0.5 to 1.5 mg daily. *Children:* 20 mcg/kg daily.

• Manganese. *Adults:* 0.15 to 0.8 mg daily. *Children:* 2 to 10 mcg/kg daily.

• Selenium. *Adults:* 20 to 40 mcg daily (100 mcg daily for 24 to 31 days with selenium deficiency resulting from long-term TPN). *Children:* 3 mcg/kg daily.

• Zinc. *Adults:* 2.5 to 4 mg daily (additional 2 mg daily in acute catabolic states; additional 12.2 mg/liter in fluid loss from the small bowel; or additional 17.1 mg/kg stool in stool or ileostomy output). *Children up to 5 years:* 100 mcg/kg daily. *Premature infants weighing up to 3 kg:* 300 mcg/kg daily.

CONTRAINDICATIONS & CAUTIONS

• Use cautiously in renal impairment because of the increased risk of trace element retention.

• Also use cautiously in biliary obstruction because copper and manganese are eliminated in bile.

• In diabetes mellitus, dosage adjustments may be necessary because chromium is important in glucose metabolism. Give cautiously.

PREPARATION & STORAGE

Multitrace available in 10-ml unit dose vials containing 4 mcg chromium, 0.4 mg copper, 0.1 mg manganese, 20 mcg selenium, and 1 mg zinc. Dilute for infusion in the appropriate TPN solution to a minimum dilution of 1:200. Chromium, copper, and manganese are available as single element products in 5, 10, and 30 ml vials. Selenium is available in 10 and 30 ml vials; and zinc is available in 5, 10, 30, and 50 ml vials. As ordered, dilute for infusion in the appropriate TPN solution.

Store at room temperature and avoid excessive heat. Don't use unless solution is clear and seal is intact. Discard unused portion within 24 hours after opening vial.

ADMINISTRATION
Direct injection: not recommended.
Intermittent infusion: not recommended.
Continuous infusion: Administer diluted solution through a patent I.V. line over the ordered duration.

INCOMPATIBILITY
No incompatibilities reported.

ADVERSE REACTIONS
All adverse reactions are signs of overdose.
Life-threatening: severe overdose.
Other: CNS damage, nausea, renal and hepatic damage, ulcers, vomiting (chromium); behavior changes, diarrhea, hypotonia, marasmus, peripheral edema, photophobia, prostration (copper); alopecia, dental defects, depression, dermatitis, garlic odor of breath and sweat, GI disorders, metallic taste, nervousness, vomiting, weakened nails (selenium); abdominal pain, dehydration, dizziness, electrolyte imbalance, incoordination, lethargy, nausea, vomiting (zinc).

INTERACTIONS
None reported.

EFFECTS ON DIAGNOSTIC TESTS
Serum chromium, copper, manganese, selenium, zinc: possible increased levels.

SPECIAL CONSIDERATIONS
• Monitor serum levels of trace elements. Use results to guide further administration, especially with high maintenance dosage.
• Don't give by direct I.V. injection (or by I.M. injection) because the solution's acidic pH (approximately 2.0) may irritate tissues.
• Watch for signs of toxicity. Calcium supplements may protect against zinc toxicity. D-penicillamine is the antidote for copper toxicity. Signs and symptoms of zinc toxicity include fever, nausea and vomiting, and diarrhea. Signs and symptoms of copper toxicity include nausea and vomiting, intestinal cramps, diarrhea, intravascular hemolysis, and renal impairment.
• Manganese toxicity is rare but may cause symptoms resembling Parkinson's disease.
• Copper deficiency in adults during total parenteral nutrition (TPN) therapy may cause anemia, leukopenia, and neutropenia.
• Signs and symptoms of chromium deficiency include weight loss, hyperglycemia, abnormal glucose tolerance, and a diabetes-like peripheral neuropathy.
• Signs and symptoms of selenium deficiency include severe muscle pain, thigh tenderness, and cardiomyopathy.

trimethaphan camsylate
Arfonad♦

Pregnancy Risk Category: C

PHARMACOKINETICS
Distribution: widespread. Drug crosses the placenta.
Metabolism: possibly metabolized by pseudocholinesterase.
Excretion: unchanged in urine. Not known if drug appears in breast milk.
Action: onset, immediate; duration, 10 to 15 minutes.

MECHANISM OF ACTION
This ganglionic blocker prevents stimulation of postsynaptic receptors by acetylcholine. It lowers blood pressure by causing peripheral vasodilation and reduced sympathetic tone.

INDICATIONS & DOSAGE
• Induction and control of hypotension during surgery (particularly vascular surgery and neurosurgery) to control bleeding. *Adults:* 3 to 4 mg/minute, then adjusted to maintain desired blood pressure. *Children:* 100 mcg/minute, then adjusted to maintain desired blood pressure.
• Rapid reduction of blood pressure in hypertensive crisis, particularly with acute dissecting aneurysm. *Adults:* 1 to 2 mg/minute initially, then p.r.n. to maintain systolic pressure of 100 to 120 mm Hg. *Children:* 100 mcg/minute, then p.r.n. to maintain desired blood pressure.
• Malignant hypertension. *Adults:* 0.5 to 1 mg/minute, gradually increased until desired blood pressure is achieved.

CONTRAINDICATIONS & CAUTIONS
• Contraindicated in anemia, asphyxia, cerebrovascular or coronary insufficiency, glaucoma, hypovolemia, and shock because of risk of hypoxia to vital organs.
• Also contraindicated in respiratory insufficiency because of risk of aggravating hypoxemia and in glaucoma because drug may precipitate glaucoma attack.
• During pregnancy, avoid use because induced hypotension may adversely affect the fetus.
• Use cautiously in hepatic or renal impairment because of reduced metabolism or excretion.
• Also use cautiously in Addison's disease and allergies because histamine-like reaction may occur along vein used for administration.
• Manufacturer recommends cautious use in patients with degenerative CNS disease or diabetes mellitus, in elderly or debilitated patients, and in patients receiving corticosteroids.

PREPARATION & STORAGE
Supplied in 10 ml ampules containing 50 mg/ml. Dilute for infusion with 500 ml of dextrose 5% in water to yield 1 mg/ml. Store ampules at 36° to 46° F. (2° to 8° C.).

After preparation, solution is stable for 24 hours at room temperature. Prepare fresh solution for each use, discarding any unused solution.

ADMINISTRATION
Direct injection: not recommended.
Intermittent infusion: not recommended.
Continuous infusion: Administer ordered dose with an infusion pump through a peripheral or a central line.

INCOMPATIBILITY

Incompatible with alkaline solutions, bromides, gallamine thiethiodide, iodides, thiopental, and tubocurarine. Manufacturer recommends against mixing with any other drug.

ADVERSE REACTIONS

Life-threatening: hypotension, respiratory arrest.
Other: angina, anorexia, blurred vision, cerebral ischemia, constipation, cycloplegia, dry mouth, impotence, mydriasis, nausea, orthostatic hypotension, paralytic ileus, pruritus, tachycardia, urine retention, urticaria, vomiting.

INTERACTIONS

Ambenonium, neostigmine, pyridostigmine: depressed antimyasthenic effects.
Anesthetics (especially spinal anesthetics): increased risk of cardiovascular collapse, severe hypotension, and shock.
Antibiotics, sulfonamides (in patients with pyelonephritis): concurrent use not advised.
Antihypertensives, diuretics, procainamide: enhanced hypotensive effects.
Neuromuscular blockers: possible increased effects.
NSAIDs: possible antagonized antihypertensive effects.
Sympathomimetics: heightened pressor response.

EFFECTS ON DIAGNOSTIC TESTS

Serum glucose: altered levels.
Serum potassium: possible decreased levels.

SPECIAL CONSIDERATIONS

• *Treatment of overdose:* Reduce dose or stop administration, as ordered. If needed, give vasopressors, phenylephrine, or mephenteramine.

Norepinephrine may be used if these drugs are ineffective.
• Monitor blood pressure every 2 minutes until stable, and monitor vital signs constantly during infusion. If catheter is in place, monitor central venous pressure.
• Assess frequently for respiratory distress, and position patient to avoid cerebral anoxia (elevate head of bed not more than 30 degrees). Provide oxygen as needed.
• Pseudotolerance may occur. Can be prevented by using a diuretic.

tromethamine
Tham, Tham-E

Pregnancy Risk Category: C

PHARMACOKINETICS

Distribution: widespread. Not known if drug crosses the placenta.
Metabolism: not appreciably metabolized.
Excretion: by kidneys. Not known if drug appears in breast milk.
Action: onset, immediately after administration; duration, 8 hours.

MECHANISM OF ACTION

Tromethamine combines with hydrogen ions from carbonic, lactic, and other metabolic acids, neutralizing acids within intracellular fluid. It increases blood pH and decreases CO_2 concentration.

INDICATIONS & DOSAGE

• Correction of metabolic acidosis resulting from cardiac arrest or cardiopulmonary bypass surgery.
Adults: Dosage depends on bicarbonate deficit. When using Tham without electrolytes, required ml of 0.3 M tromethamine solution is equivalent to weight (kg) multiplied by bicarbonate deficit (mEq/liter) then

multiplied by 1.1. When giving Tham-E, apply same formula but don't include the final step of multiplying by 1.1. Total dose for Tham or Tham-E shouldn't exceed 500 mg/kg. Average dose is 9 ml/kg or a single dose of 500 ml (150 mEq). For severe acidosis, up to 1,000 ml of solution may be given. *Children:* dosage calculated as for adults, not exceeding 40 ml/kg.

• Reduction of excess acidity in acid citrate-dextrose stored blood before transfusion. *Adults:* up to 70 ml solution added to each 500 ml unit of blood. *Children:* about 5 ml solution added to each 50 ml of blood. Usually, 55 ml (2 g) added to 500 ml of blood is adequate.

CONTRAINDICATIONS & CAUTIONS

• Contraindicated in uremia or anuria because of the risk of drug accumulation.

• Also contraindicated in chronic respiratory acidosis because drug may depress respiratory drive and exaggerate hypoxia.

• Don't use drug for more than 1 day, except in life-threatening situations.

• Use cautiously in renal dysfunction because of the risk of severe hyperkalemia.

PREPARATION & STORAGE

Supplied in 500 ml (150 mEq) single-dose containers. Use undiluted (after cardiac arrest) or dilute in required volume of blood (during bypass surgery or for transfusion). Solution concentration shouldn't exceed 0.3 M. Protect from heat and freezing, and discard unused solution within 24 hours.

ADMINISTRATION

Direct injection: not recommended.

Intermittent infusion: Administer over 1 hour (not exceeding 5 ml/minute) through an 18G needle into a central line or an antecubital vein. Use an infusion pump if possible. In children, infuse over 6 hours.

When infusing peripherally, use largest possible vein to avoid extravasation. If extravasation occurs, infiltrate area with 1% procaine and 150 units of hyaluronidase to reduce venospasm and dilute drug.

Continuous infusion: not recommended.

INCOMPATIBILITY

No incompatibilities reported.

ADVERSE REACTIONS

Life-threatening: respiratory depression.

Other: hemorrhagic liver necrosis, hyperkalemia, inflammation, I.V. thrombosis, necrosis and sloughing (with extravasation), phlebitis, prolonged hypoglycemia, venospasm.

INTERACTIONS

None significant.

EFFECTS ON DIAGNOSTIC TESTS

Serum glucose: transient depressed levels.

Serum potassium: possible elevated levels in renal impairment.

SPECIAL CONSIDERATIONS

• Assess respiratory function during and after therapy, and keep a mechanical ventilator nearby.

• Monitor ABGs and serum glucose and electrolyte levels before, during, and after therapy.

• In renal disease, monitor serum potassium closely and place patient on cardiac telemetry.

• Drug not recommended by American Heart Association for cardiac arrest.

• May be used investigationally to treat increased CSF pressure.

tubocurarine chloride (curare, d-tubocurarine chloride)
Tubarine♦

Pregnancy Risk Category: C

PHARMACOKINETICS
Distribution: throughout the body. Drug crosses the placenta. It's about 40% to 50% protein-bound.
Metabolism: minimal (1% metabolized by liver). Drug may saturate tissues and be stored for up to 24 hours after last dose.
Excretion: 38% to 75% excreted unchanged in urine within 24 hours; 12% removed unchanged in bile (40% in renal failure). Metabolite also excreted in urine. Not known if drug appears in breast milk.
Action: onset, within 1 minute; duration, 50 to 75 minutes.

MECHANISM OF ACTION
Combines with cholinergic (nicotinic) receptor sites at neuromuscular postjunctional membranes, competitively blocking depolarization of acetylcholine. Flaccid paralysis results from lack of muscle depolarization.

INDICATIONS & DOSAGE
• Adjunct to general anesthesia.
Adults: 6 to 9 mg, then 3 to 4.5 mg in 3 to 5 minutes if needed. Additional doses may be given during long procedures. *Infants and children:* 0.5 mg/kg. *Neonates up to 4 weeks:* 0.25 to 0.5 mg/kg initially, then subsequent doses of one-fifth to one-sixth initial dose.
• Aid to mechanical ventilation.
Adults: 0.0165 mg/kg; subsequent dosage determined by response.

• Diagnosis of myasthenia gravis.
Adults: 0.004 to 0.033 mg/kg as a single dose.

CONTRAINDICATIONS & CAUTIONS
• Contraindicated in conscious patients and in those hypersensitive to tubocurarine.
• Use cautiously in asthma-like respiratory conditions, bronchogenic carcinoma, and myasthenia gravis because of possible enhanced neuromuscular blockade.
• Also use cautiously in cardiovascular impairment because of potentiated cardiovascular effects and in conditions in which histamine release would be hazardous.
• Give cautiously in dehydration, endocrine imbalance, or electrolyte imbalance because of possible altered drug action.
• In hepatic failure and hyperthermia, use cautiously because of possible reduced drug effects. In hypothermia, also use cautiously because of increased drug effects.
• In hypotension, administer carefully because drug may exacerbate this condition.
• Use cautiously in pulmonary impairment and respiratory depression. Tubocurarine may deepen respiratory depression.
• In renal failure and shock, drug effects may be prolonged. Give cautiously.
• In severe obesity or neuromuscular disease, also use cautiously because of possible airway or ventilation problems.
• Use cautiously in breastfeeding women.

PREPARATION & STORAGE
Supplied in 10 ml multidose vials containing 3 mg (20 units)/ml. Store at room temperature, avoiding exces-

sive heat and freezing. Don't use if solution is discolored.

ADMINISTRATION
Tubocurarine should be given only by staff trained to administer anesthetics and to manage their adverse effects.

Direct injection: Give ordered dose over 1 to 1½ minutes. Give subsequent doses, usually 20% to 25% of initial dose, at 40- to 60-minute intervals. Lengthen intervals, as ordered, in elderly or debilitated patients.

Intermittent infusion: not recommended.

Continuous infusion: not recommended.

INCOMPATIBILITY
Incompatible with alkaline solutions, including barbiturates, sodium bicarbonate, and other drugs with high pH. Also incompatible with trimethaphan camsylate.

ADVERSE REACTIONS
Life-threatening: anaphylaxis, bronchospasm, cardiac arrest, circulatory collapse, respiratory depression, severe bradycardia, severe hypotension. Life-threatening reactions more common in premature infants and neonates.

Other: bradycardia, decreased GI motility and tone, edema, erythema, flushing, hypotension, rash, tachycardia.

INTERACTIONS
Amphotericin B, calcium salts, diazepam, lithium, magnesium sulfate, methotrimeprazine: possible prolonged neuromuscular effects.

Antibiotics: possible potentiated neuromuscular blockade.

Antimyasthenics, edrophonium: antagonized effects.

Beta-adrenergic blockers: possible enhanced or prolonged neuromuscular blockade.

Doxapram: possible masking of tubocurarine's residual effects.

Halogenated anesthetics: increased neuromuscular blockage.

Lidocaine or trimethaphan (high doses), MAO inhibitors, propranolol, quinidine salts, thiazide diuretics: possible prolonged neuromuscular effects.

Opioid analgesics: additive respiratory depression.

EFFECTS ON DIAGNOSTIC TESTS
Urine catecholamines: altered levels with fluorometric assessment.

SPECIAL CONSIDERATIONS
• *Treatment of overdose:* In early signs of paralysis (inability to keep eyelids open and eyes focused, or difficulty swallowing or speaking), notify doctor immediately. Give neostigmine or edrophonium, as ordered, to reverse the drug's effects, and provide supportive, symptomatic treatment.

• When administering tubocurarine, keep patient's airway clear and have resuscitation equipment and cholinergic antagonists, such as neostigmine or pyridostigmine, available.

• Check vital signs every 15 minutes, and notify the doctor at once of any change.

• Tubocurarine dosage is usually decreased by one-third when given with halogenated anesthetics.

• Allow succinylcholine effects to subside before giving tubocurarine.

• Monitor baseline electrolyte levels; electrolyte imbalance can potentiate neuromuscular effects. Also monitor intake and output because renal dysfunction prolongs duration of action.

• Check for bowel sounds because peristaltic action may be suppressed.

- Drug does not affect consciousness or relieve pain. Assess patient's need for analgesic or sedative.
- May contain sulfites.

urea (carbamide)
Ureaphil

Pregnancy Risk Category: C

PHARMACOKINETICS
Distribution: into extracellular and intracellular fluids, including lymph, blood, bile, and CSF. Highest concentration is in kidneys. Drug crosses the placenta and reaches the eye.
Metabolism: partially metabolized in GI tract (despite I.V. administration) by hydrolysis to ammonia and carbon dioxide. Bacterial urease resynthesizes metabolites into urea.
Excretion: by kidneys, with about 50% reabsorption. Drug probably appears in breast milk.
Action: onset, 10 minutes after start of infusion; duration, 3 to 10 hours after infusion for reduction of increased intracranial pressure and diuresis, or 5 to 6 hours for reduction of intraocular pressure.

MECHANISM OF ACTION
Produces osmotic diuresis by elevating the glomerular filtrate's osmotic pressure, hindering renal tubular reabsorption of water and solutes. Urea also elevates plasma osmolality, which enhances water flow from tissues, including the brain and eyes.

INDICATIONS & DOSAGE
- Reduction of intracranial or intraocular pressure. *Adults:* 0.5 to 1.5 g/kg infused over 30 minutes to 2 hours. *Children over 2 years:* 0.5 to 1.5 g/kg or 35 g/m² infused over 24 hours. *Children under 2 years:* 0.1

g/kg infused over 30 minutes to 2 hours.
- Rapid correction of hyponatremia in syndrome of inappropriate ADH secretion. *Adults:* 80 g infused over 6 hours.

CONTRAINDICATIONS & CAUTIONS
- Contraindicated in renal impairment and marked dehydration because of increased risk of circulatory overload and in severe hepatic impairment because of elevated serum ammonia levels.
- Also contraindicated in intracranial bleeding, except when used preoperatively for surgical control of hemorrhage, because reduction of brain edema may increase bleeding.
- Avoid use in sickle cell disease with signs of CNS involvement.
- Don't use solutions prepared with invert sugar in fructose intolerance.
- Use cautiously in cardiac disease or cardiovascular impairment because of the risk of congestive heart failure and pulmonary edema.
- Also use cautiously in hypovolemia because drug may mask symptoms.

PREPARATION & STORAGE
Supplied as a powder in 40 g vials. Add 105 ml of dextrose 5% or 10% in water or 10% invert sugar injection (unless the patient is fructose intolerant) to the 40 g vial for a solution of 30% concentration (300 mg/ml). Warm diluent to 122° F. (50° C.) to dissolve urea; cool before administration. Each dose of urea should be freshly prepared.

Before reconstitution, store drug at room temperature. Protect from heat and freezing. Use powdered drug only if seal is intact and container is undamaged, and administer solution only if it's clear and free from particles and discoloration.

Unmarked trade names available in the United States only.
♦ Also available in Canada.   ♦ ♦ Available in Canada only.

ADMINISTRATION
Direct injection: not recommended.
Intermittent infusion: Infuse diluted dose into a large vein but not into leg veins (especially in elderly patients) because of risk of phlebitis and thrombosis of superficial and deep veins. Avoid extravasation.

Infuse at prescribed rate for adults and children. Don't exceed dosage of 1.5 g/kg or 120 g/24 hours, or a rate of 4 to 6 ml (30% solution)/minute. Avoid rapid infusion, which can cause hemolysis and cerebral vasomotor symptoms.

When used preoperatively, start infusion 60 minutes before ocular surgery or at the time of scalp incision for intracranial surgery.
Continuous infusion: not recommended.

INCOMPATIBILITY
Incompatible with blood.

ADVERSE REACTIONS
Life-threatening: congestive heart failure, pulmonary edema.
Other: arterial oozing and bleeding, blurred vision, confusion, dizziness, dry mouth, faintness, fever, headache, hemolysis, hypokalemia, hyponatremia, irregular heartbeat, muscle cramps, nausea, nervousness, numbness in hands or feet, redness or swelling and pain at injection site, seizures, tachycardia, thrombosis, tiredness or weakness in legs, trembling, vomiting.

INTERACTIONS
Diuretics: possible potentiated effects.
Lithium: increased excretion. Observe patient closely.

EFFECTS ON DIAGNOSTIC TESTS
BUN: elevated levels.
Serum potassium, sodium: decreased levels.

SPECIAL CONSIDERATIONS
• Monitor blood pressure, intake and output, and serum electrolyte and BUN levels before and after administration. Also check injection site for phlebitis.
• If BUN levels are 75 to 100 mg, or if diuresis doesn't occur within 1 to 2 hours, reduce dosage or withhold drug, as ordered, until the patient can be reevaluated and renal function reassessed.
• Watch for signs of hyponatremia or hypokalemia (muscle weakness, lethargy).
• In comatose patients, insert an indwelling catheter. Use an hourly urometer collection bag to evaluate diuresis.
• Blood replacement should be adequate during urea administration.
• Stay alert for rebound intraocular and intracranial pressure elevation, which may occur 12 hours after administration.
• Urea has been used to manage acute sickle cell crisis and to help remove toxins, such as meprobamate and some barbiturates.

urokinase
Abbokinase, Abbokinase Open-Cath

Pregnancy Risk Category: B

PHARMACOKINETICS
Distribution: in plasma. Not known if drug crosses the placenta.
Metabolism: rapidly cleared in liver.
Excretion: small fractions excreted in bile and urine. Half-life is 10 to 20 minutes but may be longer in hepatic dysfunction. Not known if drug appears in breast milk.
Action: onset, immediately upon administration; duration, 12 to 24 hours.

MECHANISM OF ACTION
Promotes thrombolysis by converting plasminogen to the fibrinolytic enzyme plasmin.

INDICATIONS & DOSAGE
• Pulmonary embolism. *Adults:* 4,400 IU/kg initially by infusion, then continuous infusion of 4,400 IU/kg/hour for 12 hours.
• Venous catheter occlusion. *Adults:* 1 ml of 5,000 IU/ml solution for each clearing procedure.

CONTRAINDICATIONS & CAUTIONS
• Contraindicated in active internal bleeding; within 2 months of cerebrovascular accident, intracranial neoplasm, or intracranial or intraspinal surgery; within 10 days of major surgery, severe GI bleeding, organ biopsy, obstetric delivery, or puncture of noncompressible vessels; in severe uncontrolled hypertension; and in recent serious trauma. Thrombolytic therapy increases risk of bleeding.
• Also contraindicated in recent minor trauma (including CPR) because bleeding may occur; in high risk of left heart thrombus, pregnancy, and infectious endocarditis because of risk of systemic infection; and in cerebrovascular disease, diabetic hemorrhagic retinopathy, and hemostatic defects (including those associated with severe renal or hepatic disease) because bleeding would be difficult to control.
• Use with extreme caution in any condition in which bleeding would be hazardous or especially difficult to manage.
• Use cautiously in atrial fibrillation or other conditions with risk of cerebral embolism because of risk of bleeding into the infarcted area.
• Safe use in children hasn't been established.

PREPARATION & STORAGE
Supplied as lyophilized white powder in vials containing 250,000 units. Reconstitute with 5.2 ml of sterile water for injection (without preservatives) for a solution of 50,000 IU/ml. Don't use bacteriostatic water; it contains preservatives. Dilute solution further with 0.9% sodium chloride or dextrose 5% in water. Total volume administered shouldn't exceed 200 ml.

Reconstituted solution should be clear, practically colorless, and without particulate matter. To avoid filament formation, roll and tilt vial during reconstitution; avoid shaking. Solution may be filtered through a 0.45-micron or smaller cellulose filter.

Refrigerate vials at 35° to 47° F. (2° to 8° C.). Because urokinase contains no preservatives, reconstitute immediately before use and discard unused portion. Don't use highly colored solutions, and don't add other drugs to the solution.

ADMINISTRATION
Direct injection: To clear a venous catheter occlusion, slowly inject solution into occluded line, wait 5 minutes, then aspirate. Repeat aspiration attempts q 5 minutes for 30 minutes. If not patent after 30 minutes, cap line and let urokinase work for 30 to 60 minutes before aspirating. May require second injection.
Intermittent infusion: not recommended.
Continuous infusion: Administer initial dose of diluted solution over 10 minutes, using an infusion pump. Infuse subsequent doses, as ordered, over 12 hours.

INCOMPATIBILITY
No incompatibilities reported; however, manufacturer recommends that urokinase not be mixed with any other drugs.

Unmarked trade names available in the United States only.
♦ Also available in Canada.　　♦♦ Available in Canada only.

ADVERSE REACTIONS

Life-threatening: anaphylaxis, hemorrhage.
Other: bronchospasm, decreased hematocrit, dysrhythmias, fever, rash, superficial or surface hemorrhage.

INTERACTIONS

Anticoagulants: increased risk of hemorrhage.
Antifibrinolytic drugs (aminocaproic acid): inhibited action of urokinase.
Azlocillin, carbenicillin, dextran, ethacrynic acid, mezlocillin, moxalactam, piperacillin, sulfinpyrazone, ticarcillin, other drugs affecting platelet function: increased risk of hemorrhage because of altered platelet function.
Corticosteroids, dipyridamole, indomethacin, phenylbutazone, salicylates: enhanced risk of hemorrhage because of altered platelet function.
Thiethylene thiophosphoramide: increased efficacy in bladder cancer.

EFFECTS ON DIAGNOSTIC TESTS

Fibrin split products: elevated levels.
Hematocrit: decreased.
Plasma fibrinogen, plasminogen: reduced levels.
Thrombin time: prolonged.

SPECIAL CONSIDERATIONS

• *Treatment of overdose:* In hemorrhage, stop drug immediately. Give plasma volume expanders (other than dextrans) to replace volume deficits. For severe blood loss, give packed RBCs (rather than whole blood). For rapid reversal of hyperfibrinolysis, possibly give aminocaproic acid (efficacy isn't established).
• Monitor for bleeding every 15 minutes for the first hour, every 30 minutes for the next 7 hours, and then once each shift.

• Monitor vital signs. Also monitor pulses, color, and sensitivity of extremities every hour.
• Have typed and crossmatched RBCs and whole blood available to treat hemorrhage.
• Assess percutaneous puncture sites and cuts for oozing and for bruising or hematoma formation because urokinase may lyse fibrin deposits.
• Maintain alignment of involved extremity to prevent bleeding at infusion site.
• Avoid I.M. injections, unnecessary handling of the patient, and arterial invasive procedures. If an arterial puncture is necessary, use an upper extremity, apply pressure at site for 30 minutes, and apply a pressure dressing. Check site frequently for bleeding. Also avoid venipuncture or perform as infrequently as possible.
• Follow with heparin, usually within 1 hour after discontinuation of urokinase, to prevent recurrent thrombosis.
• Keep in mind that hematocrit, plasma fibrinogen, and plasminogen levels may decrease for 12 to 24 hours after therapy stops. Fibrin split products increase similarly. Monitor these levels.
• Watch for signs of hypersensitivity and have corticosteroids available to treat allergic reactions.
• Instruct the patient to report symptoms of bleeding.

vancomycin hydrochloride
Diatracin◆◆, Vancocin, Vancoled

Pregnancy Risk Category: C

PHARMACOKINETICS
Distribution: extensive, with therapeutic levels in serum, urine, atrial appendage tissue, and in pleural, pericardial, ascitic, and synovial fluids. Low concentrations appear in bile. Drug is 52% to 60% protein-bound, and with meningeal irritation, has some diffusion into the CSF. Drug crosses the placenta.
Metabolism: usually not metabolized; some hepatic metabolism possible.
Excretion: eliminated in urine by glomerular filtration, with 80% to 90% excreted unchanged within 24 hours. Small amounts are excreted in feces. Half-life in adults is 4 to 11 hours; in children, 2 to 3 hours; in infants, 4 to 10 hours. Half-life extends to 6 to 10 days in renal impairment. Not known if drug appears in breast milk.
Action: onset, immediate; peak effect, immediately after infusion.

MECHANISM OF ACTION
A narrow-spectrum tricyclic glycopeptide antibiotic with bactericidal action, vancomycin inhibits cell wall biosynthesis, selectively inhibits RNA, and alters bacterial cytoplasmic membrane permeability.

Susceptible organisms include *Clostridium, C. difficile, Corynebacterium,* enterococci, staphylococci (including methicillin-resistant *S. aureus*), *Streptococcus pneumoniae,* and group A beta-hemolytic streptococci.

INDICATIONS & DOSAGE
• Severe systemic infections caused by susceptible organisms when less toxic drugs are ineffective. *Adults:* 500 mg q 6 hours or 1 g q 12 hours. *Children over 1 month:* 40 mg/kg daily in divided doses. *Neonates:* 15 mg/kg initially, then 10 mg/kg q 8 hours (older than 8 days) or 10 mg/kg q 12 hours (8 days or younger).
• Prophylaxis for bacterial endocarditis in penicillin-allergic patients undergoing dental procedures or upper respiratory tract procedures. *Adults:* 1 g 30 to 60 minutes before procedure, followed by oral erythromycin. *Children:* 20 mg/kg 30 to 60 minutes before procedure, followed by oral erythromycin.
• Prophylaxis for bacterial endocarditis in penicillin-allergic patients undergoing GI or GU procedures. *Adults:* 1 g 30 to 60 minutes before procedure in combination with gentamicin. *Children:* 20 mg/kg 30 to 60 minutes before procedure in combination with gentamicin.
Note: Adjust dosage in patients with renal impairment. Initial dose is at least 15 mg/kg, even with moderate to severe renal insufficiency. Subsequent dosage is guided by creatinine clearance and serum levels of vancomycin. The following serves as an estimate:
Daily dosage is 1,545 mg for creatinine clearance rate of 100 ml/min; 1,390 mg for rate of 90 ml/min; 1,235 mg for rate of 80 ml/min; 1,080 mg for rate of 70 ml/min; 925 mg for rate of 60 ml/min; 770 mg for rate of 50 ml/min; 620 mg for rate of 40 ml/min; 465 mg for rate of 30 ml/min; 310 mg for rate of 20 ml/min; and 155 mg for rate of 10 ml/min.

For anephric patients on dialysis, initial dose is 15 mg/kg, followed by 1.9 mg/kg/24 hours or maintenance doses of 250 to 1,000 mg every few days.

CONTRAINDICATIONS & CAUTIONS

• Contraindicated in vancomycin hypersensitivity.
• Use cautiously in severe renal insufficiency because of the risk of nephrotoxicity.
• Use cautiously in elderly patients because renal function may decline.
• Use cautiously in premature neonates and young infants because of renal immaturity.
• In hearing loss, use cautiously because of the risk of ototoxicity.
• Administer cautiously in intestinal obstruction because of the increased risk of toxicity.
• Give cautiously in pregnancy because of the risk of fetal cranial nerve VIII damage.

PREPARATION & STORAGE

Available as an off-white to buff powder in 500 mg vials. Reconstitute with 10 ml of sterile water for injection for an average concentration of 50 mg/ml. Reconstituted solution is clear and light yellow to light brown. Before administration, dilute in 100 to 200 ml of dextrose 5% in water or 0.9% sodium chloride. For continuous infusion, dilute 1 to 2 g in the ordered volume for 24 hours. Inspect before administration for particulate matter or discoloration.

Before reconstitution, store vials at room temperature. Reconstituted solutions may be refrigerated for 14 days. When diluted, solutions are stable for 24 hours at room temperature.

ADMINISTRATION

Direct injection: not recommended.
Intermittent infusion: Infuse diluted dose over at least 60 minutes to reduce risk of local reactions and "red-neck" syndrome.
Continuous infusion: Use only when intermittent infusion isn't feasible. Add ordered dose to compatible solution and give by I.V. drip over 24 hours.

INCOMPATIBILITY

Incompatible with adrenosteroids, alkaline solutions, aminophylline, amobarbital sodium, chloramphenicol, chlorothiazide, heavy metals, heparin, methicillin sodium, pentobarbital, phenobarbital, secobarbital sodium, and sodium bicarbonate.

ADVERSE REACTIONS

Life-threatening: anaphylaxis, cardiac arrest, hypotension, Stevens-Johnson syndrome.
Other: anorexia, bacterial and fungal superinfection, drowsiness, eosinophilia, infusion site reaction (pain, thrombophlebitis), nausea, nephrotoxicity, ototoxicity, rash, "red-neck" syndrome (rapid infusion–related reactions including chills, dyspnea, erythematous macular rash and flushing of upper body, fever, hypotension, pain and muscle spasm of chest and back, pruritus, tachycardia, tingling, urticaria, wheezing), reversible neutropenia, thrombocytopenia.

INTERACTIONS

Aminoglycosides, amphotericin B, bacitracin, capreomycin, colistin, cyclosporin, paromomycin, polymyxin, streptozocin: enhanced ototoxicity and nephrotoxicity.
Anesthetics: increased frequency of infusion-related reactions (in children, erythema and flushing).
Antihistamines, buclizine, cyclizine, meclizine, phenothiazines, thioxanthenes, trimethobenzamide: possible masking of ototoxicity.

Bumetanide, carmustine, cisplatin, ethacrynic acid, furosemide, salicylates: enhanced ototoxicity and nephrotoxicity.

EFFECTS ON DIAGNOSTIC TESTS
BUN: possible increased levels.
CBC: eosinophilia, neutropenia, thrombocytopenia.
Serum creatinine: possible elevated levels.
Urinalysis: with nephrotoxicity, decreased specific gravity, increased protein excretion, hematuria, presence of cells or casts.

SPECIAL CONSIDERATIONS
• *Treatment of overdose:* Hemoperfusion with Amberlite XAD-4 resin may have limited value. Provide supportive and symptomatic treatment.
• Obtain specimens for culture and sensitivity tests before first dose. Therapy may begin before results are available (unless drug is being used for prophylaxis).
• When used preoperatively, give 60-minute infusion before anesthetic induction to reduce risk of infusion-related reactions.
• Watch for superinfection caused by nonsusceptible organisms.
• If "red-neck" syndrome occurs, stop infusion and notify doctor. Treat symptomatically; syndrome usually resolves within 20 minutes but may continue for several hours.
• Monitor vital signs, especially blood pressure. Check blood pressure every 5 to 10 minutes during initial therapy. Change I.V. sites frequently to help avoid extravasation.
• Obtain periodic WBC counts in prolonged therapy or with concurrent administration of other drugs that may cause neutropenia.
• Monitor renal function (BUN and serum creatinine levels, creatinine

clearance, urinalysis, output) and auditory function (audiograms, signs of ototoxicity), especially in high-risk patients.
• Also monitor serum vancomycin levels in high-risk patients. Adjust dosage or frequency, if necessary. Coordinate blood sampling and vancomycin administration with the laboratory. Obtain trough samples before next dose; obtain peak samples ½ hour after infusion. Therapeutic peak serum levels are 30 to 40 mcg/ml; trough levels are 5 to 10 mcg/ml.
• When drug is used to treat staphylococcal endocarditis, therapy should continue for at least 4 weeks.
• Drug is minimally removed (less than 30%) by peritoneal dialysis and not removed by hemodialysis. Patients receiving these treatments require usual dose only once every 5 to 7 days.

vecuronium bromide
Norcuron

Pregnancy Risk Category: C

PHARMACOKINETICS
Distribution: in extracellular fluid; rapidly reaches its site of action. 60% to 90% bound to plasma proteins. Volume of distribution is decreased in children under age 1 and may be decreased in elderly patients. Vecuronium minimally crosses the placenta.
Metabolism: in liver; rapidly and extensively metabolized. One metabolite, 3-diacetyl vecuronium, produces neuromuscular blockade and is 50% as potent as vecuronium.
Excretion: Vecuronium and its metabolites appear to be primarily excreted in feces; drug and its metabolites are also excreted in

urine. Not known if drug appears in breast milk.

Action: onset, 2½ to 3 minutes; duration, 25 to 40 minutes, depending on anesthetic used, dose, and number of doses given.

MECHANISM OF ACTION

This drug exerts skeletal muscle relaxant action by competing with acetylcholine for cholinergic receptors at the motor end plate, thus blocking depolarization.

INDICATIONS & DOSAGE

• Adjunct to general anesthesia, to facilitate endotracheal intubation and to provide skeletal muscle relaxation during surgery or mechanical ventilation. Dose depends on anesthetic used, individual needs, and response. Doses are representative and must be adjusted. *Adults:* 0.08 to 0.1 mg/kg initially. Maintenance dose 0.01 to 0.015 mg/kg 20 to 40 minutes after initial dose, then q 12 to 15 minutes p.r.n. *Children:* dosage individualized.

Note: Reduce dosage in patients with renal or hepatic impairment.

CONTRAINDICATIONS & CAUTIONS

• Contraindicated in hypersensitivity to vecuronium.

• Patients with bromide intolerance may also be sensitive to vecuronium.

• Use cautiously in neuromuscular diseases or bronchogenic carcinoma because of enhanced neuromuscular blockade.

• Also administer cautiously in elderly patients, debilitated patients, and in patients with cardiovascular impairment or edema because circulatory impairment may delay drug onset.

• In patients with electrolyte imbalance or dehydration, use cautiously because of altered neuromuscular blockade.

• Give cautiously in hepatic disease and renal failure because of prolonged neuromuscular blockade and prolonged recovery time.

• Also administer cautiously to patients with myasthenia gravis because of the profound effect of even small doses.

• In pulmonary impairment or respiratory depression, use cautiously because of deepened respiratory depression.

• In patients with severe obesity or neuromuscular disease, also use cautiously because of possible airway or ventilation problems.

PREPARATION & STORAGE

Supplied as a sterile, nonpyrogenic, freeze-dried buffered cake composed of fine crystalline particles. Available in 5 and 10 ml vials containing 10 mg drug and diluent. For infusion, dilute further by adding 10 ml of reconstituted drug to 100 ml of dextrose 5% in water, 0.9% sodium chloride, dextrose 5% in 0.9% or 0.45% sodium chloride, or dextrose 5% in Ringer's lactate. Vecuronium is compatible with all I.V. solutions.

Before reconstitution, store at room temperature and protect from light. After reconstitution with bacteriostatic water, use within 24 hours; with other solutions, use within 8 hours.

ADMINISTRATION

Vecuronium should be administered only by staff trained to give anesthetics and to manage their adverse effects.

Direct injection: Inject dose directly into tubing of an I.V. line containing a free-flowing compatible solution.

Intermittent infusion: not recommended.

Continuous infusion: Begin infusion 20 to 40 minutes after initial dose by direct injection. Determine rates by carefully observing neuromuscular blockade with a peripheral nerve stimulator. Infusion rates range from 0.008 to 0.012 ml/kg/minute with a 1:10 dilution.

INCOMPATIBILITY
No incompatibilities reported.

ADVERSE REACTIONS
Life-threatening: apnea, respiratory insufficiency.
Other: local redness, transient changes in heart rate and blood pressure (may be related to endotracheal intubation).

INTERACTIONS
Aminoglycosides, bacitracin, colistimethate sodium, colistin, polymyxin B, tetracyclines: prolonged neuromuscular blockade.
Antimyasthenics, edrophonium: antagonized effects of these drugs and of vecuronium.
Calcium salts: reversal of neuromuscular blockade.
Doxapram: possible masking of vecuronium's residual effects.
Gallamine, metocurine, pancuronium, tubocurarine: enhanced neuromuscular blockade.
Inhalation anesthetics, magnesium salts (parenteral), procainamide, quinidine: enhanced neuromuscular blockade.
Opioid analgesics: additive respiratory depression.
Succinylcholine: heightened neuromuscular blockade and prolonged duration of action of vecuronium.

EFFECTS ON DIAGNOSTIC TESTS
None reported.

SPECIAL CONSIDERATIONS
• *Treatment of overdose:* Provide mechanical ventilation with endotracheal intubation until reversal of neuromuscular blockade is adequate. As ordered, reverse blockade with acetylcholinesterase inhibitors, such as neostigmine, pyridostigmine, or edrophonium given with atropine or glycopyrrolate.
• Keep in mind that infants are especially sensitive to drug effects. Recovery time may be 1½ times that of an adult.

---

verapamil hydrochloride
Calan, Isoptin♦

Pregnancy Risk Category: C

PHARMACOKINETICS
Distribution: approximately 90% bound to plasma proteins. Drug crosses the placenta and is also distributed into CSF.
Metabolism: rapidly and completely metabolized in the liver, to demethylated metabolites.
Excretion: in urine and feces; 16% excreted within 5 days. Half-life is biphasic: 4 minutes for first phase, 2 to 5 hours for second phase. Drug also appears in breast milk in concentrations similar to those in maternal serum.
Action: onset, 1 to 5 minutes; duration, about 2 hours (antiarrhythmic effects) or about 10 to 20 minutes (hemodynamic effects).

MECHANISM OF ACTION
This drug inhibits influx of extracellular calcium ions across the membranes of myocardial and vascular smooth muscle cells, without changing serum calcium concentrations. It reduces afterload and myocardial

---

contractility and also slows SA and AV node conduction.

INDICATIONS & DOSAGE

• Supraventricular tachydysrhythmias, vasospastic angina, and conversion of reentrant paroxysmal atrial tachycardia unresponsive to vagal stimulation. *Adults:* 5 to 10 mg. If response is inadequate, give 10 mg 30 minutes later. In renal or hepatic impairment, try to avoid second dose but, if necessary, reduce amount and give 60 to 90 minutes after initial dose. *Children 1 to 15 years:* 0.1 to 0.3 mg/kg, not exceeding 5 mg. May be repeated in 30 minutes, but don't exceed 10 mg as a single dose. *Children under 1 year:* 0.1 to 0.2 mg/kg.

CONTRAINDICATIONS & CAUTIONS

• Contraindicated in hypersensitivity to verapamil.
• Also contraindicated in second- or third-degree AV block because of excessive bradycardia; in severe hypotension, cardiogenic shock, or pulmonary wedge pressure greater than 20 mm Hg because drug may exacerbate these conditions; and in Wolff-Parkinson-White syndrome because drug may precipitate severe dysrhythmias.
• Use cautiously in children (particularly neonates) because effectiveness in children is unstudied.
• Also use cautiously in Duchenne-type muscular dystrophy because of the risk of respiratory paralysis.
• In extreme bradycardia or heart failure, give cautiously because of possible reduction of sinus or AV node activity.
• Also give cautiously in hypertrophic cardiomyopathy, moderate ventricular dysfunction, and sick sinus syndrome because drug may worsen symptoms, and in mild to moderate

hypotension because drug may exacerbate condition.
• In renal impairment and renal or hepatic failure, give cautiously because the risk of toxicity rises.

PREPARATION & STORAGE

Supplied as a solution of 2.5 mg/ml. Store at room temperature and protect from light and freezing. Drug is stable for 24 hours at 77° F. (25° C.) in most common infusion solutions when protected from light. It's compatible with dextrose 5% in water, 0.9% sodium chloride, and Ringer's lactate.

ADMINISTRATION

Direct injection: Administer undiluted drug at a rate of 5 to 10 mg over at least 2 minutes. Inject directly into vein or into an I.V. line containing a free-flowing compatible solution. In elderly patients, give over at least 3 minutes to reduce adverse effects.
Intermittent infusion: not recommended.
Continuous infusion: not recommended.

INCOMPATIBILITY

Incompatible with albumin, amphotericin B, co-trimoxazole, dobutamine, hydralazine, nafcillin, sodium bicarbonate, and trimethoprim.

ADVERSE REACTIONS

Life-threatening: asystole, severe pulmonary edema, ventricular fibrillation.
Other: alopecia, atrial fibrillation, blurred vision, bradycardia, congestive heart failure, constipation, depression, diaphoresis, dizziness, drowsiness, dry mouth, dyspnea, ecchymosis, first-degree AV block, headache, hypotension, muscle fatigue, nausea, peripheral edema, purpura, vertigo.

INTERACTIONS

Anticoagulants (oral), hydantoins, salicylates, sulfonamides, sulfonylureas: decreased effectiveness because of possible displacement from binding sites.
Antihypertensive drugs: possible additive effects.
Beta-adrenergic blockers: increased risk of congestive heart failure and AV block.
Carbamazepine, cyclosporine, prazosin, theophylline, valproate: elevated serum levels of these drugs and increased risk of toxicity.
Cimetidine: possible decreased verapamil clearance.
Dantrolene (I.V.): possible cardiovascular collapse.
Digoxin: increased serum levels.
Disopyramide: additive effects and possibly fatal impairment of left ventricular function.
Estrogens, NSAIDs, sympathomimetics: possible reduced antihypertensive effects of verapamil.
Lithium: decreased serum levels.
Metoprolol: increased bioavailability.
Quinidine: heightened hypotensive effects.

EFFECTS ON DIAGNOSTIC TESTS

EKG: possible prolonged PR interval.
SGOT, SGPT: possible transient increased levels.

SPECIAL CONSIDERATIONS

• *Treatment of overdose:* Provide supportive care. If ordered, give beta agonists and I.V. calcium salts.
• Monitor EKG and arrange for periodic liver function tests.
• Give lower verapamil doses to patients with severe cardiac impairment or those receiving beta blockers. Monitor closely.

• If giving digoxin concomitantly, reduce digoxin dose by half and monitor EKG for possible AV block.
• Notify the doctor if signs of congestive heart failure, such as dependent edema or dyspnea, develop.

vidarabine monohydrate (adenine arabinoside)
Vira-A

Pregnancy Risk Category: C

PHARMACOKINETICS

Distribution: dispersed throughout most tissues, including the CSF. With intact meninges, CSF levels reach 35% of serum levels. Only trace amounts appear in aqueous humor. Drug is 20% to 30% protein-bound and may cross the placenta.
Metabolism: in peripheral tissues, to an active metabolite.
Excretion: eliminated principally by the kidneys, with 1% to 3% removed unchanged within 24 hours. Plasma half-life is 1½ hours (3 hours in renal impairment).
Action: onset, immediately upon administration; duration, unknown.

MECHANISM OF ACTION

Incorporated into viral DNA, vidarabine inhibits viral multiplication.

INDICATIONS & DOSAGE

• Herpes simplex encephalitis.
Adults and children (including neonates): 15 mg/kg daily for 10 days.
• Herpes zoster. *Adults and children:* 10 mg/kg daily for 5 to 7 days.
Note: Dosage in renal impairment reflects creatinine clearance. In adult patients with a creatinine clearance below 10 ml/min, reduce dosage by at least 25%.

CONTRAINDICATIONS & CAUTIONS
- Contraindicated in hypersensitivity to vidarabine.
- Use cautiously in renal or hepatic impairment or existing cerebral edema (CNS tumors or infections) because of the increased risk of fluid overload or cerebral edema.

PREPARATION & STORAGE
Supplied as a solution in 200 mg/ml vials. Dilute with any I.V. solution except blood products or protein solutions. Each 1 mg of drug requires 2.2 ml of I.V. solution for complete stabilization. Prewarm solution to 95° to 104° F. (35° to 40° C.) to aid drug dispersion. Shake well for uniform suspension, and use a membrane filter (0.45 micron or smaller).

Store concentrated solutions at room temperature. Dilute just before or within 48 hours of administration.

ADMINISTRATION
Direct injection: not recommended.
Intermittent infusion: not recommended.
Continuous infusion: Using an infusion pump, slowly infuse the diluted daily dose over 12 to 24 hours.

INCOMPATIBILITY
Incompatible with blood products and colloidal fluids. Don't mix vidarabine with any other drug.

ADVERSE REACTIONS
Life-threatening: anaphylaxis.
Other: anorexia, ataxia, bone marrow depression with leukopenia and thrombocytopenia (doses higher than 20 mg/kg daily), confusion, diarrhea, dizziness, hallucinations, hematemesis, malaise, nausea, pain at infusion site, pruritus, psychosis, rash, tremors, vomiting, weight loss.

INTERACTIONS
Allopurinol: possible interference with vidarabine metabolism.

EFFECTS ON DIAGNOSTIC TESTS
Hematocrit, hemoglobin: possible decreased values.
Platelet, reticulocyte, WBC counts: reduced.
Serum bilirubin, SGOT: possible increased levels.

SPECIAL CONSIDERATIONS
- Drug is effective only in immunosuppressed patients.
- Vidarabine is usually a second choice to acyclovir in the treatment of herpes simplex encephalitis. There is no evidence that vidarabine is effective in encephalitis resulting from other viruses.
- Monitor hematologic tests during therapy because of the risk of bone marrow depression. Also monitor renal and liver function studies.
- If giving theophylline concomitantly, monitor serum theophylline levels for signs of toxicity.

---

vinblastine sulfate (VLB)
Velban, Velbe♦♦

Pregnancy Risk Category: D

PHARMACOKINETICS
Distribution: rapidly distributed throughout tissues and localized in platelets and WBCs. About 75% is bound to plasma proteins. Vinblastine penetrates the blood-brain barrier poorly and doesn't appear in CSF in therapeutic concentrations. It may cross the placenta.
Metabolism: extensively metabolized in the liver to active metabolites.
Excretion: eliminated slowly, primarily in feces but also in urine.

Half-life is triphasic: alpha phase, 4 minutes; beta phase, about 2 hours; and terminal phase, about 25 hours or longer. Not known if drug appears in breast milk.

Action: onset, unknown; duration, unknown.

MECHANISM OF ACTION

Vinblastine appears to block mitosis by arresting cells in metaphase. This antineoplastic drug may also interfere with amino acid metabolism by blocking cellular glutamic acid use, thus inhibiting purine synthesis, urea formation, and citric acid cycle. Drug also exerts some immunosuppressive activity and, in high concentrations, affects nucleic acids and protein synthesis.

INDICATIONS & DOSAGE

Vinblastine may be used alone or in combination with other drugs in various schedules and regimens. Dosage reflects response to drug and degree of bone marrow depression.

• Hodgkin's and non-Hodgkin's lymphomas (including lymphocytic lymphoma and diffuse, poorly differentiated, well-differentiated, or histiocytic lymphomas); breast, testicular, renal cell, or head and neck cancer; Kaposi's sarcoma; advanced mycosis fungoides; choriocarcinoma; Letterer-Siwe disease (histiocytosis); germ-cell ovarian tumors; chronic leukemias; neuroblastoma. *Adults:* initially 0.1 mg/kg weekly or 3.7 mg/m² weekly. Successive weekly doses increased by increments of 0.05 mg/kg (or 1.8 to 1.9 mg/m²) until WBC count falls to 3,000/mm³, tumor size decreases, or maximum dose of 0.5 mg/kg (or 18.5 mg/m²) is reached (usual range 0.15 to 0.2 mg/kg or 5.5 to 7.4 mg/m²). Subsequent maintenance doses (one increment smaller than final initial dose q 7 to 14 days, or 10 mg once or twice monthly) shouldn't be given until WBC count (after preceding dose) returns to 4,000/mm³. *Children:* initially 2.5 mg/m² weekly, then successive weekly doses increased in increments of 1.25 mg/m² until WBC count falls to 3,000/mm³, tumor size decreases, or a maximum dose of 7.5 mg/m² is reached. Subsequent maintenance doses (one increment smaller than final initial dose q 7 to 14 days) are not recommended until WBC count (after preceding dose) returns to 4,000/mm³.

CONTRAINDICATIONS & CAUTIONS

• Contraindicated in hypersensitivity to the drug or a WBC count below 3,000/mm³.

• Also contraindicated in bacterial, fungal, or viral infection because of the risk of worsening infection.

• In existing or recent chicken pox or herpes zoster, vinblastine is contraindicated because of the risk of severe generalized disease.

• Use cautiously in bone marrow depression because of increased myelosuppression; in metastasis to the bone marrow because of the risk of abrupt decline in WBC or platelet counts; and with previous cytotoxic drug therapy or radiation therapy.

• Also use cautiously in debilitated or elderly patients and in patients with skin ulcers because of increased susceptibility to leukopenia.

• In hepatic impairment, give cautiously because of increased drug levels from reduced metabolism.

• Also give cautiously in patients with a history of gout or urate renal calculi because of the risk of hyperuricemia.

PREPARATION & STORAGE

To avoid mutagenic, teratogenic, and carcinogenic risks when preparing and administering drug, use a biologic containment cabinet, wear disposable gloves and mask, and use syringes with Luer-Lok fittings to prevent drug leakage. Dispose of needles, syringes, vials, and unused drug properly, and avoid contaminating work surfaces.

Avoid drug contact with eyes because severe irritation and possibly corneal ulceration may result. If contact occurs, wash the eye with water immediately.

Vinblastine is supplied in 10 mg vials. Reconstitute by adding 10 ml of 0.9% sodium chloride injection containing phenol or benzyl alcohol as a preservative to yield 1 mg/ml. Also available in 10 ml aqueous solution of 10 mg/ml. Store powder and reconstituted solution at 36° to 46° F. (2° to 8° C.). Solution is stable at these temperatures for up to 30 days without significant potency loss.

ADMINISTRATION
Direct injection: Inject dose rapidly into side port of a free-flowing patent I.V. Or inject directly into vein over 1 minute. (Avoid injecting drug into extremity veins with compromised circulation because of the enhanced risk of thrombosis.)

If extravasation occurs, stop the injection immediately and inject remaining dose into another vein. Treat the affected area immediately.
Intermittent infusion: not recommended.
Continuous infusion: not recommended.

INCOMPATIBILITY
Incompatible with furosemide.

ADVERSE REACTIONS
Life-threatening: acute bronchospasm, anaphylaxis, severe leukopenia, severe thrombocytopenia.
Other: abdominal pain, alopecia, anorexia, black tarry stools, chills, constipation, diarrhea, difficulty walking, dizziness, double vision, drooping eyelids, fever, flank or stomach pain, gonadal suppression, headache, jaw pain, joint pain, loss of deep tendon reflexes, malaise, mental depression, nausea, oral lesions, pain in fingers and toes, pain or redness at injection site, pain at tumor site, paralytic ileus, paresthesias in fingers and toes, peripheral neuritis, pharyngitis, seizures, sore throat, swelling of feet or lower legs, thrombophlebitis, unusual bleeding or bruising, vomiting, weakness.

INTERACTIONS
Allopurinol, colchicine, probenecid, sulfinpyrazone: decreased effectiveness.
Live virus vaccines: heightened risk of virus replication and adverse effects, and diminished antibody response to vaccine.
Myelosuppressive therapy: increased bone marrow depression.

EFFECTS ON DIAGNOSTIC TESTS
Platelet count: possible decrease.
Serum and urine uric acid: possible elevated levels.
WBC count and differential: decreased.

SPECIAL CONSIDERATIONS
● Before and during therapy, monitor hematocrit, platelet count, total and differential WBC count, SGOT, SGPT, and serum bilirubin, creatinine, LDH, BUN, and uric acid levels. WBC nadir occurs 5 to 10 days after administration; recovery is usually complete within another 7 to 14 days.
● Monitor for life-threatening acute bronchospasm. If this occurs, notify the doctor immediately.
● Discontinue therapy in marked leukopenia (particularly granulocytopenia) or thrombocytopenia. Resume

therapy when WBC counts return to satisfactory levels.
• Give antibiotics, as ordered, to patients with leukopenia who develop infection.
• Advise patient to use stool softener to avoid constipation when taking drug.
• Provide adequate oral hydration and, as ordered, also give allopurinol, to alkalinize urine. These steps may prevent uric acid nephropathy.
• Weekly drug doses are associated with less risk of serious toxicity than long-term daily doses. Give vinblastine at intervals of at least 7 days to allow monitoring of each dose's full effect on WBC count.
• Therapy should continue for 4 to 6 weeks or longer. Some patients (especially those with carcinomas) require a trial of at least 12 weeks.
• Tell the patient to contact the doctor if he develops fever, sore throat, or unusual bleeding or bruising, especially if he's receiving myelosuppressive drugs. Also have patient report symptoms of neurotoxicity (such as paresthesias or loss of deep tendon reflexes).

vincristine sulfate
Oncovin♦

Pregnancy Risk Category: D

PHARMACOKINETICS
Distribution: rapidly dispersed throughout the body, with peak biliary concentration 2 to 4 hours after administration. Drug is extensively tissue-bound and protein-bound. It penetrates the blood-brain barrier poorly and usually doesn't appear in CSF in cytotoxic concentrations.
Metabolism: drug may be metabolized extensively (probably in liver)

but also appears to undergo decomposition within the body.
Excretion: principally removed in feces (about 67%). The rest is excreted in urine. Half-life is triphasic: alpha phase, about 1 hour; beta phase, about 2 hours; gamma phase, 85 hours. Not known if drug appears in breast milk.
Action: peak serum level, immediately after administration.

MECHANISM OF ACTION
Vincristine appears to arrest mitosis in metaphase, prohibiting cell division. It may also interfere with amino acid metabolism and, in high concentrations, may impair nucleic acid and protein synthesis. It has some immunosuppressive activity.

INDICATIONS & DOSAGE
Dosage adjustment (usually reduced) may be necessary. Vincristine may be used in combination with other drugs, altering incidence or severity of adverse effects.
• Leukemias (especially acute lymphoblastic leukemia); Hodgkin's and non-Hodgkin's lymphomas; osteogenic and other sarcomas; Wilms' tumor; rhabdomyosarcoma; multiple myeloma; brain medulloblastoma; neuroblastoma; mycosis fungoides; lung, breast, reticular cell, renal cell, and ovarian carcinoma. *Adults:* depending on protocol, 0.01 to 0.03 mg/kg weekly as single dose or 0.4 mg to 1.4 mg/m² weekly as single dose. *Children:* 1.5 to 2 mg/m² weekly as single dose.

CONTRAINDICATIONS & CAUTIONS
• Contraindicated in hypersensitivity to vincristine.

• Also contraindicated in existing or recent exposure to chicken pox or herpes zoster because of the risk of severe generalized disease.

• Use cautiously in hepatic impairment because of decreased drug metabolism; in infection because of decreased resistance; and in neuromuscular disease because of the increased risk of neurotoxicity.

• Also use cautiously when large fluid intake is required because of risk of inappropriate secretion of antidiuretic hormone (ADH).

PREPARATION & STORAGE

Use extreme caution when preparing and administering vincristine to avoid mutagenic, teratogenic, and carcinogenic risks. Use a biological containment cabinet, wear disposable gloves and mask, and use syringes with Luer-Lok fittings to prevent drug leakage. Dispose of needles, syringes, vials, and unused drug properly, and avoid contaminating work surfaces.

Avoid drug contact with eyes because severe irritation and possibly corneal ulceration may result. If contact occurs, wash eye immediately with water.

Vincristine is supplied in 1, 2, and 5 ml vials containing 1 mg/ml. For infusion, dilute to ordered concentration and volume with a compatible I.V. solution, such as dextrose 5% in water or 0.9% sodium chloride injection. Undiluted drug is best stored at 36° to 46° F. (2° to 8° C.); however, it's stable at room temperature for at least 1 month. Protect from light to prevent degradation.

Because vincristine is a vesicant, assemble necessary supplies for managing extravasation before administration. Also ensure a patent I.V. line.

ADMINISTRATION

Direct injection: Inject dose over 1 minute directly into vein or into side port of a newly started I.V. line. Use a 23G or 25G winged-tip infusion set. If possible, use distal rather than major veins, which allows for repeated venipuncture if necessary.

If extravasation occurs, stop the injection immediately and inject the remaining dose into another vein. Give a local injection of hyaluronidase and apply moderate heat or cold compresses to minimize discomfort and cellulitis.

Intermittent infusion: not recommended; however, drug has been diluted and given as a slow infusion over 4 to 8 hours.

Continuous infusion: not recommended.

INCOMPATIBILITY

Incompatible with furosemide.

ADVERSE REACTIONS

Life-threatening: anaphylaxis, severe leukopenia, severe thrombocytopenia.

Other: agitation, alopecia, anhidrosis, anorexia, bloating, blurred or double vision, chills, confusion, constipation, depression, diarrhea, difficulty walking, dizziness, drooping eyelids, fever, flank pain, hallucinations, headache, insomnia, jaw pain, joint pain, nausea, painful or difficult urination, pain in fingers and toes, pain or redness at injection site, paresthesias in fingers and toes, rash, seizures, sore throat, stomach cramps and pain, stomatitis, swollen feet or lower legs, testicular pain, thrombocytopenia, unconsciousness, unusual bleeding or bruising, unusual increases or decreases in urination, urinary incontinence, vomiting, weakness, weight loss.

INTERACTIONS

Allopurinol, colchicine, probenecid, sulfinpyrazone: decreased effectiveness.

Asparaginase: additive neurotoxicity.

Bleomycin: synergistic effects.

Digoxin: decreased effects (several days after vincristine administration).

Doxorubicin: enhanced myelosuppression.

Live virus vaccines: heightened risk of virus replication.

Myelosuppressive therapy: additive bone marrow depression and cytotoxic effects.

Neurotoxic drugs, spinal cord irradiation: increased neurotoxicity.

EFFECTS ON DIAGNOSTIC TESTS

Platelet count: possibly decreased (minimal) or increased.

Serum and urine uric acid: possible elevated levels.

WBC count and differential: possibly decreased.

SPECIAL CONSIDERATIONS

• *Treatment of overdose:* As ordered, administer anticonvulsant doses of phenobarbital and give enemas to prevent ileus. Monitor cardiovascular function and hematologic studies. Treatment is usually symptomatic.

• Start a prophylactic bowel regimen before treatment and continue throughout treatment to prevent severe constipation and paralytic ileus. A stool softener may prevent upper colon impaction.

• Perform a complete physical exam before administration. Check for numbness, tingling, altered walking pattern, and depressed tendon reflexes. If these signs of hypotension develop after administration, notify the doctor and expect to reduce dosage or discontinue drug.

• Hematologic toxicity with vincristine is less than that with other antineoplastic agents. Mild leukopenia, anemia, and thrombocytopenia are rare at usual doses. However, drug is highly toxic with a low therapeutic index.

• Before and during therapy, monitor hematocrit, platelet count, SGPT, SGOT, total and differential leukocyte counts, WBC counts, and serum bilirubin, creatinine, LDH, BUN, and uric acid levels. Leukopenia usually reaches nadir within 4 days.

• Provide adequate oral hydration and give allopurinol, as ordered, to alkalinize urine. These steps may prevent or minimize development of uric acid nephropathy.

• Temporarily discontinue drug if signs of hyponatremia or inappropriate ADH secretion appear. Restrict fluids and, if needed, give a diuretic affecting the loop of Henle and the distal tubule.

• In hepatic impairment, expect to lower vincristine dosage.

vindesine sulfate
Eldisine♦♦

Pregnancy Risk Category: D

PHARMACOKINETICS

Distribution: rapidly dispersed in plasma, with extensive tissue binding. Not known if drug crosses the placenta.

Metabolism: partially metabolized in the liver.

Excretion: 13% eliminated in urine within 24 hours. Remainder is sequestered in the body or eliminated in bile. Half-life is triphasic: alpha phase, about 3 minutes; beta phase, about 2 hours; gamma phase, about

---

Unmarked trade names available in the United States only.
♦Also available in Canada.   ♦♦Available in Canada only.

20 hours. Not known if drug appears in breast milk.
Action: onset, unknown; duration, unknown.

MECHANISM OF ACTION
An investigational anticancer drug, vindesine is derived from vinblastine sulfate, but its activity resembles that of vincristine sulfate. Drug arrests cell division at metaphase, causing cell death. Drug also interferes with synthesis of nucleic acids, proteins, and lipids. Full extent of activity hasn't been determined.

INDICATIONS & DOSAGE
Indications and dosages may vary. Check current literature for latest protocols.
• Lymphoma; leukemias; metastatic breast cancer; lung, esophageal, and colorectal cancer. *Adults and children:* 3 to 4.5 mg/m² q 1 to 2 weeks, or 1 to 2 mg/m² daily for 2 to 10 days q 2 to 3 weeks. Adjust dosage in patients with impaired liver function.

CONTRAINDICATIONS & CAUTIONS
• Contraindicated in hypersensitivity to vindesine.
• Also contraindicated in severe leukopenia or thrombocytopenia because of the risk of increased hematologic toxicity.
• Avoid use in bacterial infection because of the risk of widespread infection, and in existing or recent chicken pox or herpes zoster because of risk of generalized disease.
• Use cautiously in bone marrow depression because drug may cause severe leukopenia.
• Also use cautiously in hepatic impairment because of reduced drug metabolism leading to increased drug levels.

• In elderly or debilitated patients or in patients with skin ulcers, give cautiously because of heightened susceptibility to leukopenia.

PREPARATION & STORAGE
Use extreme caution when preparing and administering vindesine to avoid mutagenic, teratogenic, and carcinogenic risks. Use a biologic containment cabinet, wear disposable gloves and mask, and use syringes with Luer-Lok fittings to prevent drug leakage. Dispose of needles, syringes, vials, and unused drug properly, and avoid contaminating work surfaces.

Avoid vindesine contact with eyes because this drug can cause corneal ulceration. In accidental contact, flush eye with copious amounts of water.

Vindesine is supplied in 5 mg vials with enclosed 5 ml diluent. For injection, reconstitute with the 5 ml of sterile diluent provided to yield a 1 mg/ml solution. For infusion, dilute prescribed amount of reconstituted solution in ordered amount of dextrose 5% in water or 0.9% sodium chloride. Store intact vials and reconstituted solution in refrigerator. Reconstituted solution is stable for 30 days when refrigerated. Diluted solution is stable in dextrose 5% in water or 0.9% sodium chloride for 24 hours at room temperature.

ADMINISTRATION
Direct injection: Give as I.V. bolus directly into vein, using a 21G or 23G needle, or into infusion port of a primary I.V. line containing a compatible solution. Flush line before administration with 10 ml of 0.9% sodium chloride to establish vein patency. Afterward, flush line with another 10 ml of 0.9% sodium chloride to remove residual drug.

Intermittent infusion: not recommended.

Continuous infusion: Infuse diluted drug over ordered duration (usually several hours) into a patent I.V. line containing a compatible solution.

INCOMPATIBILITY

Incompatible with solutions having a pH greater than 6.0, including multielectrolyte solutions, such as Ringer's injection. Don't mix with other drugs.

ADVERSE REACTIONS

Life-threatening: acute bronchospasm, anaphylaxis, severe leukopenia, severe thrombocytopenia.
Other: abdominal pain, alopecia, anemia (rare), anorexia, bleeding from old peptic ulcers, cellulitis, constipation, diarrhea, dizziness, fever, headache, hemorrhagic enterocolitis, hoarseness, inappropriate ADH secretion, jaw pain, loss of deep tendon reflexes, malaise, mental depression, nausea, oral vesicles, paralytic ileus, paresthesias, peripheral neuritis or neuropathy, pharyngitis, phlebitis, rash, rectal bleeding, seizures, vomiting, weakness.

INTERACTIONS

Cytotoxic drugs, radiation therapy: increased cytotoxic effects.
Vinblastine sulfate, other vinca alkaloids: heightened risk of neurotoxicity.

EFFECTS ON DIAGNOSTIC TESTS

Platelet count: possibly decreased.
Serum and urine uric acid: possible elevated levels.
WBC count and differential: reduced.

SPECIAL CONSIDERATIONS

• Avoid extravasation. If it occurs, treat locally with ice packs and, possibly, hydrocortisone.

• Monitor for life-threatening acute bronchospasm after administration (most common in patients also receiving mitomycin). Notify the doctor immediately.
• Before and during therapy, monitor hematocrit, platelet count, SGOT, SGPT, total and differential WBC count, and serum bilirubin, creatinine, LDH, BUN, and uric acid levels.
• Patients with cachexia or ulceration of the skin may be more susceptible to the drug's leukopenic effect. If leukopenia develops, watch for signs of infection. Leukopenia nadir is 7 to 11 days after administration.
• Monitor closely for neurotoxicity. Record the patient's signature before each course of therapy and observe for deteriorated handwriting. Tell patient to report numbness or tingling of extremities, jaw pain, or constipation. Assess for footdrop, wristdrop, and depressed tendon reflexes.
• To prevent paralytic ileus, administer stool softeners and encourage fluids and ambulation.
• Maintain good oral hydration, and if ordered, give allopurinol to alkalinize urine.

warfarin sodium
Coumadin

Pregnancy Risk Category: D

PHARMACOKINETICS

Distribution: dispersed to the liver, lungs, spleen, and kidneys. At least 97% is bound to plasma proteins, primarily albumin; uptake by erythrocytes is variable. Drug crosses the placenta.

Metabolism: hydroxylated by hepatic microsomal enzymes to inactive metabolites.

Excretion: in bile, as inactive metabolites that are reabsorbed in urine. Drug doesn't appear in breast milk.

Action: onset, 12 to 72 hours; duration, 2 to 5 days.

MECHANISM OF ACTION

This indirect-acting anticoagulant interferes with hepatic synthesis of vitamin K–dependent clotting factors, depleting Factors II (prothrombin), VII, IX, and X. These factors must be fully depleted before warfarin effects become apparent.

INDICATIONS & DOSAGE

• Venous thrombosis, pulmonary emboli, atrial fibrillation with embolization, coronary occlusion. (Nonlabelled uses: after orthopedic or coronary bypass surgery, thromboembolism with prosthetic heart valves, acute MI and transient ischemic attack, progressive cerebrovascular accident, and small-cell lung cancer.) *Adults:* 10 to 15 mg daily for 2 to 5 days for induction of anticoagulation; thereafter, dosage based on prothrombin time (PT). Therapeutic range is 1½ to 2½ times PT control value in seconds; dosage must be individualized. Alternatively, a single dose of 40 to 60 mg (20 to 30 mg for elderly or debilitated patients) may be given. Maintenance dose of 2 to 10 mg daily is based on PT.

CONTRAINDICATIONS & CAUTIONS

• Contraindicated in bleeding; hemorrhagic dyscrasias; history of hemorrhagic tendencies; open GI, GU, or respiratory wounds or ulcers; cerebrovascular hemorrhage; aneurysms; pericarditis or pericardial effusions; subacute bacterial endocarditis; and pregnancy.

• Because of the increased risk of bleeding, avoid use in diverticulitis, vasculitis, severe uncontrolled or malignant hypertension, severe renal or hepatic impairment, polyarthritis, visceral carcinoma, bleeding granuloma, severe diabetes mellitus, severe allergic or anaphylactic disorders, and vitamin C or vitamin K deficiency.

• Also avoid use in any diagnostic or therapeutic procedure with potential for uncontrolled bleeding, such as eye, brain, or spinal cord surgery.

• Give cautiously in active tuberculosis, in GI ulcers, and during menstruation and postpartum period because of the risk of hemorrhage.

• Also give cautiously in conditions that may enhance warfarin's anticoagulant effect, including steatorrhea, diarrhea, infectious hepatitis, congestive heart failure, scurvy, poor nutrition, cachexia, collagen disease, thyrotoxicosis, and hypermetabolic states, such as fever and hyperthyroidism.

• In women, elderly patients, and patients with small bodies, use cautiously because of increased sensitivity to warfarin effects.

• Also use cautiously in conditions that may decrease warfarin's anticoagulant effect, such as increased intake or absorption of vitamin K, hyperlipidemia, hypothyroidism, and edema.

PREPARATION & STORAGE

Available as a powder in a 50 mg vial. Reconstitute by adding 2 ml of sterile water for injection for a solution of 25 mg/ml. Use immediately after reconstitution; solution contains no preservatives. Compatible I.V. solutions include Dextran 6% and 0.9% sodium chloride, dextrose 2.5% in half-strength Ringer's injection, dextrose 2.5% in water, Ionosol

B with dextrose 5%, Ionosol D-CM, Ionosol MB with dextrose 5%, Ionosol PSL, Ringer's injection, 0.45% sodium chloride, 0.9% sodium chloride, and ⅙ M sodium lactate.

Protect warfarin sodium from light and store at room temperature, always below 104° F. (40° C.).

ADMINISTRATION
Direct injection: Inject desired dose into I.V. tubing containing a free-flowing compatible solution.
Intermittent infusion: not recommended.
Continuous infusion: not recommended.

INCOMPATIBILITY
Incompatible with amikacin, ammonium chloride, ascorbic acid injection, Dextran 6% in dextrose 5%, epinephrine hydrochloride, metaraminol, oxytocin, promazine, tetracycline hydrochloride, vancomycin, and vitamin B complex with C.

ADVERSE REACTIONS
Life-threatening: hemorrhage, necrosis or gangrene of skin or other tissues (most common in abdomen, breast, thighs, and buttocks).
Other: abdominal cramps, agranulocytosis, alopecia, dermatitis, diarrhea, fever, hypersensitivity reactions, leukopenia, mouth ulcers, nausea, priapism (rare), purple-toe syndrome, urticaria, vomiting.

INTERACTIONS
Acetaminophen, indomethacin, meclofenamate sodium, mefenamic acid, phenylbutazone, salicylates: heightened anticoagulant effects.
Adrenocorticosteroids, antimetabolites, dipyridamole, potassium, quinidine, quinine: enhanced bleeding tendencies.

Alcohol (acute ingestion), propoxyphene, sulindac: enhanced anticoagulant effects.
Alcohol (chronic abuse), barbiturates, ethchlorvynol, glutethimide: decreased anticoagulant effects.
Allopurinol, amiodarone, chloral hydrate, diflunisal (large doses), disulfiram, glucagon, inhalation anesthetics, influenza vaccine: enhanced anticoagulant effects.
Anabolic steroids, clofibrate, dextrothyroxine, diazoxide, ethyacrynic acid, gemfibrozil, danazol, thyroid drugs: increased anticoagulant effects.
Ascorbic acid (large doses), carbamazepine, griseofulvin: decreased anticoagulant effects.
Azlocillin, carbenicillin, dextrans, dipyridamole: inhibited platelet aggregation.
Cephalosporins, penicillin (parenteral), sulfinpyrazone: enhanced bleeding tendencies.
Chloramphenicol, co-trimoxazole, erythromycin, isoniazid, ketoconazole, miconazole, sulfonamides: enhanced anticoagulant effects.
Cholestyramine, colestipol, cyclophosphamide, estrogens, mercaptopurine, oral contraceptives, phenytoin: decreased anticoagulant effects.
Cimetidine, methylphenidate, methylthiouracil, ranitidine: enhanced anticoagulant effects.
Indomethacin, oxyphenbutazone, phenylbutazone, salicylates, streptokinase, urokinase: increased bleeding tendencies.
Methaqualone, nafcillin, oral antidiabetics (continued use), rifampin, spironolactone, vitamin K: decreased anticoagulant effects.
Nalidixic acid, neomycin (oral), oral antidiabetics, phenytoin, propylthiouracil, sulfonylureas, triclofos, vitamin E: increased anticoagulant effects.

EFFECTS ON DIAGNOSTIC TESTS

Coagulation factors: decreased levels of vitamin K–dependent factors.
Prothrombin time, activated partial thromboplastin time: prolonged.
Serum theophylline: falsely decreased levels with Schack and Waxler ultraviolet method.
Urinalysis: altered urine color (may turn orange).

SPECIAL CONSIDERATIONS

• *Treatment of overdose:* In moderate to severe hemorrhage, discontinue drug and give phytonadione (vitamin K₁) orally or I.V., as ordered. Effects may not appear for several hours. If bleeding is severe and immediate restoration of vitamin K–dependent coagulation is needed, give fresh whole blood or plasma concurrently.
• Monitor closely for signs of bleeding. Test all exudates for microscopic blood, and observe bleeding precautions.
• Tell the patient to report signs of bleeding, such as hematuria, ecchymoses, melena, excessive menstrual bleeding, petechiae, bleeding from gums or other mucous membranes, or oozing from minor cuts. Also tell him to avoid taking any other drugs unless he consults his doctor, and to wear Medic Alert identification.
• Monitor PT periodically, and keep in mind that changes in diet, environment, physical condition, and concurrent drug use may alter response to warfarin.
• If the patient needs dental care or surgery, adjust warfarin dose.
• Avoid abrupt discontinuation. Taper dose gradually over 3 to 4 weeks.

whole blood

Pregnancy Risk Category: Not applicable

COMPOSITION

One unit (513 ml) of whole blood contains approximately 180 to 240 ml of RBCs, 235 to 295 ml of plasma, and 63 ml of an anticoagulant and preservative. Whole blood may be homologous (collected from a random donor and tested for hepatitis and human immunodeficiency virus [HIV]), or it may be autologous (collected from the patient and saved for future use, or salvaged during surgery or after trauma). Because autologous blood eliminates the risk of alloimmunization and the transmission of blood-borne diseases, it's used whenever possible, before homologous blood.

INDICATIONS & DOSAGE

• Acute, massive blood loss (greater than 25% of total blood volume) requiring oxygen-carrying properties of RBCs as well as volume expansion of plasma. *Adults:* number of units depends on patient's condition. *Children:* 20 ml/kg initially followed by volume required for stabilization.

CONTRAINDICATIONS & CAUTIONS

• Because of the risk of disease transmission and adverse reactions, don't transfuse homologous blood if crystalloid or colloid solutions can treat the condition sufficiently. Acute loss of up to one-third of total blood volume (3 to 4 units) can usually be treated effectively without blood transfusion.

PREPARATION & STORAGE

Available in a sterile pack containing 475 ml of blood and 63 ml of an anticoagulant and preservative, such as citrate phosphate dextrose adenine (CPDA-1), which prevents clotting and provides nutrients for long-term cell survival. Store at 34° to 43° F. (1° to 6° C.) in a continuously monitored refrigerator—temperatures above or below this range may cause decreased viability, hemolysis, and bacterial proliferation. After removing whole blood from refrigerator and breaking sterile seal, infuse within 4 hours.

ADMINISTRATION

Direct injection: Appropriate for neonates only. Draw prefiltered blood into a syringe and inject slowly through a 19G to 21G needle or catheter.

Intermittent infusion: not recommended.

Continuous infusion: Administer through a Y-type or straight infusion set with a minimum 170-micron filter at a rate rapid enough to stabilize hemodynamic status. Use 0.9% sodium chloride to prime and clear tubing. Also keep this solution available for possible adverse reactions. Use automatic infusion devices only if they've been tested and approved for transfusion by the manufacturer. Don't inflate manual pressure cuffs above 300 mm Hg.

Begin infusing blood slowly while remaining at the bedside. Take vital signs. If patient shows no evidence of a transfusion reaction, adjust flow to the prescribed rate.

If rapid, massive transfusion is necessary, you may use microaggregate filter (20- to 40-micron) to remove WBC particulates. Microaggregates may migrate to the lungs and cause dyspnea.

INCOMPATIBILITY

Incompatible with all drugs and solutions except 0.9% sodium chloride.

ADVERSE REACTIONS

Life-threatening: acute hemolytic reaction; graft-versus-host disease (GVHD); and viral diseases, such as non-A or non-B hepatitis, hepatitis B, cytomegalovirus, and AIDS.

Other: alloimmunization, febrile nonhemolytic reactions, skin reactions, volume overload.

INTERACTIONS

None reported.

EFFECTS ON DIAGNOSTIC TESTS

Direct Coombs' test: possible positive result, from antibodies bound to RBCs.

Hematocrit: increased over pretransfusion levels once bleeding has resolved (for adults, 3% increase/unit).

Hemoglobin: increased over pretransfusion levels once bleeding has resolved (for adults, 1 g/dl increase/ unit).

Indirect Coombs' test: possible positive result, from antibodies formed in plasma after exposure to minor RBC antigens.

SPECIAL CONSIDERATIONS

• Take vital signs, record results, and establish a patent venous catheter before requesting release of blood from the blood bank.

• Confirm the recipient's identity by comparing the name and ID number on blood bag tag with that on the patient's bracelet. Verify blood compatibility by comparing blood group and type on bag to chart or other blood bank record. Have another authorized staff member perform this check, too. Accurate identification of the recipient before drawing the crossmatch sample and beginning the infusion can help prevent acute hemolytic reactions.

• Keep in mind that the ABO type of whole blood must be identical to that of the recipient, but that Rh-negative blood (lacking the D antigen) may be given to an Rh-positive patient.

• Warm blood to body temperature with an approved blood-warming device to prevent dysrhythmias associated with rapid, massive infusions of cold blood.

• Monitor vital signs every 15 minutes (may vary according to hospital protocol) until 1 hour after transfusion. Record vital signs, product number, starting and ending times, volume infused, and response to transfusion.

• If an acute hemolytic reaction occurs, stop the transfusion at the needle hub and rapidly infuse 0.9% sodium chloride. Contact the doctor and the blood bank and begin symptomatic treatment to maintain renal blood flow. Arrange a serologic evaluation of blood and urine.

• If a febrile nonhemolytic reaction occurs, stop the transfusion and keep the vein open with 0.9% sodium chloride. Confirm the recipient's identity and contact the doctor and the blood bank. Arrange a serologic evaluation of blood and urine, and start symptomatic treatment. If ordered, give antipyretics.

• If a skin reaction occurs, give antihistamines, as ordered.

• Watch for signs of volume overload (cough, dyspnea, crackles at lung bases, distended neck veins). If these occur, stop the transfusion and keep the vein open with a slow infusion of 0.9% sodium chloride. Contact the doctor and begin treatment as ordered, including diuretics and other measures to reduce fluid volume. Whenever possible, prevent volume overload by administering concentrated blood components.

• Tell the patient to report signs of GVHD (fever, rash, hepatitis), which may appear 2 to 3 weeks after transfusion. No effective therapy exists, but GVHD can be prevented by exposing blood to ionizing radiation (1,500 rad) before transfusion.

• Whole blood stored for more than 24 hours contains insignificant amounts of platelets and labile clotting Factors V and VIII. Treat specific clotting deficiencies with component therapy.

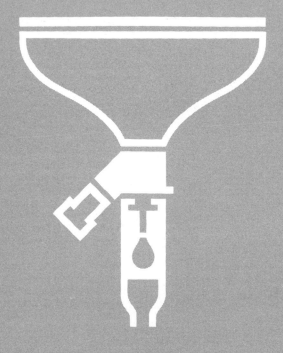

Appendices and Index

Converting units of measure

This table provides approximate dose equivalents using the apothecary and metric systems of weights and measures. If the doctor prescribes a dosage form in the apothecary system, the pharmacist may supply a corresponding metric equivalent, and vice versa. Most medications are prepackaged and ready to administer, but it's useful to know what the equivalents are if you must calculate dosages yourself.

APOTHECARY EQUIVALENTS	METRIC EQUIVALENTS
Liquid measure	
1 quart	1,000 ml
1 1/2 pints	750 ml
1 pint	500 ml
8 fluid ounces	250 ml
7 fluid ounces	200 ml
3 1/2 fluid ounces	100 ml
1 3/4 fluid ounces	50 ml
1 fluid ounce	30 ml
4 fluid drams	15 ml
2 1/2 fluid drams	10 ml
2 fluid drams	8 ml
1 1/4 fluid drams	5 ml
1 fluid dram	4 ml
45 minims	3 ml
30 minims	2 ml
15 minims	1 ml
12 minims	0.75 ml
10 minims	0.6 ml
8 minims	0.5 ml
5 minims	0.3 ml
4 minims	0.25 ml
3 minims	0.2 ml
1 1/2 minims	0.1 ml
1 minim	0.06 ml
3/4 minim	0.05 ml
1/2 minim	0.03 ml

Converting weight
To begin, 1 lb equals 0.453592 kg. Conversely, 1 kg equals 2.2 lb. To convert pounds to kilograms, divide the number of pounds by 2.2. To convert kilograms to pounds, multiply the number of kilograms by 2.2.

Converting temperature
To convert Centigrade to Fahrenheit:
$$(°C \times 1.8) + 32 = °F$$

To convert Fahrenheit to Centigrade:
$$(°F - 32) \div 1.8 = °C$$

Major electrolyte components of I.V. solutions

SOLUTION	SODIUM (mEq/liter)	POTASSIUM (mEq/liter)
Acetated Ringer's solution	131	4
Acetated Ringer's solution with dextrose 5%	131	4
Aminosyn 3.5% M	47	13
Aminosyn 7% with electrolytes	70	66
Aminosyn 8.5% with electrolytes	70	66
Ammonium chloride 2.14%		
Dextrose 2.5% in half-strength lactated Ringer's solution	65	2
Dextrose 4% in modified lactated Ringer's solution	26	<1
Dextrose 5% in electrolyte no. 48	25	20
Dextrose 5% in electrolyte no. 75	40	35
Dextrose 5% in sodium chloride 0.11%	19	
Dextrose 5% in sodium chloride 0.2%	34 or 38.5	
Dextrose 5% in sodium chloride 0.3%	51 or 56	
Dextrose 38% with electrolyte pattern T	49	46
Dextrose 50% with electrolyte pattern A	84	40
Dextrose 50% with electrolyte pattern B	32	
Dextrose 50% with electrolyte pattern N	90	80
Dextrose 50% with electrolytes and acetate 60 mEq/liter	80	40
Dextrose 50% with electrolytes	110	80
FreAmine III 3% with electrolytes	35	24.5
Invert Sugar 5% and electrolyte No. 2	56	25
Ionosol B in dextrose 5% in water	57	25

CALCIUM (mEq/liter)	MAGNESIUM (mEq/liter)	CHLORIDE (mEq/liter)	ACETATE (mEq/liter)	PHOSPHATE (millimoles)	OTHER (mEq/liter)
3		109	28		
3		122	28		
	3	40			
	10	96	124	30	
	10	98	142	30	
		400			ammonium 400
1.4		54			lactate 14
<1		22			lactate 6
	3	24		3	lactate 23
		48		15	lactate 20
		19			
		34 or 38.5			
		51 or 56			
	7.7	54	37	35	
10	16	115			gluconate 13 sulfate 16
9	16	32			gluconate 4.2 sulfate 16
	16	150		28	sulfate 16
9.6	16	70	60		gluconate 9.6 sulfate 16
	16	140	36	24	
	5	40	44	3.5	amino acids 3%
	6	25		12.5	lactate 25
	5	49		7 or 13	lactate 25

(continued)

Major electrolyte components of I.V. solutions *(continued)*

SOLUTION	SODIUM (mEq/liter)	POTASSIUM (mEq/liter)
Ionosol D with invert sugar 10%	80	36
Ionosol G in 10% invert sugar	60	17
Ionosol MB in dextrose 5% in water	25	20
Ionosol T in dextrose 5% in water	40	35
Isolyte E	140	10
Isolyte G with dextrose 5%	65	17
Lactated Ringer's solution	130	4
Normosol M in dextrose 5% in water	40	13
Plasma-Lyte A	140	5
Plasma-Lyte R	140	10
ProcalAmine	35	24
Ringer's solution	147 or 147.5	4
Sodium bicarbonate	598	
Sodium chloride 0.45%	77	
Sodium chloride 0.9%	154	
Sodium chloride 3%	513	
Sodium chloride 5%	855	
Sodium lactate ⅙ M	167	
Travasol M 3.5% with electrolyte no. 45	25	15
Travasol 5.5% with electrolytes	70	60
Travasol 8.5% with electrolytes	70	60

CALCIUM (mEq/liter)	MAGNESIUM (mEq/liter)	CHLORIDE (mEq/liter)	ACETATE (mEq/liter)	PHOSPHATE (millimoles)	OTHER (mEq/liter)
5	3	64			lactate 60
		147			ammonium 70
	3	22		3	
		40		15	lactate 20
5	3	103	49		citrate
		149			ammonium 70
3		109 or 110			lactate 28
	3	40	16		
	3	98	27		gluconate 23
5	3	103	47		lactate 8
3	5	41	47	3.5	amino acids 3% glycerin 3%
4 or 4.5		156			
		77			
		154			
		513			
		855			
					lactate 167
	5	25	54	7.5	
	10	70	100	30	
	10	70	141	30	

Identifying and treating toxic drug reactions

TOXIC REACTION	CLINICAL EFFECTS
Anemia, aplastic A deficiency of all of the formed elements of the blood, representing a failure of the cell-generating capacity of the bone marrow	• Bleeding from mucous membranes, ecchymoses, petechiae • Fatigue, pallor, progressive weakness, shortness of breath, tachycardia progressing to congestive heart failure (CHF) • Fever, oral and rectal ulcers, sore throat without characteristic inflammation
Anemia, hemolytic A disorder characterized by the premature destruction of RBCs; common in people with glucose-6-phosphate deficiency	• Chills, fever, pain in the back and abdomen (hemolytic crisis) • Jaundice, malaise, splenomegaly • Signs of shock
Bone marrow toxicity, agranulocytosis An abnormal condition of the blood characterized by a severe reduction in the number of granulocytes (basophils, eosinophils, and neutrophils)	• Enlarged lymph nodes, spleen, and tonsils • Septicemia leading to shock • Slowly progressing fatigue followed by sudden onset of overwhelming infection with chills, fever, headache, and tachycardia • Pneumonia • Ulcers in the colon, mouth, and pharynx
Bone marrow toxicity, thrombocytopenia An abnormal condition in which the number of platelets is reduced, usually by destruction of erythroid tissue in bone marrow (associated with certain neoplastic diseases) or by an immune response to a drug	• Fatigue, general weakness, lethargy, and malaise • Hemorrhage, loss of consciousness, shortness of breath, tachycardia • Sudden onset of ecchymoses or petechiae, large blood-filled bullae in the mouth
Cardiotoxicity Damage to the heart	• Acute hypertensive reaction • Atrial and ventricular dysrhythmias • Chest pain • CHF • Chronic cardiomyopathy • Pericarditis-myocarditis syndrome
Dermatologic toxicity Damage to the skin	• May vary from phototoxicity to acneiform eruptions, alopecia, exfoliative dermatitis, lupus erythematosus-like reactions, toxic epidermal necrolysis

INTERVENTIONS	SELECTED CAUSATIVE DRUGS
• Discontinue drug if possible. • Provide vigorous supportive care including transfusion therapy, neutropenic isolation, antibiotics, and oxygen therapy, particularly if hemoglobin level is low. • In severe cases, bone marrow transplantation may be necessary.	Carbamazepine, chloramphenicol, co-trimoxazole, gold salts, mephenytoin, penicillamine, phenylbutazone
• Discontinue drug. • Provide supportive care including transfusion therapy and oxygen therapy. • If autoimmune etiology is suspected, obtain a blood sample for direct and indirect Coombs' test.	Mefenamic acid, penicillins, phenazopyridine, primaquine, sulfonamides, vitamin K derivatives
• Discontinue drug therapy. • Begin antibiotic therapy while awaiting blood culture and sensitivity results. • Provide supportive therapy including neutropenic isolation, warm saline gargles, and good oral hygiene.	Carbamazepine, flucytosine, gold salts, nitrofurantoin, penicillamine, phenothiazines, phenylbutazone, phenytoin, procainamide, propylthiouracil
• Discontinue drug or reduce dosage. • Administer corticosteroids and platelet transfusions.	Etretinate, floxuridine, flucytosine, gold salts, heparin, interferons, methotrexate, penicillamine, phenylbutazone, tetracyclines, valproic acid
• Institute cardiac monitoring at earliest sign of problems. Discontinue drug therapy if possible. • If patient is receiving doxorubicin, limit cumulative dose to less than 500 mg/m^2. • Closely monitor patients receiving concurrent radiation therapy.	Cyclophosphamide, daunorubicin, doxorubicin, estramustine, ifosfamide
• Discontinue drug. • Administer topical antihistamines and analgesics, as ordered.	Androgens, barbiturates, corticosteroids, diuretics (particularly thiazides), hydralazine, iodides, pentamidine isethionate, phenothiazines, phenylbutazone, procainamide, psoralens, sulfonamides, sulfonylureas *(continued)*

Identifying and treating toxic drug reactions *(continued)*

TOXIC REACTION	CLINICAL EFFECTS
Hepatotoxicity Damage to or destruction of liver cells	• Abdominal pain, hepatomegaly • Abnormal alanine aminotransferase (ALT), formerly SGPT; aspartate aminotransferase (AST), formerly SGOT; lactic dehydrogenase; and serum bilirubin levels • Bleeding, low-grade fever, mental changes, weight loss • Dry skin, pruritus, rash • Jaundice
Nephrotoxicity Damage to or destruction of kidney cells	• Albumin, casts, or RBCs or WBCs in urine • Altered creatinine clearance, elevated blood urea nitrogen • Blurred vision, dehydration (depending on part of kidney affected), edema, mild headache, pallor • Dizziness, fatigue, irritability, slowed mental processes • Electrolyte imbalance, oliguria
Neurotoxicity Damage to or destruction of cells in any part of the nervous system	• Akathisia, bilateral or unilateral palsies, cerebral infarction, dystonia, fasciculation, muscle twitching, tremor, paresthesia, strokelike syndrome, unsteady gait, weakness • Apnea, depressed respirations • Hypertensive crisis, intracerebral or subarachnoid hemorrhage
Ocular toxicity Damage to or destruction of eye cells	• Acute glaucoma • Blurred, colored, or flickering vision • Cataracts • Corneal deposits • Diplopia • Miosis • Mydriasis • Optic neuritis • Scotomata • Vision loss
Ototoxicity Damage to cranial nerve VIII or to the organs of hearing and balance	• Ataxia • Hearing loss • Tinnitus • Vertigo

INTERVENTIONS	SELECTED CAUSATIVE DRUGS
• Reduce dosage or discontinue drug. • Monitor vital signs, blood levels, weight, intake and output, and fluid and electrolyte balance. • Promote rest. • Assist with hemodialysis, if needed. • Provide symptomatic care: vitamins; potassium supplements to correct alkalosis; salt-poor albumin to maintain fluid and electrolyte balance; aspiration of blood from the stomach; reduction of dietary protein; and administration of lactulose or neomycin to reduce blood ammonia levels.	Amiodarone, antineoplastics, asparaginase, carbamazepine, chlorpromazine, chlorpropamide, dantrolene, erythromycin estolate, ketoconazole, methotrexate, methyldopa, niacin, plicamycin
• Reduce dosage or discontinue drug. • Assist with hemodialysis, if needed. • Monitor vital signs, weight changes, and urine volume. • Provide symptomatic care: Fluid restriction and loop diuretics to reduce fluid retention, I.V. solutions to correct electrolyte imbalance.	Aminoglycosides, antineoplastics, contrast media, corticosteroids, gallium, gold products (parenteral), nonsteroidal anti-inflammatory drugs, penicillin, pentamidine, vasopressors
• Notify doctor as soon as changes appear. • Reduce dosage or discontinue drug. • Provide symptomatic care: Remain with the patient, reassure him, and protect him during seizures. Provide a quiet environment, draw shades, speak in soft tones. Maintain airway and ventilate the patient as needed.	Analeptics, antibacterials, anticonvulsants, antihistamines, CNS depressants, phenothiazines, rauwolfia alkaloids, tricyclic antidepressants, vasopressors
• Notify doctor as soon as changes appear. • Stop drug, as ordered. (Some oculotoxic drugs used to treat serious conditions may be given again at a reduced dosage after the eyes are rested and have returned to near normal.) • Monitor carefully for changes in symptoms. • Treat effects symptomatically.	Amiodarone, anticholinergic agents, antineoplastics, cardiac glycosides, chloramphenicol, clomiphene, corticosteroids, cyclophosphamide, cytarabine, ethambutol, methotrexate, phenothiazines, quinine, quinine, rifampin, tamoxifen, vinblastine, vincristine
• Notify doctor as soon as changes appear. • Discontinue drug or reduce dosage, as ordered. • Monitor carefully for symptomatic changes.	Aminoglycosides, chloroquine, cisplatin, colistimethate sodium, loop diuretics, minocycline, quinidine, quinine, salicylates, vancomycin

Transfusing blood components

Whenever you administer blood components, you should take great care to avoid mistakes. Proper identifying and matching procedures are crucial. Also be sure to consider use of filters and blood warmers, needle size, and administration rate. Stay alert, too, for potential complications.

Checking compatibility

Before administering any blood component requiring ABO and Rh compatibility, you'll need to confirm the patient's identity. (If you infuse blood that doesn't match the patient's blood, results could be fatal.) After obtaining blood from the blood bank and before hanging each unit, you and another nurse at the patient's bedside must identify each unit and check the patient's name (ask the patient his name if he's lucid and can speak); then identify the name and I.D. number on his wristband. (When blood is drawn for typing and cross-matching, the patient receives an I.D. bracelet including his full name, hospital number, room number, date and time blood was drawn, the number of the blood component compatibility tag, and the name or initials of the person performing the blood collection.)

After confirming the patient's identity, examine the compatibility tag attached to the blood bag and the information printed on the bag to verify that the ABO group, Rh type, and unit number match. Also check the expiration date on the blood component bag.

Report any discrepancies to the blood bank, and delay transfusion until they're cleared up.

Determining filter use

Ordinarily, a 170-micron blood filter is used for blood transfusions. Albumin, though, comes packaged with its own filter tubing. Blood tubing has a large screen filter, which removes fibrin clots and other debris. Microaggregate filters of 20 to 40 microns are used for patients with pulmonary impairment, although some hospitals use them routinely for multiple transfusions. These filters remove WBCs and smaller microaggregates. They're used only for whole blood or packed RBCs, never for plasma or platelets (they screen out platelets). If used to remove WBCs from packed cells, microaggregate filters eliminate the need to wash RBCs. These filters produce a slower flow rate than a standard filter.

Selecting needle size

Use a 16G, 18G, or 20G needle or cannula to administer whole blood or packed RBCs. If vein access is poor, you may infuse blood using a 22G or 24G cannula, but a blood pump may be needed to ensure an adequate rate. A 21G or 23G winged administration set can be used for small veins and in infants. However, small-gauge plastic cannulas are preferred; they have a lower risk of infiltration. When pumps aren't used, dilute packed cells with 0.9% sodium chloride and increase head pressure by raising the I.V. pole to aid blood flow when using smaller-gauge needles.

Giving the transfusion

At the start, use 0.9% sodium chloride to clear the Y tubing and dilute packed RBCs. Attach the saline solution to one leg of the Y tubing and the blood bag to the other, keeping the saline higher than the blood and both Y clamps open. After allowing about 50 to 75 ml of saline to backflow into the blood bag, clamp the tubings. Mix the blood bag to distribute the normal saline, then start the transfusion. Diluted packed RBCs will infuse at an even rate. Infuse blood slowly, 5 to 10 drops/minute for 15 minutes, increasing to 21 drops/minute (125 ml/hour). One unit of blood or packed RBCs should be infused in 2 hours. If you're infusing at a slower rate, don't exceed 4 hours.

Using blood warmers

When rapid, multiple infusions are needed in severe blood loss, you'll need to warm whole blood and packed RBCs to prevent hypothermia. Commercial blood warmers electronically maintain blood at normal body temperature. Blood warming can also prevent dysrhythmias when blood is given via a central line (cold blood can affect the heart's conduction system). What's more, blood warming can avert reactions to cold agglutinins, which have been identified during crossmatching.

Dealing with complications

Despite increasingly accurate crossmatching precautions, transfusion reactions can still occur. Possible complications are febrile reactions, hypersensitivity reactions (urticarial reaction, acute hemolytic reaction, and anaphylaxis), circulatory overload, and viral contamination.

• *Febrile reaction.* The most common reaction to either packed RBCs or whole blood, febrile nonhemolytic blood reactions occur in 1% to 2% of blood transfusions. This follows an antigen-antibody reaction to WBCs or platelets in the blood component. Patients with a history of transfusions or multiple pregnancies are most susceptible. A leukocyte-removing blood set with a built-in filter (cell saver) is available to provide leukocyte-poor blood.

Although a febrile reaction usually occurs after transfusion, it can occur any time during (or several hours after) the transfusion as well. Obtain pretransfusion vital signs for baseline comparison and monitor the patient closely. Typical symptoms include fever and chills, commonly with severe shaking. Other symptoms may include chest pain, dyspnea, headache, hypotension, and nausea and vomiting. If such symptoms occur, stop the transfusion and notify the doctor and the blood bank. Treat symptomatically.

• *Hypersensitivity (allergic) reactions.* An *urticarial* allergic reaction caused by a plasma-soluble antigen in the plasma is less common with packed RBCs because most of the plasma has been removed. Such reactions also account for about 1% to 2% of all blood reactions and are usually mild. Like febrile reactions, allergic reactions may occur during the transfusion or within a few hours after its completion. Generally, the reaction consists of hives or an urticarial rash, pruritus, and possibly fever.

If the patient develops an urticarial reaction, stop the transfusion and keep the vein open with 0.9% sodium chloride or dextrose 5% in water. Notify the doctor and the blood bank. After giving an antihistamine (usually diphenhydramine), resume the transfusion.

Other hypersensitivity reactions include acute hemolysis and anaphylaxis, either of which may occur early during the transfusion. Monitor patients closely during the first 20 minutes.

• *Acute hemolytic reaction.* This reaction is possible within minutes of administration but can also develop during or immediately after (delayed hemolytic reaction) transfusion. Symptoms may include back pain, chest pain, chills and fever, dyspnea, flushing, nausea and vomiting, oliguria and, later, hypotension, shock and disseminated intravascular coagulation (DIC). A life-threatening reaction, DIC is caused by ABO incompatibility.

If the patient develops signs and symptoms of acute hemolytic reaction, stop the transfusion at once and notify the doctor and the laboratory. Disconnect the blood set, and keep the vein open with 0.9% sodium chloride, using a new administration set. Send a blood and urine specimen to the laboratory. Initiate supportive treatment for hypotension and shock. To promote

(continued)

Transfusing blood components *(continued)*

urine flow, administer I.V. fluids and furosemide. These patients are at high risk of renal damage; dialysis may be necessary.

• *Anaphylaxis.* Rarely, life-threatening anaphylaxis may occur in patients with immunoglobulin A (IgA) deficiency who are sensitized to IgA as a result of previous transfusions or pregnancies. The reaction may begin with infusion of the first few milliliters of blood. It causes respiratory and cardiovascular collapse and severe GI symptoms (abdominal cramps, vomiting, and diarrhea).

If anaphylaxis occurs, stop the transfusion at once, call the doctor, and initiate emergency resuscitation measures. Send blood samples to the laboratory. Give 0.4 ml of 1:1,000 epinephrine subcutaneously. Treat hypotension with 0.1 ml of 1:1,000 epinephrine in 10 ml of saline given I.V. over 5 minutes. Intubate the patient and give oxygen, I.V. fluids, steroids, and vasopressors as needed.

Future blood needs may be met with frozen deglycerolized blood cells. Anaphylactic reactions don't result from red cell incompatibilities and thus can't be anticipated by pretransfusion testing.

• *Circulatory overload.* Caused by excessive or rapid blood transfusion over a short time, circulatory overload occurs most commonly in elderly and debilitated patients. Symptoms include chest pain, cough, cyanosis, distended neck veins, dyspnea, frothy sputum, hemoptysis, crackles, and tachycardia. If symptoms occur, keep the vein open with dextrose 5% in water, and notify the doctor. As ordered, administer diuretics.

• *Viral contamination.* While not common, transmission of hepatitis B virus and human immunodeficiency virus (HIV) is possible during blood transfusion. Symptoms of these disorders may not appear for weeks (hepatitis) to years (HIV) after transfusion.

• Rare complications include *hypokalemia,* caused by leakage of potassium from the cells during prolonged storage, and *hypocalcemia,* which can follow massive transfusions of citrated blood because of citrate binding with plasma calcium.

Antidotes for vesicant extravasation

Most antidotes are instilled through the existing I.V. line, to purposely infiltrate the area, or with a 1-ml tuberculin syringe, where small amounts are injected subcutaneously in a circle around the infiltrated area. The needle is changed before each injection of antidote. Some of these drugs are used in combination with one another.

ANTIDOTE	DOSE	EXTRAVASATED DRUG
Hyaluronidase **15 units/ml** Mix a 150-unit vial with 1 ml normal saline for injection. Withdraw 0.1 ml and dilute with 0.9 ml saline to get 15 units/ml.	0.2 ml × 5 subcutaneous injections around site	aminophylline calcium solutions contrast media dextrose solutions (concentrations of 10% or more) hyperalimentation solutions nafcillin potassium solutions vinblastine vincristine vindesine
Sodium bicarbonate 8.4%	5 ml	carmustine daunorubicin doxorubicin vinblastine vincristine
Phentolamine Dilute 5 to 10 mg with 10 ml of sterile saline for injection.	5 to 10 mg	dobutamine dopamine epinephrine metaraminol bitartrate norepinephrine
Sodium thiosulfate 10% Dilute 4 ml with 6 ml sterile water for injection.	10 ml	dactinomycin mechlorethamine mitomycin
Hydrocortisone sodium succinate 100 mg/ml Usually followed by topical application of hydrocortisone cream 1%.	50 to 200 mg 25 to 50 mg/ml of extravasate	doxorubicin vincristine
Ascorbic acid injection	50 mg	dactinomycin
Sodium edetate	150 mg	plicamycin

Prevention and emergency treatment of extravasation

Extravasation—the infiltration of a drug into the surrounding tissue—can result from a punctured vein or from leakage around a venipuncture site. If vesicant (blistering) drugs or fluids extravasate, severe local tissue damage often results. This may cause prolonged healing, infection, multiple debridements, cosmetic disfigurement, loss of function, and possibly amputation.

Preventing extravasation
To avoid extravasation when giving vesicants, adhere strictly to proper administration techniques and follow these guidelines:
• Don't use an existing I.V. line unless its patency is assured. Perform a new venipuncture to ensure correct needle placement and vein patency.
• Select the site carefully. Use a distal vein that allows successive proximal venipunctures. To avoid tendon and nerve damage through possible extravasation, avoid using the dorsum of the hand. Also avoid the wrist and digits (they're hard to immobilize) and areas previously damaged or with compromised circulation.
• If you need to probe for a vein, you may cause trauma. Stop and begin again at another site.
• Start the infusion with D_5W or NSS.
• Use a transparent dressing to allow inspection.
• Check for extravasation before starting the infusion. Apply a tourniquet above the needle to occlude the vein and see if the flow continues. If the flow stops, the solution isn't infiltrating. Another method is to lower the I.V. container and watch for blood backflow. This is less reliable because the needle may have punctured the opposite vein wall yet still rest partially in the vein. Flush the needle to ensure patency. If swelling occurs at the I.V.

site, the solution is infiltrating.
• Give by slow I.V. push through a free-flowing I.V. line or by small-volume infusion (50 to 100 ml).
• During administration, observe the infusion site for erythema or infiltration. Tell the patient to report burning, stinging, pain, pruritus, or temperature changes.
• After drug administration, instill several milliliters of D_5W or NSS to flush the drug from the vein and to preclude drug leakage when the needle is removed.
• Give vesicants last when multiple drugs are ordered.
• If possible, avoid using an infusion pump to administer vesicants. A pump will continue the infusion if infiltration occurs.

Treating extravasation
Extravasation of vesicant drugs requires emergency treatment. Follow your hospital's protocol. Essential steps include:
• Stop the I.V. flow and remove the I.V. line, unless you need the needle to infiltrate the antidote.
• Estimate the amount of extravasated solution and notify the doctor.
• Instill the appropriate antidote according to hospital protocol.
• Elevate the extremity.
• Record the extravasation site, the patient's symptoms, the estimated amount of infiltrated solution, and the treatment. Also record the time you notified the doctor and his name. Continue documenting the site's appearance and associated symptoms.
• Follow hospital protocol, and apply either ice packs or warm compresses to the affected area.
• If skin breakdown occurs, apply silver sulfadiazine cream and gauze dressings or wet-to-dry povidone-iodine dressings, as ordered.
• If severe debridement occurs, plastic surgery and physical therapy may be needed.

Home I.V. therapy

Today, more and more patients are receiving I.V. therapy at home, rather than in the hospital. Home therapy is more comfortable and convenient for patients and costs less than hospital-based I.V. therapy. It's used most commonly for patients who require I.V. therapy but need no special monitoring.

Home I.V. therapy differs little from hospital-based I.V. therapy. The preparation of drugs is the same and any of the various delivery methods can be adopted for home use. Nearly all drugs administered intravenously in the hospital — including fluids, antibiotics, antifungals, chemotherapeutic agents, insulin, chelating agents, analgesics, even some blood products — can also be given intravenously at home. The only exceptions are drugs that are used in emergencies and require meticulous patient monitoring, such as lidocaine or nitroprusside.

Home I.V. therapy does present a nursing challenge, however. First of all, patients must be chosen carefully and receive extensive teaching. Not only must they, a caregiver, or family member be able to care for the I.V. site and maintain the equipment, they must be able to recognize potentially serious complications, such as drug hypersensitivity.

Because home care is usually supervised by a home health care agency, referral to such an agency and coordination of third-party payments are also important aspects of initiating home therapy.

Home care patients are usually supervised by a home health care agency that specializes in home I.V. therapy. Besides administering drugs and checking equipment, the agency typically provides necessary supplies.

Choosing patients for home I.V. therapy

Patients with long-term or chronic medical conditions are especially well-suited to receive home I.V. therapy. For example, patients with infectious disorders that have a protracted recovery period, such as osteomyelitis, can be readily treated at home. Patients who require prolonged chemotherapy, continuous pain control, or long-term parenteral nutrition can also be treated at home.

Candidates for home I.V. therapy must be willing and able to administer therapy safely, learn the potential complications and interventions, understand the basics of asepsis, and be able to obtain the necessary supplies. Patients who need help must enlist a home caregiver, such as a family member or friend, to assist them in administering therapy.

Home therapy devices

As in the hospital, I.V. drugs can be given at home by direct injection, intermittent infusion, or continuous infusion. Specialized infusion pumps, such as the ambulatory infusion pump, implantable infusion pumps, implantable access device, and patient-controlled analgesia (PCA) pumps, permit the patient to move about during treatment and are especially useful for home I.V. therapy.

Whatever equipment the patient will be using, ensure that both he and his caregiver know how to set up, maintain, and monitor it. Review specific precautions. For example, explain that most systems cannot be immersed in water and must be protected from temperature extremes. Because a home care patient won't receive the same close monitoring he would in the hospital, select control devices that will prevent him from administering fluids incorrectly. Describe malfunctions that will activate an alarm, and instruct the patient to contact his home health care agency or medi-

(continued)

Home I.V. therapy *(continued)*

cal equipment supplier if an alarm is activated.

Initiating home I.V. therapy

Effective patient teaching is critical to the success of home I.V. therapy. Teaching should begin in the hospital. If a family member or other caregiver will be assisting the patient, include him in the teaching sessions.

• Teach the patient how to care for the I.V. site and how to recognize complications such as infection, irritation, or extravasation. For example, instruct him to contact his doctor or home health care nurse if redness, swelling, or pain develop, if the dressing becomes moist, or if blood is visible in the tubing.

• Review symptoms of drug hypersensitivity and toxicity. Remember that allergic reactions to some drugs may be delayed for weeks after administration.

• If the patient has a peripheral I.V. line, explain that the access site must be changed at established intervals. Set up a schedule for changing access sites with the home health care agency. Similarly, for patients with an ambulatory infusion device (such as a PCA pump or an implantable access device), establish a schedule for refilling the pump or medication cassette.

• If the patient is using an intermittent infusion device, such as a heparin lock, teach him how and when to flush it. Stress the importance of monitoring the site daily for signs of local infection.

• When appropriate, teach the patient with an implantable access device how to access it for drug delivery, flushing, and heparinization. Emphasize the importance of aseptic technique; instruct the patient to begin by thoroughly washing his hands and putting on sterile gloves. Show him how to locate and stabilize the port by palpation and how to clean the site with povidone-iodine, working outward in concentric circles from the site. Demonstrate how to attach a Huber (noncoring) needle to the appropriate syringe, extension, or I.V. tubing; insert the syringe into the port; and apply a sterile dressing to the site during drug administration. Finally, demonstrate how to regulate, monitor, and discontinue the infusion, as well as how to flush the port with 0.9% sodium chloride and heparin.

Pain control

Continuous narcotic infusion (CNI) or PCA may be used at home to deliver narcotic analgesics in patients with chronic severe pain (such as intractable cancer pain). These methods commonly afford superior pain relief compared to conventional narcotic administration.

Continuous narcotic infusion

Delivered by an ambulatory or implantable infusion pump, CNI produces stable analgesic blood levels, resulting in continuous pain control, few adverse reactions, and a reduction in patient anxiety. Initially, several boluses of the drug may be required to achieve effective pain relief. Thereafter, the infusion rate is typically adjusted to deliver the lowest effective dose.

The patient's caregiver should monitor his comfort level by observing the patient for signs of pain, including restlessness, grimacing, guarded positioning, and increased blood pressure and pulse rate. If the patient is controlling his own administration, he can monitor his own comfort level. Keeping a pain diary can help the patient document the effectiveness of CNI. Stress, however, the importance of contacting the doctor before making any adjustments in the prescribed drug dosage.

Demonstrate for the caregiver how to monitor breathing rate and level of alertness, especially during initial treatment and after dosage increases. Tell him to notify the doctor immediately if respiratory depression or other adverse reactions occur.

Patient-controlled analgesia

In PCA, the patient controls delivery of the analgesic by pressing a button on the PCA pump. A timing unit imposes a lock-out time between doses — usually 5 to 10 minutes — to prevent accidental overdose. Typically, PCA systems can be programmed to deliver narcotics three ways: at a continuous rate, at a continuous rate with intermittent boluses, or by bolus only. Specific systems, however, may vary.

A PCA system is especially effective for terminal cancer patients. To receive PCA therapy, a patient must be mentally alert, able to understand and comply with instructions and procedures, and have no history of allergy to the analgesic. Ineligible patients include those with limited respiratory reserve, a history of drug abuse or chronic sedative or tranquilizer use, or a psychiatric disorder.

Before the patient begins using the PCA system, make it clear that while the system will provide increased comfort, it doesn't guarantee total pain relief. Then, teach him how the PCA pump works. Demonstrate how to change the medication cassettes and lock them into the pump, as well as how to attach the tubing to the pump, prime the pump, piggyback the tubing to the I.V. or vascular access port, and secure the delivery unit. Encourage the patient to practice with a sample device. Explain that he should administer enough analgesic to relieve pain without inducing drowsiness.

Instruct the patient's caregiver how to monitor his respiratory rate and level of pain control. If the patient reports insufficient pain relief,

notify the doctor or home health care nurse.

Home parenteral nutrition

Home parenteral nutrition (HPN) enables prolonged or indefinite I.V. total parenteral nutrition (TPN). This technique has dramatically improved the health of patients with such chronic conditions as Crohn's disease and malabsorption syndrome, and with such acute conditions as incomplete bowel obstruction and antineoplastic therapy. In addition, it has also shortened hospital stays for such patients.

Although short-term parenteral nutrition can be administered using a peripheral I.V. line, long-term administration of nutrient infusions containing high amounts of glucose requires access to a central vein. To prepare for HPN, a barium-impregnated silicone rubber catheter with a Dacron cuff is implanted in the superior vena cava, with an entrance site on the abdomen. The extravascular portion of the catheter is reinforced with Teflon to reduce the risk of catheter fracture. About 2 to 3 weeks after implantation, firm tissue covers the catheter cuff to provide a physical barrier to microbial contamination.

Usually, HPN patients can ingest part of their caloric requirements and require 10 to 14 hours of infusion nightly to supply the remaining nutrients. If all the patient's nutrition must be received intravenously, a continuous infusion may be necessary. The exact composition of the infusion solution is tailored to the patient's specific caloric and metabolic needs. A standard parenteral nutrition solution consists of 50% dextrose in water, supplemented as necessary with amino acids, lipids, vitamins, and minerals (see *Composition of parenteral nutrition solutions,* page 582).

(continued)

Home I.V. therapy *(continued)*

Composition of parenteral nutrition solutions

Common components of parenteral nutrition solutions include 50% dextrose in water, amino acids, and any of the additives listed below. Additives may treat specific metabolic deficiencies.

ADDITIVE	PURPOSE
Acetate	• prevents metabolic acidosis
Amino acids	• provide protein for tissue repair • maintain positive nitrogen balance
Biotin	• required for fat synthesis, amino acid metabolism, and glycogen formation
Calcium	• promotes proper bone growth and remodeling • aids in blood clotting
Chloride	• maintains acid-base equilibrium and osmotic pressure
Essential fatty acids	• provide calories • required for synthesis of fats and cell membranes
Folic acid	• required for DNA synthesis
Magnesium	• promotes carbohydrate and protein absorption
Micronutrients (such as zinc, manganese, and cobalt)	• promote wound healing and RBC synthesis
Pantothenic acid	• required for energy metabolism
Phosphate	• reduces risk of peripheral paresthesia
Potassium	• required for cellular activity and tissue synthesis
Sodium	• regulates water distribution and fluid balance
Vitamin B complex	• promotes carbohydrate and protein absorption
Vitamin C	• promotes wound healing
Vitamin D	• required for normal bone growth • maintains serum calcium levels
Vitamin E	• antioxidant; preserves other fat-soluble vitamins • preserves integrity of cell membranes
Vitamin K	• prevents bleeding disorders

Before initiating HPN, assess the patient's or caregiver's ability to perform the necessary care routines. Consider the patient's motivation, mental aptitude, job or other daily activities, home environment, and the accessibility of health care support systems, including a suitable home health care agency.

The patient and caregiver must know how to care for the catheter site correctly and how to recognize infection. This is especially important if the patient has a multilumen catheter; such catheters are associated with a two or three times greater incidence of sepsis compared with single-lumen catheters. Remind the patient to change the site dressing once a week or whenever it becomes soiled or nonocclusive and to change administration tubing as scheduled. Tell him that after the implanted catheter has been in place for 1 month or longer, he may be allowed to remove his dressing and bathe or shower. Also remind the patient to prevent contact between the catheter and granular or lint-producing surfaces to avoid local tissue reaction from airborne particles and surface contaminants.

Confirm a suitable TPN schedule with the patient, taking into account life-style as well as nutritional needs. Emphasize adherence to the prescribed schedule and volume to prevent glucose imbalance. Teach family members and caregivers to recognize signs of fluid overload, high or low blood glucose, and electrolyte imbalance. Finally, at discharge, arrange for a follow-up physical examination; specimens for laboratory analysis must be obtained to detect metabolic complications.

INDEX

W

X

Y

Z